Freudian Dictionary

The *Freudian Dictionary* provides a comprehensive and accessible guide to essential Freudian terms and concepts. Organized conceptually, the book is grounded in detailed and meticulous readings, and covers the full range of Freud's writings and subjects. It also provides an overview of the development, vicissitudes, and syntheses of Freud's unique lines of thought.

Contemporary developments in psychoanalytic thought have aspired to surpass their Freudian origins. But this comprehensive guide to Freud's work provides a touchstone for those wishing to clarify these roots, and the foundations of the discipline itself. It will be a valuable companion to psychoanalysts in practice and training across a range of schools, as well as a reference work for sociologists, artists, philosophers, historians, and other scholars.

José Luis Valls is a Member of the International Psychoanalytical Association (IPA) and a Member of the Argentine Psychoanalytic Association (APA) with Training Function. He has served as Director of the APA's journal *Revista de Psicoanálisis*, Coordinator of the APA Committee on Ethics, and Director of the APA History Department for two administrations. He has lectured and taught internationally and has published numerous articles on Freudian metapsychology and clinical cases. The first edition of the *Diccionario Freudiano* [*Freudian Dictionary*] (2005) was published by Editorial J. Yébenes. His book, *Metapsicología y Modernidad, el Proyecto Freudiano* [*Metapsychology and Modernity, the Freudian Project*] (2004), was published by Editorial Lugar.

Freudian Dictionary

A Comprehensive Guide to Freudian Concepts

José Luis Valls
Translated by Susan H. Rogers

Routledge
Taylor & Francis Group
LONDON AND NEW YORK

First published 2019
by Routledge
2 Park Square, Milton Park, Abingdon, Oxon OX14 4RN

and by Routledge
52 Vanderbilt Avenue, New York, NY 10017

Routledge is an imprint of the Taylor & Francis Group, an informa business

British Library Cataloguing-in-Publication Data
A catalogue record for this book is available from the British Library

Library of Congress Cataloging-in-Publication Data
A catalog record has been requested for this book

ISBN: 978-0-367-15100-3 (hbk)
ISBN: 978-0-367-15103-4 (pbk)
ISBN: 978-0-429-05504-1 (ebk)

Typeset in Times New Roman
by Swales & Willis, Exeter, Devon, UK

To Sari, my wife.
To José,
Gaby,
Ceci,
and Manuel,
our children.

Contents

Foreword to the first edition

Freud's works, a major contribution in the field of science, extend from the late nineteenth to well into the twentieth century. The best proof of this contribution is the growing number of Freud scholars and exegetes, and also of detractors who announce his death, time and again, thereby paradoxically demonstrating his perpetuity.

José Luis Valls is one of those who have dedicated their life to the study of Freudian thought, and his *Dictionary* is evidence of an obstinate and reflective passion placed in the service of understanding and explaining it.

In order to accomplish the enormous task of presenting the full complexity of his teacher's thought, Valls has preferred the form of the dictionary in which each of Freud's concepts is elucidated rigorously within the fabric of its limitless connections, part of a theoretical corpus that awes us, as he says, by its "theoretical consistency, audacity, and freedom of spirit", as much as by its practical effects. Re-thinking clinical work by reviewing implicit and explicit assumptions that guide it is doubtless a major task for every analyst, from the beginner to the most experienced. In this effort of constant revision, contact with the numerous aspects of Freud's ideas which emerge from the also abundant difficulties presented by his clinical work occupies as fundamental a place now as it did then.

In his Prologue, Valls tells us that he wants to study Freud by following in his wake, and we must thank him for this. After many years of returning to the source from the clinical base with an attitude of respectful meditation, Valls attempts, and in my opinion renders, a faithful approximation to the creator's vicissitudes without aiming to impose his own way of thinking.

Valls approaches Freud *per via di levare*, refusing to subjugate Freud to his own concepts or to update him for the benefit of any fashionable ideology. The result is the erudition and honesty this book exudes, which does not imply ignoring that, as Croce said, all history is contemporary history; consequently, any approach to Freud inevitably proceeds from problems encountered in our times.

Aware of the difficulty of his endeavour and the deviations that could steer him off his course, Valls offers us his vision of his teacher by situating himself within the works themselves, a position from which he strives for consistency with their totality.

R. Horacio Etchegoyen
March 3, 1995

Preface to the English edition

Since Argentine psychoanalysts do not usually publish their books in English, I am proud to do so. This pride doubtless stems from the unique subject of my text: the works of Freud; that is to say, this pride is due to him and what he did. Perhaps my innovation is the way I view and think about these works. Despite the large amount of reading that flies about my head at this point in my life, opening windows and doors, it has been useful neither to "surpass" nor to forget Freud's works but instead to re-think them, work on them, and put them to the test; with the knowledge that his texts, products of Illuminist Modernity, generate a gap in this scientific positivism; that they are in reality a profound critique of reason which proceeds from reason itself. The unconscious, his major discovery, shows us the irrational part of our psyche, not as something interesting simply to think about as an abstract object of curiosity, but as the principal agent of human actions that is operating in the shadows.

Paradoxically, I consider the origins of psychoanalytic theory to stretch farther back than usually thought; that is to say, I find these beginnings neither in the Preliminary Communication to the *Studies on Hysteria* nor in *The Interpretation of Dreams*, although the latter could be seen as the origin of Freudian clinical works (in which Freud always develops theoretical positions fundamental for understanding the functioning of the human soul). I place the dawn of a theory that develops and becomes more complex, with constant comings and goings, somewhat more removed in time. I begin with his letters to Fliess and a text later rejected by Freud but saved by the action of one of his patients and followers, Princess Marie Bonaparte; I share her view that his works transcended him – she compared him to Plato – and that his writing therefore no longer belonged to him but to humanity. On this point I agree with her, and I proceed in consequence. The paradox is that, in searching through the oldest part, we find weapons that enable us to return to the circulation of what is newest. When we dive into the nineteenth century, we illuminate everything produced in the twentieth, and generate a road to better understanding of twenty-first-century human beings.

Therefore, the Freudian text with which I begin is the *Project for a Scientific Psychology*, an eminently positivist manuscript written in 1895, a theoretical biological-philosophical essay on the human mind, perhaps excessively ambitious for a young physiologist; I take some of his outstandingly psychological concepts from this text and place them into the subsequent logic of Freud's works. This work is therefore not only clinical but also possesses a theory that, if examined deeply, may reach unsuspected heights of knowledge of psychical functioning and therefore of human beings. This dictionary contains the main concepts in this text, described in such a way that the reader may connect and integrate them with the rest of Freud's works, since their participation may be read between the lines in his later manner of thinking on a new level. Hence, concepts such as the experience of satisfaction, his conception of perception, and others participate in this dictionary, since they are too valuable to be left aside. The same may be said regarding the numbered Fliess papers including the famed Letter 52 to Fliess. I have also summarized each of Freud's cases, basically cases of hysteria, from the first period, as well as many well-known and less famous Freudian concepts, perhaps giving them a new perspective.

Why turn to Freud in our developing twenty-first century? Because we think that the acuity and profundity of his thinking on the human soul have not been surpassed; further, his concepts may help us to understand the relation between the biological and the social, thereby giving psychology a new dimension as a product of this dialectic. If this dictionary serves to promote and rekindle the reading and re-reading of Freud rather than replacing it, it will have accomplished its principal task. Now we reach English-language psychoanalysts and others interested in these topics, people of culture. The works of Freud are presently indispensable for understanding human beings; four editions of this text have been published in my native language, Spanish, in which I can sometimes think. Words serve us, as Freud tells us, not only to communicate with each other, but also to communicate with ourselves, to know ourselves better. We work with the words of our patients and with our own. Like the symptoms and suffering of our patients and ourselves, the words that circulate in this dictionary seek their meaning. The Freudian theory of the human soul gives us an accurate instrument for refinding this lost meaning. We need only to know it better, then put it to use.

José Luis Valls

Preface to the first edition

> Here again you yourself have said almost all there is to say on the subject. But though you have taken the wind out of my sails I shall be glad to follow in your wake and content myself with confirming all you have said by amplifying it to the best of my knowledge – or conjecture.
>
> (*Why War?*, Einstein and Freud, 1933, p. 203)

Geniuses always take the wind out of our sails, and Freud is no exception. He is by now nearly a century ahead of us and still gaining ground. His works are quite alive and fresh today, participating in all serious discussions on human nature in general and on our psyche in particular. The depth of the conceptualizations, the excellence of the investigations and meticulous observations, the truth and intellectual honesty they show us, their logical consistency, audacity, and freedom of spirit, and perhaps most importantly, the practicality of their effects, have made psychoanalysis, his creation, one of the major scientific contributions of the twentieth century.

Therefore, how could we fail to follow in his wake? One of the objectives of this book is to return to the source, just as Freud does with his patients, but to return at this time to him; he is now the source, through his works. This is extremely complex. Therefore, I give the reader my conceptual elaboration of this enormous complexity in the simplest terms possible while also trying to remain faithful to the spirit of Freudian letters, "amplifying it to the best of my knowledge – or conjecture".

Psychoanalysis has grown, probably more than Freud may have imagined and perhaps less than he would have liked. It has become more complex, has suffered crises, and confusions have been generated: some theoretical, others political, and even theoretical-political confusions (within the psychoanalytic movement, of course). At least this is what I experienced as a psychoanalyst. There are diverse tendencies in psychoanalytic thought today, born from Freudian developments and aspiring to surpass them; they obviously do in some way, although it is sometimes unclear in what way. On this difficult road, reading Freud has always handed me a "torch in the darkness".

I wish to express my gratitude for this, and to offer a sincere tribute to the works that have largely charted the course of my life.

This text is therefore intended to be a dictionary on the works of Freud, organized conceptually. The conceptualization is mine, of course; it is the way I understand what Freud writes. It probably includes elaborations of my own regarding the way of understanding and interrelating different concepts; I'm sure it does, and this is also doubtless a means of generating movements in science. I hope that this movement of review will lead to an advance, unlike so many apparent advances which result in intellectual steps backwards. At the same time, I aim to present an overview of the development, vicissitudes, entries and cross-entries, and syntheses of the unique thinking I consider Freud's own; from the *Project* … to his *Moses* …, doing my best to thread together the multiplicity of meanings in the works he wrote, some apparently unconnected.

This means that my intention is not only to provide a detailed list of the places or works in which Freud mentioned a certain subject, or to what he was referring when he did. It is not to be a priest or the owner of the truth, but instead to display what I consider essential in Freudian thought, bringing it into competition with other lines of thought on equal terms and at the same table.

This book is not meant to be a monograph on what Freud wrote on diverse subjects in various parts of his works, although this may sometimes be inevitable, but rather to give the solidest impression possible of how I conceptualize it after a very long time spent reading, re-reading, thinking, and rethinking his works, having to answer my students' questioning, which certainly always provided an incentive; of how I understand, therefore, certain concepts that may be interpreted diversely (especially by readers outside the field who are unfamiliar with the logic Freud develops throughout his works) by taking a position hopefully consistent with the totality of his works; that is to say, by situating myself inside the theory developed by Freud.

I therefore aim to make my position on these subjects especially clear. For this purpose, I include them within a global logic of Freudian thought, which leads me to need to define all of his concepts or at least those I think are most important.

However, this conceptualization is not a result of whim but is grounded in my detailed and meticulous reading which involves the greatest respect for Freud's writing on each particular subject. For this reason, I have included quotes whenever they seemed necessary. The quotes from Freud's text have quotation marks followed by a parenthesis containing the reference to the work in *The Standard Edition of the Complete Psychological Works of Sigmund Freud*, the year of publication, and the page number.

The references are essentially to works of Freud. The entries [in the English edition] utilize the terms chosen by James Strachey for the above-mentioned English translation from the original German, with the exception of "Trieb" which has now been left in German to distinguish it from "instinct". It is commonly referred to as "drive", although Strachey rejected this term.

These works, however, are not the only influence on my thinking. I believe that the contribution of other authors may doubtless enrich Freud's thought; this is my intention as an author, although in writing this book in particular, as I do when "I teach Freud", I consciously attempt to remove all influence from my elaboration and make an effort to understand the particular logic of Freudian thought; although I recognize that this goal is impossible, my intention stands firm.

Internal references to other articles in this work are marked with an asterisk (*); I advise the reader to consult them in order to grasp more clearly the way I interconnect these concepts.

The overall summary of the development of the concepts discussed by Freud is partly self-evident (or so I hope) and partly arguable (and I also hope so): it is for the reader to decide how well I have succeeded.

My highest objective for this book is to destroy the myth surrounding the Freudian creation for psychoanalysts and others, considering it just as I would any other scientific work: neither absolute truth nor absolute falsehood, but rather a scientific hypothesis having levels of truth and error and its own profound logic; and from this position, to discuss it exhaustively, "in his wake", attempting to preserve its creator's conceptual clarity, deepening its depth, delving into it, but never jumping over it.

In conclusion, my objectives are quite ambitious, probably excessively so. If some are attained, I believe my endeavour to be fully justified.

José Luis Valls

A

ABASIA

Ger.: Abasie. – Sp.: abasia. – Fr.: abasie. – It.: abasia. – Port.: abasia.

This term refers to a type of affection characteristic of conversion hysteria*, although it is also found in some neurological disorders. It consists of great difficulty in walking which may even make it absolutely impossible even without paralysis of the lower limbs, the patient being able to perform correctly other types of movement. It is the predominant symptom* of Elisabeth von R.*, one of the most famous patients of Freud's early period.

> [Fräulein Elisabeth von R.] … had been suffering for more than two years from pains in her legs and … had difficulties in walking … She walked with the upper part of her body bent forward, but without making use of any support. Her gait was not of any recognized pathological type, and moreover was by no means strikingly bad. All that was apparent was that she complained of great pain in walking and of being quickly overcome by fatigue both in walking and in standing, and that after a short time she had to rest, which lessened the pains but did not do away with them altogether. The pain was of an indefinite character; I gathered that it was something in the nature of a painful fatigue. A fairly large, ill-defined area of the anterior surface of the right thigh was indicated as the focus of the pains, from which they most often radiated and where they reached their greatest intensity. In this area the skin and muscles were also particularly sensitive to pressure and pinching (though the prick of a needle was, if anything, met with a certain amount of unconcern). This hyperalgesia of the skin and muscles was not restricted to this area but could be observed more or less over the whole of both legs. The muscles were perhaps even more sensitive to pain than the skin; but there could be no question that the thighs were the parts most sensitive to both these kinds of pain. The motor power of the legs could not be described as small, and the reflexes were of medium strength. There were no other symptoms, so that there was no ground for suspecting the presence of any serious organic affection. The disorder had developed gradually during the previous two years and varied greatly in intensity.
>
> (1895*d*, pp. 135–6)

In the case history of "Elisabeth von R.", Freud was able to reconstruct quite exhaustively each element of hysterical conversion corresponding to its associative part and to connect them with different moments in which, through those elements, hysterogenic zones* had formed a certain type of connection with her sister's husband. All formed part of a global incestuous phantasy, far from the conscious, in the relationship with this brother-in-law towards which her paralysis symbolically expressed a linguistic expression: "not being able to take a single step forward" (1895*d*, p. 176).

During treatment the cure of hysterical symptoms is produced when all these traumatic events (in this case conflictive rather than traumatic) return to conscious memory cathected with moments of libidinal hyperexcitation (the subject's hyperexcitability could make them traumatic) as proof of their participation in a global incestuous idea (hyperexcitation is therefore produced by the incestuous character of primarily repressed infantile sexuality*).

Through analysis, the symptom's meaning enters the secondary process*, after which the wish* may be expressed in words and discharged by abreaction*. Consequently, symptomatic bodily expression is no longer necessary.

The symptom's meaning has two aspects: as a mnemic symbol* of events that produced excitation or contiguities with it, leaving behind hyperalgesia or anaesthesia in these hysterogenic zones. The other aspect is its global quality, its blocking action as an anticathexis* of the incestuous wish of which love for her brother-in-law is a derivative too close for the patient's psyche. Her astasia-abasia, a motor disorder opposing the repressed wish, corresponds to this fact. It is a metaphor whose meaning is the opposite of satisfaction of the wish, in favour of defensive ego repression*.

ABREACTION

Ger.: Abreagieren. – Sp.: abreacción. – Fr.: abréaction. – It.: abreazione. – Port.: ab-reação.
This is the major mechanism of the psychotherapeutic cure proposed by Breuer and Freud in the "Preliminary Communication" (*On the Psychical Mechanism of Hysterical Phenomena: Preliminary Communication*, 1893).

The cure consisted basically of verbal expression of the repressed traumatic event associated with liberation of the affect* repressed at the time of the trauma*, neither of which was accessible to memory* in normal waking life. To induce their re-experience, the technique most utilized was hypnosis:

> each individual hysterical symptom immediately and permanently disappeared when we had succeeded in bringing clearly to light the memory of the event by which it was provoked and in arousing its accompanying affect, and when the patient had described that event in the greatest possible detail and had put the affect into words.
>
> (S.E. 2, p. 6)

Abreaction consisted of discharge of the retained affect together with the presentation* responsible for it, which had been separated from the conscious* when the symptom* formed, at which time it was relegated to a "second consciousness". It was retrieved through hypnosis. When the traumatic scene was then remembered and verbalized, the corresponding affect that for different causes had not been discharged at the time was "abreacted".

Once the affect has been obtained, the traumatic scene loses its pathogenic value, becoming identical to another presentation, and the symptom consequently ceases.

We therefore define abreaction as an actual affective discharge produced during the cure of an affect corresponding to a psychical trauma from the past, not discharged at that time but meanwhile persisting in a second consciousness, far from associative commerce, a position from which it generated symptoms and hysterical attacks*.

The basic scheme, though mainly centred on re-experiencing the traumatic scene with affective discharge and recollection*, did not include its working through since the concept of unconscious* had not yet acquired conceptual clarity (it is mistaken for the preconscious*, for example) but operated instead through what he calls the "second consciousness"; it is nevertheless quite similar to Freud's elaborations in the first and even the second topic.

It also follows important psychoanalytic rules such as making conscious the unconscious and filling in some mnemic lacunae.

The centre of the scene is occupied by symptomatic relief, a place from which it was removed over time, perhaps too far, so that now it is important to recall this modification in order to restore it to its proper place in the mechanism of the cure by a new "turn of the screw".

ABSTINENCE

Ger.: Abstinenz. – Sp.: abstinencia. – Fr.: abstinence. – It.: astinenza. – Port.: abstinência.

This refers to a fundamental technical rule of psychoanalysis by which the psychoanalyst must avoid any action that may serve to satisfy the patient's repressed wishes* during and within the analytic process. Freud stipulates: "Analytic treatment should be carried through, as far as is possible, under privation – in a state of abstinence" (*Lines of Advance in Psycho-Analytic Therapy*, 1919, p. 162).

The psychoanalytic function is to induce the patient to speak and to help the patient to make conscious these unconscious wishes. The terrain of the cure must remain in the domain of words. The wish* must remain in the terrain of unconscious fantasy* and not be put into action; the analytic function is to transform it into words and thereby make it apt for thinking and working through. A part of it always remains unsatisfied and provides a motor for analysis. If it were put into action without words, it would become a repetition* of a repressed scene of infantile sexuality* and would most likely be traumatic for the patient. But most importantly, it would lead to impossibility for the cure.

The strictest abstinence is recommended when transference love* appears at some moment in a person's analysis, and the analyst seemingly faces two possible alternatives: (1) to interrupt the treatment (only a momentary solution, but not for the patient's cure, since the patient will probably repeat the same situation with another therapist, having missed this opportunity to understand unconscious complexes that have determined his or her history, which is no less than the history of psychical structuring); (2) to respond affirmatively to the patient's demands (with which a new love match could be formed, but the possibility of cure would be interrupted as it would be in the first alternative). Freud describes a third alternative for this awkward situation that may arise. This third solution is simply to continue with the analysis, considering the patient's demand as simply another element of resistance*, also unconscious to the patient's conscious knowledge. Transference love is not the only situation of this kind that may arise and may require abstinence. Any situation that would involve any degree of intimacy or that belongs more to the terrain of action* than of words requires it as well. It depends on the analyst's skill in each particular case to recognize it and bring it back to the terrain of words, thereby returning it to psychoanalytic terrain *par excellence*. Therefore, the rule of abstinence pertains to psychoanalytic technique* and hence to the ethics* of treatment.

ABSTRACT THOUGHT

Ger.: Abstraktes Denken. – Sp.: pensamiento abstracto. – Fr.: pensée abstraite. – It.: pensiero astratto. – Port.: pensamento abstrato.

This type of thought* is first achieved with the appearance of words and later when their degree of binding* is greater (compared to common thought*). It is the highest level of theoretical thought, rising above action and words, and separating from what it represents, sometimes so much so that it risks loss of its distinction from the thing as in schizophrenic thought (*The Unconscious*, 1915).

This type of thought gives priority to metaphors and symbols in its functioning, and ignores more concrete and direct meanings, choosing others that encompass the former but take them further and expand them.

The ability for abstraction, the most complex level of thought activity, is acquired in adolescence; although it is separate from immediate action, it may promote and produce it in the long term in an individual or human group. The person who has thought it needs to dedicate arduous ego work to make it understood on this level due to the high levels of complexity it may reach. It may also come to nothing, especially when the distance from concrete meanings is very great. Or it may be utilized as rationalization* attempting to withdraw from what is real. What is real is generated by experiences with things* and traces left by them in the psychical apparatus*: thing-presentations* which must ultimately provide the underpinnings for all levels of thought.

ACTION

Ger.: Aktion. – Sp.: acción. – Fr.: action. – It.: azione. – Port.: ação.

The psychic process is a presentational path that must conclude in action which may be immediate or mediate. This action was carried out first by the neuromuscular system previous to the introduction of any "prostheses" that mankind may have invented to extend our range of power and possibilities.

In any case, also from the beginning of life, the child performs other types of action in relation to immediate affective discharge (internal change*) with no particular aim other than affective discharge itself; the second step in this determination may be reached by screaming, this action gradually acquiring characteristics of language*. In these cases, in spite of progress, previous stages persist and affective expression continues as such: it is partly action but not action such as to "change the face of the Earth". That is to say, it aims to change the internal medium of the body and the psyche but not the external medium (although it may also act on it indirectly).

The other type of action is specific action* which we discuss separately.

Thought* activity is planning for action*, directly or indirectly, although it does not replace it (except in obsessional thought* but only as part of this pathology) and must conclude with it, either before or afterwards, with the exception perhaps of reproductive thought: conscious recollection in which the act of remembering may not require an action, although it does not necessarily dispense with it. Action may be purely sexual; in this case it is the culmination of love* for the object*, or may be desexualized, creating culture*, as in the case of sublimation*.

Repression* greatly restricts possibilities of action or, even worse, diverts it from its aim since the possibility to access the repressed presentation* is lost. Psychoanalysis recovers these repressed presentations and enables the ego to think about them and lead them to action, or not, as a product of conscious thought, in which case problems of ethics* intervene. When the thing-presentation* is repressed – that is to say, does not find any word-presentation to access the conscious*, since this presentation is decathected* and anticathected* – subjects may perform actions that are not products of thought but instead repetition compulsions*. Hence, in regard to scenes corresponding to traumatic* situations or to anticathexes against them, preconscious* ego* thought* is unable to correct or control them since their meaning and even their existence is unknown.

ACTIVITY AND PASSIVITY

Ger.: Aktivität und Passivität. – Sp.: activo-pasivo. – Fr.: actif-passif. – It.: attivo-passivo. – Port.: ativo-passivo.

We may discuss several polarities in psychical life: subject (ego*)–object* (external world) and pleasure*–unpleasure*; active–passive is one of these.

Activity is a universal characteristic of Trieb* related to pressure (*Drang*); that is to say, its motor factor, the sum of force or measure of demand of work that it represents. All Trieb, in this sense, is a fragment of activity.

But are there passive Triebe?

Trieb is active in its pressure, peremptory quality, and motor factor, but may be active or passive in relation to its aim.

Vicissitudes of Trieb previous to repression* allude to the aim: for example, turning round upon the subject's own self* and reversal into the opposite*. The clearest examples are the pairs: sadism*–masochism and to look at–to be looked at, in which those with an active aim (sadism, to look at) pass over to a passive aim (masochism, to be looked at).

In the subject's life, especially in infantile prehistory, traumatic situations* may occur which fixate to the Trieb or its aim, transforming it from active into passive, which later becomes a character trait* or other pathology.

In his analysis of the "Wolf Man", Freud showed how in the initially ambivalent Trieb (both active and passive) the active tendency predominated at first. Following a traumatic event (seduction by his sister), preceded by a threat of castration, Trieb returned from its incipient and precocious genitality to the anal-sadistic phase with a passive aim, which produced a change in his character from kind to naughty, masochistically seeking paternal punishment. This passivity remained fixated and led to a character trait of the adult "Wolf Man". It also appeared in one of his most unruly hysterical symptoms, his constipation.

In Little Hans we find some examples of an alternating pair "to look at–to be looked at" which are deferred* and repressed*, transformed into the dam against Trieb that is shame*.

Triebe with an active or passive aim are present in both boys and girls. Most commonly, the passive ones predominate in girls and the active in boys, to which cultural customs of course effectively contribute.

After puberty they practically take on a masculine (active) or feminine (passive) quality.

Trieb with a passive aim retains the narcissistic object (the ego) unlike the active whose aim is the object.

From this differentiation derive differences in manners of masculine falling in love* (an active wish* to love the object) and of feminine* love* (the passive wish to be loved by the object) as masculine and feminine characteristics in general.

Sexual Trieb is therefore, in regard to its aim, active or passive (although variants may result from traumatic events experienced by the subject) from the beginning. With the advent of the phallic stage, phallic–castrated differentiation is added, which becomes masculine–feminine in the period of pubertal development.

ACTUAL NEUROSIS

Ger.: Aktualneurose. – Sp.: neurosis actual. – Fr.: névrose actuelle. – It.: nevrosi attuale. – Port.: neurose atual.

This type of neurosis with neuro-vegetative symptoms* is caused by actual (not historical) problems. Freud describes alterations in the mode of discharge of somatic sexual tension. There are two types of actual neurosis: neurasthenia* and anxiety neurosis*. They are distinguished by the mechanical factor of discharge, either its excess or lack. For example, if orgasm is interrupted (*coitus interruptus*), especially if it is practised frequently, somatic sexual tension accumulates, and this exaggerated accumulation of quantity of excitation* automatically becomes anxiety*.

This theoretical explanation, presented by Freud in his works on anxiety neurosis, is subsequently supported throughout his works.

We may extend this accumulation of quantity of excitation to other periods of life (adolescence and menopause) when it becomes excessive. Somatic sexual tension sent by the biological body to the psychical apparatus* increases; the latter is unprepared or unable, psychically or mechanically, to respond to this demand, and is unable to adequately reach specific action*. If the tension of need does not find relief, whether for mechanical or psychical reasons, it becomes automatic anxiety*. Then, it manifests as an attack of anxiety without presentation* or with a presentation adopted at a later moment, in the sphere of preconscious rationalization.

There are other psychical causes of penetration of a quantity of excitation unprocessed by a presentation into the psychical apparatus. For example, if cathexis* is withdrawn from the unconscious thing-presentation* (as occurs in narcissistic libidinal withdrawal*), the quantity of excitation penetrates the psychical apparatus in pure form, upon which the latter perceives it automatically as anxiety and then as an experience of the end of the world. However, here we are observing schizophrenia*, which is very far from actual neuroses. This common ground also reveals the richness of this conceptualization, which intertwines the biological with action and the psychological in order to account for an affect* such as anxiety which presents in its pure form in such apparently dissimilar affections.

In neurasthenia the cause is the opposite: an excess of abnormal discharge. Masturbation* is an excessive producer of symptomatology of asthenia. This explains the actual mechanical effect of the alteration, which has no direct relation with the psychical (presentations), memory* or repression*. When it does, we are on the terrain of transference neuroses*, which may in turn aid the establishment of actual neuroses (hysteria* with anxiety neurosis, a product of sexual repression in an indirect manner), forming mixed neuroses. Every transference neurosis contains an actual-neurotic core around which the symptom of historical origin is established.

ADHESIVENESS OF THE LIBIDO

Ger.: Klebrigkeit der Libido. – Sp.: viscosidad de la libido. – Fr.: viscosité de la libido. – It.: vischiosità della libido. – Port.: viscosidade da libido.

This term describes the degree to which the libido* in some individuals adheres to presentations* or to the "pathways" of their interrelations.

When adhesiveness is intense, it is difficulty for displacement*, as difficult as a fixation*. The opposite case is found in subjects who possess an almost absolutely displaceable libido, something akin to "writing on water" of libidinal cathexes.

It is also called psychical inertia*, and may be a serious difficulty for the cure at both ends of the spectrum.

It is an "id resistance" which on the one hand clings to its inherited schemes and on the other hand functions with the pleasure principle*, one of whose major characteristics is free displacement of libido among presentations.

However, the concept of adhesiveness of the libido always refers to cases with more adhesiveness and more difficulty for psychical changes or changes of wished-for objects by the psyche (Freud also called it "entropy").

It is one of the causes of prolongation which makes some analyses interminable, as if these patients were clinging to their psychoanalyst just as they were once clinging to their illness.

AFFECT

Ger.: Affekt. – Sp.: afecto. – Fr.: affect. – It.: affetto. – Port.: afeto.

This is a feeling noticed by the conscious* (Pcpt.-Cs. or perceptual-conscious system, 1915–17) corresponding to increase or decrease in the time unit (rhythm, 1924) of quantities of libidinal excitation* coming from beneath the body surface.

Increases are generally registered as unpleasure* and decreases as pleasure*; other, different, pleasurable or unpleasurable affects are located in qualitative variations (produced by the form and time lapse in which these increases or decreases are produced) between each of these extremes. One of the unpleasurable affects is taken as a reference or standard for the rest: anxiety*.

In his *Project for a Scientific Psychology* (1895) Freud explicitly discussed affect in reference to memory* of the experience of pain*, which leaves increased quantitative tension Qη in ψ and also motivates compelling discharge.

Following the experience of pain, emergence of affect is left as a sequela (Freud was clearly referring to fear or real anxiety) in response to any subsequent event similar to the experience that once produced pain.

In the same text, when he discusses internal change* – a bodily form of it, essentially vascular and respiratory, to express feelings that accompany prototypical screaming, the safety valve previous to learning the specific action* – he was also explaining the origin of affect or affective discharge as a sentiment that announces the wish* for the object*.

In his 1915 metapsychological papers, he describes a psyche composed of thing-presentations* and word-presentations* with a quantity of libidinal energy (sexual Trieb*) cathecting them (this represents peremptoriness, *Drang*, or pressure of work of Trieb* and also "ignites" the presentation*, converting it into a wish*).

He also refers to this amount of libidinal energy as quantum of affect*; it corresponds to the quantitative factor of Trieb (cathecting the presentation and in turn being cathected by it) and is perceived as such by the perceptual-conscious end (Pcpt.-Cs.). As long as there is no discharge of the Trieb source, it is perceived by way of internal change as different types of unpleasurable affect. When total or partial discharge is produced through the specific action, affects, now pleasurable and also of a different type, are felt.

The unconscious* contains presentations*. Their degree of cathexis is registered directly by the Pcpt.-Cs. as affect. Therefore, affect is never strictly unconscious given that it is something felt by the conscious. What may be unconscious is the presentation it sometimes produces. This refers to affect produced by presentational causes which are therefore psychical and consequently historical.

Some affects are produced by biological or mechanical causes (as in the case of anxiety in actual neuroses*) produced by an accumulation of somatic sexual tension (1894–1925), in which case the problem does not refer to the presentational, or at least not directly. Anxiety is also conscious in this case.

When Freud describes the anxiety signal* in *Inhibitions, Symptoms and Anxiety* (1926d), he explains that anxiety in this case is not produced from repression* as something new but rather as an affective state following a pre-extant image: the memory of traumatic situations* in infancy which have now become situations of danger*, signs of danger that compel the unconscious ego* to use defence mechanisms* (or presentations in the broad sense) in an automatic manner.

Affective states are also incorporated into mental life as sediments of ancient traumatic experiences that awaken as mnemic symbols* in similar situations. In the same way, the birth trauma* provides a model later taken up by the ego as the mnemic symbol* of anxiety* which it uses as a signal to lead the id* where the ego wishes; in other words, it applies its unconscious defence mechanisms*.

The anxiety signal* in this case has no economic explanation since it consists of a reproduction of memory: a memory, a mnemic symbol, of a situation once traumatic and now dangerous. It is only a signal. It is more presentation than mere quantum of affect; its results are only a jot of everything that could be perceived if id* Trieb continued in the same direction it had taken, entering the preconscious ego with all this material, and had gone on to the possibility of action. This type of anxiety gives the ego power, since it enables the ego to dominate the id by using the omnipotent pleasure–unpleasure principle to its advantage, utilizing defence mechanisms governed by the same principle to achieve this success.

The explanation is: what was once part of a specific action may later participate as a symbol of affect.

For example, what was necessary for the baby's self-preservation – heavy breathing, tachycardia, hyper-perspiration, and so on – are bodily components of anxiety that express sensations of a very particular unpleasure whose memory is used as a signal by the unconscious ego in order to defend itself from the id.

In a broader definition of the concept of affect, sentiments in general could be included, each of which has a more complex and specific explanation (cf. love, hate, aggression, pain, and others). Their common bodily root is internal change (expression of emotions, screaming, vascular innervation) whose psychological dimensions grow as experiences of satisfaction* and pain* are experienced with the object. Traces left by these experiences* form thing-presentation complexes composed of the image of an object that subsequently generates a wish for the object and also the image of the action to be carried out with the object in order to obtain a feeling (affect) that constitutes the essence of what is wished for.

The thing-presentation cathected by and cathecting affective quantum forms the foundation of the unconscious psyche. Cathexis is mutual: the meeting point between quantity of excitation and the strictly psychical representative.

AFFECTIVE STRUCTURE

Ger.: Affektentwicklung. – Sp.: formación de afecto. – Fr.: formation de l'affect. – It.: formazione d'affetto. – Port.: formação de afeto.

Freud utilizes this concept when he needs to explain the problem of unconscious feelings in his metapsychological papers of 1915 (p. 178).

How is it possible to relate presentation and affect*? By definition, feelings are something felt and therefore conscious (cf. consciousness*). In this perspective, it is absurd to postulate unconscious feelings or affects.

However, preconscious presentations cause affect and are generally joined to affect. We also know that presentations may be unconscious (thing-presentations*), especially those that are repressed. Consequently, affect is in some way included in them and therefore, if libidinal cathexis* of presentations continues its path to the ego's preconscious on the way to action, it will produce affective expressions in the ego.

In this sense, Freud describes affective structures remaining in the unconscious. This affect is destined to presentation: it is suffocated* when the presentation is repressed*, which could lead to discharge if the ego accepted this result.

AGGRESSION

Ger.: Aggression. – Sp.: agresión. – Fr.: agression. – It.: aggressione. – Port.: agressão.

This tendency to destroy or humiliate sometimes leads to the action of damaging the object* or, in other cases, the rival.

At the outset of mental functioning, governed mainly by the "purified pleasure ego", the relation with what is considered the object (the source of sensations of unpleasure*, such as stimuli) is indifference or hate*. The latter is a tendency which aims to increase the distance between the object and the ego*. "Repulsion" is felt towards what is considered the object, and it is hated. This feeling may become more intense and become an inclination to be aggressive towards the object for the purpose of destroying it.

The hate that generates aggression is therefore a form of the ego's link with the object.

In its origins it is mixed with and not distinguished from love: for example, the oral tendency to incorporate or devour. Freud observes:

> As the first of these aims we recognize the phase of incorporating or devouring – a type of love which is consistent with abolishing the object's separate existence and which may therefore be described as ambivalent. At a higher stage of the pregenital anal-sadistic organization, the striving for the object appears in the form of an urge for mastery, to which injury or annihilation of the object is a matter of indifference. Love in this form and at this preliminary stage is hardly to be distinguished from hate in its attitude towards the object.
>
> (1915*c*, pp. 138–9)

In the phallic phase (cf.: phallic-urethral erotism) the difference between love* and hate is clearer. At that point the former is the type of link with the object and the latter with the (oedipal) rival.

Therefore, hate is mixed with or is a part of sexual Trieb. It separates from the latter as its definite opposite only in the phallic phase. Another part of hate (which leads to aggression) comes from self-preservative ego* Trieb (the struggle for life).

When Freud formulated his second Trieb theory in 1920, he postulated the existence of death Trieb*, which added complexity to the panorama since this death Trieb is a fundamental part of the mixture* of Trieb composing aggression. The latter consists in a mixture of Eros* with death Trieb by virtue of which the muscles are able to liberate the subject from the tendency to return to the inorganic.

Death Trieb is characterized mainly by the tendency to return to the inorganic. The living organism defends itself from this tendency in different ways; the first is by deflecting it through the use of muscles, being aggressive and thereby transforming death Trieb into destructive Trieb* or aggression. In this way the tendency to return to the inorganic is passed on to another subject in the external world. Death Trieb always acts more or less in a fused state with sexual Trieb* (sadism*, Trieb for mastery*).

Even when aggression appears to be more de-eroticized, as if pure, its discharge produces the omnipotent satisfaction of narcissism, the pleasure* of mastery over even the life and death of others. This type of narcissistic satisfaction is what reveals its erotic roots.

Death Trieb not deflected to the outside remains in the subject as primary or erotogenic masochism*.

Trieb for aggression or destruction is reintrojected from outside; it forms feminine and moral masochism*, in both cases bound by the superego* and aimed against the ego* but less eroticized in moral masochism than in feminine masochism.

We place the "neuroses of destiny" in the category of moral masochism and its unconscious sense of guilt* or need for punishment*.

When the sense of guilt is conscious, as in melancholia*, there may be a major defusion* of Triebe and the superego may become a "pure culture of death Trieb". In obsessional neurosis* the aggressive Trieb originating in libidinal regression (anal-sadistic) is bound by the superego and turned against the ego, although in this case there is less defusion; aggression is expressed as self-reproaches*, compulsions* to aggressive ideas or actions (foreign to the ego), or a tendency to mastery (adequate to the ego as a character trait) in which aggression is mistakenly considered a way to show love.

AGORAPHOBIA

Ger.: Agoraphobie. – Sp.: agorafobia – Fr.: agoraphobie. – It.: agorafobia. – Port.: agorafobia.
This type of phobia* consists in the fear of being in open spaces (fear of going "outside" or to "the street"). It is more common in adults than in children.

Freud attributes it to an unconscious defence of neurotic subjects in response to the temptation to succumb to erotic concupiscence, which would bring up, as it did in childhood, the danger of castration or something analogous. He presents the example of a young man who was afraid of surrendering to the charms of prostitutes and contracting syphilis as punishment.

Like all phobias, agoraphobia progressively gains ground, and imposes increasing limitations on the ego* in order to keep it far from the dangers of Trieb. These impositions may lead the subject to reclusion and social isolation (libidinal introversion) in order to avoid the dangers of "the street".

Agoraphobia includes a temporal regression* to the subject's childhood when it was possible to "go out to the street" only in the care of a protector. Now, this companion takes care of the subject, shielding not from real dangers but from the subject's own Trieb temptations; by virtue of displacement* and projection* they are felt to be dangers from "outside", from "the street", something that was "real" in childhood.

This symptomatic formation manifests the influence of childhood factors which govern adults on account of their neurosis*. Apparently the opposite of agoraphobia, the "fear of being alone", is a form of claustrophobia explained by Freud as the wish to escape the temptation of solitary onanism. Agoraphobia usually becomes established as an illness after the subject has experienced an attack of anxiety in precipitating circumstances, afterwards feared, which the subject will endeavour to avoid. When this is not possible, an attack of anxiety reappears.

ALLOPLASTIC (BEHAVIOUR)

Ger.: Alloplastich. – Sp.: aloplástico. – Fr.: alloplastique. – It.: alloplastico. – Port.: alloplástica.
Alloplastic behaviour is adequate to aims and in turn endeavours to modify reality* without disavowing* it, in work upon the external world that modifies the latter.

It includes all types of specific action*: actions that discharge the source of Trieb* in the most complete manner possible. We include the production or capture of food, possession of the sexual object*, and sublimations* that generate culture* and are generated by it.

"Alloplastic" describes a type of behaviour that leads to discharge of Trieb. Because it functions according to the reality principle*, producing changes in the external world, as for example the facts of culture itself, we may relate it to the concept of health.

When these endeavours are desexualized, a product of identifications* with attributes of entities previously cathected as objects, they are sublimations. Paranoiac individuals lose their capacity to sublimate by re-sexualizing homosexual links with objects, the ego* generating a defence against these newly sexualized ties. Desexualized homosexual libido* is what composes social ties.

ALTERATION OF THE EGO

Ger.: Ichveränderung. – Sp.: alteración del yo. – Fr.: altération du moi. – It.: modificazione dell'io. – Port.: alteração do ego.

This concept is discussed by Freud in *Analysis Terminable and Interminable* (1937*c*) and *An Outline of Psycho-analysis* (1940*a*), in which he explains that the patient's cooperative ego* is an ideal fiction. The ego is directly "altered" in relation to marks left by personal experiences, especially traumatic situations (the more traumatic and the less developed the ego at the moment of this experiencing, the more altered or more defended the ego will be, with more extreme defences* intervening, to which the unconscious ego will be fixated) and situations of danger* in which these defences were useful. Although these defences may remain active in the present, they partly form an unconscious ego infrastructure on which a preconscious ego superstructure is formed which knows nothing of the previous one but whose actions may be more or less modelled by the unconscious ego, in some cases altering the entire functioning of the ego. Particularly when ego defences are firmly consolidated, they constitute a difficulty for progress of treatment since instead of cooperating, they present real obstacles.

> Every normal person, in fact, is only normal on the average. His ego approximates to that of the psychotic in some part or other and to a greater or lesser extent; and the degree of its remoteness from one end of the series and of its proximity to the other will furnish us with a provisional measure of what we have so indefinitely termed an "alteration of the ego".
>
> (1940, p. 235)

It is among the factors that prolong the period of analysis, creating inconveniences and resistances* or directly generating impossibilities of cure.

"Alteration of the ego" is formed, therefore, mainly by the different unconscious defence mechanisms* of the ego, which may be more or less regressive, more or less involving ego cathexes. The ego's unconscious defence mechanisms generate, apart from their specific function and when their defensive role particularly against Trieb becomes rigid or extreme, diverse types of disorder that alter the ego. This includes pathological character traits*, homosexual perversions* (when fixations* produced by primary repressions occur in the period of the first level of recognition of sexual differences, in the phallic period, when fixation is based on disavowal* of the difference, for example), and even the phenomena of psychotic restitution.

The function of ego defence mechanisms, despite alterations of the ego they may produce, is to defend the ego from danger generated for it by Trieb*.

They generally succeed in doing so by ignoring it and sending it back to the unconscious id*.

Since the analyst proposes precisely (or rather, accepts the proposal arising from the preconscious ego of the patient's thought and also the unconscious wish) to act as an investigator and consequently someone who seeks to learn and to show patients their Trieb, the defence mechanism pertaining to the analysand's unconscious ego in turn generates ego resistance against the progress of the analysis. Let us not forget that the ego calls on the "omnipotent pleasure principle" for help in order to generate its unconscious defence mechanisms and that these are therefore governed by the same principle. From this perspective, we see that ignorance of Trieb protects the ego from anxiety* and therefore it would be strange if it failed to put up some sort of resistance against learning about the history of this Trieb. When it is absolutely predominant and thereby dominates the ego, we say that the ego is altered.

The defence mechanism is partly a system of ignorance of itself, Trieb, and the wish*, "the core of our being" (*The Interpretation of Dreams*, 1900, p. 603).

This mechanism on the one hand protects the ego, forming its unconscious part and giving it a certain degree of binding that suppresses the wish and essentially prevents it from reaching action, apart from turning away from it and transforming it into "internal foreign territory" (1933*a*, p. 57). On the other hand or on the same hand, it impoverishes the ego since everything that becomes unconscious is then felt not to be its own: that is to say, it cannot think, sublimate, or enjoy it. It actually stops pertaining to the preconscious ego and joins the ranks of the repressed in the much-feared id.

It is also true that it accomplishes its main objective: Trieb is inaccessible to the ego and therefore to action, constituting an unconscious ego infrastructure that enables the preconscious superstructure to function with less pressure from Trieb, although when the defensive infrastructure is too large it takes up most of the energetic cathexis, altering the ego to the point that it becomes very difficult to modify.

Overcoming "alterations of the ego" and their concomitant resistances thus becomes one of the objectives of psychoanalysis, particularly of analysis of the patient's ego and character.

An ego that functions under the domination of its unconscious defence mechanisms is an impoverished ego, an ego whose capacity to face the difficulties of reality, its essence, is altered.

This ego is enriched when it gains knowledge of the internal world from which it defends itself automatically and when it realizes that it is defending itself. Then it is able to choose whether to defend itself or to decide whether it is worth defending itself. The defence may become a part of associative commerce or thought* activity, thereby achieving a higher level of mastery* of Trieb and becoming richer.

It is interesting to recall that, in Draft K*, 1896, Freud discusses alteration of the ego as one of the means of symptom formation* of the ego, which symptoms gradually alter. This alteration consists of delusion* generated by the patient on the basis of primary symptoms (distrust) and symptoms of the return of the repressed* (hallucinations*). In this conceptualization delusion is considered an alteration of the ego, which in any case is evident. All defence alters what it is defending; if the defence is extreme, it makes it difficult or impossible to return things to their original position.

AMBIVALENCE

Ger.: Ambivalenz. – Sp.: ambivalencia. – Fr.: ambivalence. – It.: ambivalenza. – Port.: ambivalencia.

This term refers to a psychical state characterized by the simultaneous presence of contrary emotions and sentiments towards the object*.

It is produced in relation to sexual Trieb* in the active–passive* pair, barely mentioned by Freud, or in the love–hate pair which he developed more fully.

In *Instincts and Their Vicissitudes* (1915*c*) he explains:

> Preliminary stages of love emerge as provisional sexual aims while the sexual instincts are passing through their complicated development. As the first of these aims we recognize the phase of incorporating or devouring – a type of love which is consistent with abolishing the object's separate existence and which may therefore be described as ambivalent. At the higher stage of the pregenital anal-sadistic organization, the striving for the object appears in the form of an urge for mastery, to which injury or annihilation of the object is a matter of indifference. Love in this form and at this preliminary stage is hardly to be distinguished from hate in its attitude towards the object.
>
> (pp. 138–9)

Once the difference between love* and hate* has been recognized (in the genital* stage), regression* to previous libidinal stages may occur (libidinal regression, as in obsessional neurosis, in which regression is to the anal-sadistic stage), and ambivalence of Trieb may reappear in relation to the same object.

Sometimes, ego regression tends to occur, in which case the ego has not only Trieb ambivalence but also ego* ambivalence in relation to the object as well as regression of Trieb.

If ego ambivalence predominates, a character* pathology results whereas if Trieb ambivalence predominates, it may become neurosis.

When synthesis of sexual Trieb* is complete and the genital stage is established (cf. genital*), love becomes the opposite of hate and coincides with the total sexual aspiration.

We observe a broad spectrum of possibilities in the phenomenon of love. During the period of the Oedipus complex*, the child finds a first object of love in one of the progenitors; all the sexual Trieb that demands satisfaction comes together on this object. Repression*, which occurs later, obliges the child to renounce most of these infantile sexual aims and leaves a sequel: a deep modification of the relation with the parents. After this effect, the child remains tied to them but with Trieb that is necessarily called "aim inhibited". The child's feelings towards these loved persons receive the term "tender".

This "aim-inhibited" love or tenderness is the affect able to create more enduring ties between human beings, which is explained by the fact that they cannot be fully satisfied.

Sensual love is destined to be extinguished by satisfaction; in order to persist it must be admixed from the outset with purely tender components – that is to say, aim inhibited – or undergo a change in this direction.

Aim-inhibited love is what binds members of the group* and is an essential factor in the generation of culture*. Sensual love is antisocial in this sense; the sexual couple requires intimacy and does not share its love; if it does so, we speak of sexual perversion*.

Freud also observed that children (and adolescents)

> derived their sexual objects from their experiences of satisfaction. The first autoerotic sexual satisfactions are experienced in connection with vital functions which serve the purpose of self-preservation. The sexual instincts are at the outset attached to the satisfaction of the ego-instincts; only later do they become independent of them, and even then we have an indication of that original attachment in the fact that the persons who are concerned with a child's feeding, care, and protection become his earliest sexual objects; that is to say, in the first instance his mother or a substitute for her.
>
> (1914*c*, p. 87)

In other cases, he notes, the object is not chosen on the model of the mother but of the subject: "We say that a human being has originally two sexual objects – himself and the woman who nurses him" (1914*c*, p. 88). From these two derive the models of object choice*: the anaclitic* type (most commonly masculine*) and the narcissistic type (more typically feminine*).

Therefore, we could say that love derives from the growing complexity of the ego accomplished by the vicissitudes of sexual Trieb. This produces in turn complex mixtures with a tendency to return to the inorganic inherent to death Trieb*.

The main obstacle – we could almost say the only one – that death Trieb encounters in its path towards the inorganic is this complication that arises for it with the phenomena of life, of which the principal exponent is love.

As complexity grows, different phenomena appear; sexual Trieb admixes with death Trieb, and by so doing is able to master it, though only partially. The genital sexual act carried to its genital aim, sensual love, is the principal form of mastery* of pure quantity (cf. quantity of excitation*), of non-quality, and death Trieb.

Culture is edified basically on suppression* of sexual Trieb, specifically of incest. Repression* makes a beachhead in the repression of incest and then extends over all possible sexuality, using for this expansion the laws of association* between presentations*. The destructive Trieb* which results from a first level of mixture with sexual Trieb in which hate is not distinguished from love is also suffocated; they are also not well distinguished in some types of aggression or in mastery (in the former the domination of the destructive tendency over the loving tendency is perhaps more clearly seen at times, but we must remember that in order to conquer the object of love a certain level of aggression is needed; in the latter, the object of love is retained without consideration of the harm to the object involved in this retention).

The libidinal ties on which cultural groups are based are aim inhibited. All cultural creations are products of this libido that we could call sublimated. There is less mastery of death Trieb in these creations since some death Trieb remains unmixed. Thus, a paradox arises: this complication encountered by the inorganic generated by the phenomena of life, from which in turn culture was born, carries within itself fairly free and unmastered death Trieb in the very essence of the creation of the cultural fact. Therefore, in this culture it seems that sometimes the destructive tendencies of human beings predominate over those of love.

ANACLISIS

Ger.: Anlehnung. – Sp.: apuntalamiento. – Fr.: étayage. – It.: apoggio o anaclisi. – Port.: apoio.
A path to sexual Trieb* facilitated by Trieb of self-preservation of the ego* in order to choose the predominance of its erotogenic zones* and object choices.

"To begin with, sexual activity attaches itself to functions serving the purpose of self-preservation and does not become independent of them until later" (*Three Essays on the Theory of Sexuality*, 1905*d* [added in 1915], p. 182).

At first, some feelings corresponding to the experience of satisfaction* with the mother separate; this additional pleasure*, initially united to self-preservative Trieb, breaks away and sexual Trieb gradually separates, independent of the fact that in early times, in relation to sexual Trieb, the pleasure ego*, which does not distinguish the mother as an object, dominates. However, even at first, the initial reality ego* is functioning for self-preservative Trieb. This is why the object can be recognized as such while in another sense it is not entirely, and autoerotism* begins to predominate. When the incipient ego* cathected with sexual Trieb starts to recognize or fully recognizes the object as the source of its pleasure, it decides to have* it; for this reason, the first object chosen is the mother for both girls and boys.

Following the Oedipus complex*, once the prohibition of incest is internalized by the formation of the superego*, in spite of this fact and unknown to the ego, the sexual object chosen tends to possess attributes in some way similar to the first objects, satisfiers of self-preservative Trieb. In this way, the choice follows the models of the nurturing mother or the protective father. However, if autoerotism or the "pleasure ego" predominated more absolutely and it was therefore not possible to fully accept sexual difference, object choice* will probably be of a more or less narcissistic type.

However, we could also say that in both cases sexual Trieb is always "supported" by self-preservative Trieb, especially in relation to the attributes of primary objects; but even more so in the case of choosing an object with attributes of the subject's own ego.

ANAL (CF. ANAL EROTISM)

ANAL EROTISM

Ger.: Analerotik. – Sp.: erotismo anal.: – Fr.: érotisme anal. – It.: erotismo anale. – Port.: erotismo anal.
This term refers to a means to obtain pleasure* by stimulation of the anal sphincter, anal mucous membrane, the muscle tissue surrounding the anus (such as the buttocks), and the muscular system in general, as well as everything related to excrements expelled by the anus. These forms predominate in the anal period of infantile sexuality* when movements of the striate muscles begin to be mastered, the child learns to train the sphincters, the first signs of language* appear, and the first anxieties around object loss* and a strong wish* to master the object appear; sadism* and masochism* also develop in this stage.

The forms of anal pleasure begin to acquire active–passive* polarity. Active pleasure coincides with development and mastery of muscular activity, which is simultaneously the main path by which death Triebe* become destructive

Trieb* and Trieb of mastery*, which leads active muscular Trieb to acquire sadistic, cruel characteristics; anal erotism in general is connected to sadism.

Although anal erotism is connected to sadism, it is also related to masochism, which is a passive way to obtain pleasure from this highly important erotogenic zone*. The child often retains faeces during this period when, through mastery of the striate muscles, the child learns to control sphincters. Thus, the child acquires higher levels of culturalization, but also erotization of intestinal functions in relation to an object*, now more clearly recognized as a source of pleasure which the individual therefore tries to subjugate.

Retention of faeces produces pleasure in the anal mucous membrane when defecation is painful. Pleasure obtained in this way is passive. Other connotations are gradually added: defecation acquires the meaning of something valuable, a "gift" for the mother; through a symbolic equation and supported by the infantile sexual theory*, the cloacal theory*, it subsequently means a child, and so on. At the same time, rebellions typical of this period, which tend to lead to a spanking, reveal additional passive-masochistic pleasures. We recall that, as Freud describes it in *A Child Is Being Beaten: A Contribution to the Study of the Origin of Sexual Perversions* (1919), the phantasy of a beating* tends to generate masochistic masturbatory pleasure in adults.

In both sadism and masochism, objects begin to be necessary to obtain pleasure, and in this sense they interrupt autoerotism* (we recall that in adult masturbation, the object is present in phantasy), which nonetheless continues to be central, as in all infantile sexuality.

The stage of predominance of the anal erotogenic zone as a source of pleasure and mastery of muscles is also the stage of initial babbling, language learning, infantile play, and early levels of culturalization.

Sublimation* of anal erotism originates characteristic ego* character traits* such as a tendency towards saving, order, and persistence, so important to culture*. However, when fixation* points are generated with anticathexes*, these traits may become pathological if they are made more rigid and exaggerated (through reaction formation*). Primary repression of anal erotism also generates a change of affect* with respect to adult satisfaction of this Trieb.

The affect of disgust* emerges in this way as a dam against all excremental functions and products in general, but particularly against the anal function. Following the Oedipus complex, disgust extends to everything sexual (incestuous) when the phallic zone takes supremacy over all the erotogenic zones.

In libidinal regressions* such as those of obsessional neuroses* and especially in some types of perversion*, the anaclisis* of original anal erotic pleasure on the intestinal excremental function is clearly observed.

In the stage of predominance of the anal zone, curiosity also emerges, and with it infantile sexual theories in which sexual differences are not recognized (all human beings have an anus). Thus, threats of castration possibly heard at this time are disavowed* as being unimportant. The child thinks that all human beings are able to have children through the anus.

As mentioned above, if anal erotism is sublimated, it may be transformed into character traits; however, if the mechanism of anticathexis predominates in its formation, character disorders may result. It will partly be repressed to the unconscious (from which it may return in symptoms*, mainly of obsessional neurosis); another part will be a constituent of normal sexuality, and if it continues to be the predominant pleasure, it may generate perversions in adulthood.

ANALOGY

Ger.: Analogisch. – Sp.: analogía. – Fr.: analogie. – It.: analogia. – Port.: analogia.

One of the laws of association*, together with contiguity, opposition*, and cause–effect, it marks a relation of similarity between different things. Described since Aristotle, it gained importance with the associationist school of psychology which explained all psychical phenomena as forms of association* governed only by the type of association. This school enjoyed some acceptance between the late eighteenth and early nineteenth centuries. One of its most outstanding members was John Stuart Mill, some of whose works Freud translated and also quoted in his paper on the conception of *Aphasias* (1891), a paper which includes a discussion of very interesting ideas regarding thing-presentations* and word-presentations*.

Although Freud did not embrace this philosophy, he took up some of its concepts that he considered useful for his own reasoning and discoveries.

He conceives of a psyche composed of presentations* and energy. This energy circulates among the presentations, cathecting them (this energy acquires the name of libido* when it cathects the presentation or is cathected by it) in search of discharge.

The laws by which the libido passes from the cathexis* of one presentation to another are those of association. One of these is the law of analogy. Primary process* uses analogies in order to produce identities more easily; that is to say, it mistakes analogies for identities. When there is an ego* with secondary process*, this is moderated. In other words, thought* activity enables distinction between contiguity and identity (cf. perceptual identity* and thought identity*), the analogy of identity and even of opposition approximating cause–effect.

Association by analogy is the major generator of universal symbols* previous to or simultaneous with the acquisition of language* according to the Freudian hypothesis; it is then forgotten and pertains to the unconscious*. These symbols reappear in dreams*, in myths* of peoples, and even in some neurotic symptoms*.

The mechanism of repression* exercised by the unconscious part of the ego also chooses its substitute formation* by using analogical laws (also by contiguity and even opposition) with the repressed presentation, in such a way that their similarity is unnoticed by consciousness*.

This similarity or analogy is produced in connection with one of the attributes of the presentation. When this characteristic of the presentation is mistaken for the whole of it, the identity achieved is apparently total when in reality it is partial.

The ego has to use secondary process for the process of discrimination by thought, thereby distinguishing between analogy and identity, attribute and thing*.

ANIMISM

Ger.: Animismus. – Sp.: animismo. – Fr.: animisme. – It.: animismo. – Port.: animismo.

It means in general the belief that objects of Nature are alive; it may refer to a particular thing* or to Nature as a whole. It coexists in primitive peoples with anthropomorphism, by which things of Nature are considered to possess a soul similar to the human soul.

Animism is a thought* system of primitive individuals, children, and some neurotics. It may constitute a thought system or cosmovision, one of the three created by humanity: (a) animistic (mythology); (b) religious; and (c) scientific. Animism is not actually a religion but does meet all the requisites of religion.

The practical need to master the world must have had an essential role in the creation by primitive individuals of their first cosmological system. In children it also involves the Trieb of mastery*. As they gradually recognize the object as a source of their pleasure* and its presence as being indispensable to avoid invasion by tension due to need, the Trieb of mastery also grows, not only as a defence against fear of object loss* but also to be able, by virtue of animistic techniques and strategies (such as magic*), to influence the object either directly or indirectly.

Primitive individuals aim to control Nature, their enemies, or their objects of pleasure through analogous or similar things, objects that receive the aggression*, plea, or adoration addressed to the former. A child's playing* is similar. Although fantasy*, daydreams, or even dreams* are modes of wish fulfilment*, playing goes a step further: it acts on a real object, a substitute for the original one; this is the origin of symbolization.

Behind animism is omnipotence of thought*. "At the animistic stage men ascribe omnipotence to *themselves.*" By analogy, this corresponds to infantile narcissism*. "At the religious stage they transfer it to the gods but do not seriously abandon it themselves, for they reserve the power of influencing the gods in a variety of ways according to their wishes." This corresponds to children's infantile period with their parents. "The scientific view of the universe no longer affords any room for human omnipotence; men have acknowledged their smallness and submitted resignedly to death" (*Totem and Taboo*, 1913, p. 88). This last system or cosmovision (obviously, in regard to its relative preponderance over the others; the three are always present, although one predominates) corresponds to the state of maturity of the individual who has renounced the domination of the pleasure principle in personal actions and, having recognized the limitations presented by the existence of reality*, seeks an object in this external world. Animism is based on the projection of impulses of feeling of primitive people or children on to the external world. "He turns his emotional cathexes into persons, he peoples the world with them and meets his internal mental processes again outside himself" (1913, p. 92).

Animistic, religious, and scientific systems may coexist in the same period, in the same society, and (as forms of mental functioning or different coexisting logics) in the same person, at different times and also in the same instant (splitting of the ego*, isolation*).

ANTICATHEXIS

Ger.: Gegenbesetzung. – Sp.: contrainvestidura. – Fr.: contre-investissement. – It.: controcarica o contrainvestimento. – Port.: contra-carga o contrainvestimento.

This is the ego's* defensive cathexis* of a presentation* whose attributes are opposite to those of a quantity of excitation* which penetrates the psychical apparatus*, sometimes from the external world, breaking through the protective shield* (an experience of pain*, an actual traumatic situation*), and sometimes from inside (sexual Triebe*, which must be deferred* in order to be traumatic).

The formation of the anticathexis, an extreme defence, the only mechanism of primary repression (pressure to disoccupy), leaves a fixation* and in some cases, as in reaction formation* – the prototype of anticathexis – the inversion of the form of satisfaction, or rather, the disorder of the affect*, in relation to the original Trieb satisfaction.

Primary repression (fixation) is the final corollary of multiple defensive anticathexes in response to external or internal traumatic facts occurring during infantile sexuality*. It is consolidated definitively with repression of the Oedipus complex* and establishment of the superego*. Of the latter we could also say that it is an enormous anticathexis that completes the establishment of primary repression by unifying all previous anticathexes formed during the periods of predominance of each erotogenic zone* (more anticathexes are formed in some of these than in others, depending on experiences with objects* and originating different fixation points). Each previous fixation – when primary oedipal repression, origin of infantile amnesia*, is consolidated, culminating in splitting of the apparatus into an unconscious* and a preconscious* – and all previously repressed infantile sexuality are re-signified in a deferred manner in light of the Oedipus complex, now in a state of repression. It will always push to return from the repressed as an unconscious wish*, and succeeds whenever it finds weak points in repression.

Following the definitive institution of primary repression and the structuring of the superego, repression is exerted on derivatives of the original incestuous and parricidal Trieb. It is then called secondary repression or repression proper. This is the repression observable in clinical work with adults; it is found in subjects with a psychical apparatus already fully constituted, with an unconscious id*, an ego, and a superego with unconscious, preconscious, and conscious parts.

Secondary repression (pressure to pursue) consists of three mechanisms: removal of the preconscious cathexis (from the word-presentation); attraction exerted from primary repression towards the unconscious; and a new anticathexis.

In secondary repression, anticathexis is utilized to reinforce preconscious decathectization*; with the quantity of libidinal cathexis provided by this removal, another presentation is cathected which thereby dislodges the unconscious derivative of the repressed, acting as a stopper which prevents access to the preconscious.

This anticathexis is also established in the perceptual-conscious system (Pcpt.-Cs.). External stimuli of sexual Trieb (for example, disgust* in response to sexual stimuli) may be perceived, and sometimes they are not perceived (as in the case of moderate hysterical blindness).

Secondary repression anticathexis is in turn a force working against the advance of analysis which is observed in psychoanalytical clinical work as one of the ego resistances*.

Anticathexis is defined from the three metapsychological perspectives: the economic, the presentational, and the dynamic. It is the cathexis of a presentation that is different and may even be opposite to the original presentation; a change in the presentation displaces the former one; its success depends on the quantitative energetic cathexis, and its maintenance depends on a constant expenditure of effort. The original presentation is thus dislodged from the unconscious from which it cannot return as long as the new presentation is acting as an anticathexis and the unconscious ego is trying to "capture" any other presentation that approximates or resembles the presentation of the wish that is thereby repressed.

In pain* or external traumatic events, the painful or damaged organ is anticathected narcissistically. Great effort by the ego is perceived. The ego withdraws libido* from all other psychical places and places it in the damaged part of the body, also endeavouring to flee what is traumatic. This explanation shows how the anticathexis functions within the pleasure principle*. If the quantity of excitation in the traumatic fact surpasses its possibilities, the "beyond" of death Trieb* may come into play, aiming this entire phenomenon towards the tendency to repetition of the traumatic as marked by fixation. This repetition is due to the need* to repeat the experience of the traumatic situation in order to work it through* and recover it for the pleasure principle on the one hand, or for mere repetition on the other.

ANXIETY (SEE: STRACHEY, J., 1962, APPENDIX, THE TERM "ANGST" AND ITS ENGLISH TRANSLATION, IN *THE STANDARD EDITION OF THE COMPLETE PSYCHOLOGICAL WORKS OF SIGMUND FREUD*, VOL. 3, PP. 116–17)

Ger.: Angst. – Sp.: angustia. – Fr.: angoisse. – It.: angoscia. – Port.: angústia.

This affect* or particular, unpleasurable affective state is associated with a type of process of bodily discharge, also typical, and perception of this mode of discharge. The bodily process consists predominantly of hyperventilation, tachycardia, increased sweating, and secretions in general.

This model of bodily response is taken on the one hand from the human infant's first type of reaction to the birth trauma – a trauma produced essentially but not only by the steep increase in quantity of bodily excitation* produced in passing from omphalo-mesenteric oxygenation to pulmonary breathing – and, on the other hand, is a relic of what once were actions adequate to an aim in humanity's prehistory that now remain simply as internal changes* or affective expressions.

At birth, the infant expresses internal change (expression of emotions, screaming, vascular innervations); this kind of response is adequate at the outset, since the body thereby receives necessary oxygenation. However, following this manifestation, it is adopted by the ego* as the prototypical reaction to danger. For the rest of the subject's life, the initial reaction to a situation of danger*, whether internal or external, is always anxiety.

At some points in his works – the Fliess papers* and his papers on anxiety neurosis – Freud considers another model of anxiety: reactions produced during the sexual act. These two models complement each other.

The model of reaction to danger is generally closer to the concept of a signal and of toxic accumulation than to equivalence with sexual excitation (although all sexual excitation also involves danger).

Anxiety is the unpleasurable affect *par excellence*, the common denominator to which all other unpleasurable affects refer. The ego does not want to feel it. It defends itself from it, and the neuroses derive from this.

ANXIETY, THEORY OF

Ger.: Angst Theorie. – Sp.: angustia, teoría de la. – Fr.: théorie de l'angoisse. – It.: teoría de l'angoscia. – Port.: angústia, teoria da.

Freud is usually said to have postulated two theories of anxiety*, and this is partly true. However, we shall follow the hypothesis of a single theory which grows more complex as knowledge of psychical functioning deepens. In this way, we may advance without discarding the early theory but instead by adding further complexity, as the creator of psychoanalysis always did in relation to his theory.

Basically, all anxiety is one and the same; its variants reside in the motives that provoke it or different explanations of it.

In his papers on anxiety neurosis*, he explains it as a product of accumulated somatic sexual tension (quantity of excitation* not transformed into libido* or sexual desire* since it is not bound to presentations*).

When for some non-psychical reason (the cause not being repression* of psychical presentations* but an actual mechanical effect produced in the very fact of sexual action; for example, in unsatisfactory sexual relations in which discharge is habitually interrupted or postponed), an inadequate sexual discharge is produced, the amount of accumulated excitation without psychical binding automatically becoming anxiety.

This theory involves the previous conception that not all action is united to presentations or has a psychical correlate; or that if this were so, it would not cancel the fact that each action has a mechanical correlate foreign to the psychical (in the sense of presentations) or which runs parallel to it by a different path, producing bodily effects and thereby generating affects* (automatic anxiety*). These unpleasurable feelings, in some cases quite intense and in others composed almost entirely of bodily affections, are perceived by the conscious perceptual end (Pcpt.-Cs.) where they acquire the quality* of unpleasure* so that the ego* subsequently seeks to find binding for it in preconscious* word-presentations* and thereby give it presentational quality, something difficult to achieve except by way of rationalization.

The outcome is that the quantity of accumulated excitation is perceived automatically by the perceptual apparatus as anxiety.

Until 1925, this theoretical base influences the theory of repression and with it the theory of anxiety of the first topic. In this period, Freud states that repression generates anxiety since it separates the presentation from its cathexis* which is transformed into affect and principally into anxiety; also because it distorts all the psychical values through the action of anticathexis which transforms what was pleasurable into something now producing anxiety.

As he deepens his knowledge of the ego and after describing his second topic or structural theory in 1923 in *The Ego and the Id*, he relates the explanation of neurotic symptom formation* to defence mechanisms* against anxiety, as well as differentiating and relating fear of Triebe* to fear of external dangers. With this development he interlinks all these hitherto mutually contradictory theories. This brilliant synthesis is discussed in *Inhibitions, Symptoms and Anxiety* (1925). He preserves his first explanation: "We see, then, that it is not so much a question of taking back our earlier findings as of bringing them into line with more recent discoveries" (p. 141). It is still useful for explaining actual neuroses* or the actual-neurotic factor in all psychoneurosis, even the automatic anxiety in schizophrenic crises, to which we could add traumatic neuroses* and some psychosomatic pathologies.

The accumulation of quantity of excitation explains the birth trauma* which is the maximum feeling of fear of defencelessness*. It is quite approximately reproduced when automatic anxiety is a symptom*.

To defend itself against this automatic anxiety, the ego generates mediations by making the pathway more complex and by reaching new levels and characteristics of anxiety; the ego is thereby able to dominate the id.

The ego is the "seedbed of anxiety". It cultivates it in its own earth, transforms it into a signal, and presents it both to Trieb coming from the id and also to the unconscious portion of the ego in such a way that the ego defence mechanism under the guidance of the pleasure principle* represses Trieb, thereby avoiding unpleasure to which its satisfaction could lead.

This type of "cultivated" anxiety is the anxiety signal*, a signal the ego uses to succeed in repressing Trieb and thereby manage it or at least prevent it from reaching action or discharge.

It is therefore the anxiety signal that generates repression and not the opposite. This anxiety needs no explanation by quantitative accumulation; it is a procedure, a memory* of "what might occur if …", which manages to force Trieb to back away and detain the process (when repression is successful, obviously, since when it fails automatic anxiety may return, in which case an economical explanation is necessary).

The anxiety signal originates from an intimate relation with reality*, since it is based on real facts or facts experienced as real (cf. historical truth*) at certain moments in life, such as object* loss, threat of castration, or loss of love.

We may say that castration anxiety* is the prototype of anxiety signals to which the other anxieties refer: such as object* loss, loss of love, fear of the superego*, and social anxiety*.

As we have seen, all these anxiety signals and their respective defences may fail – due to some psychical (schizophrenia) or non-psychical cause (actual neurosis) – in which case the psychical apparatus* is invaded by quantity of excitation, automatic anxiety then flooding the panorama.

ANXIETY DREAMS

Ger.: Angsttraum. – Sp.: sueños de angustia. – Fr.: rêves d'angoisse. – It.: sogni d'angoscia. – Port.: sonhos de angústia.

In these dreams*, disguised repressed unconscious wish fulfilment* is grasped by the preconscious ego*, producing anxiety*. The cause of anxiety is not the wish fulfilment itself, which is not real but only hallucinatory, but what it implies: for example, punishment* by castration*.

What is pleasurable for one system may not be pleasurable for another, since fulfilment of the wish (if it is repressed, it is because it was infantile: incestuous or parricidal or an unconscious derivative of these) might be pleasurable for id* Triebe whereas the ego would be anxious about it; what is decisive is the sensation experienced by the ego, which is the agency that feels anxiety.

The dream content may more or less justify this anxiety from a preconscious viewpoint, but anxiety may also be caused by unconscious factors; for example, when castration anxiety*, appearing in disguise in the dream, gives the preconscious an apparent reason to think that the causes of its anxieties are present in the dream's manifest content.

However, since there is no reason in real life, the dream's content is rejected and forgotten (repressed). Patients with a certain level of omnipotence of thought*, for example obsessional neurotics*, tend to experience this as premonition.

A prototypical example of an anxiety dream is the "Wolf Man's" famous dream when he was a child. It fulfilled the repressed wish for passive coitus with his father, to receive a gift-child from him, reviving and resignifying the primal scene* of the parents apparently perceived in his earliest infancy; this scene was given representation in the day's residues* based on memories* and children's stories (the wolves), which could partly justify a rational cause for the quantity of anxiety from the preconscious viewpoint. However,

from the unconscious viewpoint, it was related with castration anxiety, since this anxiety is part of the wish for passive coitus itself, a first degree of recognition of sexual difference based on that period of phallic predominance in which the differentiation recognized is castrated–not castrated; thus, the passive wish involves the element of castration.

This is an intolerable wound for this patient's ego (his bedrock*) which at this level of libidinal development centres its narcissism* on the phallus, on account of the magnitude of pleasurable sensations it provides; for this reason it is integrated into a unit with all the previous pleasurable sensations and also constitutes what he is loved for and what enables him to love the object*.

When this ego perceives the castration implicit in fulfilment of the passive feminine wish in the dream, it experiences anxiety in its "bedrock", the degree of participation and conceptualization of the "masculine protest" (Alfred Adler's concept) that could be accepted.

ANXIETY FOR LOSS OF LOVE

Ger.: Angst vor Liebersverlust. – Sp.: angustia de pérdida de amor. – Fr.: angoisse de la perte d'amour. – It.: angoscia di perdita d'amore. – Port.: angústia de perda de amor.

This type of anxiety signal* is perceived mainly by girls when they enter the phallic period; therefore, it is part of the castration complex*.

When they understand the difference between their body and the boy's, which they understand as that of an uncastrated child, they understand it as if they were missing the genital and not as their female sex (a process to which the ego* has to arrive with difficulty after an effort of complex thought activity* at which they arrive in puberty in the best of cases). Therefore, upon this crucial discovery, they succumb to penis envy*. This anatomical difference is aggravated by disequality in comparison to boys in the constitution of the ego since the phallus does not in their case gain sufficient primacy (cf. phallic primacy) over the other erotogenic zones* (their phallus is the clitoris in any case, and this is cause for envy). In the period of the castration complex, what girls understand as a lack of genital is gradually replaced by the erotogenic body as a whole and the vagina in particular (we may think about the diffuse quality of female orgasm). For this reason, narcissism* in women is not constituted from a principle such as "self-love" but from what predominates in them which is a need to be loved, which makes them more dependent on the object*. This may also be an element contributing to the fact that some women constitute their ego more as an object than as a subject.

In the period of the castration complex in girls, the need to be loved (at first by the mother) becomes acute, and therefore the fear of losing her love is quite intense.

A time usually comes then when she blames her mother for her handicap, separates from her, then wants to have a child, a symbol of the wished-for penis (this passage is called the symbolic equation). By this path leading to her femininity she finds her father as an object and then is fearful of losing his love, since he is now the object from which she expects her penis-child.

Later, in adolescence, she makes her definitive exogamic* object choice*, a choice that carries within it her history with primary objects and its corresponding fears.

The constitution of the female superego* takes longer than the male superego; its form of structuring is also less dramatic. Female fear of loss of love is more prolonged, which quite probably influences the generation of differences in relation to later anxieties: fear of the superego and social anxiety*.

Fear of loss of love "plays much the same part in hysteria as the threat of castration does in phobias and fear of the superego in obsessional neurosis" (1925, p. 143), which is certain to have some relation to the fact that hysteria is predominantly female.

ANXIETY FOR OBJECT LOSS

Ger.: Angst vor Objektverlust. – Sp.: angustia de pérdida de objeto. – Fr.: angoisse de la perte d'objet. – It.: angoscia di perdita d'oggetto. – Port.: angústia de perda de objeto.

This anxiety* is felt by the baby in the process of leaving behind the pleasure ego* (in which the object*, since it produced pleasure, was considered ego*). The infant gradually recognizes the mother as an object of pleasure*, as not-I, and begins to desire her, is no longer her (we recall that in the pleasure ego everything hated is recognized as not-I).

In this way, the child passes from the category of being* to the category of having*, and consequently the possibility of not having; this possibility is a source of anxiety since the presence of the object has proven to be highly important, even indispensable, among other reasons in order to protect from invasion by tension due to need* or quantity of excitation*; in other words, by automatic anxiety* similar to the anxiety of the birth trauma*.

This fear of object loss is the first anxiety that functions as a signal activating ego defence mechanisms*, most of them unconscious, and other forms of defence* that, although not included in these mechanisms, are perhaps the most efficient ones possible for the ego. As products of this type of anxiety, infantile play, language*, and other symbolic attempts to retain the object of pleasure spring up; in this way, the subject may at least succeed in having it.

Anxiety for object loss is expressed in clinical work basically as fear of loneliness, of the dark, of the presence of strangers, and others. In any case, the background of this anxiety is castration anxiety* although the latter appears later in the subject's life and is more complex on the level of recognition of the object as a source of pleasure.

Anxiety for object loss consists in a signal produced by the ego in a minute quantity, which automatically and unconsciously calls up the defence mechanism that originates a substitute formation*, a compromise, which produces the effect being sought: to make Trieb* unconscious; in this sense, the ego's defence is effective. This form of anxiety needs no economic explanation: it is produced by the ego (like all anxiety signals) in minute quantities and is based on memory*, the dangerous presentation*. The result of the defence mechanism may be the generation of symptoms*, character traits*, and so on. In adults it may be produced by ego regression*, since it is more primitive (in the infantile period in which this type of anxiety predominates the distinction between ego and object of pleasure is unclear) than castration anxiety, fear of the superego*, and social anxiety*, although they may be mixed and therefore hard to distinguish. This type of anxiety predominates in defence mechanisms (disavowal) in Meynert's amentia*.

If for some reason ego defence mechanisms fail, an anxiety attack may occur, producing automatic anxiety which does have an economic explanation since it is generated by the quantity of excitation or its equivalent: invasion of tension due to need.

ANXIETY HYSTERIA

Ger.: Angsthysterie. – Sp.: histeria de angustia. – Fr.: hystérie d'angoisse. – It.: isteria d'angoscia. – Port.: histeria de angústia.

In this type of hysteria, the main symptom is anxiety* expressed in response to a certain type of perception*. It is better known in the history of psychoanalysis by the name of phobia*. Freud considers the latter only one of its components, secondary mechanisms of inhibition* emerging from the ego* in order to avoid confrontation with conflicts provoking the appearance of symptoms*.

It is a hysteria because its fixation point* is in phallic-urethral erotism*, carrying its conflictive themes. Since its predominant anxiety is castration anxiety*, it is more common in men than in women. Its problem is the oedipal problem, intimately related to the level of recognition of sexual difference possible in the phallic phase (phallic–castrated).

The boy's oedipal phantasies* may reflect the positive Oedipus (loving towards the mother, murderous towards the father) with its concomitant castration anxiety, or the negative Oedipus (homosexually loving towards the father, a failed attempt to disavow* sexual difference). When he places himself in the feminine position in relation to his father, this position itself involves his own castration, which may generate the "male protest" from the ego's "bedrock"* and also cause the ego castration anxiety.

In both positive and negative Oedipus, the father is the feared castrator; this figure is based on phylogeny since the prehistory of the human family is inherited (repeated) in primal phantasies* of castration.

The phylogenetic also intervenes in infantile animal phobias as a legacy of totemism*.

Anxiety hysteria is one of the neuroses of defence*, precisely because anxiety is the main symptom. It is anxiety* neurosis because its anxiety is indeterminate, produced by an invasion of quantity of excitation* in the psychical apparatus*.

Anxiety hysteria involves several steps. Perhaps at the onset, the tendency to flee from the stimulus predominates; perhaps we could deduce primary repression from the appearance of the dam which is shame in response to exhibitionistic and voyeuristic tendencies. When children enter the Oedipus complex* (positive or negative), they fear castration which may be executed by the father. This anxiety is realistic*. For children, reality* is given, not only by threats but by the sight of the female genital and by understanding* what these threats mean. This process is not usually conscious. To keep it from becoming conscious, the ego utilizes libidinal displacement* on to the presentation of an animal, which causes the animal phobia. Therefore, anxiety strikes when the chosen animal enters the perceptual field. In contrast, the child is calm when it is not near.

A substitute formation has been achieved: the phobogenic object*. Other substitute formations are derived from it according to laws of association* (contiguity*, analogy*, opposition). The phobia's territory spreads in this way. The ego secondarily inhibits its activities in order to prevent encounters with the phobogenic object; it also resorts to a certain regression* to the infantile stage in which it needed the parents' protective company. A companion is needed in order to feel safe behind the phobic rampart* constructed in this manner, to avoid emergence of the repressed phantasy.

When the repressed returns*, anxiety and phobia appear in all their splendour. At other moments, secondary defence* predominates, evidencing an evasive character, with some roots in shame which characterizes the phobic rampart*. The substitute formation is relatively stable. Animal phobia in childhood may become a phobia in adulthood of travelling, airplanes, open or closed spaces, or others.

The anxiety of anxiety hysteria is therefore an anxiety signal* in response to the danger of castration. This anxiety was realistic in childhood, to which the ego fixated to the phallic erotogenic zone* returns; therefore, when the substitute formation and the consequent anxiety signal of castration appear, the ego resorts to new displacements extending throughout the subject's environment, together with inhibitions, avoidance, and companions, which acquire all the characteristics of anxiety neurosis, neurosis, or even a phobic character.

Because of the quantity of inhibitions the phobic is driven to avoid meeting objects causing anxiety, and the ego is impoverished. The problem then changes: anxiety in response to a substitute formation advances to an avoidance phobia. In this way, the phobic person succeeds in avoiding anxiety by virtue of a secondary defence that progressively dominates the panorama. This change lowers anxiety hysteria as such but raises the defensive phobic rampart, which is not secure and may fracture again in response to new frustrations*. Then, anxiety reappears.

Both female anxiety hysteria (which may also consist in animal phobias, usually pests: rats, snakes, cockroaches) and agoraphobias* or claustrophobias (generally in males but also in females) are explained as anxiety in response to the temptation to give in to erotic Trieb tendencies. Small animals usually represent the male genital; open spaces, an invitation to exhibitionistic tendencies, and closed spaces, to masturbatory temptations. However, they are specific to each individual and possess singular meanings in function of the person's history.

ANXIETY NEUROSIS

Ger.: Angstneurose. – Sp.: neurosis de angustia. – Fr.: névrose d'angoisse. – It.: nevrosi d'angoscia. – Port.: neurose de angustia.

This type of actual neurosis* was originally described by Freud, who differentiated it from neurasthenia*. Its origin is not in the past, which now corresponds to psychical presentations*, but in actual events, usually occurring in a mechanism of sexual discharge which stagnates somatic sexual tension.

Anxiety* produced in these neuroses is not directly connected with relations between presentations, and therefore also not with the subject's history or the repression* of Triebe*.

However, in some cases abnormal discharge may derive from neuroses of defence* or transference* neuroses, although in these cases anxiety has an actual explanation. These are mixed neuroses, probably the most common type.

The symptoms of pure anxiety neurosis described by Freud are general irritability, anxious expectation (the core symptom of this neurosis), and attacks of anxiety, either by itself or with a fear of going mad or a sensation of imminent death; also bodily alterations; breathing, cardiac activity, vasomotor activity, and glandular activity. The patient may complain of "spasms in the heart", "breathlessness", "waves of sweating", or "insatiable hunger" in which the feeling of anxiety may even become secondary. In the latter, it is equivalent to an attack of anxiety: (a) alterations of cardiac activity, brief arrhythmia, persistent tachycardia, pseudo-angina pectoris; (b) breathing difficulties; nervous dyspnoea, asthma-like attacks; (c) surges of sweating; (d) trembling and shuddering; (e) attacks of insatiable hunger; (f) sudden attacks of diarrhoea; (g) attacks of loss of balance; (h) vasomotor neurasthenia; (i) attacks of paraesthesia.

Nocturnal terror is quite frequent, usually associated with anxiety, dyspnoea, perspiration, and other symptoms. Several of the symptoms associated with or substituting attacks of anxiety may also manifest chronically. As we see, anxiety neurosis is not only actual in relation to the patient but is also common in the present age, especially in stages of life with excessive excitation, as in adolescence and menopause. Therefore, it is a clinical picture that should be revaluated and studied in depth. We know its major cause: a relative increase of quantity of excitation*.

ANXIETY SIGNAL

Ger.: Angstsignal. – Sp.: angustia señal. – Fr.: signal d'angoisse. – It.: segnale d'angoscia. – Port.: sinal de angustia.

This signal is produced and felt by the ego* which utilizes it to dominate Trieb*. It does so by means of defence mechanisms* in response to the latter. It then utilizes the pleasure principle* against Trieb satisfaction, paradoxically, since following the installation of primary repression the possibility of Trieb satisfaction generates unpleasure* (anxiety*) in the ego. When the id* sends the cathexis of an unconscious Trieb wish (or in other terms, a cathected thing-presentation* seeking a word-presentation* in order to make it known to consciousness* and therefore to the ego), the ego may not accept it as its own and therefore produce the anxiety signal, for which it utilizes the memory* of moments of anxiety that were real in childhood; for example, the sight of female genitals in the case of castration anxiety*.

The anxiety signal is therefore based on experience. This is the case of fear of object loss* when the baby begins to recognize the object* as such, and with it, its importance to him or her. It is also true for the castration anxiety that arises in the boy's phallic state; its counterpart in women is fear of losing the object's love*. In non-neurotic adults (in neurotics also, especially obsessional neurotics), they tend to be fear of the superego* and social anxiety*.

The anxiety signal is a highly effective resource for the ego to dominate Trieb, although it is frequently very costly; damage to its structure is an unwanted effect (at least for the psychical portion of the pleasure principle) that cannot be attributed to the anxiety signal but rather to defence mechanisms produced by the ego in response to it. Even so, it is worthwhile to underscore defensive efficacy; after the signal, the presentation appears (word- or thing- depending on the case, which also indicates the level of severity of pathology or the degree of alteration of the ego*) and Trieb, now "de-activated", loses its efficacy.

ANXIOUS EXPECTATION

Ger.: Enwartungs angst. – Sp.: apronte angustiado. – Fr.: expectation angoissée. – It.: appronto angosciato. – Port.: aprontamento angustiado.

A state of hyper-cathexis* with quiescent (bound) energy* of the perceptual apparatus or the perceptual-conscious system (Pcpt.-Cs.) of the ego* (attention*) that is prepared against danger. It is in reality the last bastion of the protective shield*. Freud considers that this might have been the permanent state of the primitive individual in response to the dangers of Nature (1915).

An external event is traumatic if it is able to overcome the protective shield; or if this hyper-cathexis of attention does not exist at the moment of the event, the invasion of stimuli occurred, and consequently the psychical apparatus was unable to bind them with past presentations*, resulting in the feeling of terror*.

An effect of the traumatic event may be traumatic neurosis* with its typical symptoms* such as repetitive dreams* of the traumatic event. These repetitions are not directly at the service of wish fulfilment* but "are endeavouring to master the stimulus retrospectively, by developing the anxiety whose omission was the cause of the traumatic neurosis" (1920*g*, p. 32). If some binding of the stimulus is attained, it then pertains to the pleasure principle* and the search for wish fulfilment.

The conscious perceptual end (Pcpt.-Cs.) needs to be cathected in order to endure external stimuli; once it has been exceeded, the psychical apparatus repeats the event (usually in dreams but sometimes in actions) by virtue of repetition compulsion* on the one hand, and on the other hand, in order to effect the anxious hyper-cathexis and bind the quantity of excitation* to other presentations of the subject's previous history.

It is interesting to add that in the case of actual neuroses* and also anxiety neurosis*, Freud describes a basic state that he names "expectant anxiety": a permanent state of alertness to danger; of course the danger (for the psychical apparatus) in this case is a quantity of somatic sexual excitation, not discharged or not properly discharged, rather than the external world; however, this expectant state, with a perceptual end hyper-cathected with hyper-cathexis of attention, a producer of anxiety*, is similar.

ART

Ger.: Kunst. – Sp.: arte. – Fr.: art. – It.: arte. – Port.: arte.

One of the supreme creations of human culture*, a product of sublimation* of the childhood sexual Trieb* rejected by this culture. Art is able, by taking a certain roundabout way, to reconcile the pleasure principle* with the reality principle*. Artists originally reject reality* when they cannot accept renouncement of Trieb satisfaction imposed on them by reality. They then devote themselves to their object fantasies* (erotic and ambitious); up to this point they are no different from the common neurotic, but unlike the latter, they are able to return to reality by virtue of their own gifts, transforming their fantasies into a new type of reality valued by others: works of art. In this way they succeed in becoming heroes*, rulers, and creators, pampered by fortune as they had wished (for which they must be successful artists), without need of making deep changes in the external world. Their spectators, readers, or listeners (all consumers of art), with their own Triebe* unsatisfied, identify with this new reality created by artists and participate in its enjoyment through this identification. Art, like child's playing, is a "fantasy acted out" which involves action and scenification (*Formulations on the Two Principles of Mental Functioning*, 1911*b*).

Primitive art probably originated in magic*, a technique of the animistic conception of the universe included in omnipotence of thought*; the first artistic objects emerged as an expression of the Trieb of mastery* in order to dominate enemies or objects of nature, or to fulfil their wishes* by creating objects analogous to those they wished for or feared (*Totem and Taboo*, 1912–13). This animistic period also exists in children, and their first reactions probably have similar meanings for them. In children as well as artists, the defence* against fear of object loss* is present when the object* begins to be recognized as a source of pleasure. In this case children endeavour to possess the object or to be loved by it; artists strive for the same in the derivatives of those childhood parents (their admirers). But artists are also heroes who in mythical fantasy killed the father; they are Oedipus at the crossroads to Thebes, as are all children during the period that carries his name.

Children play at being grown-up, executing all the specific actions* that they assume grown-ups do. Artists are grown-ups that unknowingly go back to playing as when they were children without leaving adulthood.

ARTIFICIAL GROUP

Ger.: Künstliche masse. – Sp.: masa artificial. – Fr.: masse artificielle. – It.: massa artificiale. – Port.: massa artificial.

This highly organized type of human group possesses hierarchical orders and solid structures which guard against its breakdown; it therefore persists through time and survives its members' individual existence. The basic structure of artificial groups is their own history and traditions. Any individual, by being a member of a group of this type, becomes part of its history and leaves aside individual history to be one more link in the history of the group to which the subject belongs.

It refers to institutions like the Church and the army which utilize a certain type of external compulsion to prevent their dissolution and prevent changes in their structure.

In the above examples, an individual may even be incorporated into this type of group against the person's wishes, and any attempt to separate from it tends to be obstructed or severely punished or is subject to certain conditions.

The basic structure of these groups shares a feature with ephemeral groups*: an idealized leader. They also have two types of link: between the members and the leader and among members.

Unlike ephemeral groups, certain differences between members of the artificial group are expressed in hierarchies established among them.

ASSOCIATION

Ger.: Assoziation. – Sp.: asociación. – Fr.: association. – It.: associazione. – Port.: associação.

A mechanism for linking one presentation* to another, produced by displacement* of libidinal energy* (which Freud also calls quantum of affect*). This displacement may be produced in two ways: by free displacement in which libidinal quantities may pass from one presentation to another by means of the laws of association: analogy, contiguity, and opposition. These displacements are mistaken for identities and therefore function with perceptual identity* and primary process*. They are predominantly visual thing-presentations corresponding to the unconscious and are those seen in dreams.

When cathexis is stronger and displacement weaker, since a higher level of binding makes association between presentations more complex, other mechanisms intervene. In this form of association, the reasons for it and its identity are differentiated (since it is not enough for something to have an attribute that is analogous, contiguous, or opposite to something else for the former to be wished for). Although it also endeavours to find identity with what is wished for, it does so by utilizing thought*: it seeks identity of thought* which corresponds to the preconscious ego*, thought activity, and secondary process*.

The concept of association is derived from associationism, the philosophical school of which Freud read John Stuart Mill, from whom he extracted the laws of relation between presentations; Freud added directionality, a tendency characterizing the pleasure principle*, and Trieb* wishes. Hence, association acquired the characteristics of the means of interrelation between presentations, but with an objective (the Trieb wish or the defence against it), which takes association a step further.

Hybrid word-presentations tend towards a certain freedom of association that generates fantasy and daydreaming. These associations involve more displacement than in thought activity. Words are governed especially by the pleasure principle and even a certain level of perceptual identity. However, the business of passage of quantum of affect between presentations is more rigorous in thought* in which displacement is weak, the principle of reality* governs, and identity with what is wished for is sought instead by thinking about thought identity* (by calibrating to what extent it is and is not identity and by studying the attributes of the perceptum and the presentation, comparing them, and subjecting them to reality testing*). Free fantasy is generally rejected by conscious censorship*. If these fantasies* become derivatives of repressed presentations, they may then be repressed by unconscious censorship, thereby forming the basis for parapraxes*, neurotic symptoms*, dreams*, and so on.

ATTENTION

Ger.: Aufmerksamkeit. – Sp.: atención. – Fr.: attention. – It.: attenzione. – Port.: atenção.

Libidinal energy (in the broad sense including the ego's* self-preservative interest* which in reality comes from the id* but is bound and "stored" in and by the ego) which cathects the perceptual-conscious system (Pcpt.-Cs.). Its cathexis is indispensable for the register of anything by consciousness*.

It functions on two levels: a freely floating level which despite its weak cathexis registers equally all possible perceptions; the second level, copious and heavily cathected, gives clarity to perception. When a perception connected with something either wished for or feared is discovered, the Pcpt.-Cs. receives a strong cathexis of attention, with which it acquires conscious clarity.

Although attention serves to perceive the external world, it also registers thought* activity coming from the internal world by virtue of word-presentations*.

To make a thought conscious, the preconscious (Prec) word-presentation must be cathected by attention which makes it conscious. This cathexis is managed by the conscious ego, especially through conscious censorship*.

When we ask patients to associate freely, we are in reality asking their ego to cathect their word associations* with attention, to postpone conscious critical censorship which might attempt to decathect them in order to avoid conflicts that generate anxiety*. We are asking them to stop utilizing conscious censorship for reinforcement of unconscious repression* from which the return of the repressed may bring about symptoms* and neurosis*.

Perception* is not passive. Cathexis of attention includes the cathexis of unconscious wishes*, mediated by the ego, which like feelers (*A Note Upon the "Mystic Writing Pad"*, 1925*a*, p. 231 and *Negation*, 1925) register all possible perceptions, since what is wished for or feared may be among them.

AUTOEROTISM

Ger.: Autoerotismus. – Sp.: autoerotismo. – Fr.: auto-érotisme. – It.: auto-erotismo. – Port.: auto-erotismo.

The predominant characteristic or modality of libido* satisfaction of infantile sexuality* by means of self-stimulation (touching, rhythmic stroking, compression of mucous membranes, visualization of erotogenic zones*) of the subject's own body, which produces organ pleasure*.

Although it predominates as we said in early stages, it extends in part over the entire lifetime. Because it predominates in infantile sexuality, it is said to be autoerotic.

Autoerotism is previous to constitution of the reality ego*. Although this ego* originates in the body and is based in part on the body image, it gradually becomes a complex entity or psychical structure that exceeds the body on another level with increasingly sophisticated functions. Libido that seeks satisfaction in this psychical structure that is the ego constitutes narcissism*.

Once narcissism is established, autoerotism follows a modality of narcissistic libido satisfaction. However, it subsequently becomes more complex; for example, in adolescent masturbation, object libido may be satisfied through masturbatory fantasies. In this case, masturbation may be a form of autoerotic satisfaction that discharges both narcissistic libido through action and also, through fantasy, object libido introverted (cf. introversion*) from reality that has taken refuge in fantasy. This complexity is even greater since narcissistic object choice* involves both object libido and narcissistic libido or an intermediate stage between them: homosexual libido.

Schizophrenia* involves total libidinal withdrawal (in relation to wished-for objects or wishing for objects). There is no refuge in fantasy (since its existence requires the wish for an object) but only an overload of libido in the ego; consequently, the loss of any wish for an object is expressed clinically as an experience of the end of the world due to this withdrawal; and hypochondria* or megalomania* due to hyper-cathexis* of the ego. Libidinal regression* may, in the "simple" form of schizophrenia, reach autoerotism; in this case, libido cathects the body although the latter does not configure an ego, or does so with its last remnant (the body) in relation to its libidinal cathexes, having thereby been degraded to the utmost as a psychical entity.

AUTOMATIC ANXIETY

Ger.: automatische Angst. – Sp.: angustia automática – Fr.: angoisse automatique. – It.: angoscia automatica. – Port.: angústia automática.

This anxiety* is produced by an excessive quantity of excitation* in the psychical apparatus* which may be partly libidinal* (if it acquires some type of presentation*) or pure quantity (in which case we speak of Trieb defusion* in the manner of free death Trieb). It is similar to a repetition of the birth trauma in the sense of great defencelessness* of the psyche in response to tension due to need.

It has different causes. It is the only actual neurosis* that is a manifestation of a quantity of excitation unbound by the psychical apparatus (or only very slightly bound to presentations, something solely or predominantly actual), although a few presentations may utilize this quantity to make a quantity of libido; for this reason, Freud mentions retained libido in actual neuroses as a generator of anxiety; their salient feature is that the quantitative strongly dominates the presentational; it may also provide proof of the actual-neurotic in all transference neurosis* regarding the portion of excitation not bound to presentations. It also appears when, for some reason, the ego's anxiety signal* fails or its defence mechanisms* have not responded to the anxiety signal, leaving the ego devastated by excitation, which generates anxiety attacks in historical or transference neuroses.

In schizophrenic psychosis*, given the deep alteration of the ego and the withdrawal of cathexis from the unconscious thing-presentation* (and since this cathexis generates Trieb and the unconscious object wish, both are lost), the quantity of excitation* is left without any possibility of binding, or can only be bound by words, a weak binding to be sure. Given this relative and also extreme liberty, this quantity of excitation, lacking the qualification that would be provided by a thing-presentation, is expressed automatically as anxiety.

AUTOPLASTIC (BEHAVIOUR)

Ger.: Autoplastiche. – Sp.: autoplástica (conducta). – Fr.: autoplastique. – It.: autoplastica. – Port.: autoplástica.

This term refers to a type of behaviour characteristic of psychosis* and in part of neurosis* in which the endeavour to modify an unacceptable reality* is limited to internal changes* that at most modify perception* (hallucination*) or the conception of reality* (delusion*), or produce alterations in the subject's own body (neurotic symptoms, some equivalent to anxiety and anxiety* itself), but not reality.

Freud utilizes this adjective in reference to behaviour in his article of 1924(*e*): *The Loss of Reality in Neurosis and Psychosis.*

B

BEATING PHANTASIES

Ger.: Schlag phantasien. – Sp.: fantasías de paliza. – Fr.: fantasmes de raclée. – It.: fantasie di picchiare. – Port.: fantasias de sova.

These are sado-masochistic masturbatory phantasies* usually presenting in female patients, although they are not absent in men. A scene is fancied: "a child is being beaten", associated with intense sexual pleasure*.

The way phantasies are composed is complex and comprises several stages; their study clarifies the genesis of perversions*, particularly masochism* and the role of sexual difference in the dynamics of the neuroses*.

Among the different stages, the most pleasurable in both women and men is unconscious* and masochistic (the child being beaten is the fancier him- or herself, unknown to the subject). In women beating phantasies are also feminine, as in men, and therefore correspond in men to the negative Oedipus complex* and in women to the positive.

These phantasies condense* a number of meanings such as jealousy* of the siblings of infantile sexuality (formally, it is boys who are being beaten) and expiation of guilt* (these boys are siblings and the subject as well), which is included in the masochistic part, though it is unconscious.

BEDROCK

Ger.: gewachsenen Fels. – Sp.: roca de base. – Fr.: roc de base. – It.: rocca di base. – Port.: rocha de base.

This is a place in psychical fabric, a moment reached during a treatment, and also a "concept" discussed by Freud in *Analysis Terminable and Interminable* (1937) as a nearly final limit to the therapeutic possibilities of psychoanalysis.

The theme of bedrock is composed of two sub-themes, both related to sexual difference; one is produced in men and the other in women. These two themes are: penis envy* in women and, in men, the revolt against the possibility of having a passive or feminine attitude towards another man.

Thus, they are ultimately a kind of last defence* against "being castrated" in both sexes, which in this case appears comparable to the feminine, as it is in the phallic period of childhood. For this reason, the individual's bedrock depends on the magnitude of the subject's unconscious castration complex*.

At entry into the phallic period of infantile sexuality*, the problem emerges of the first level of recognition of sexual difference, which is phallic–castrated. Some beings have a penis and others have been dispossessed of it. Those who possess one suffer anxiety* for being able to lose it; those who do not, the complex involving the narcissistic wound of feeling handicapped.

Establishment of the superego* erases this problem during the latency* period, but it resurges in adolescence in a symbolic, displaced, or disguised way.

On this road, all types of defence emerge: some may be useful to avoid facing the problem originating in sexual difference and others are for facing it in the most adequate way possible;

the degree of predominance of each of these defences depends on the reality principle*, and growth of the ego* and its preconscious word-presentations*, language*, thought activity*, and so on, dominant in each person.

Depending on the results of differentiation recognized during the phallic phase, the second level of sexual differentiation is worked through: masculine–feminine.

In any case, in the unconscious*, the former differentiation (phallic–castrated) partly remains standing in different degrees in each person. This forms the limit it is possible to reach in analysing these themes.

> At no other point in analytic work does one suffer more from an oppressive feeling that all one's repeated efforts have been in vain, and from a suspicion that one has been "preaching to the winds", than when one is trying to persuade a woman to abandon her wish for a penis on the ground of its being unrealizable or when one is seeking to convince a man that a passive attitude to men does not always signify castration ... The decisive thing remains that the resistance prevents any change from taking place – that everything stays as it was. We often have the impression that with the wish for a penis and the masculine protest we have penetrated through all the psychological strata and have reached bedrock, and that thus our activities are at an end. This is probably true, since, for the psychical field, the biological field does in fact play the part of the underlying bedrock.
>
> (*Analysis Terminable and Interminable*, 1937, p. 252)

Anatomical sexual differentiation, decisive in the phallic period to the development of the oedipal drama, acts to support the maintenance, in the unconscious, of the horror of castration. Therefore, at bottom, in different forms and quantities, it is not accepted or, the opposite, it is accepted only up to a certain point.

This limit is each individual's "bedrock": the point to which the existence of castration is acceptable. Past this point, the ego must split, and therefore also thought activity. Then, contradictions are accepted and primary process* begins to infiltrate thought*; this is the origin of phenomena ranging from simple "eccentricities of normal people" to ego splitting characteristic of fetishism* or homosexuality*.

BEING

Ger.: Sein. – Sp.: ser. – Fr.: être. – It.: essere. – Port.: ser.

In Freud's works, the idea concerning being is technical-theoretical; it refers to a primitive category of ego functioning of the psychical apparatus, the opposite of having*, another type which gradually emerges in subsequent development.

Therefore, the category of being predominates at the outset of mental functioning, essentially with respect to sexual Trieb*, especially related to the pure pleasure ego* for which the object* of pleasure* is not recognized as such but rather as "being" part of the ego.

If pleasure belongs to the ego, or rather *is* the ego, it is impossible to conceive of its inexistence or lack.

> "Having" and "being" in children. Children like expressing an object relation by an identification: "I am the object". "Having" is the later of the two; after loss of the object it relapses into "being". Example: the breast. "The breast is a part of me, I am the breast". Only later: "I have it" – that is, "I am not it".
>
> (*Findings, Ideas, Problems*, 1941, p. 299)

The pleasurable is thus categorized as ego, and what is unpleasurable or indifferent as not-ego.

It is a criterion of psychical functioning from which a first level of conception of the world is born from the pure pleasure ego. This is perhaps the only one possible until muscle activity can be handled adequately and specific activities tending towards the Trieb* satisfaction attempted by the incipient ego (which must develop into a definitive reality ego* or beyond in order to succeed) put into action.

The notion of identification* (being identical to the other, *being* the other) is implicit in this conception as "the earliest expression of an emotional tie with another person" (*Group Psychology and the Analysis of the Ego*, 1921, p. 105); that is to say, direct, primary identification* without previous recognition of the object as the source of wished-for pleasure.

"At the very beginning, in the individual's primitive oral phase, object cathexis and identification are no doubt indistinguishable from each other" (*The Ego and the Id*, 1923, p. 29). However, subsequent secondary identifications* also participate in this "being the object" when regression returns to it on account of different causes, once again *being* the object after having recognized it as the wished-for object.

Thus, in secondary identifications it is possible to *be* attributes of the object, either consciously or unconsciously.

This description fits the terms of normality (the ego's character* or the superego* or in mourning*, for example) or of neurosis (classical hysterical identification), as well as group phenomena and identification with the artist's work of art.

In the psychoses* it is even more complex (cf. different types of identification*, psychosis*, melancholia*; also the constitution of the ego and the superego, group psychology*, art*, and others).

We could say that the problem of being is the problem of narcissism* *par excellence*: when the ego functions in this category, it does not recognize anything it could wish for that it *is* not.

In this sense, we could consider the object link with the mother or her substitutes predominantly narcissistic, almost indistinguishable from autoerotism*, to which it is also intimately connected, since in practice it initiates it (*Three Essays on the Theory of Sexuality*, 1905), and with its anaclisis* in self-preservative Triebe* very slowly comes to recognize the object as something external that one desires but does not have (although the ego is distinguished from the object nearly from the outset by the initial reality ego*, which corresponds mainly to self-preservative Triebe). Consequently, recognition of the object's absence generates anxiety* (fear of object loss*, which the ego utilizes later as one of the signals to defend itself against attacks by Triebe), and the wish* seeks to "refind" the object and to "master" it.

That is to say, for the pure pleasure ego, everything wished for is ego. However, at the same time, bodily limits manifest the existence of different bodies, at first in relation to self-preservative Trieb. With respect to sexual Triebe, they are recognized especially when the erotogenic zones* are united under phallic primacy*, added to the history of each of these zones, and inscribed as traces of experiences with objects through them. This body attains the first levels of unity by virtue of the predominance of sight as the erotogenic zone in a certain period and the subsequent appearance of language*. This process culminates in the phallic phase, which then brings together the dispersed erotogenic zones, subsuming them to the search for a sensation that surpasses and also includes them.

At this time it definitively acquires the name "ego", concluding the construction of narcissism which in practice was already functioning.

> This would seem to imply an important amplification of the theory of narcissism. At the very beginning, all the libido is accumulated in the id, while the ego is still in process of formation or is still feeble. The id sends part of this libido out into erotic object cathexes, whereupon the ego, now grown stronger, tries to get hold of this object libido and to force itself on the id as a love-object. The narcissism of the ego is thus a secondary one, which has been withdrawn from objects.
>
> (*The Ego and the Id*, 1923, p. 46)

Thus, two apparently opposite conceptions are united: an objectless primary narcissism on the one hand and, on the other, narcissism which in reality proceeds from objects.

These are different conceptions of the world of a developing ego which emerges from *being* objects; it is partly real and partly historical truth*, hallucinatory satisfaction of wishes*.

The latter mechanism must be inhibited by the definitive reality ego in order to enter the category of *having*, which implies not *being*.

As this not *being* objects is gradually accepted, and they are recognized as being foreign to the ego, the object world is, so to speak, born. This world collapses in schizophrenics; since they cannot bear *having* (which involves frustrations for not *having*), they regress to *being*, and from there to the end of the world experience.

BELIEF IN REALITY

Ger.: Glaube. – Sp.: creencia. – Fr.: croyance de la realité. – It.: credenza nella realtà. – Port.: crença na realidade.

The ego* is said to believe that something is real when it is perceived by the senses; it believes in them and in what they show regarding reality*. For this reason the ego hypercathects (cf. hyper-cathexis*) the perceptual-consciousness apparatus (Pcpt.-Cs.) with attention energy. It may even test reality* for which it needs to move and study the perceived from different angles. When cathexis* is withdrawn from the perceptual apparatus (as in dreams* or in some psychoses* such as Meynert's amentia or hysterical psychosis), topical regression from thought activity with words may occur. In this case there is a passage from word-presentation* to thing-presentation (mainly an image) and, since the perceptual end is meagrely cathected, the wish* is perceived – or the anticathexis against it, as in hysterical psychosis – as real: as a hallucination (in these cases, visual).

In this case, the perceptual end (Pcpt.-Cs.) registers perception. The ego believes in this perception, feels that it is real, and its affects* are expressed in consequence. In dreams, the immobility of the muscular apparatus leads the ego to omit reality testing (the ego wishes to sleep and therefore permits the hallucination and even believes in it), which resumes its work upon waking.

In the above psychoses – amentia and hysterical psychosis – decathexis* of the perceptual apparatus on the one hand results in the register of what is in reality a wish-fulfilling fantasy as a perception and, on the other hand, the force of the wish fulfilled by the hallucination together with the ego's lack of strength to inhibit this hallucination lead the ego to omit "reality testing"*. However, in schizophrenia*, there is no regression from word-presentation to thing-presentation. These hallucinations are predominantly words heard as coming from outside. In this disorder, the ego* and superego* have been projected to this outside, or rather, returned to their original place (by identification* with external objects*). However, they return as words heard. In advanced degrees of schizophrenia, the psychical apparatus* is nearly destroyed. This means that, for example, wish-presentations, cathexes of thing-presentations, are decathected and psychical structures are projected. Although the unprojected remainder of the ego attempts to test reality, its effort is too weak to distinguish inside from outside because of the enormity of its alteration (cf. alteration of the ego*) and alienation (the ego is more external than internal, as in infancy).

For the psychical apparatus, everything perceived by the perceptual-consciousness system is real. It does not move in search of reality but rather seeks identity with what is wished for. Or rather, it aims to "refind" what is wished for in reality (*Project for a Scientific Psychology*, 1950; *Negation*, 1925). For this reason, everything perceived is studied by thought*, which judges existence* and attribution*. The conclusion is that the object exists and possesses certain characteristics. It is precisely by virtue of these characteristics that the ego tries to find identity of thought*. It utilizes thought and meticulous study of its attributes to discover to what extent the object, whose existence was believed because it was perceived, tallies with what is wished for. Thus, with this complexity created by the fact that what is sought is what is wished for (including the fact that what is not sought is what is feared), we may speak in terms of reality testing. It becomes more complex when death Trieb* is included, since wishes then involve their Trieb fusion with it;

in any case, reality testing does not vary, although what is sought in reality may do so.

BELLE INDIFFÉRENCE

A characteristic of patients (generally women, since hysteria is more typically feminine and their indifference is accordingly beautiful) with conversion hysteria mainly suffering from motor disorders but also when major symptoms* reside in the sensory area. It refers to the patient's attitude of indifference in relation to the symptom.

It was described by Charcot.

In conversion hysteria*, repression* of derivatives of incestuous presentations* is successful since it is able to make both the presentation and the quantity of affect* disappear, whereas in anxiety hysteria* and in obsessional neurosis*, anxiety* is present.

The presentational content of Trieb* has withdrawn radically from consciousness*. No kind of word-presentation remains there which can "speak" of the repressed. In its place, as a substitute formation* (and also as a symptom), a hyperintense (somatic) innervation has arisen, sometimes sensory and sometimes motor, in the form of either excitation or inhibition.

When the disappearance of the quantum of affect is successful, the patient's indifference towards a bodily symptom becomes remarkable; this may be the paralysis of a member which in the case of organic illness would at least arouse realistic anxiety*.

BINDING

Ger.: Bindung. – Sp.: ligadura. – Fr.: liaison. – It.: legame. – Port.: ligadura.

Energy or quantity of excitation* entering the psychical apparatus* acquires psychical quality* when it is bound with memory traces* that remain in the unconscious*; through the latter's characteristic processes (condensation* and displacement*) and after diverse types of transcription, they are transformed into conceptual images or thing-presentations*. At this moment, when energy is bound to the presentation*, psychical categories such as object* wish*, libido*, and Trieb* are constituted. This first level of binding (energy with thing-presentations) functions from that point forward ruled by the pleasure principle* with primary process* and perceptual identity*. Freud refers to this level of binding with the presentation as "free energy"*, given the extreme mobility of passages of energy from one presentation to another, which produces their condensations and displacements, all of which is typical of unconscious functioning.

However, precisely to prevent frustration*, inevitable when the dawning psychical apparatus is ruled by perceptual identity, an ego* must appear, product of primary identifications*, and must endeavour to moderate movements of energy through cathexes of presentations* located collaterally in relation to the facilitated associative path, thereby founding the initial outlines of secondary process* (reproductive thought). Secondary process is "finally" established with the appearance of word-presentations* inherent to speech* and thought* activity in general, progressing in this way in the formation of a preconscious ego which acquires a more definitive level at the end of the phallic phase, during and after the period of the Oedipus complex*. At these levels, binding is produced by the word-presentation, which represents the thing-presentation in consciousness*; this opens the possibility to be thought and related logically by consciousness, on account of its relation with other presentations, also taking into account data provided by reality testing* and then forming a synthesis in order to end (or not) in action (which may be rejected by emitting a judgement of condemnation*) if the ego after thinking decides to do so. This type of binding, a transformation of free energy into bound energy, is what Freud considers *stricto sensu*: it is "strong cathexis with weak displacement", increased complexity of movements of passage of libidinal energy from one presentation to another. Energy thus bound is located in the preconscious ego.

When for some reason energy unbinds from the presentation, it becomes pure energy without psychical presentation; in this situation we observe phenomena related to what is traumatic for the psychical apparatus, something "beyond the pleasure principle" (cf. death Trieb*, repetition compulsion*, Trieb fusion and defusion*, Nirvana principle*).

BISEXUALITY

Ger.: Bisexualität. – Sp.: bisexualidad. – Fr.: bisexualité. – It.: bisessualitá. – Port.: bi-sexualidade.

An originary and universal disposition of human sexuality* outlined by W. Fliess from a psychological perspective, its base is biological. According to Fliess, both sexes exist potentially in men and women. One of them gradually represses the other until it becomes predominant. A person of the male sex has all the feminine repressed and vice versa. However, according to A. Adler, all individuals resist remaining in the feminine, inferior line of development and direct their efforts towards the masculine, the only satisfactory one; in this case, it is always the feminine that is repressed in both sexes (Adler's "masculine protest" stems from this idea).

Freud's version is different. Nearly all infantile sexuality* is repressed when the Oedipus complex* arrives and sexual Triebe* clash with ideals (among other things). Sexuality is totally repressed (presentations* of events in infantile sexuality form the primarily repressed unconscious* whereas subsequent derivatives are repressed secondarily), both masculine and feminine, when the incestuous idea is repressed. However, in a stricter sense, we may say that the level of sexual differentiation to which a five-year-old child has access is primarily repressed; that is to say, the phallic–castrated level; this level does not become masculine–feminine until puberty, although even at that time it alludes by analogy to the primarily repressed level.

Is the feminine depreciated? We should say that it is in the unconscious, since in oedipal boys and girls, what is later to be feminine is mistaken by analogy for castration, the anxious affect and its subsequent derivations in this regard passing from the repressed unconscious into ulterior adult transferences and object choices. In any case there is in reality no repression of the feminine but rather of infantile sexual Trieb, since it may bring on danger of castration. The category of the feminine as such is a result of later developments in puberty and adolescence which carry the mark of castration left by infantile sexuality present in the unconscious.

In *The Ego and the Id* (1923), Freud considers bisexuality highly important since it is responsible for the type of resolution and outcome of the Oedipus complex, which in each individual is normally one of two types: positive (referring to the predominance of the subject's own sex, having identified [cf. identification*] with the parent of the same sex) or negative (the opposite). Bisexuality is part of the cause of ambivalence* in the subject's relation with the parents (positive and negative Oedipus), which adds complexity to phallic phase rivalry as described up to that point in his works.

Rivalry with the opposite-sex parent that appears in the phallic and/or genital phase now becomes only an exponent of the positive Oedipus complex. In the negative Oedipus complex, the boy identifies with his mother and wishes for passive coitus with his father as a way to disavow* castration; however, this attempt fails since the very conception of passive coitus reveals acceptance as a premise of sexual differentiation which at that time consists of phallic–castrated; therefore, castration anxiety* is also felt. The father executes this castration. In response to this unsolvable conflict the Oedipus complex is repressed or dissolved* and the superego* is established as a "commemorative monument" to it. In adolescence, the conflict re-emerges, bearing the marks of the subject's history; with it comes bisexuality with its unique and complex history.

In girls the pathway to the feminine is different. The initial tie with the mother is prolonged and passes from a pre-oedipal to a negative oedipal bond, after which the daughter must confront her mother in order to separate from her; the motivating cause is the protest against her mother for having made her castrated. Transference is then established with the father, which converts the Oedipus into a positive complex in which she expects the father to give her the penis-child her mother failed to give her at first; based on the father's oedipal refusal (which defines him as a father), her sexuality turns towards other men.

BODY

Ger.: Leib. – Sp.: cuerpo. – Fr.: corps. – It.: corpo. – Port.: corpo.

Our body corresponds to the part of nature that we are; in this sense it is something external to the psychical apparatus*. It is also part of external reality* in the sense that Trieb* stimuli originate in it, enter the psychical apparatus, and make it function. It is also on the periphery of this apparatus (where it receives news of stimuli from the external world by means of its erotogenic zones*), and the psychical apparatus* also belongs to it. Perception* corresponds to the periphery of this body. It is also what carries out action. It is the most intimate part of our being and the most concrete and immediate "image" of our ego*; it is therefore a libidinized, "psychologized" body.

The subject of the body and its place in Freudian theory may be approached from different perspectives which inevitably intermingle, since Freud considers the division between mind and body artificial. The soul* and the body are things that differ but are within the same unit.

On the one hand, we have a dynamic conception of the relation between the biological (somatic sexual energy and tension of need which generate need of sexual discharge and of nourishment by the body's cells; to this we should add "preparedness to understand" reality; that is to say, phylogenetic schemas inherited from the experience of our species), the social (objects* and their language*), and the mark left by this relation in this body. This mark is nothing less than the memory trace* left in memory by experiences of satisfaction* and pain* with the object, from which derives the presentation* of these objects and of experience with them. This is the way in which energy whose origin is biological becomes psychical and is then called Trieb, libido*, or desire* (these three are different types of binding between quantity of energy and the presentation).

Thus we have the dynamic result in Freudian thought that each experience leaves a trace of this experience with the object and thereby becomes psychical (the relation with the first object forms in a basic way, through and in the subject's and the object's body; it is a bodily relation that leaves a trace, a presentation – including an identification – which may then intervene in bodily innervations and thereby lead to action). What is purely psychical (the ontogenic) is therefore a product of this relation; this experience is complex from the first moment since it really leaves three traces or parts of the same one: one is the object's image (of the object's body), another of the object's movements and the subject's body, and the third, perhaps the most important: the sensation felt (in the body) in this encounter. Therefore the same psychical presentation originates in the body (or a part of it: the breast), the subject's body (the mouth and the act of sucking in the first experiences), and the other's body, and is the memory of this relation between bodies, partial at first, until they attain unity, a relation that is now wished for, bodies that in this way become desiring and desired, erotogenic bodies.

The link with the object then becomes more complex, changing erotogenic zones* and their histories in the link with it, language* intervenes, relations over distances may be established by virtue of words; in these, in any case, bodily relations are symbolized. Words also originate in thought, geometrically increasing complexity. Since the link with the object is always stronger through the body, this object and its body near us, with the possibility of action, is always the most wished-for object.

Something else may also occur: part of the tension of need is not bound to any presentation* and remains unbound – a possibility maintained despite the existence of the psychical – thereby becoming the actual-neurotic factor of ulterior neuroses.

Is the central relation with the object therefore only body to body? For sexual Trieb*, although the body is initially autoerotic (in two ways: it is satisfied either in the subject's own body or in the object's body but without recognition of it as an object), it is satisfied by organ pleasure. Concordantly with its growing recognition of the object's existence as a separate body, it libidinizes the object by cathecting its presentation or by desiring it.

Something similar occurs with the subject's own body in relation to its libidinization, not so much in terms of desire (whereas what is wished for is what is recognized as lacking, the subject not only has its own body but is it; narcissism can only wish in relation to the ideal's aspirations; however, this is just one element within a growing complexity unnecessary to include in this definition which proposes to focus on the theme of the body).

The libidinization of the subject's own body and its history (with itself and with the object) is what we call ego*, an ego that becomes progressively more complex. In the relation with this object through the erotogenic zones and their symbolization in words, all this is then called narcissism*.

Narcissism and recognition of the object* generate an erotogenic body impregnated with desire*: sexual desire. Recognition of the object and of the ego gradually evolves from partial (the different erotogenic zones) to total (with the arrival of phallic predominance); once it is totalized, to castrated-phallic, and finally to masculine–feminine in adolescence and sexual maturity.

The body is the seat of the erotogenic zones (the body surface and even internal organs) and consequently, sensations of pleasure and unpleasure and also of pain* interwoven with sexuality*. External and internal sensations and the mirror image of the subject's own body configure an image of the psychical ego based on this body scheme. Love of this body, seat of this ego, is narcissism.

Affects are felt and expressed in the body; in actual neuroses*, symptoms are predominantly bodily.

The source of Triebe for Freud is in the body's organs; from there they arrive to the psychical apparatus as quantity of excitation* which acquires characteristics of Trieb*: libido* and psychical desire* when it is bound with the presentation of the object from which it seeks satisfaction; this presentation was left by previous experiences of satisfaction searched for in reality; when they are refound, they leave new presentation-traces that broaden the desiring circuit and consequently action, which is mainly bodily.

Affects* are felt in the body; they are qualifications made by the conscious out of quantitative changes in the energy originating in the body; they are considered bodily reactions corresponding initially to internal change* (expression of emotions, screaming, vascular innervation), the path by which language is learned in the link with the mother. As experience with the object becomes its presentation, affects begin to develop a close relation with presentations, acquiring an increasing psychical dimension.

The theme of the body image reaches a higher level of complexity, aside from being what it is: part of the "ought to be" of the ego ideal* and of the "ought not to be" of moral conscience* (both belonging to the superego*); in this sense the body image, as the seat for example of the subject's superficial beauty, may act on the subject's self-esteem* and constitute a new source of conflicts (this is very important in our times when the image has acquired such relevance and originates conflicts, especially in adolescence, raising or lowering self-esteem depending on individual problems); that is to say, the subject's narcissism (especially in women, for whom bodily beauty may offer a way to alleviate castration*). In these cases the body image is welded to the ego image. There is also psychical beauty of the ego, beauty of the soul; of course, this is more connected with ethics* and wisdom, values currently depreciated in our culture, although they are also idealized.

The body is therefore the base of all Freudian thinking: the psyche grows out of it and later, through language and thought, it leads action, aimed basically towards other bodies with their oedipal history, psyche, and language: other human beings.

What is most fascinating about development in Freud is the dynamic process he describes by which the biological body (a product of the prehistory of the species) needs the object (the maternal object is the first representative of the social), given its helplessness, in order to satisfy its Triebe*; the trace left by this object (its presentation) then produces psychical desire (thereby generating the psyche itself); wish for the object slowly becomes exogamic and social with the appearance of the father, and the social again becomes psychical with the establishment of the superego*, in a spiral that becomes more and more complex in which the bodily root of everything may even be lost, especially in view of the quantity of growingly sophisticated "prostheses" of the body continually created by culture*, complexity that ends only when the body's cycle ends in death.

BOUND ENERGY

Ger.: gebundene Energie. – Sp.: energía ligada. – Fr.: énergie liée. – It.: energia legata. – Port.: energia ligada.

When this state of psychical energy (whose source is bodily needs) is bound to a thing-presentation* and its consequent word-presentation*, which represents it to consciousness so that it can be thought and therefore related to other words, then all this course taken with it by the psyche may succeed in reaching discharge. Thus, it may find endless relations with other presentations* belonging to the world of thought* and, through this inhibitory (cf. inhibition of the ego*) elaboration, moderate its passage into action.

By virtue of this type of energy, the unconscious, the preconscious*, the id*, and the ego* are intimately joined.

This is the state of energy the analyst seeks as the patient comes to know the unconscious better, connecting it with the preconscious ego's thought activity in order to tame this energy and to carry out the specific action at the adequate moment in reality*. Bound energy is the state energy should achieve in order to make specific action* possible. This state is reached relatively and indirectly, since in sessions we do not access energy but instead word-presentations* (bound in turn to thing-presentations*) to which the energy binds. When the patient's presentational world expands, analytic work acts on the possibilities of binding biological bodily energy.

BROTHER-COMPLEX

Ger.: Brüder Komplex. – Sp.: complejo fraterno. – Fr.: complexe fraternel. – It.: complesso fraterno. – Port.: complexo fraternal.

What we refer to as the brother-complex in Freud's works does not possess the foundational influence on the psychical apparatus that we attribute to the Oedipus complex and its derivates, the father-complex* and the mother-complex*. We may say that it is not as important since it does not originate the structure of the psychical apparatus, although it integrates it entirely; for example, it may originate fixations and consequently, modalities of defence or even the subject's character*. It corresponds more to problems among siblings and not directly with their parents; in this sense, it remains on a second, more individual than universal level, although its importance is often far from trivial. The central theme tends to be jealousy for the parents' love; the latter thereby enter indirectly. It is expressed by obvious sibling rivalry or the opposite: its apparent absence (cf. defence mechanism: stepping aside*).

However, it is interesting that Freud marked the origin of humanity at the appearance of the law stipulating the fraternal alliance*, after the brothers had killed and eaten their powerful, ubiquitous father. That is to say that union among brothers is given a special place in relation to access to culture in his theory as something to be attained: an ideal.

In other terms, the arrival of a sibling in the family is in itself a narcissistic wound for children who are building their narcissism* upon maternal love, a love that must suddenly be shared and therefore desexualized. Freud underscores how traumatic this is in the life of any child (for example, Little Hans, the young homosexual woman, *Constructions in Analysis*), and that it therefore generates fixations* and later, possibly pathological disorders such as neurotic symptoms or character traits*.

The link between siblings is a model of eventual social links, charged with ambivalence and sexualized peaks, although desexualization is its essence.

C

CASES OF HYSTERIA FROM THE FIRST PERIOD

Ger.: Hysterie fälle von der Erstenzeit. – Sp.: casos de histeria de la primera época. – Fr.: cas d'hystérie de la première époque. – It.: casi d'isteria della prima epoca. – Port.: casos de histeria de primeira época.

Anna O.

The pseudonym of the first patient treated by the method that originated what would later be psychoanalysis. This treatment was carried out by J. Breuer between 1880 and 1882. It is one of the case histories published by Breuer and Freud in their *Studies on Hysteria* (1895).

This is the case of a hysterical psychosis* in a young lady aged twenty-one, highly intelligent, capable of reasoning, with energetic and tenacious will power, one of whose character traits* was "sympathetic kindness".

Her major symptoms* were paraphasia, strabismus convergens, severe disturbances of the vision, contracture paralysis which was total in the right upper extremity (with some anaesthesia, especially of the elbow) and in both lower extremities, partial in the left upper extremity, paresia of the cervical muscles; also, visual hallucinations*, somnambulism, tussis nervosa, disgust* for food, inability to drink despite thirst, and attacks of sleep at certain times of the day. As her treatment progressed, new symptoms emerged: progressive alterations of speech, first the dwindling of words, then loss of grammar and syntaxis as well as conjugation of verbs (utilization of an infinitive created from weak forms of the participle and the preterite without the article). Later, when words were almost totally lacking, she painfully searched for them in four or five languages; then, she could barely be understood. She also wrote in this difficult dialect. There was a period (two weeks) when she fell completely mute.

Breuer understood that something had offended her very deeply, and that she had decided not to say anything at all. When he told this to the patient, some of her muscle contractures loosened and she began to speak English and to understand German without realizing that she was answering in English.

This symptomatology was not constant but appeared only at some times of day (in the morning or the afternoon). After speaking with Breuer about herself, she felt cheerful and jovial but remembered nothing about the previous episode, a fact that Breuer referred to as a "secondary state". This young lady was fragmented into two personalities: sometimes she was psychically normal and at other times entered the "secondary state" and was then alienated. Provoking causes of her illness were the discovery of a serious condition in her father and his later death. She nursed her father when he was ill, but when she began to present a picture of weakness with contractures, coughing, glottal spasms, and other symptoms, she was separated from her father, who died some time afterwards.

In his session with her, Breuer reconstructed all the facts and fantasies* Anna O. had had. In relation to the symptoms, he determined the motive of their origin. For example, in a hypnotic state induced by Breuer, the patient remembered that the contracture with paralysis and anaesthesia in the right arm had begun one night when she was nursing her bed-ridden father; she was half-asleep and had a hallucination: she

> saw a black snake coming towards the sick man from the wall to bite him. (It is most likely that there were in fact snakes in the field behind the house …) She tried to keep the snake off, but it was as though she was paralysed. Her right arm, over the back of the chair, had gone to sleep and had become anaesthetic and paretic; and when she looked at it the fingers turned into little snakes with death's heads (the nails). (It seems probable that she had tried to use her paralysed right arm to drive off the snake and that its anaesthesia and paralysis had consequently become associated with the hallucination of the snake.) When the snake vanished, in her terror she tried to pray. But language failed her: she could find no tongue in which to speak, till at last she thought of some children's verses in English and then found herself able to think and pray in that language.
>
> (1893–5, pp. 38–9)

Following these reconstructions*, the severity of the symptoms diminished. Then, others came to the surface until the same type of cure was applied. In the period before the memory* was found (when she talked about it with the therapist, she improved), there was sometimes a worsening of symptoms, and these symptoms entered the conversation.

After two years of treatment, this talented patient was cured of her hysterical psychosis and all the associated neurotic symptoms. She is to be credited for the apt term, "talking cure", and the humorous term, "chimney sweeping", to describe Breuer's work.

In her case history, the symptoms that emerged in the secondary state are compared to dream* mechanisms. This patient's habitual dreaming awake or daydreaming is also discussed as a predisposition to hysteria and a generator of symptoms. The patient referred to her fantasies as her "private theatre".

Breuer describes:

> I used to visit her in the evening, when I knew I should find her in her hypnosis, and I then relieved her of the whole stock of imaginative products which she had accumulated since my last visit. It was essential that this should be effected completely if good results were to follow. When this was done she became perfectly calm, and next day she would be agreeable, easy to manage, industrious and even cheerful.
>
> (1893–5, p. 30)

But later she would return insistently to the previous state.

This case history also mentions associations* by analogy* and contiguity* as provoking factors of her "secondary state" and the consequent appearance of symptoms. Other multiple symptoms and theoretical interpretations* also discussed merit reconsideration and further study.

Cäcilie M.

She is a hysterical patient often mentioned in *Studies on Hysteria* (1893–5). Freud explains that he got to know her far better than the others, but that personal considerations prevented him from reporting her clinical history in detail.

In a footnote on false connections*, he presents the example of Cäcilie M. He says that "the mood attaching to an experience and the subject-matter of that experience … come into different relations to the primary consciousness" (1893, p. 69). This appreciation is apparently directed at rationalizations as a form of false connection, but when he discusses the mood and the presentation* as a passage from one scene to another, he is referring to the problem of transference* and to the phenomenon of repression*. He describes the appearance of reminiscences, as if scenes repeated were preceded by a corresponding mood. The patient became irritable, anxious, or desperate, always unaware that this humour did not belong to the present but to the state she was about to suffer. It was in this transition period that she made the "false connection".

In another footnote, he gives examples of narrations in which she remembers a symptom surmounted some time previously which reappears when it is remembered, as if this were a kind of suspicion or anticipation, which was relatively frequent in Cäcilie.

> On each occasion what was already present as a finished product in the unconscious was beginning to show through indistinctly. This idea … was worked over by the unsuspecting "official" consciousness (to use Charcot's term) into a feeling of satisfaction, which swiftly and invariably turned out to be unjustified.
>
> (Ibid., p. 76)

Then, "we do not boast of our happiness until unhappiness is in the offing" (Ibid.).

The subject of anticipations or suspicion, I think, is taken up again much later in theory in a footnote to the article on *Negation* (1925).

Finally, Cäcilie M. is presented as an example of symbolic symptom formation*. The patient suffers from very violent facial neuralgia that suddenly emerges two or three times a year. When Freud attempts to evoke the traumatic scene,

> the patient saw herself back in a period of great mental irritability towards her husband. She described a conversation which she had had with him and a remark of his which she had felt as a bitter insult. Suddenly she put her hand to her cheek, gave a loud cry of pain and said: "It was like a slap in the face".
>
> (Ibid., p. 178)

This ended her pain* and the attack. "[T]his neuralgia had come to be indicative of a particular psychical excitation by the usual method of conversion, but … afterwards it could be set going through associative reverberations from her mental life, or symbolic conversion" (Ibid., p. 179).

At another time, Cäcilie M. was afflicted with violent pain in her right heel, a sharp pain with each step that prevented her from walking. Analysis evoked a time in a clinical hospitalization when she had told the doctor of her fear of "not being on the right footing" in the company of people she didn't know.

Freud notes that no other patient has given such a generous sample of symbolization, but that it must be extended to hysteria in general and that conversion symptoms only give life to feelings whose linguistic expression justifies them. Thus, for example, the phrases "it stabbed me to the heart" or "I shall have to swallow this" (Ibid., p. 180) are metaphors of concrete bodily facts that may express pain or some kind of submission. In hysteria, these fantasies are not expressed as verbal metaphors but are instead felt again, staged, and represented, as if the metaphor had become the (unconscious*) script of a performance that is somewhat "theatrical". These feelings, actions, or bodily difficulties in action thereby "symbolize" these verbal metaphors although consciousness* does not realize their meaning.

Word-presentations* may normally express affects* metaphorically, as in these examples, which correspond to wish*-presentations. In hysteria, these word-presentations are decathected by repression, and the unconscious wish can only express the same metaphoric phrase in a bodily form, utilizing the body in a sense that symbolizes something that was once concrete in order to override repression and return from the repressed (cf. return of the repressed*). This is supported by Darwin's theory that "expression of emotions" consists of operations that were originally meaningful and adequate to an aim, although they are now in most cases weakened to the point that their linguistic expression seems a figurative transference. It is highly probable that all this was once understood literally, and that hysteria is correct when it reconnects the original meaning of words to their most intense innervations.

Elisabeth von R.

Elisabeth is the last and most important of the cases in *Studies on Hysteria* (1893). Freud considers this treatment his "first full-length analysis of a hysteria" (1893, p. 139).

Hysteria is in this case hysterical neurosis; that is to say, the return of the repressed: the emergence of the symptom.

Freud undertakes a detailed and exhaustive study of the meaning of the symptoms, linking them in the smallest detail with traumatic facts that globally point to a similar meaning which is the repressed or, as he also refers to it at that time, the "incompatible idea" (p. 157): the idea expressed by the symptoms.

With Elisabeth, Freud leaves aside hypnosis and uses pressure on the head as a "momentary hypnotic order" in order to overcome resistance* to knowledge of the repressed.

The patient was twenty-four when Freud was consulted about her pains in both legs and difficulty in walking (astasia-abasia* but not paralysis). Her attitude towards the symptom was also a typical example of *belle indifférence**. Pinching and pressure on the legs produced an attitude of both disturbance and pleasure (as if it was tickling) that led her to arch her body slightly backwards in a mini *arc de cercle*.

Shortly before this, her father and a married sister had died. Her sister had died after giving birth, due to an old cardiac ailment.

She was the youngest of three sisters and was quite attached to her father. Her mother suffered from a chronic eye condition. Elisabeth was intelligent, somewhat too "cheeky" and "cock-sure" (p. 140) for the feminine social ideal of the times. In this sense, she was unhappy with being a woman. She was ambitious: she wanted to study or to receive a musical education. She was indignant at the idea of sacrificing her inclinations and freedom of judgement to marriage.

Her father had fallen gravely ill from a cardiac condition that he had kept a secret, and Elisabeth had been nursing him since the first day, all the time. At that time, she felt the first pains in her right leg. Her father died. After a year of mourning, her elder sister married a talented and hard-working man with whom Elisabeth did not get along well, and with whom she argued over the care of her ailing mother. At that time, Elisabeth felt helpless and powerless to provide her mother with a substitute for her loss.

Shortly afterwards, her second sister married. Her new brother-in-law, a cordial man, reconciled Elisabeth with the institution of marriage. They lived near the mother and had a child who made the new grandmother happy again.

At a certain time her mother had to have an eye operation. During her convalescence, the three families were reunited in a summer resort, and at this time Elisabeth's pains "exploded" along with her difficulty for walking. Since they appeared after a long walk in the area, they were attributed to exhaustion or having gotten chilled. After this, Elisabeth became the ill member of the family.

Meanwhile, the second sister was pregnant again and was not well after the delivery; two weeks later, her condition was worse, and Elisabeth and her mother needed to travel to see her. During this trip, the pains raged together with anxiety* regarding her sister's fate. Unfortunately, when they arrived they found that she had already died. This provoked a new rupture in the family, since the brother-in-law separated from the family group and kept his son away from the grandmother, which made Elisabeth angry.

This chronological sequence of events does not in any way describe Elisabeth's specific alteration: astasia-abasia. Freud looks for the explanation by exploring the deepest strata of memories* and the interconnection of their meanings. Eventually, the memory of a young man for whom Elisabeth had felt some attraction at the time of her father's illness appeared; even the memory of a party which she had enjoyed intensely with him and from which she had returned in a whirl of emotions. Unfortunately, this moment coincided with a turn for the worse in her father's health, and Elisabeth never saw this young man again.

With the progress of Elisabeth's treatment, it occurs to her that the pains always started in her right thigh and were more intense there because this was the place where her father's leg lay while the bandages around them were replaced, since they were quite swollen. This had occurred hundreds of times. Freud takes this fact as a good explanation for the genesis of an atypical hysterogenic zone*. At that time, Elisabeth's legs began to "answer" (participate in the conversation: *mitsprechen*). When a memory was called up, a painful feeling appeared which increased as she went on with the description, and relented when she finished. In this period of abreaction* the symptoms obviously improve. Freud finds that relapses are connected with associations produced by events of the day. Thus, the right leg hurt when memories related to nursing her sick father or to her relationship with a companion from her youth, and other things that fell within the first pathogenic period. The pains in the left leg were awakened by a memory of her dead sister and of the two brothers-in-law; in sum, impressions from the second half of her history of suffering.

> The original painful spot in her right thigh had related to her nursing her father; the area of pain had extended from this spot to neighbouring regions as a result of fresh traumas. Here, therefore, what we were dealing with was not strictly speaking a single physical symptom, linked with a variety of mnemic complexes in the mind, but a number of similar symptoms which appeared, on a superficial view, to be merged into one symptom.
>
> (1895, p. 150)

Then, with Freud, the patient proceeded to divide

> all the scenes with painful impressions attached to them into groups for me, according as she had experienced them while she was sitting or standing, and so on. For instance, she was standing by a door when her father was brought home with his heart attack, and in her fright she stood stock still as though she was rooted to the ground.
>
> (Ibid.)

Elisabeth then remembered the terrible scene when she was again standing, as if spellbound, by her dead sister's bed.

In relation to her pain in walking, she underscored a scene. This walk had presumably been too long. When Freud gets her to give more details, she recognizes that she was in a sentimental mood. She had gone off happily with her friends, it was a beautiful day, and neither her mother nor her sister had gone, but her brother-in-law had gone along. She returned from the walk with violent pains. During the walk she had been pained by the contrast between her sister's married happiness, evident in her brother-in-law's attitude, and her own loneliness.

Another scene brought new meaning to the connection between her pains and sitting. A few days after her sister and brother-in-law had left, she went for a walk, alone and yearning, to a little hill where they used to go together and sat down. She again thought about her loneliness, her family's fate, and her ardent wish to be happy as her sister was. She returned from this morning meditation with great pains which, after a bath, became established permanently.

At first her pains were relieved when she lay down, but after the urgent train trip (when she found her sister dead), the connection was established between lying down and pains, and this became more painful than standing or walking: the painful zone expanded with each new traumatic event. The patient said that painfulness was the feeling of helplessness*, the feeling of not taking a step forward, and with this she sought symbolic expression for her pain-tinged thoughts (mourning*).

In any case, what predominated and generated the abasia was the psychical associative functional paralysis, reinforced by a symbolic functional paralysis.

At this time, the patient felt better, psychically relieved and productive, but her pains returned from time to time.

Meanwhile, based on her narrative, Freud has a suspicion. It intensifies when Elisabeth hears a noise during a session and, thinking that it is her brother-in-law who has arrived, tries to leave. She then has intense pains.

Freud goes more deeply into the memory of the scene when the pains started. Elisabeth tells him again, adding more detail. She highlights the relationship with her brother-in-law and her wish to get a man like him. She remembers the trip to see her sick sister. Freud asks her if the possibility of her death had occurred to her. Elisabeth says that she had carefully avoided this thought. Then the memory appears in her dead sister's house. When she was lamenting that she had died without saying goodbye, "at that very moment another thought had shot through Elisabeth's mind, and now forced itself irresistibly upon her once more, like a flash of lightning in the dark: 'Now he is free again and I can be his wife'" (Ibid., p. 156).

This was the incompatible idea from which she defended herself by transforming it into a separate psychical group* by the act of will* which led to the defence. Elisabeth loved her brother-in-law and had spared herself the painful certainty this love* produced in her by instead creating bodily pains.

"The resistance with which she had repeatedly met the reproduction of scenes which operated traumatically corresponded in fact to the energy with which the incompatible idea had been forced out of her associations" (Ibid., p. 157).

The effect of the recovery of this repressed presentation was shattering for Elisabeth: she cried aloud, felt intense pains, rejected it, and so on.

Freud then attempted to alleviate by abreaction* the excitation stored up for such a long time. He was able to get the patient to talk about each of the circumstances in which this tendency had been kept unconscious, which relieved her greatly. He also investigated her family reality* in order to learn to what point his patient's wishes could possibly be realized.

Elisabeth no longer had symptoms and her treatment was considered finished.

Emma

This case is mentioned in the second part, "Psychopathology", of the *Project for a Scientific Psychology* ([1895] 1950), in the fourth section: The hysterical proton pseudos.

Here, Freud explains that hysterical compulsion* originates in a type of displacement* of energy that is a primary process*. The force that moves this process is an ego defence* that exceeds the normal. He then offers the example of Emma who could not go into a shop alone. Emma bases this attitude on a memory from when she was twelve years old (shortly after the beginning of puberty). She had gone into a shop to buy something, saw two shop assistants laughing, and ran out in a fright. She thinks that they were laughing at her clothes and that one of the assistants had pleased her sexually.

Freud finds this explanation incomprehensible. A second memory comes up: when she was eight, she had gone twice into a pastry shop and the man had groped her genitals through her clothes. The baker had grinned at her: Emma reproaches herself for having gone in a second time, as if she had wanted to provoke the assault. Freud maintains that by connecting one scene with the other, her fright is more understandable. The associative connection between the two scenes (the one that explains it and the "incomprehensible" one) resides in the laughter (of the shop assistants and the baker).

One scene evokes the other, but in the meantime she has become pubertal: the memory of the first scene awakens sexual release which is transformed into anxiety. It is as if the actual bodily feeling "understood" (cf. understanding*) the earlier scene, anxiety emerging as an ego defence against this conflictive understanding.

Then Freud shows a presentational chain in which some presentations (the most innocuous) reach consciousness* and others remain unconscious. He explains clearly and well the process of pathological repression and the concept of the deferred* traumatic sexual event which he develops more deeply many years later in the case history of the "Wolf Man" (1917); there, he includes the already discovered infantile sexuality* with little variation but a higher level of complexity, the basic ideas of which are presented in this case.

Emmy von N.

The first patient to which Freud applied Breuer's method of cathartic hypnosis. Emmy was forty years old, a widow, and the mother of two adolescent daughters. Her clinical picture is that of a mixed neurosis, with symptoms* of anxiety neurosis*, phobias*, with hallucinations*, which the patient does not remember afterwards; she also suffers from permanent symptoms such as nervous tics and stuttering, and few conversions.

Freud's interpretation of her material is fairly superficial compared to those that followed. We are especially interested in it to appreciate Freud's gradual process of discovery, since the evolution of the treatment is described day by day. Besides applying cathartic hypnosis, Freud analysed the symptom during hypnosis until he reached the conclusion that improvement was more complete and lasting with the latter system. At this time he explains tics and stuttering as a result of contrasting presentations*, the expression of oppositional will.

Emmy's treatment in two periods was able to suppress the patient's symptoms, albeit without producing structural changes that would have given her the preparation necessary for her to dispense with becoming ill after fresh traumatic events.

Mathilde H.

A patient mentioned by Freud in a footnote to *Studies on Hysteria*, in reference to "festivals of remembrance" (1895, p. 163); that is to say, the repetition of neurotic symptomatology on the anniversary of a traumatic event. Freud wonders whether in these festivals that return year after year the same scenes are repeated or whether different details are presented for their abreaction*. He decides that the latter occurs. Then he presents the example of Mathilde, a pretty girl of nineteen, whom he treated on two occasions, first for a partial paralysis of the legs and then, a few months later, for an alteration of the character*: irritated to the point of apathy for living, she was inconsiderate to her mother, irritable, and surly.

By means of hypnosis, he discovers the cause of her irritation: the breaking off of her engagement several months before. In the relationship with her fiancé, many things had come up that were disagreeable to her and her mother, although the marriage would offer many economic advantages, which generated a state of indecisiveness and great apathy. At last, her mother instead of the patient gave the decisive "no". Sometime later, she awoke as if from a dream and thought over the decision that had already been made for a long time, weighing the pros against the cons, and so on. It was a long period of doubt, with animosity towards her mother based on that occasion of the decision. Compared to this thought* activity, life seemed a pseudo-existence, something dreamed.

One day near the anniversary of her engagement, all this state of irritation ceased. This was interpreted by Freud as a state of "reparational abreaction"; the content of a neurosis, otherwise enigmatic, in which the festival of remembrance had been the cause of the effect of reparation.

Katharina

When Freud was on holiday, Katharina, a girl of about eighteen, consults him for difficulties in breathing. Freud diagnoses a hysterical attack* with anxiety-producing content. Katharina also feels oppression in her eyes, buzzing in her ears, heaviness of the head, dizziness, oppression of the chest, and fear of death and of being attacked from behind. She also sees a horrible face that threatens and frightens her.

Freud is attentive and lets her talk. In the narrow frame of only one interview (held in these special conditions), Freud learns the origin of the frightening face. For ethical reasons, her narrative disguises events in the patient's life, some of which are conscious memories and others became conscious during the "conversation" with Freud; in no case were they recognized before this conversation as having any relation to her symptomatology.

Then, a story comes up with an uncle (actually her father, as he explains at the end of the case history) with tendencies to commit incestuous acts, even to having sexual relations with his niece (daughter).

He shows clearly in this case history how traumatic events are understood in a deferred* way, and how the incompatibility of this understanding forces the ego to repress and to derive libido* involved into a conversive symptom*. When it is abreacted in this "conversation" with Freud, symptomatic relief is obtained.

Freud learns that a series of traumatic events had occurred (incestuous insinuations by the father) that the patient did not fully understand. She does understand them (cf. understanding*) when she witnesses a sexual scene between her father and her cousin; this scene, considered auxiliary, is in turn traumatic in itself and provokes the neurosis that had been incubating since the earlier traumatic situations*.

Katharina's anxiety does not correspond to anxiety neurosis*; it is hysteria; that is to say, an exacerbated reproduction of anxiety that emerged in each sexual trauma*.

Miss Lucy R.

This case history may be read in *Studies on Hysteria*. Lucy's is a light hysteria with few symptoms, the archetype of hysteria acquired without "hereditary taint" (Ibid., p. 122).

Lucy is a thirty-year-old Englishwoman who works as a governess in charge of two little girls in the household of a factory director. (Their mother had died a few years before.) Her symptoms are: irritability and fatigue, general analgesia, nasal mucous membranes without reflexes and – her most bothersome symptom – subjective sensations consisting of "the smell of burnt pudding".

Since the patient did not respond to hypnosis, Freud gave it up, which meant that the analysis took place in a context very much like a normal conversation. This fact provoked a difficulty, since hypnosis produced a "somnambulistic extension of memory" (Ibid., p. 109); "it is precisely the pathogenic memories which … are 'absent from the patients' memory, when they are in a normal psychical state" (Ibid.). This fact materializes when patients cut off their occurrences and stop associating. Freud then resorts to an artifice: he presses their forehead with his hand and asks them to continue, which usually occurs. Freud considers this technical artifice "a momentarily intensified hypnosis" (Ibid., p. 271) which overcomes resistance* and leaves the way free for occurrences and memories* to pass through.

In this case, he utilizes this method to reach the memory of the traumatic situation* when the patient really perceived this smell. Lucy recalls a letter from her mother asking her to return, a tender scene with the girls and her guilty fantasies of having to abandon them in spite of having promised their mother never to do so. She could no longer bear the atmosphere in the house (she was on bad terms with the rest of the staff). Simultaneous with this scene, the girls had forgotten that they were cooking pudding and its burning was perceived. Is this the traumatic scene: did the smell take the place of a mnemic symbol* and is this what is being repeated?

Freud is not satisfied. An indispensable condition for the acquisition of hysteria is that a presentation* is deliberately repressed from consciousness*, and this factor is missing. Freud risks an interpretation*: Lucy is in love with her employer and is afraid that her workmates may laugh at her. Lucy answers, "Yes, I think that's true … I didn't know – or rather I didn't want to know. I wanted to drive it out of my head" (Ibid., p. 117).

In the following days this symptom disappears and is replaced by another: the smell of cigar-smoke. Freud insists. The memory emerges of a visitor who kisses the girls, and the father angrily forbids him from doing so while Miss Lucy feels a stab at her heart. Since the gentlemen were smoking, her conscious memory retains the smell of cigar-smoke.

In real chronology, this second scene actually occurs before the first one when she reads the letter from her mother. Analysis continues. A third scene, still earlier, appears: the director had gotten angry with Lucy and had even threatened to let her go. This new scene had crushed her amorous hopes and was quite probably the real pathogenic nucleus, since from that time on, the symptoms disappeared and Miss Lucy resigned herself and accepted her reality.

The smell of cigar-smoke, the mnemic symbol of the second scene, served as an anticathexis* of the third scene (the real traumatic scene: her employer's rejection).

This treatment took place in an irregular way, apparently in the interval between patients, over nine weeks, which was quite a lot at that time. There was absolute remission of all the symptoms, which had not returned four months later.

Rosalía H.

This patient is mentioned by Freud in *Studies on Hysteria* when he discusses symptoms generated with a deferred* (Nachträglich) effect. That is to say, conversion is not a response to fresh impressions but to the memory of them.

Rosalia is twenty-three years old and is training to be a singer. She complains that her beautiful voice does not obey her in certain registers, and also of her feelings of choking and constriction in her throat and that the notes sound strangled, to the extent that she has not been able to sing in public. This imperfection, which only affects her middle register and is not constant, cannot be explained by any defect of the vocal cords.

By hypnosis, Freud learns that she was orphaned when she was small and had been taken in by an aunt, the mother of many children, married to a man who abused her and their children brutally, and who openly had sexual relations with the servants in the house. When her aunt died, Rosalia became her cousins' protector. She made an effort to suffocate expressions of the hate* and contempt she felt towards her uncle. It was at this time that the constriction in her throat appeared.

Afterwards, she found a singing teacher who encouraged her and with whom she secretly took lessons. Since she often arrived burdened by scenes at home, a relation between singing and her hysterical paraesthesia was consolidated. Even after having left her uncle's house, she continued to feel constriction in her throat, mainly when singing.

Freud tried to abreact her hatred for her uncle by inviting her to insult him in session and other similar things, which did her good. Meanwhile, she went to live as a guest in the home of another uncle, which her aunt resented, thinking that her husband had some special interest in Rosalia, and therefore tried to ruin her stay in Vienna. She also envied her artistic inclinations. For this reason, her niece never dared to sing or play the piano if her aunt was at home.

As we see, as Freud progressed in the analysis, new situations of excitation were being created.

At this time a new symptom appeared: a disagreeable tingling sensation at the tips of her fingers compelled her to make twitching movements. Although Freud thought that the analysis of a recent symptom would be easier, he was surprised by the emergence of a number of memories of scenes from early childhood, all of which had something in common: she had tolerated an injustice without defending herself, when her hand would have been able to act.

Then, another memory appeared with the first uncle: he had asked her to massage his back, and while she was doing this, he had thrown off the covers, jumped up, and tried to catch her. She was able to escape. She didn't like to remember this situation, but when she did, the more recent memory came up, after which the feeling and the twitching in her fingers had been established as a recurring mnemic symbol*. The uncle in whose house she was now living had asked her to sing a song. Since she was sure that her aunt had gone out, she played the piano and sang. But the aunt returned, and Rosalia jumped up and slammed the piano closed. The music fell. Then, the memory traces* of previous injustices, analogous to the actual one, were removed; but because of this one, she had to leave Vienna, a painful circumstance since she had nowhere to live. As she told Freud about this scene, Rosalia moved her fingers as if she were flicking something away or rejecting an offer (a symbolic presentation of the ego's rejection of the repressed wish* that is pressing to return).

Therefore, the recent experience had awakened first the memory of similar previous contents, and the mnemic symbol formed provided validity for all the others in a condensed way.

Conversion was supported in part by what she had recently experienced and in part by a remembered affect.

Thus, Freud concludes that a process like this one, in which past and present are connected by a mnemic symbol that unites them in a symptom*, must be the rule in the genesis of hysterical symptoms.

The symptom appears at two different times until it is finally installed after the second trauma which is a reminder of the first.

CASTRATION (CF. CASTRATION ANXIETY AND CASTRATION COMPLEX)

CASTRATION ANXIETY

Ger.: Kastration Angst. – Sp.: angustia de castración. – Fr.: angoisse de castration. – It.: angoscia di castrazione. – Port.: angústia de castração.

This anxiety* is felt by boys when they understand the difference between the sexes in terms of phallic–castrated.

In this period (phallic) boys understand the female genital, mistaking it for a lack of the male genital, by virtue of judgement based on perception* (perception of a lack), which generates the realistic anxiety* that there is a true possibility that this danger could befall them.

Afterwards, it becomes the anxiety signal* *par excellence* (following the dissolution* or repression* of the Oedipus complex* and the installation of the superego* in the psychical apparatus*.)

Castration anxiety therefore appears at the height of the Oedipus complex and generates infantile neuroses (Little Hans, the "Wolf Man"), generally animal phobias* as relics of totemism*; later they acquire the characteristics of this mnemic symbol* cultivated by the ego* in its seedbed in order to produce its defence mechanisms* against what it feels to be Trieb danger.

Castration anxiety is also a level of anxiety signal, even more complex than in object loss. It is felt basically in relation to the father, the Oedipal rival, and is the result, in Freud's phylogenetic hypothesis, of the epoch of the primal horde* when the primal father castrated his sons in order to possess all the women of the horde.

In *Inhibitions, Symptoms and Anxiety* (1925) Freud explains that castration anxiety refers to anxiety for object loss, since possession of the penis is the condition for experiencing the latter anxiety. Definitive recognition of sexual difference with all the new conflicts it brings up makes the link with the object* more complex.

Lack of object refers ultimately to the danger of relapsing into tension due to need and automatic anxiety*. Castration anxiety is an anxiety signal that leads the ego to automatically put its defence mechanisms into action, thereby generating new mediations that progressively remove it away from the danger of automatic anxiety.

In adults, castration anxiety is generally replaced by anxiety before the superego* and social anxiety*; it is basically their substrate. However, these anxieties involve an even greater degree of mediation and complexity. Castration anxiety is the main factor in the creation of neurotic symptoms in clinical pictures known as historical or transference neuroses, particularly anxiety hysteria* and its phobias*.

It is interesting to note that the reality ego* culminates its constitution in the phallic period when the phallus whose supremacy dominates the rest of the erotogenic zones* gives them a unity that is later called the ego. This is another demonstration of the importance of castration anxiety in the constitution of the male psychical apparatus (a heavier categorical imperative, more dramatic and quicker to form the superego which is completely installed directly following the end of the Oedipus complex rather than in puberty as in the case of females; also, men have a more unconscious superego than women).

This anxiety is also realistic in boys during the period of the Oedipus complex; it afterwards becomes an anxiety signal cultivated by the ego and utilized as a mnemic symbol in response to Trieb* that attempts to return from the repressed to satisfy primarily repressed infantile sexuality*, from which the adult ego now defends itself with its secondary repressions or defence mechanisms.

CASTRATION COMPLEX

Ger.: Kastration Komplex. – Sp.: complejo de castración. – Fr.: castration, complexe de. – It.: complesso di castrazione. – Port.: complexo de castração.

Excitations and effects related to loss of the penis.

The child's sexual development takes place in two phases. The first, from birth to the age of five or six, is infantile sexuality* which falls beneath the blanket of repression*, followed by a period of latency*, after which the second phase emerges in its definitive form in puberty and then adolescence.

At the culmination of the infantile sexual period, the predominant erotogenic zone* is the phallic-urethral* zone; with awareness of the predominance of this zone, a number of things occur simultaneously. First, divergent paths open up in the evolution of boys compared to girls.

On the infantile level of knowledge, sexual differences are noticed and experienced in reality as possession or non-possession of genitals (the individual not possessing them has been castrated and the one that does possess them is in danger of being castrated).

This reality, in itself difficult to face and to resolve, there being no alternative at that time of life, even more so considering the incomplete infantile psychical apparatus*, is partly accepted, originating castration anxiety* in boys and phallic envy in girls. It may also be disavowed* in both cases, signalling a path to sexual perversion* which may include some type of psychosis*.

In both girls and boys, this infantile level of thought* does not fully recognize the existence of the vagina as a genital organ (however, we may assume that the still incomplete reality ego* partly does, as well as object sexual Triebe*; we have only to observe its universal symbols* in dreams* originating in the unconscious*), which must be accepted definitively, in both cases, on the long road to puberty and adolescence.

In the phallic phase, the vagina and the clitoris are experienced by both sexes as castration of the only genital ultimately considered as such at this infantile level: the phallus.

The boy's fear of possible castration, proven when the boy views the female genital, is called castration anxiety; it is from this anxiety that the ego of the adult neurotic defends itself with unconscious defence mechanisms*, the origin of character traits*, and neurotic symptoms*.

In girls, acceptance of the existence of castration originates the castration complex *par excellence*. She bases her ego on what she feels is a mutilation. This situation leads to feelings of depreciation and extreme dependence. The constitution of her superego* is slower and closer to consciousness, not hastened by the urgency of castration.

In regard to this process, Freud points out that the sexual evolution of women may take one of three major paths: repression of sexuality* in general; nonacceptance of castration, leading to masculinity in the character or to homosexuality* as a perversion; or passage to femininity with acceptance of the difference between female and male genitals and between masculinity and femininity, each with its own characteristics, rather than as castration of a single form of genital (the phallus).

The third step, reached after puberty, is obviously the normal path, although it partly includes the previous steps, which are repressed.

CATHARSIS

Ger.: Abfuhr (Ablauf). – Sp.: Catharsis. – Fr.: catharsis. – It.: catarsi. – Port.: catarse.

A phenomenon of discharge of quantity of excitation*, this discharge may occur simultaneously with the traumatic event; in this case, the psychical apparatus* acts almost only as a reflex arc by virtue of the principle of inertia*, returning immediately to the previous state (of level of stimulus).

In other cases, the affect* may be retained, for example when an erotogenic zone* is stimulated at a time of life when it is not yet equipped for discharge. When this erotogenic zone and its psychical correspondences become preeminent, the traumatic event returns in a deferred* manner, producing feelings that were not produced before, against which the ego* now defends itself with repression* and its eventual generation of symptoms* (when it is not successful and allows the return of the repressed*).

Here, psychoanalysis tries to retrieve traumatic memories* against which the ego retained affect at that time, in order to abreact* it by means of catharsis, thereby discharging it; it will then propose to bind these memories by means of their working through, which thereby allows more passage to the ego's* preconscious*. The abreaction (acting only once, without subsequent working through, so that repression tended to return and the symptom to reappear), producer of catharsis, was the first method that replaced hypnotic orders, in comparison to which it was much more effective. It was therefore an anticipation or initial level of analysis that Freud never left aside but included as a step in the cure.

CATHEXIS

Ger.: Besetzung. – Sp.: investidura. – Fr.: investissement. – It.: carica o investimento. – Port.: carga ou investimento.

In Spanish, according to the Dictionary of the Royal Spanish Academy, the term "investidura" means the action and effect of investing: to invest or confer dignity or an important position. Quantity of excitation* is invested [cathected] by the presentation*, which thereby bestows upon it the "dignity" necessary to become psychical and to receive new names: libido* and quantum of affect*. In this case it is the presentation that invests [cathects] quantity of excitation, bestows the "worthy vestments". The presentation is also invested [cathected] by quantity (which at this instant acquires the category of libido); in the case of the thing-presentation*, it forms unconscious desire* and Trieb* (the latter concept at the boundary between the biological and the psychical). In preconscious* investment or cathexis (of attention) of word-presentations*, these word-presentations are informed to consciousness*. For this reason, we say that cathexis is a "bifrontal" concept: it is both libido that cathects a presentation and also the latter that cathects libidinal energy; in both cases, produced in unison, the phenomenon acquires a new category: psychical "dignity".

Both decathexis* and anticathexis* are phenomena contrary to this process of cathecting; decathexis of the thing-presentation, a typical phenomenon in schizophrenia*, produces loss of presentational "dignity" (at least in phenomena at the outset of this illness: disaggregation, experience of the end of the world, and libidinal withdrawal*), the psychical apparatus being left helpless (cf. helplessness*) due to an excessive quantity of excitation (automatic anxiety*). Anticathexis is the mechanism of primary repression by which fixation* to a certain erotogenic zone is produced, the splitting also generated leading to an unconscious now repressed from a preconscious. Anticathexis is also a component of secondary repression or defence mechanisms*; in this case, it is what produces the resistance* of repression.

If the thing-presentation is to reach a higher (or worthier) level, it must be hyper-cathected (cf. hyper-cathexis*) with the word-presentation and the latter in turn hyper-cathected with attention from consciousness in order to be thought by virtue of the strong cathexis and weak displacement* characteristic of secondary process*. Thus, we see that each new level of presentational complexity ("dignity") requires stronger cathexis or investment.

CENSORSHIP

Ger.: Zensur. – Sp.: censura. – Fr.: censure. – It.: censura. – Port.: censura.

This concept goes through a certain evolution in Freud's works. It is the process in which a derivative-presentation (of another presentation* repressed primarily) is denied access to a higher level of the psyche (to words or the preconscious*) or is allowed access only if it is well disguised and not recognized by the ego* as its own.

Freud first defines dream censorship. Its function is to disfigure the presentation* intolerable for consciousness*. In Chapter 7 of *The Interpretation of Dreams* (1900) and in the metapsychological papers of 1915, it is referred to as "repression" (Verdrängung) which is in reality a very specific form of censorship. This repression splits the psychical apparatus* into unconscious and preconscious, and takes place in two steps: primary repression which is gradually installed following different traumatic moments of infantile sexuality*, creating fixations* which culminate in the period of the Oedipus complex* and generate subsequent infantile amnesia*; and secondary repression which seeks to hunt down derivatives of infantile sexuality, already repressed and attempting to return through them from the repressed*; when successful, it generates neurotic symptoms* and other products entering from the unconscious through defects in repression; thus, they configure its third step: the return of the repressed*.

Freud also describes conscious censorship which blocks the passage of preconscious word-presentations* into consciousness (Cc) by depreciating them because they produce shame and so on. This censorship's mechanism is to remove hyper-cathexis* of attention* from the word-presentation which it needs in order to access consciousness*; this is what the patient is asked to set aside when complying with the "fundamental rule"* of "free association"*.

In the terms of the second topic (which adds complexity to the first topic in this respect but does not suppress it), censorship is in this case exercised by the superego* on an ego* that has not reached the level of the ego ideal* required of it by the superego. It then takes the form of self-reproaches* or self-censorship: expressions of the sense of guilt*, a feeling that has no complete metapsychological explanation in the first topic except as Trieb turning against itself. For this reason, the connection between censorship and guilt is more complex (although they occur at different times since in adults they sum up and condense) and explains more psychical phenomena more completely.

The superego may also punish the ego for giving the id* certain liberties (acted out or fancied) not accepted by moral conscience*. It is a remnant of parental censorship during upbringing; censorship that therefore refers in an unconscious transference manner to the threat of castration (cf. castration anxiety*).

The ego automatically censures a Trieb impulse when its thing-presentation* seeks a word-presentation* somehow associated by the ego with something not accepted by the superego, since it has produced an anxiety signal* in the ego. The ego defends itself from this anxiety by utilizing defence mechanisms* against Trieb*, although it does not make Trieb disappear, at least in neurosis, but simply takes away the "passport" or permit to circulate in consciousness (words*), without which the preconscious ego cannot think or bind it. These defence mechanisms are therefore progressively sophisticated forms of intrapsychical censorship.

CHANCE

Ger.: Zufall. – Sp.: azar. – Fr.: hazard. – It.: alea. – Port.: acaso.

Freud adheres to psychical determinism* throughout his works. His central concept, the unconscious*, determines the action that the subject believes to choose freely in consciousness*. This does not mean that Freud does not believe in the existence of chance in reality* outside the psyche. Actually, we are born by chance (we do not choose either our parents or our place of birth, which in turn determine us) and we suffer childhood trauma* unavoidably, but the psychical apparatus* later ensures that memory traces* left behind by these events are determinants of the subject's ulterior behaviour. That is to say that what occurred by chance from our viewpoint at a certain time later becomes a determinant. What occurred by chance in the external world is determinant once it becomes a psychical presentation. However, chance may also act in events of the subject's later life; not all are determined; in any case, the psychical apparatus tries to bind them, to relate them to previous events, and to find analogy or contiguity and even logical relations among presentations. Superstition considers that external events are motivated by psychical events. Animism* and anthropomorphism interpret the world through a human vision in which psychical functioning is in everything; this idea is based on a need to appropriate nature for wish fulfilment. Science tries to define the scope of all this. In some situations it is difficult to judge how much is chance and how much unconscious motivation: accidents and somatic illness, for example. This is also the endeavour of science in general and of psychoanalysis in particular.

CHARACTER

Ger.: Charakter. – Sp.: character. – Fr.: caractère. – It.: carattere. – Port.: caráter.

A person's character is essentially the manner in which the person's ego* functions, its way of carrying out or not carrying out specific action*, its points of fixation*, defence mechanisms*, attitudes, and attributes; in sum, the salient characteristics of this ego. Therefore, character is formed gradually, in the same way and in the same measure, as a person's ego.

Freud describes the ego as being formed out of the individual's "surface" (*The Ego and the Id*, 1923); that is to say, produced in contact with external reality*, in the link with it.

How does external reality penetrate the individual's psychical apparatus*? Of course, it enters at first through the perceptual end* (Pcpt.-Cs.). But when, how, and why does a perception* become the individual's ego?

This occurs because the psychical apparatus seeks identity. The ego introduces reality into itself, becoming the same, identical to it, identifying (cf. identification*) with it. What is external reality? It is basically any source of experiences of pleasure or pain*; that is to say, object* reality, the reality in which objects are wished-for sources of pleasure (which is recognized gradually, precisely in the same measure as the formation of the ego).

Identification is "the earliest expression of an emotional tie with another person" (*Group Psychology and Analysis of the Ego*, 1921, p. 105). The complete name of this identification and the first in time is primary identification*, also because it is previous to recognition of the object of pleasure as something foreign to the ego. Although the object's attributes are not recognized as such, they come to integrate the ego and become its own attributes: the way it handles action. The object's fixation points, defence mechanisms, and other traits are also included as tendencies. These primary identifications are produced in a psychical apparatus functioning with the category of being*.

As objects are progressively recognized as a source of pleasure, different types of links with them are established. Some of these are object choices* in which the category of having* predominates.

These choices take place by virtue of anaclisis* of sexual Trieb* over self-preservative Trieb. In some identification with these objects and others, the category of being is maintained.

Object choice and identification with the same object later become opposites, especially following definitive recognition of sexual difference.

After the Oedipus complex*, attraction to objects belonging to this period declines (they are now felt to be incestuous); a large part of their attributes finally becomes part of the ego, and "thus reinforces the primary" identification (*The Ego and the Id*, 1923, p. 31), and by secondary identification* comes to form a part of the ego that is the superego*. In boys it reinforces or gives official origin to their masculinity; their character also becomes firmer and acquires a more definitive modality in which defence mechanisms or secondary repression are more solidly integrated; if they are very intense and/or become rigid, they generate an alteration of the ego* or of the boy's character, constituting a character pathology.

The ego is an eminently defensive entity against Triebe coming from the id*; the characteristics of these methods of defence also constitute certain idiosyncrasies of different character types.

One of the major and most successful ways the ego may defend itself from invasion of Trieb is sublimation*; that is to say, by transforming Trieb into a socially acceptable (therefore more or less desexualized) action, therefore also acceptable to the ego and superego. The transformation of sexual Trieb with predominantly anal erotogenicity and a tendency to order, thrift, or tenacity is one of many examples (*Character and Anal Erotism*, 1908); also that of phallic-urethral Trieb into ambition and so on. In these cases, sublimations are not simply isolated satisfactory acts, at least not alone, but acquire the form of an ego characteristic, a way of doing things. Hence, they become character traits.

In relation to defence mechanisms, the paradigm of generators of character traits is reaction formation* which attains "*apparent* health, but actually … successful defence" (*Further Remarks on the Neuro-Psychoses of Defence*, 1896, p. 170) typical of the period of latency* in general and of the obsessional character in particular. As defence mechanisms become more rigid, including disavowal* of sexual difference, a characteristic of so-called sexual perversions, they generate more or less pathological character traits, usually related to bearing a certain wounded narcissism (haughtiness, arrogance).

Briefly, character is not a structure in itself but rather the attributes of a structure called the ego, which includes a specialized part, the superego.

These defensive attributes of an ego structure against id Trieb originate in external reality and are in turn pressured by another structure that arises from the psychical apparatus following the Oedipus complex and splits off from the ego, reinforcing the constitution of character: the superego.

Character is therefore ultimately a person's way of being: the precipitate of a singular history, traumatic events, fixations, repetition compulsion*, links and object choices, defence mechanisms, all these factors intimately related to particular types of identification.

A person's character helps the individual to maintain "normality". It is not necessarily pathological but takes this direction when it becomes definitively rigid and has few variables for dealing with the frustrations* of reality. It then becomes a character pathology which may in turn lay the foundation for eventual neuroses* or other pathological pictures.

Psychoanalysis may produce changes in character by deep analysis of the ego and its defences*, also by reconstructing their history which is mainly the history of the formation of the ego; this history returns vividly to the present in the phenomenon of transference*.

Character is a triumph of the ego over Trieb, which becomes integrated into it. Where there is character, there is no return of the repressed*, no symptoms*, no neurosis. It could even be said that there is (apparently) no psychical conflict*. What occurs is that Trieb is suffocated*, which creates an illusion of lack of conflict. However, any rise in quantity of excitation easily generates decompensation, with which the repressed returns and neurosis reappears with its subjacent conflict.

CLOACAL THEORY

Ger.: Kloakentheorie. – Sp.: cloaca, teoría de la. – Fr.: théorie cloacale. – It.: cloaca, teoria della. – Port.: cloaca, teoria da.

This is the second of the three principal infantile sexual theories*. The first attributes a penis to all human beings and the third is the sadistic conception of coitus. The theory of the cloaca stems from the child's ignorance of the existence of a vagina as a genital organ or from disavowal* of sexual difference embodied by boys and girls. Therefore, children attribute birth to evacuation rather than to delivery. If children are born through the anus, men can give birth as women do (this corresponds to the first theory according to which women have a penis). In reality, this theory includes two sexes only based on secondary sexual traits, a function in the family, the type of preferences, or a way of being, and so on, but not based on the essential.

Once the difference between the sexes is recognized, at least on an initial level (phallic–castrated opposition), the cloacal theory is discarded. However, it may remain in the repressed unconscious* or even in the ego* by virtue of a mechanism of ego splitting (which partly recognizes the fact of castration and partly does not). Ego splitting* occurs characteristically as a consequence of disavowal* of sexual difference produced in sexual perversion*.

In the "Wolf Man" case history (1918), Freud discusses this problem and the complex manner in which it appears in the case. The patient took three different attitudes towards castration: in his "masculine protest" which generated his phobic anxiety (castration anxiety*), he detested it; a second tendency accepted castration and was consoled by substitutive femininity, the origin of his symptoms* of constipation as hysterical conversion*; a third, older and deeper, which could still be activated, is doubtless the theory of the cloaca which disavows castration, and could reemerge transiently during acute conflict.

The cloacal theory interconnects the transmutation of anal Triebe* through the symbolic equation: faeces-penis-child-gift-money, all identical in the unconscious.

COGNITIVE OR OBSERVING THOUGHT

Ger.: Bewustes Denken. – Sp.: pensamiento observador. – Fr.: pensée observante ou cognitive. – It.: pensiero osservatore o cognoscitivo. – Port.: pensamento observador ou cognitivo.

This type of thought* arises when perception* is cathected* with attention* and receives the signal of the presence of a perception. The ego* wants to know about it. It wonders: what does it mean? Where does it lead? It now associates more intensely, advances farther along its associative path to determine how similar the perceived is to what is desired or which desired object it resembles. That is to say, it tries to "re-cognize" it.

Signs of quality* emanate from the perception. Observing thought needs these signs of quality* in order to place cathexis* correctly. Therefore, the associative path must be converted into a perception. This is achieved through verbal associations binding thing-presentations* with sounds (word-presentations*) that both signify them and are associated with motor verbal images. That is to say, conscious observing thought is directed by attention and attention by the wish* which attempts to unite what the subject is now perceiving with previous perceptions; it does so through verbal associations, through words, which is the way to perceive associations and give them perceptual quality. It is therefore composed of attention directed to verbal associations perceived in consciousness* through language* which is already motor discharge, a type of internal change*. Perception involves more psychical quantity, more cathexis of attention, than common thought*, since it is hyper-cathected*.

The thought process consists in a displacement* of quantities regulated by association with quality. In any case, the quantities displaced are relatively small; although thought is a movement, it is not real movement (it is not specific action* but rather a rehearsal for it). The basic difference is that the quantity of energy (desexualized libido) discharged through thought is quite small. There is an economic reason for this. If the ego spent large quantities of energy (as occurs in obsessional* thinking) on observing thought, very little would remain for specific action which requires so much.

Thought reconciles strong cathexis* with weak displacement*, a state Freud referred to as binding.

A bit of history: the tension of need following the experience of satisfaction* became a desire to repeat this experience. For this purpose, perception of the external world and of the course of thought itself were cathected with attention; thought enters perception by virtue of the creation of language*, with little displacement but an intense cathexis. This "state of binding" constitutes secondary process*. (However, in primary process*, associations are more fluid, freer, and of course also signed by wishes, but less effective for specific action since they are closer to perceptual identity* or hallucinations*.)

Binding is therefore a secondary process at the service of what is eventually the reality principle* which is a modified pleasure principle*, which means that it takes this reality into account.

COLLECTIVE FIGURE

Ger.: Mischbildung. – Sp.: formación mixta. – Fr.: formation mixte. – It.: formazione mista. – Port.: formação mista.

This type of dream condensation* expresses similarity, concordance, or community among various elements of a dream*. It creates a new figure condensing these elements. They tend to be things, but may also be persons. When a collective figure joins persons, certain individual features of each, not held in common, are brought together. For example, one person's name belongs to another person, or has another's visual traits or gestures, words said, and even another person's situation. What they have in common may or may not appear in the dream's manifest content*.

Condensation by identification* or collective figures may serve precisely to save figuration of common elements in different presentations*.

Collective figures enable dream work* to evade dream censorship* by disguising presentations that would otherwise have had to be more energetically repressed.

COMIC, THE

Ger.: Komisch (witzig). – Sp.: cómico. – Fr.: comique. – It.: comico. – Port.: cômico.

A pleasurable psychical operation whose path of discharge is laughter, it originates as something found but not necessarily sought in social relations between human beings; it may include the appreciation of certain animals, inanimate objects, or situations presenting exaggerated or caricaturesque aspects. Their description generally corresponds to events that occur to adults or to persons whose psychical apparatus* is fully established: with an id*, an ego*, and a superego*, and also well-defined limits between the unconscious*, preconscious*, and consciousness*.

The comic is an operation of the preconscious (Prec) part of the ego belonging to thought* activity, judgement, and secondary process*. The unconscious does not intervene in its creation as it does in the case of jokes*.

The comic is something observed in persons: their movements, forms, actions, and character traits*; at first, it may only involve body movements, and later include intellectual movements or their manifestations. As we said, it may focus on animals, things, or situations. We laugh at the exaggerated and aimless antics of clowns because they remind us of infantile awkwardness. We laugh at any exaggerated expenditure of energy: from the comic of movement the comical may branch out into comical body shapes and facial expressions.

Why does exaggerated and aimless movement produce a comical effect which may even lead to other situations? Freud attributes it to the comparison (drawn automatically as a form of understanding*) between movement observed in another and what the subject would have done instead. Through the process of judgement and the complex of the fellow being*,

> I have acquired the idea of a movement of a particular size by carrying the movement out myself or by imitating it, and through this action I have learnt a standard for this movement in my innervatory sensations.
>
> (*Jokes and Their Relation to the Unconscious*, 1905, p. 191)

We understand a fellow human being who is carrying out the same actions; then, once we are familiar with them, we can proceed to compare them to our own. The process is simplified by the intervention of memory which saves us from repeating the same procedure each time by substituting it with an expenditure of presentation* cathexis*. When we see a fellow human being acting exaggeratedly or aimlessly – in our automatic comparison, to understand, with the action we would carry out in the same situation – presentation cathexis is saved. The energy saved is discharged by the pleasurable mechanism of laughter.

> This would be the way in which, other circumstances being favourable, pleasure in a comical movement is generated – an innervatory expenditure which has become an unusable surplus when a comparison is made with a movement of one's own.
>
> (Ibid., p. 194)

The pleasure of the comic therefore arises from an expenditure of presentation cathexis that the disproportion of the other person's movement saves us.

COMPLEMENTAL SERIES

Ger.: Ergänzungsreibe. – Sp.: serie complementaria. – Fr.: série complémentaire. – It.: serie complementare. – Port.: série complementar.

This is Freud's dynamic explanation of the causes of neurotic symptoms* and of psychical pathology in general, which includes the formation and changes arising in the psychical apparatus* and its structural parts at different moments in life.

The first series is constituted by everything inherited and by experiences of infantile prehistory; that is to say, anything previous to the dissolution of the Oedipus complex*. He refers to the sum of these two as the constitutional or disposition*.

If actual frustration* (the second series) is added to disposition, then neurosis or some other form of psychopathological decompensation (the third series) is triggered.

Since these series complement each other, all three are necessary to produce an alteration.

Those proceeding from disposition related to fixation points* are generally causal factors of the choice of neurosis. The greater the dispositional factor, especially the inherited, the more difficult it makes the cure.

In actual* or traumatic neuroses*, the actual factor predominates, and therapeutic work must centre especially on it, perhaps by searching for connections with the patient's history; that is to say, making it psychological, re-transforming it into a transference neurosis*; for this task, the previous constitutional factor is necessary. These patients may thereby enter the domains of the pleasure principle*, memory, and also the thinkable, the presentational world (thing-presentations* and word-presentations*) with all their complexity, and thought* activity (especially word-presentations, signifiers of thing-presentations) belonging to the preconscious ego*.

COMPLEX OF THE FELLOW BEING

Ger.: Komplex des Nebenmeschen. – Sp.: complejo del semejante. – Fr.: complexe du semblable. – It.: complesso del simile. – Port.: complexo do semelhante.

A concept discussed in the *Project for a Scientific Psychology* (1895–1950), it is a reflection on the origin of understanding* of the expressive acts of others. Freud considers that in the act of perception* the perceptive concept is classified. It is divided into two basic parts: a central part, unchanging, which is essentially what is sought, called the thing*, and another, changing and susceptible of being related to characteristics of its own; the latter corresponds to the thing's attributes. Freud extends this mechanism of judgement to fellow human beings. In them, some parts characterize them and cannot be understood: they are simply that way. This is the central, unchanging aspect of the object* (facial features, for example), the "thing" of the object. Fellow human beings also have attributes: the movement of their hands, their screams, their attitudes in general. Their attributes, however, may be understood when related to observations of the subject's own body by moving one's own hands, for example screaming, or remembering one's own screams and what they meant or what they were related to. This is the way to understand the fellow human being: by putting the other's attributes through one's own body, putting oneself "in the other's place", or by bringing this "place" to oneself. It is the identificatory "imitative value" (cf. identification* and narcissism*) in all perception.

The complex of the fellow being corresponds to secondary process*, to thought activity*, although affect* (screams, laughter) is also involved. Word-presentations* are not indispensable for this type of thinking, since it functions in babies almost only with reproductive thought based on images or thing-presentations* and certain bodily movements (cf. ego*). Obviously, language* acquisition, with its word-presentation*, adds exponentially greater complexity.

The complex of the fellow being therefore consists in the emission of a judgement of existence* and a judgement of attribution* regarding the fellow human being. It is carried out by the budding reality ego* and belongs in part to reality testing*.

COMPULSION

Ger.: Zwang. – Sp.: compulsión. – Fr.: compulsión. – It.: coazione. – Port.: compulsão.

An uncontrollable characteristic inherent to some acts, ideas, phantasies*, symptoms*, and affects*; even character traits* or weaknesses of the ego*; due to great psychical intensity together with intense displacement among presentations*. That is to say, uninhibited presentations (cf. inhibition*) not bound by the secondary process* of the preconscious ego, which therefore perceives them as foreign to it, something imposed on it from within itself. Compulsions also show broad independence from the organization of other psychical processes corresponding to the preconscious ego; the latter usually remain adapted to the demands of the external world and obey the laws of logical thinking.

An action is compulsive when its logic responds to the pleasure principle*; that is to say, non-existence of time, space, and contradiction, in sum, the laws of the reality principle*. Compulsion originates in Triebe* or defence* against them: superego anticathexis*; or, more commonly, in both simultaneously. This is the case of obsessional symptoms such as ceremonials and obsessions themselves.

Patients tend to get along badly with their compulsions, criticizing them and complaining about them, until they are taken into the character by the ego, at which point they lose their ego-dystonia, which is a triumph of primary process* over secondary process, of the pleasure principle over the reality principle, and of the id* or the superego* over the ego*. This success may also be seen as the opposite: a Pyrrhic victory of the ego in which it disowns something that is satisfied excluding reason, whether it is Trieb satisfaction, superego punishment, or a compromise between the two.

Another example of this type of act is compulsive masturbation*, generally in adolescence, with its typical cycle of self-prohibition, masturbation, guilt, self-prohibition, and repetition.

Kleptomania and some addictions such as the tendency to gamble, alcoholism, and drug addictions are unconscious derivatives of this compulsive masturbatory cycle (*Dostoevsky and Parricide*, 1928).

COMPULSION TO REPEAT OR REPETITION COMPULSION

Ger.: Wiederholungzwang. – Sp.: compulsión de repetición. – Fr.: compulsion de répétition. – It.: coazione o ripetere. – Port.: compulsão de repetição.

A universal characteristic of Triebe* pressing to return to a former state, it is an expression of the principle of inertia*, the first law of movement of classical physics, applied here to organic life in general and to psychical life in particular. It is expressed clinically as a tendency to repeat a certain type of complex action, to involuntarily re-create situations more or less painful or frustrating to the subject, who is unable to prevent it.

What is the former state to which it returns? It is the state of the organism before the organism's own existence (death Trieb*; between these two extremes we find all the variations of repetition and all possible proportions of Trieb fusion or defusion*.

Repetition compulsion is observed in psychoanalytic treatment as a neurotic symptom* (typically in obsessional neurosis* although also in phobia* and hysteria*), as a character trait*, and also as sexual perversion*. It may even be detected in psychotic delusions*. When the traumatic event is actual, it generates traumatic neuroses* with their typical repetitive dreams*. In "normal" individuals it may appear as a "neurosis of fate or destiny".

Also, especially since this is the most important point for therapeutic possibilities, the patient also "repeats" in transference* established with the psychoanalyst. Sometimes patients "act out" episodes of their childhood in transference; they are generally repressed traumatic facts to which they are "fixated" (cf. fixation*), whether they are converted from passive to active or are repeated just as they are. That neurosis is transformed into this neurosis: a transference* neurosis, transferred on to the analyst; it is an artificial neurosis, an intermediate situation between illness and life on which the psychoanalyst may now exert influence "in vivo" by learning about it and showing the patient's ego* the Trieb* from which it is defending itself, the reason for which it is doing so, and the way in which it is doing it.

Repetition compulsion is a model of the type of functioning of the unconscious* with its facilitations* and its search for perceptual identity*, sometimes wanting to satisfy the pleasure principle* and others to go beyond it, almost always mixing both aims in diverse proportions.

What is most characteristic is therefore this search for identity: an identical situation, whether pleasurable or a traumatic experience.

It is also a form of "remembering" following the forgetting* produced by repression*. For this reason, it becomes one of the strongest resistances* to the cure: resistance from the id*. The id wants to repeat (a form of remembering*), not to remember (in the sense of remembering through thought* activity). The agency that wants to remember with words is the preconscious ego which seeks to be cured.

The principal therapeutic aim in this case is working through* by the preconscious ego of the repeated situation that has become actual in transference by utilizing this working through based on constructions* of the histories of infantile sexuality* with their traumatic situations*. In this way, these forgotten and disguised events reappear in their word-presentations*, making repetitions thinkable, understandable, and linkable to other presentations by the preconscious ego and its thought activity; thereby recovering for the ego's consciousness* the "forgotten" past that returned as mere repetition.

Freud mentions a "demonic repetition", the most resistant to the cure. It is probably the one whose mixture contains a larger proportion of the tendency to return to the inorganic or to anything that approximates it (death Trieb). Demonic repetition is considered to motivate the patient to abandon treatment halfway through, to fall ill after the neurosis has been cured with more or less severe somatic affections, or to begin to have accidents. It is sometimes synonymous with the negative therapeutic reaction* when the patient's symptoms worsen in spite of progress in the treatment.

In these last cases, an unconscious sense of guilt* or a need for punishment* participates, composed of destructive Trieb* bound by the superego* and turned against the ego.

CONDENSATION

Ger.: Verdichtung. – Sp.: condensación. – Fr.: condensation. – It.: condensazione. – Port.: condensação.

One of the characteristic forms of primary process* functioning in regard to thing-presentations*, though sometimes also with respect to word-presentations. It originates in the tendency to perceptual identity* with which the unconscious* functions. It is a type of mechanism observed clinically in dreams*, in some symptoms*, parapraxes*, myths*, and so on.

In condensation, different elements are joined together by virtue of attributes that enable connections, either by analogy* or contiguity*. These connections are mistaken by primary process for identities. In this way, one element, because it is near another, is itself and the other one at the same instant, or because one of its attributes is similar to another, it is the same thing.

There are different types of condensations: a single element is several at the same time (a common intermediate element in dreams*). The union of several elements generates a new figure possessing attributes of each of those elements (an accumulation person).

Summing up all the characteristics, the elements in common stand out whereas differing characteristics are vague (mixed person).

Condensation is part of dream work* and also serves the aims of censorship* since the condensed elements that appear in the dream are not understandable to consciousness*.

Through condensation the manifest content* of the dream is scanty in comparison to its latent content* (the associations* that spring from it).

Symptoms* also undergo condensation, especially hysterical symptoms, as well as nearly all products of the unconscious* such as jokes* and parapraxes*.

Condensation is produced from free energy*, with a level of binding between cathectic* and presentational* energy which enables free displacement* of energy from one presentation to another. By virtue of condensation a presentation is many at the same time (which allows over-determination) and is therefore hypercathected*, or many presentations are mixed together.

CONSCIENCE

Ger.: Gewissen. – Sp.: conciencia moral. – Fr.: conscience morale. – It.: coscienza morale. – Port.: consciência moral.

One of the parts or functions of the superego* is the "judging" function. This position in infantile prehistory and especially during the development of the Oedipus complex* was held by the father figure, once admired as an object of wished-for identification* and later seen as a rival for possession of the object* which has become incestuous (in the boy's positive complex); in the negative, it is formed by the father-complex*; in girls, it is formed in a different manner, slower and more consciously, culminating no earlier than puberty.

The figure of this father, already clearly recognized as an object, with the characteristics of a rival (hate* of the rival, a product of defusion of death Trieb*, is the origin of the extreme sturdiness reached by the superego and the aggressiveness of the "categorical imperative" towards the ego*), is enthroned in the son's psychical apparatus*, generating the superego structure in charge of showing the ego how it must be and how it must not be; therefore, what is good and what is bad, nothing less than ethical limitations.

Conscience is generally dedicated to prohibitions (in reality, repressions*, which is not the same since the latter mechanism is unconscious*) of which the prohibition of incest and parricide are the most important and the origin of all the rest.

The other part, substructure, or function of the superego is the ego ideal*. It is generated from a different aspect emerging from infantile narcissism*. It demands omnipotence, perfection (a way to counteract the infantile defencelessness of its origins and the primordial source of all moral motives [*Project for a Scientific Psychology*, [1895] 1950, p. 318]).

Being parts of the same structure – the superego – moral conscience and the ego ideal work together. Conscience keeps watch to make sure the ego complies with the requirements of the ideal. If it does, it rewards the ego with a raise in self-esteem*. If not, it punishes the ego with guilt*.

Conscience is the heir of the Oedipus complex. It becomes established in the psychical apparatus and results from secondary identification* with the castrating father which belongs to the same complex. In this sense it is a vicissitude of human sexual Trieb* or a special form of anticathexis* gestated in the psychical apparatus in order to prevent direct satisfaction of Trieb*. In another sense it is a form of binding the psychical apparatus utilizes for destructive Trieb* (also a deflection of the death Trieb*) to control both anticultural sexual Trieb and aggression*, a product of the deflection of death Trieb.

In early childhood, the parents observe, give orders, judge, and threaten the child with punishment. Following establishment of the superego, the latter takes over these functions with the adult ego.

Another aspect of the superego, as we said, has its source in infantile narcissism. It is the ego ideal. Conscience demands perfection of the ego as did the infantile ideal ego*, and now the ego ideal, since the ego aspires to this perfection itself.

If the ego's actions approach the ideal, criticism from moral conscience dissipates and self-esteem grows. The ego feels esteemed by its ego ideal. However, if the distance between the ego and the ego ideal is large, criticism of moral conscience grows and self-esteem drops; this produces a sense of guilt.

Conscience is formed mainly of words: parental advice, threats, and reprimands. It originates in conscious perception*; one part remains in preconscious memory and the other takes root firmly in the id*, first the phylogenetic and Trieb that is fruit of fusion and defusion of its component life and death Triebe*.

Therefore, an unconscious part of conscience also includes its thing-presentations* (feared presentations). However, the unconscious includes not only the lowest but also the "most sublime".

CONSCIENCE, GUILTY OR SOCIAL ANXIETY

Ger.: Schuld-bewusstsein. – Sp. culpa, conciencia de. – Fr.: culpabilité, conscience de. – It.: colpa, coscienza di. – Port.: culpa, consciência de.

A type of guilt, also called social anxiety*, produced when the subject behaves unacceptably or commits acts prohibited by the authorities. When the superego* has not yet been established in children, this is the only type of guilt possible.

In adults, it is joined by the anxiety of moral conscience* or of the superego*: a sense of guilt* whenever acts against the laws governing the social community are committed. The individual feels condemned by the community, which increases the subject's narcissistic isolation; or these individuals may attempt to counter it by seeking to be accepted by the community, either by adopting conciliatory attitudes or arrogant and defiant attitudes. This is the case of persons who commit conscious crimes against social laws which they later regret.

The sense of guilt is expiated through repentance by virtue of which the love* of authorities is recovered by children, and reinsertion into the community by adults who must also serve the sentences imposed by human society for the crime committed.

CONSCIOUSNESS

Ger.: Bewusstein. – Sp.: conciencia. – Fr.: conscience. – It.: coscienza. – Port.: consciência.

Freud defines this in *The Interpretation of Dreams* (1900) as "a sense-organ for the perception of psychical qualities" (p. 615). It is located throughout the entire body surface; it is therefore the limit between the body and the world outside. It corresponds to the concepts of perceptual end* (cf. scheme in Chapter 7 of this work) and perception-consciousness pole (Pcpt.-Cs.) of *A Metapsychological Supplement to the Theory of Dreams* (1917).

Consciousness registers the qualities* of stimuli from the external world but has no memory, retains no trace of them, and is always available to register new qualities. Traces are "filed" in other psychical places (preconscious, unconscious).

Aside from registering external stimuli as qualities, consciousness also recognizes sensations belonging to the inside of the body in a range that spans from displeasure* to pleasure*. Increases of quantity of internal excitation* are usually felt as a displeasurable quality whereas decreases are felt as a pleasurable quality.

At first, there is no qualitative register of the internal world, except the hallucination* that arises when the baby's tension of need is very great and the baby most probably tends to momentarily perceive conditions of satisfaction. However, real frustration teaches the baby to inhibit* hallucinatory satisfaction of wishes*, from which an inhibiting ego* is born, the antecedent or first form of the reality ego*.

Freud describes the psychical apparatus* in several ways (encompassing them all). In what has been called the first topic, consciousness is one of the three "psychical places": unconscious*, preconscious*, and consciousness. In what is called the second topic (1923) it becomes part of the ego, of which it is the core.

In his *Project for a Scientific Psychology* (1950 [1887–1902]) he had discussed consciousness, perhaps more than in any other work. He described it at that time as being composed of two types of neurones* that perceive the external world: ϕ neurones, which register quantities, and ω neurones which register the quality of these quantities: the period* of the quantity. The latter type of neurone belongs to consciousness.

After the *Metapsychological Supplement to the Theory of Dreams* (1917), perception and consciousness are the same, which leads to the term "perception-consciousness" (Pcpt.-Cs.).

In *A Note upon the Mystic Writing Pad* (1925), the unconscious, through the Pcpt.-Cs. system, sends out antennae to the external world in order to take samples of it, then immediately draws them in again. They are feeler innervations that show consciousness influenced by the rest of the psychical apparatus, basically by its unconscious wishes* (although in another article, *Negation* [also 1925], he explains that these innervations reach consciousness by way of the ego). In any case, consciousness is thus no longer simply a passive registrar of perceptions* but actively seeks certain perceptions and avoids others. This activity is intimately connected with different magnitudes of attention* sent by the ego to consciousness. Schematically, there are two levels of magnitude: a low level of cathexis* and another with copious attention. The latter makes consciousness sharp and is the antonomastic conscious register.

If consciousness has acquired a higher level in human beings, it is because memory traces were registered in the same way as the external world in general. Memory traces could then be related in more or less complex ways and among themselves by virtue of language*. Words are felt again as a perceptual quality (they are heard). This new type of presentation* (word-presentation*) represents to consciousness the presentation of material things. As the psychical apparatus grows more complex, word-presentations also signify chains of other (preconscious) word-presentations whose ultimate meanings are thing-presentations*.

Words, first emitted, then remembered, made it possible for individuals to know their own thoughts* and, of course, to communicate them to others.

When words are perceived, not only signifiers of thing-presentations are perceived, but also different types of logical relations between them (also with word-presentations); when utilized by the preconscious ego, it acquired a very efficient means to perfect the action that changed "the face of the Earth".

Consciousness is a part of the ego that is also in charge of reality testing* by which an internal wish is distinguished from an external perception.

In contact with the external world, it functions as a protective layer against stimuli* which, after being moderated by it, may then be processed by the psychical apparatus.

To summarize: the official ego is formed from the outside towards the inside of the psychical apparatus and possesses the Pcpt.-Cs. in its outer portion, on its periphery. This perception-consciousness end searches the external world for certain registers on the one hand (what is wished for and what is feared, the latter in order to escape from it) and registers everything it perceives on the other (since the wished for and the feared may be in any perception). This demonstrates unconscious influence on conscious perceptions. It is done with a low level of general cathexis (evenly suspended attention, we could say). When something that attracts the ego more intensely appears in the perceptual field, the ego sends the perceptive apparatus (Pcpt.-Cs.) a higher degree of attention cathexis (Freud refers to it as reflex attention); at this point conscious perceptive quality is registered more sharply.

Concerning thoughts, in order to reach consciousness clearly, they need emission of words first and the memory of this later. In any case they must be cathected with attention since a word-presentation lacking attention cathexis or having very little remains in the preconscious.

If the word-presentation, representative of the thing-presentation before ego consciousness, is deprived of preconscious cathexis and displaced (cf. displacement*) on to another word having an analogous or opposite meaning or on to a body cathexis, for example, this other presentation functions as an anticathexis*, the former going into a state of repression* by which it no longer belongs to the ego, with which its access to consciousness becomes impossible if repression is not lifted.

For preconscious presentations there is also censorship* of consciousness (which functions by minimizing, prohibiting, hiding them out of shame, and so on). In reality, this censorship belongs to the preconscious ego, and is therefore easily made conscious by means of a simple attention cathexis. For this reason the analyst asks the patient to suppress it as far as possible (cf. free association*), to allow derivatives of the repressed to show repressed presentations the way to consciousness.

CONSTANCY (CF. PRINCIPLE OF CONSTANCY)

CONSTRUCTION

Ger.: Konstruktion. – Sp.: construcción. – Fr.: construction. – It.: costruzione. – Port.: construção.

One of the major weapons in the psychoanalytic therapeutic arsenal, it is the logical reassembly of historical truths* experienced by a subject through meticulous and exhaustive analysis of a dream*, a symptom*, a parapraxis*, and so on.

The term construction refers in general to non-recordable facts. Therefore, constructions are hypotheses, though hypotheses that emerge from valid proof extracted from data arising in the analysis, for example of a dream. This logical sequence functions as a clarifying explanation for a number of subsequent behaviours, facts, and symptoms. New logical relations are found for presentational contents the patient possesses in dispersed form, unrelated among themselves, or apparently forgotten, which reappear in a symptom or other unconscious* product.

Therefore, constructions are made from history: principally from infantile prehistory previous to the Oedipus complex*, even previous to language acquisition.

However, constructions are also made from later periods, forgotten because they were traumatic (certain periods of adolescence, for example).

A construction is made by the analyst on the basis of data contributed by the patient; sometimes the patient may sketch it out in previous associations*. It is one way to lift repression*, to refind the forgotten, victim of the former. The construction itself tends to awaken memories* and these in turn may be the genesis of new constructions, a new way to understand* historical truth*.

The construction puts the repressed into words, and these words may be thought and bound. What was repressed becomes a part of the preconscious ego*, which is thereby strengthened. A construction does not always evoke memories. However, if the patient accepts it and feels it is real, it opens a new panorama on understanding of him- or herself; in order to lift repression, it may be something similar to remembering. What is important is that a good construction produced during the analytic process may cause symptoms to disappear and may also modify the ego* and its character traits*, generating deep changes in it.

However, the opposite may occur, for example after the conclusion of a construction: the symptomatology of a person with negative therapeutic reaction* may worsen since the unconscious sense of guilt* or need for punishment* forces the individual to cling to illness. In these cases, the same tends to occur with any other therapeutic weapon, such as interpretation*, analysis of transference*, and others.

Another important element in putting together a construction is repetition compulsion* generated in psychoanalytic treatment. Patients repeat experiences from their forgotten past which are transferred on to their analyst. When transference neurosis* is produced to a moderate degree with the analyst, construction continues, and now includes transference repetition to understand it, in the manner of actual proof. The fact that it is repetition shows that its origin is historical and that the meaning of what is actual lies in this history. Construction is thus built up with the emergence of associations and memories of similar scenes experienced with primary objects* or subsequent scenes belonging to the period of latency* or adolescence, which had already taken place on other occasions, referring, however, to different situations. When this occurs now in the therapeutic relation, they offer a complete impression of what was experienced before by the patient in the forgotten past, and the meaning that up to this moment had not appeared is thus found. This forgotten past is present in transference and can now be understood and put to use by the ego's secondary process*.

Construction is therefore a therapeutic weapon to make conscious* the unconscious*; it has deep theoretical connotations, becoming nearly synonymous with the thought process*; thought applied in this case to primary process* elements, thereby recovering primary process and transforming it into secondary process, into ego, the objective of psychoanalysis.

The word construction also has a broader sense that approximates it to that of interpretation*. For example, in the analysis of a symptom, when many past facts are reconstructed in connection with it, which contributed to its genesis, its repressed meaning is found. These facts may be remembered and yet this is still the work of construction.

It happens that, in continuing to work by following the revelation of the pathogenic core of a symptom, other pathogenic cores are found in connection with the former. If the history of certain ways of being, characteristics of the patient's ego, is analysed in the same way, new meanings are discovered and other memories come to light, even including other, more or less pathological, character traits that had not yet appeared which also bring in new meanings. Analysis consequently becomes more and more complex.

However, at some moments no more memories are found; some pieces of the puzzle are missing. Then, hypotheses are drawn which "fit" into all the previous work. These hypotheses are certain to be closer to historical truth when they are assembled in a logical way with more pieces of analysis previously done, when it has been the most complete possible.

CONTACT-BARRIERS

Ger.: Kontaktschänken. – Sp.: barreras-contacto. – Fr.: barrières-contact. – It.: barriere-contatto. – Port.: barreiras-contato.

In his *Project for a Scientific Psychology* of 1895 (1950), this is a form of connection between ψ neurones* that also acts as a barrier between them for the passage of quantity of stimulus. By virtue of this barrier function, each ψ neurone obtains a certain quantity of accumulated energy, and through that of the constant connection between them is kept at a constant level, circulating within the whole ψ circuit. In this way, a certain quantity of energy can be stored that is necessary for carrying out, at the appropriate time, the specific action*.

In order to carry out the specific action, a larger quantity of energy than what is provided by stimuli seeking discharge is usually needed, since the individual is exposed to the 'exigencies of life'*. Therefore, contact-barriers correspond to secondary function. The psychical apparatus thereby passes from the principle of inertia* to the principle of constancy* since these bridge-barriers make a constant quantity in this apparatus possible (at this point the ego* no less is constituted), which is indispensable for production of discharge after the stimulus has entered it. However, this is not all; their existence enables associations between neurones and the construction of thought (secondary process) in order to choose an action. This is therefore the main way in which instinctual repetition compulsion in human beings is overcome, seen in this perspective which we could consider neurological or theoretical-neuronal. In any case, although Freud soon discarded this scheme, it might be very interesting to find its corresponding points in subsequent explanations. It also manages to include both the secondary function (principle of constancy) and the primary function (principle of inertia), and joins them, since the secondary function is necessary for carrying out the primary function.

We could add that contact-barriers participate in one explanation of memory (and with it, of the whole psyche), which is defined here as the aptitude of neurones to be changed durably by a single process (the change takes place in a different manner of discharge or in different ways of being travelled by the stimulus). When a stimulus passes from one neurone to another, it does so in a certain way; this type of passage indicates ('facilitates', Cf. facilitation*) the path for subsequent passages (by the principle of inertia). However, for diverse reasons, it sometimes takes a different direction, leaving new traces and facilitations.

Memory is therefore constituted by facilitations between ψ neurones, although differences in facilitation between ψ neurones create different passages which generate the complexity of their existence.

The quantity of stimulus allowed to pass through the contact barrier depends on the following factors: a) whether the stimulus is more or less facilitated (a facilitation produced in turn by the quantity of stimulus that passed and the number of repetitions of the process: the larger the quantity that passes each time or the greatest number of times, the higher the facilitation); b) the quantity of actual stimulus (the actual quantity also facilitates passage); c) the presence of quantity in a contiguous neurone (at this point we should now call the quantity of excitation 'cathexis'*), which acts as a pole that attracts (this is the mechanism used by the ego* when it places collateral cathexes that divert the circulation of energy, thereby managing to direct it).

Contact-barriers are a mechanism created in the context of a neurological scheme and in this sense is mentioned by J. Lacan:

> "In 1895 the theory of neurones did not exist. Freud's ideas regarding the synapsis are entirely new: Freud takes the view of the synapsis as such, that is to say, the rupture of continuity between one nerve cell and the next. *(Seminar 2)*."

For us, they are valid principally as psychological models, particularly if we substitute neurones for representations (as Freud also does in the course of the text of the *Project…*) and the contact-barriers as models of forms of connection between them, for example the different forms of association* or of logical relations. Is not the passage to secondary process* produced by these contact- barriers? Is this not constructed from logical relations between representations? Does this type of relation between representations not need strong cathexis and weak displacement? Through what are displacements produced? They are produced by these bridges. These contact-barriers are the same 'bridges' that the obsessional neurotic tries to break with the mechanism of isolation*.

CONTIGUITY

Ger.: Aneinandergrenzen. – Sp.: contigüidad. – Fr.: contigüité. – It.: contiguità. – Port.: contigüidade.
One of the laws of association*, probably the oldest in the psychical apparatus*; contiguity may be in space or in time; the latter is also called simultaneity.

A fact is associated with another which occurs simultaneously or is located next to what occurs. Stored in memory accordingly, one of them may be remembered by the other.

In the unconscious*, contiguity is transformed into identity, after which a fact is not remembered for having been next to another meaningful one but instead becomes meaningful in itself.

Thus, in the "dream of the injection to Irma" in *The Interpretation of Dreams* (1900), Irma is the friend (preferred as a patient by Freud because she is docile) because she figures in the dream* as being under the contiguous window where Irma's friend was seen. Also in fetishism* for furs or women's underwear, Freud attributes the choice of fetish to the moment previous, therefore contiguous, to discovery of female castration; for this reason they are not genuine penis symbols (its analogies*), but are able to somehow retrieve things at moments previous to knowledge of sexual difference, when the infantile sexual theory* of the phallic mother* was valid.

Preconscious* thought* work resides in distinguishing between contiguity and identity whenever the unconscious utilizes one of them to bring up a derivative of the repressed wish.

Contiguity may serve as a means of establishing other phenomena such as transference*, neurotic symptoms*, or even paranoid delusions*. Every delusion contains displacements*, and one of the laws by which libido* is displaced among presentations* is that of contiguity. The same occurs in the phenomenon of transference, a product of "false connections"*, some established by analogy and others by contiguity. Sometimes patients remain silent. If asked, they say that "nothing important" occurs to them. Afterwards, they usually admit that their thoughts had turned to objects in the analyst's office, the furniture and other furnishings:

everything contiguous to the analyst, which in their unconscious is the psychoanalyst.

CONVERSION

Ger.: Conversion. – Sp.: conversión. – Fr.: conversion. – It.: conversione. – Port.: conversão.
This symptom, characteristic of hysteria, is the reason for the term "conversion hysteria"*; it is a product of the repression* of a wishful* phantasy*, derivative of another wish belonging to infantile sexual Trieb* and repressed primarily, later an effect of the return of the repressed*. It generates a hyperintense somatic innervation, sometimes sensory and sometimes motor, either excitation or inhibition, as both a substitute formation* and a symptom*.

The hyper-innervated place is revealed as a portion of the repressed presentation* that has attracted the entire cathexis to itself by condensation*. By condensing Trieb wish fulfilment with the anticathexis*, conversion constitutes a compromise formation from which the conversion symptom results.

Condensation predominates in hysterical conversion. One symptom represents a number of fantasies referring to different scenes in which situations connected with repressed wish fantasies were experienced.

Conversion may be formed by mechanisms of association* (cf. cases of hysteria from the first period*, Elisabeth von R.): contiguity*, analogy*, and others, or as a mnemic symbol*. In the latter case, there is no need to resort to the patient's associations for their interpretation (the fantasy of the slap on the cheek in Cäcilie M.'s facial neuralgia).

Conversion usually produces one of the main effects sought by repression (produced by the ego* by utilizing the anxiety signal* to conduct energy): to not feel displeasure*.

"Here the salient point is that … the patient displays towards his symptoms what Charcot called 'la belle indifférence des hystériques'" (*Repression*, 1915, pp. 155–6).

The repressive process of conversion hysteria ends in symptom formation*. However, anxiety hysteria* and obsessional neurosis* need to recommence at a second moment.

Conversion also involves important ego regression*: return to a phase with no separation between preconscious and unconscious and therefore without language* or censorship* (previously unpublished 1915 manuscript: *Overview of the Transference Neuroses*, 1987). In this phase, the only level of language possible was bodily, expressed through mimicry. The theme of mimicry was also discussed by Freud in *Jokes and Their Relation to the Unconscious* (1905) when he describes the phenomenon of the comic*. Conversion hysteria also involves a certain degree of libidinal regression to the phallic state* with its incestuous objects and oedipal problems related to the phallic–castrated, the level of sexual differentiation attainable at that time.

CONVERSION HYSTERIA

Ger.: Konversionhysterie. – Sp.: histeria de conversión. – Fr.: hystérie de conversión. – It.: isteria di conversione. – Port.: histeria de conversão.
This illness was the departure point for developments in which psychoanalysis gradually took shape as a method to treat mental affections, as well as a theory and science of psychical functioning.

"Hysteria" (hysteria *par excellence*) is characterized by functional somatic disorders in the muscular innervations, in sensitive and sensory organs, based on their bodily presentations. These disorders do not follow the systems of organic central and peripheral innervations. Their lines are fanciful and changing. They usually follow commonplace presentations of certain actions, sensations, or sensory perceptions*.

Perhaps the most significant Freudian discovery in this area was that each motor, sensitive or sensory alteration corresponds, by association or as a memory* symbol, to unconscious meanings; that is to say, meanings repressed by the subject's ego.

Triebe* originating in the id*, fixated to primarily repressed incestuous presentations, partly due to hereditary and partly to traumatic causes, return from the repressed* through derivatives sharing associative routes with them (contiguity*, analogy*, or memory symbol). However, these derivatives sometimes come too close to the primarily repressed presentation, and therefore the cathexis* is removed from preconscious word-presentations* that would enable their access to consciousness*. This cathexis enters a somatic innervation which acts as a substitute formation*, a compromise formation permitting satisfaction of an incestuous phantasy* while the conscious ego does not feel it as such.

In conversion hysteria, repression is successful in dealing with the affect of anxiety. It is able to ignore the repressed presentation and also to drain off part of the cathexis by somatic conversion. Perhaps for this reason, anxiety* is barely present. This description corresponds to lasting organic symptoms*, but also highlights a hysterical character trait*, the so-called *belle indifférence** (symptoms that would be severe for any somatic patient do not produce realistic anxiety* since the repressed Trieb or wish is being discharged precisely through the symptom).

Aside from lasting organic symptoms such as paralysis, anesthesias, hyperesthesias, neuralgias, gastrointestinal disorders, and sensory disorders, the famous hysterical attack* is an acute form of this illness and was already described by Charcot. Freud interprets it as phantasies projected on to motility in the form of a pantomime, disfigured as in dreams* and which may conclude in tonic-clonic convulsions in the manner of an autoerotic orgasm, a dramatic experience for the patient as well as observers.

As mentioned, hysterical repression is successful in the sense that the return of the repressed does not cause anxiety. There are some exceptions: acute periods or attacks may present complete with all their phases or in frustrated forms, any of the phases separately, or even as psychotic breakdowns which may be part of attacks or may present separately with unpleasurable visual hallucinations* (Anna O.'s snakes) or hysterical delusions* (such as N. Hanold's in *Gradiva*).

Substitute formations coincide with symptoms in conversion hysteria, and also with anticathexis* and a compromise formation whose presentation is not the direct opposite of Trieb. In these cases there is little anxiety. Then, some of the features of the hysterical character are generated. The anticathexis of secondary repression is established in the sensitive and sensory apparatus, aimed at not perceiving allusions to repressed presentations. This may generate the contradictory character of an eroticized personality with seductive but ingenuous behaviour, that "does not see" (Laforgue refers to it as a "scotoma") anything erotic, especially if it involves an incestuous nuance.

In conversion hysteria as in other neuroses, there are two types of regression*: libidinal regression to incestuous wish* presentations from the phallic phase and intense ego regression to a phase previous to language* acquisition and therefore without any separation between preconscious and unconscious, without censorship*, when bodily mimicry was the form of expression ("Panorama of the Transference Neuroses", 1915 manuscript). Phallic regression is the origin of the incestuous wish phantasy. The second type of regression, ego regression, facilitates the specificity of hysterical substitute formation (conversion into a bodily symptom expressing this phantasy, defence against it, punishment for it, or all of this in condensed form) in a way consciousness* does not understand. If we add the anticathexis of secondary repression that generates character traits (ego resistances*) and the situation of constant seduction associated with ingenuousness and acute hysterical attacks*, we describe the typical clinical picture of conversion hysteria.

Although conversion hysteria is more common in women, it is not limited to them. The prototypical anxiety is for object* loss more than castration* anxiety. This type of anxiety is more characteristic of women because of the particular formation of their psychical apparatus*, especially their superego*. Traumatic situations*, generators of fixations, are sometimes produced by scenes of passive seduction suffered by the infant in relation to an adult. This scene may correspond to a real experience (historical truth*) or to indicators misinterpreted by the child through the child's inherited "categories", in this case primal phantasies* of seduction (also historical truth). In the former case, the traumatic cause predominates and in the latter, the hereditary cause. Freud considers the former more accessible to psychoanalytical treatment and offering a better prognosis.

This treatment leads bodily innervations back to the wish phantasies signified by them, thereby recovering the word-presentations of the unconscious wishes. These are brought into associative commerce, into thought* in the conscious ego, to be put into action, or condemned by judgement*. To explain it the three ways Freud does, the unconscious* is made conscious, memory lacunae are filled in, and what was id* becomes ego.

"Hysteria" is the neurosis with which psychoanalysis was born and for which it continues to be the most effective, especially in curing its symptoms, but also, clearly more difficult, its typical character traits.

COUNTER-TRANSFERENCE

Ger.: Gegenübertragung. – Sp.: contratransferencia. – Fr.: contre-transfert. – It.: controtransfert. – Port.: contratransferência.

This is the psychoanalyst's unconscious* affective response in connection with unconscious or conscious contents of the patient's material.

Freud advises psychoanalysts to discern and master it in themselves (*Observations on Transference-Love (Further Recommendations on the Technique of Psycho-Analysis III)*, 1915). An example in psychoanalytic treatment: when transference love* for the analyst develops in a patient (independent of the patient's gender; in this regard, I consider that all possible situations may arise), it should be discerned by the analyst as repetition compulsion* in the patient's transference* rather than an effect of the analyst's personal aptitudes or charms. It is on this base that the possibility of the patient's cure is built; that is to say, conscious knowledge of the hitherto unconscious pathogenic nucleus and the consequent possibility to work it through and bind it psychically with secondary process.

Freud states that no psychoanalyst is able to go further in the analyst than what his or her own complexes allow. He therefore also recommends analysts to deepen their own psychoanalyses, especially with respect to these points.

The subject of counter-transference was later developed by Sandor Ferenczi, and also received special emphasis in the works of Melanie Klein and her disciples, for example Wilfred Bion. In Argentina, it was developed especially by Heinrich Racker.

CRIMINALS FROM A SENSE OF GUILT

Ger.: Die Verbreche aus Schuld-bewusstsein. – Sp.: los que delinquen por sentimiento de culpa. – Fr.: les délinquants par sentiment de culpabilité. – It.: quelli che delinquono per sentimento di colpa. – Port.: os que delinquen por sentimento de culpa.

This type of character* is observed in persons whose sense of guilt* impels them to commit misdeeds, after which they find some mental relief. A person who has never experienced psychoanalysis or studied its theory may be surprised to learn that this sense of guilt antecedes and even causes the criminal action, but this is the case.

The sense of guilt proceeds from the Oedipus complex*. It is a reaction to the child's criminal wishes* to kill the father and have sexual relations with the mother during the period when phallic-urethral* erotism predominates. Since any misdemeanour is minimal compared to those desired during the Oedipus complex, committing crime is a relief. The superego* which arose in order to impede crimes, now established, paradoxically generates them.

This problem is linked to masochism* when the "misdeed" in reality is committed as a means to be punished: masochists, like naughty children, are calmed when they receive the father's "beating" (the change in the "Wolf Man's" character, 1914–18).

In all these cases, the sense of guilt is conscious whereas its cause is unconscious.

CRITICAL THOUGHT

Ger.: Kritisches Denken. – Sp.: pensamiento crítico. – Fr.: pensée critique. – It.: pensiero critico. – Port.: pensamento crítico.

This is thought* about thoughts when an error is found after any complete thought activity. It is the capacity for self-criticism of ego* activity in order to correct errors of thought.

Critical thought reaches a higher level when repressions* are lifted during the psychoanalytic process, and the patient learns the unconscious meaning of some "errors" (for example, some parapraxes*); the ego may correct them or may become aware of new meanings these errors reveal, since the patient now has adequate word-presentations* with which to do so. In this way, unconscious repetition compulsions* that have led to this error may be corrected, thereby enriching the preconscious ego's presentational resources.

CULTURE (HUMAN)

Ger.: Kultur. – Sp.: cultura (humana). – Fr.: culture (humaine). – It.: cultura (umana). – Port.: cultura (humana).

Freud defines this as every way in which human life has risen above its animal conditions, and is distinguished from animal life.

It has two aspects: on the one hand, all the knowledge and ability to do that humankind has acquired in order to dominate the forces of nature and to take from it goods to satisfy its needs; on the other hand, it encompasses all the norms necessary for the regulation of reciprocal links among human beings and, in particular, the distribution of acquirable goods.

Culture is therefore a creation of humankind; it is edified on a compulsion* and also a renouncement of Trieb*. Paradoxically, although it is a human creation, the worst enemy of culture is humankind itself.

Freud hypothesizes on the origin of culture in the development of the Oedipus complex*. It has a background: bipedestation; that is to say, the use of the vertical posture which draws the person away from olfactory stimuli, and the consequent separation from menstrual periods as a form of attraction of the sexual object*. Visual stimuli (direct vision of the genitals), and later, auditory stimuli, begin to become relevant. (Internal alteration* as an expression of emotions through screams which evolve into a call to the object, the sounds of the primal scene*, and finally, the appearance of language* which makes conscious and preconscious thought* possible through words and their meaning.)

Another step to access culture is learning to control the sphincters, from which cultural concern with cleanliness springs (*Civilization and Its Discontent*, 1930).

In *The Acquisition and Control of Fire* (1932), he proposes that culture is also structured on the Trieb renouncement of the pleasure* of extinguishing fire with a stream of urine.

The Freudian hypothesis presented in *Totem and Taboo* (1913) explains the final arrival of culture through the repression* of sexual and aggressive wishes* arising from the Oedipus complex. The sons cannot bear the omnimode chief of the primitive horde*. They band together. They rebel against him. They murder him. They eat him. The guilt-ridden fraternal alliance* establishes the prohibition of incest. The superego* is born in the psychic structure. All culture is built on these two basic prohibitions: of incest and of murder. Human beings are ready to enter culture once they have repressed their infantile sexuality*, once a superego has been installed in their psychic apparatus*.

The history of humankind since its origin is a list of struggles and killings for power. Even so, culture endures. How does culture manage to dominate Triebe*? It assigns them a representative in the psychic apparatus of each individual, which we call the superego, whose function is to suppress sexual and destructive Triebe*, even resorting to ever more destructive weapons. This superego connects destructive Trieb* and death Trieb* within it in order to defend itself from sexual Trieb. Perhaps with the objective of bringing it into line with culture?

Human groups* link together through aim-inhibited homosexual Triebe* (tenderness, friendship), which establish cultural ties. The great creations of culture also arise from inhibition* of the aim of sexual Triebe to make them socially acceptable. This product and process are what we call sublimation*. Whether or not humankind has an "original sin", culture has an "original problem". It has been built upon the suppression* of Triebe. This suppression can only generate discontent, as well as the existence of neurosis and mental illness in general, as forms of human suffering, moving away from the possibility of happiness.

Sublimation de-sexualizes Trieb. This involves the unmixing of Trieb* and therefore the liberation of death and destruction Trieb, with which culture tends radically to destruction (*The Ego and the Id*, 1923; *Civilization and Its Discontent*, 1930). It is in this dialectic contradiction that culture moves, a human creation that changes nature and provides human beings with prostheses to make them more powerful. This very power may generate their own destruction.

CURE BY LOVE

Ger.: Liebes Genesung / Heilung durch Liebe: – Sp.: cura por amor. – Fr.: cure par amour. – It.: cura per via dell'amore. – Port.: cura pelo amor.

The fantasy* of cure (the opposite of the analytic cure and often used as resistance* against the treatment) of the neurotic who "seeks a way back to narcissism from his prodigal expenditure of libido upon objects, by choosing a sexual ideal after the narcissistic type which possesses the excellences to which he cannot attain" (1914, *S.E.*, p. 101).

In these cases, what is loved is what possesses the excellence lacking the ego* in order to attain the ideal, a characteristic of the neurotic who excessively cathects object presentations to the detriment of those of the ego. Sometimes, patients come to treatment in search of this: to obtain the object's* love. If they are successful, through the transitory lifting of repression*, they think they are cured. Sometimes this aim materializes in the person of the analyst. In this case, transference love* is generated, which is one of the strongest resistances to treatment.

"The patient's incapacity for love, resulting from his extensive repressions, naturally stands in the way of a therapeutic plan of this kind" (Ibid.).

During treatment, when some repressions are lifted, these patients tend to choose an idealized love-object, and entrust their complete recovery to the satisfaction of this love.

This is not a psychoanalytic cure. If the greater part of repressions is not lifted, and all the period of infantile sexuality* and the constitution of the ego reconstructed, the objectives of psychoanalysis are not completed. They continue to be the lifting of repressions, including the primary* repressions, and the working through* of the repressed, the filling in of mnemic lacunae – produced by the repression – and the advent of the ego over the id* (the mastery* of id Trieb* by the ego, learning about it and accepting it). We could be content with the outcome of the cure by love "if it did not bring with it all the dangers of a crippling dependence upon his helper in need" (Ibid.).

The psychoanalytic cure proposes the development of secondary process* through knowledge of primary process*, and the mastery of Triebe through knowledge of them and their binding.

The possibility to experience and express love, different from this "cure by love", is sought by treatment. A true relaxation of the repression in infantile sexuality and its working through enables the ego, for example, to love the object without needing to repress unconscious incestuous wishes*. In fact, the ego is strong in part because of its capacity to love, and because it does not need so much to be loved in order to preserve its self-esteem*; it is freer of the object, although it also needs to love it and be loved, being enriched through this love.

D

DANGER-SITUATION

Ger.: gefahr Zustand. – Sp.: situación de peligro. – Fr.: situation de risque. – It.: situazione di pericolo. – Port.: situação de perigo.

Following the birth trauma and subsequent traumatic* situations, any situation similar to or reminiscent of one of them; that is to say, which suggests that it may occur again, is a danger-situation.

The danger-situation generates fear of danger (realistic anxiety*), the danger of repetition of the traumatic situation.

However, in the development of the human psychical apparatus* in which satisfaction of sexual Trieb* becomes so complex, Trieb also becoming more complex, danger-situations diversify when the ego* acquires them as danger signals in order to suppress or repress sexual Triebe that have become antisocial (incestuous, for example).

Danger-situations then become warnings that, if Trieb struggling to access the preconscious ego succeeds in doing so, what was felt during the traumatic situation will be experienced again; that is to say, a fresh invasion of quantity of excitation* into the psychical apparatus, overwhelming presentations* of the object* wish* and all possibility of binding*.

As the object is gradually recognized as the principal seat of pleasure*, danger-situations are produced around it. Therefore, when the object departs, or someone else appears in its place, or when it is dark and cannot be seen, the affect* corresponding to this danger appears: fear of object loss*. When the first levels of sexual difference are recognized and the Oedipus complex* unfolds, a new type of danger arises, generating a special type of anxiety in response to a new danger, the castration* complex.

> Let us call a situation which contains the determinants for such an expectation a danger-situation. It is in this situation that the signal of anxiety is given. The signal announces: "I am expecting a situation of helplessness to set in", or: "The present situation reminds me of one of the traumatic experiences I have had before. Therefore I will anticipate the trauma and behave as though it had already come, while there is yet time to turn it aside". Anxiety is therefore on the one hand an expectation of a trauma, and on the other a repetition of it in a mitigated form.
>
> (*Inhibitions, Symptoms and Anxiety*, 1925, p. 166)

The danger-situation is therefore the danger of repetition of the traumatic situation when the subject felt helpless*. However, it is not this situation itself but danger of it happening, a mediation that may have different levels of complexity in the psychical apparatus and may be more or less distant from the traumatic situation which is nonetheless always behind it.

DAY'S RESIDUES

Ger.: Tagesreste / Traumtag. – Sp.: restos diurnos. – Fr.: restes diurnes. – It.: resti diurni. – Port.: restos diurnos.

These preconscious presentations* of unimportant events experienced or phantasies produced, usually the day before the dream*, retain for some reason a degree of cathexis* and participate in assembling the dream's manifest content*.

They constitute the working partner in the society that manufactures the dream's manifest content: the capitalist partner is the repressed unconscious wish*. The role of the day's residue is secondary: it is a kind of "front man" for the unconscious wish, and offers to accept the cathexis of the unconscious presentation.

Freud mentions several groups of these

> thought-impulses which persist while we sleep, we may divide them into the following groups: (1) what has not been carried to a conclusion during the day owing to some chance hindrance; (2) what has not been dealt with owing to the insufficiency of our intellectual power – what is unsolved; (3) what has been rejected and suppressed during the daytime. To these we must add (4) a powerful group consisting of what has been set in action in our unconscious by the activity of the preconscious in the course of the day; and finally (5) the group of daytime impressions which are indifferent and have for that reason not been dealt with.
>
> (*The Interpretation of Dreams*, 1900, p. 554)

We may add (6): in *Notes upon a Case of Obsessional Neurosis* (1909) he adds preconscious phantasies during the day. In any case, the psychical intensities of these day's residues must not be underestimated; they are instigating causes of the dream, although in adults their manufacture cannot be done alone: only in cooperation with the unconscious wish.

When day's residues are worrying, dream work* may produce a pure wish dream in which all the worries of the day are solved, or alternatively, may be woven into the wishes of the superego*, originating dreams that produce suffering for the ego* as in "dreams* of punishment".

The dreams of traumatic neurosis* are an exception to dream theory since both their capitalist partner and their businessman seem to be the day's residue. A traumatic event in reality has overwhelmed the protective shield* against stimuli. Great quantities of excitation* entered which the apparatus was unable to bind, not even with preparedness anxiety* which is its last bastion. Through the dream, the psychical apparatus remembers the traumatic event over and over again, partly because it remained outside the pleasure principle* and tends to repeat itself compulsively; also because when preparedness anxiety is felt, the protective shield against stimuli is recovered, and consequently the situation may return to the pleasure principle (even though it may be in the form of unpleasure*, but now having possibilities of presentation and affect in order to relate it with other presentations and thereby find new levels of binding for it).

DEATH TRIEB

Ger.: Todestrieb. – Sp.: pulsión de muerte. – Fr.: pulsion de mort. – It.: istinto o pulsione di morte. – Port.: pulsão de morte.

This term denotes the tendency of multicellular beings and even all organic matter to return to the inanimate. In human beings its path is specific and complex.

Freud advances his first and greatest approaches in his hypotheses on this Trieb* in his paper, *Beyond the Pleasure Principle* (1920).

Based on his observations of phenomena of repetition compulsion* in human behaviour, and especially the repetition of events which were never pleasurable for any of the different systems of the psychical apparatus*, repetitions presenting a daemonic character, he concludes that they do not belong to the pleasure principle*. They are instead governed by what Barbara Low called the "Nirvana principle"*: the tendency to return to the absolute repose characteristic of inorganic matter.

In this paper, Freud states: "'the aim of all life is death' and retrospectively: 'inanimate things existed before living ones'" (p. 38).

> The attributes of life were at some time evoked in inanimate matter by the action of a force of whose nature we can form no conception. It may perhaps have been a process similar in type to that which later caused the development of consciousness in a particular stratum of living matter. The tension which then arose in what had hitherto been an inanimate substance endeavoured to cancel itself out. In this way the first instinct came into being: the instinct to return to the inanimate state.
>
> (Ibid.)

Death Trieb would then result from a tension of living substance, especially in the most complex beings such as the multicellular, which leads to the absolute end of this tension, which we call death. Phenomena of life arise on this path to which all Triebe, all of them preservative, also seek to return in order to reduce tension generated by the appearance in the psychical apparatus of life Trieb which now also seeks to return, but to these phenomena previous to life: this type of return is therefore different from the former one; it is even opposed to it, since this is a return to a moment previous to life, to some previous experience of satisfaction* or pleasure*, not to death.

The existence of life therefore results from growing complexity of the path of living matter towards the inorganic, from the search which endeavours to prolong this path.

This tendency to return to the inorganic must not succeed if phenomena of life are to exist. It must be deflected towards the outside, mainly through the muscular system, and be transformed into destructive* or aggressive* Trieb, sadism*, or Trieb for mastery*; depending on the different forms and degrees of fusion* with Eros* or life Trieb.

Death Trieb is only seen by means of these fusions with Eros, since in itself it is "mute" (has no unconscious presentation, since death was never experienced and therefore there is no memory trace* of it), not joined to thing-presentations* (these are what remains of the subject's own experiences in the psychical apparatus), and instead seeks to unbind libido* from them.

Presentations give life Trieb presentational quality* (through the memory of the perceptual quality experienced at the moment of the experience). It is in this growing complexity that the world of the psychical is born. Death Trieb seeks to break this connection, thereby returning to pure quantity of excitation*, which is closest to the inorganic.

One part of death Trieb cannot be deflected; it remains as such within the psychical apparatus, while also fusing with Eros and generating primary or erotogenic masochism*: the pleasure of receiving pain*.

Another part, as mentioned, is expelled through aggression, but also returns to the psychical apparatus, bound by the superego* and generating either the sense of guilt* or moral masochism. The superego takes in presentations corresponding to masochistic phantasies of Eros*. The second takes those of sadism, aggression, or mastery, also belonging to fusion with Eros. In the third, aggression is reintrojected through secondary identification*, origin of the superego, and from there, also desexualized*, turns against the ego*, which the superego utilizes to enforce its "categorical imperative". This produces the paradox that the more heavily suppressed* Triebe have been, the more intense the sense of guilt (conscious or unconscious) will be.

In feminine masochism, fusion of reintrojected aggression with Eros is more sexualized, which generates masochistic sexual pleasure, although some superego binding is involved, contributing the quantity of sense of guilt that is satisfied by masochistic sexual pleasure.

Death Trieb together with Eros (life Trieb including sexual, object, narcissistic, and self-preservative Triebe*) is referred to as the "second Trieb theory"; although in reality it is the culmination of a complex trajectory involving all the previous advances in its progress, which it neither opposes nor surpasses but rather makes more complex, thereby accounting for phenomena not previously observed which, without it, would be left unexplained or only very incompletely explained.

DEBASEMENT OF THE EROTIC (OR SEXUAL) OBJECT

Ger.: Erniedrigung des Sexual Objekt. – Sp.: degradación del objeto erótico (o sexual). – Fr.: dégradation de l'objet érotique. – It.: degradazione del oggetto erotico. – Port.: degradação do objeto erótico.

This process is produced by the separation of tender from sensual currents in the course of an individual's libidinal development.

The sensual current, totally repressed during the period of the Oedipus complex*, reappears in puberty, displaced on to other objects*. Since they retain their unconscious* fixation* to incestuous objects, the ego* defends itself from them by restricting object choice*.

The sensual current seeks only objects that do not recall the prohibited incestuous figures, idealized and therefore overvalued. This leads to psychical debasement of the sexual object when an object opposite to the "pure mother" or "nourishing mother" is sought sexually. As soon as the condition of debasement is fulfilled, sensuality can be freely expressed, and important sexual capacities and a high degree of pleasure can develop (*On the Universal Tendency to Debasement in the Sphere of Love*, 1912, p. 183).

Perverse sexual aims may even be sought whose absence is felt as a loss of pleasure* and whose attainment is only possible with the debased, depreciated sexual object.

Sometimes the splitting of love life is so great that if these individuals establish a tender relationship, they are sexually impotent, sexual potency returning only when the tender link is impossible.

This type of disorder is more common in men than in women and is also more common than it seems. Freud proposes: "I shall put forward the view that psychical impotence is much more widespread than is supposed, and that a certain amount of this behavior does in fact characterize the love of civilized man" (Ibid., p. 184).

In women we observe little need to debase the sexual object. Women are more attracted to what is secret or prohibited. This condition of the forbidden in female love life is comparable to debasement of the sexual object in men.

An individual that has successfully overcome the Oedipus complex with few or relatively weak or transitory incestuous fixations is more likely to feel tenderness and sensuality for the same person, thereby evading the debasement that perhaps remains in some other part of the psyche but may return at moments of frustration* or quantitative increase of libido and Trieb (in adolescence and menopause).

DECATHEXIS (WITHDRAWAL OF THE CATHEXIS)

Ger.: Entziehung der Besetzung. – Sp.: desinvestidura (sustracción de la investidura). – Fr.: désinvestissement. – It.: disinvestimento (sottrazione dell'investimento. – Port.: desinvestimento.

This is the mode of functioning of all defence mechanisms* by which psychical energy* (libido*) is withdrawn: from preconscious word-presentations* in neuroses*; from unconscious thing-presentations* in narcissistic psychoses*; from the conscious perception system (Pcpt.-Cs.) in acute hallucinatory psychoses, hysterical psychoses, and, in part, fetishism* and other sexual perversions*; or from the entire psychical apparatus* in the case of dreams*. Cathexis corresponds to the second step of secondary repression or more precisely, the complement of primary repression whose only mechanism is anticathexis*. The latter acts again in secondary repression by reinforcing and sustaining decathexis, aided by the attraction exerted by the primarily repressed.

When bodily energy cathects a thing-presentation*, it becomes psychical. Then it is called either Trieb* or wish*, depending on the placement of emphasis: whether on the quantitative force that pushes (*Drang*) or on the presentation. If the energy is sexual (a characteristic ultimately acquired from the presentation) it is called libido, the major representative of life Triebe*.

When in addition to cathexis of the thing-presentation the word-presentation is also cathected, conditions are created for mastery* of Trieb.

If the word-presentation is decathected, the wish is repressed, and unconscious cathexis remains in the thing-presentation in a state of repression (repressed unconscious wish).

In narcissistic psychoses, cathexis is withdrawn from unconscious thing-presentation, which leaves the psychical apparatus without unconscious wishes, without life Trieb (or very little, the ego being almost obligatorily libidinized instead of seeking objects), and with a quantity of pure excitation* unbound to any presentation (automatic anxiety experienced as the end of the world); this is a liberation of death Trieb*, a tendency to return to the inorganic, to pure quantity. However, word-presentations remain cathected and serve as a very weak bridge to restitution* of the object world, now a delusional world, but at least a world.

DEFENCE

Ger.: Abwehr. – Sp.: defensa. – Fr.: défense. – It.: difesa. – Port.: defesa.

All beings are exposed to continuous stimuli which, in the case of complex organisms, originate both in the external world and in their own internal physical world (Triebe*). Human beings possess a psychical apparatus* that defends them from continuous stimuli to which they are subjected and which generate in them an impulse to return to the state previous to arrival of the stimulus. Defence, in this sense, is something akin to the reason for the existence of the psyche. The psyche wishes above all else to defend itself from stimuli. The best way to do this is by performing specific actions* to end them: if they are exterior, by escaping from or destroying them; if they are internal stimuli (that is to say, Triebe), by satisfying them. To do this, its functioning must include the reality principle* and the establishment of an ego* which thinks and also directs appropriate action. However, during human development, serious problems arise satisfaction of these Triebe (sexual* and destructive*) meets with serious problems, since they clash first with cultural ideals and then with those in the subject's own psychical apparatus (ego ideal* and superego*). For this reason, other types of defence develop whose aim is to block satisfaction of Trieb or to ignore it. The unconscious mechanisms in charge of preventing the preconscious ego from discovering the existence in itself of Triebe incompatible with it are called ego defence mechanisms* inherent to the unconscious ego. The latter defends the preconscious ego, without its knowledge, from harassment of Triebe. Nonetheless, this defence has a price: character traits* and – when these fail – neurosis* (in the broad sense, including the concept of psychosis*).

Some types of defence mechanism permit certain forms of Trieb pleasure*, for example, defence mechanisms pertaining to the perversions*. This type of affection is able to satisfy sexual, part, infantile, homosexual, and narcissistic Triebe. It does so by having sexual relations beyond those accepted by society (these individuals consequently suffer social anxiety* from which they also defend themselves). The pleasurable act includes certain ego defence mechanisms against dangers deriving from the Oedipus complex*; they try to spare themselves castration anxiety* by disavowing* sexual difference. Disavowal therefore proves the absence of castration with each sexual act (fetishist, homosexual, exhibitionist, and so on). It is not totally successful, and therefore the ego splits (cf.: splitting of the ego*); it partly accepts castration and partly does not, thereby losing its synthetic function and becoming two egos, two opposite thoughts thereby able to coexist in unison in secondary process.

Therefore, the most adequate means of defence against Trieb stimulus is necessarily the synthesis the ego must attain in the face of pressures from the id*, the superego, and reality*, and action consistent with this synthesis (cf.: specific action*).

Regarding stimuli from the external world, the organism establishes a barrier of protection against stimuli* in the conscious perception system (Pcpt.-Cs.) and its cathexis* of attention* which is in reality (as an anxiety signal*) the last level of this barrier. If this point is passed, organic pain* is felt, which may lead to establishment of a traumatic neurosis* if the quantity of stimulus penetrating the psychical apparatus exceeds its possibilities of binding*. In traumatic neuroses, a compulsion* to repeat the scene remains, first in dreams*, and may even come to action, in an effort to induce the psychical apparatus, through repetition, to feel the anxiety signal it did not feel when the last barrier was breached. It may also do the same merely to repeat, in a demonic (death Trieb*) manner.

DEFENCE MECHANISMS

Ger.: Abwehr mechanismus. – Sp.: mecanismos de defensa. – Fr.: mécanismes de défense. – It.: difesa, meccanismi di. – Port.: defesa, mecanismos de.

These automatic operations by the unconscious part of the ego* defend it from Triebe*, or rather, from potential dangers that could derive from their satisfaction.

When the presentation* of an incestuous or parricidal Trieb or their derivative appears, the unconscious ego resorts to a signal, a small sample of anxiety. This anxiety signal* changes the course of the associative path between presentations, guided by the pleasure principle*, and the path leading to what the anxiety signal warns against is abandoned. The original Trieb or its derivatives are thus sent back to the unconscious id* where they enter the state of repression*. In this way, the ego defence* is momentarily effective in freeing the ego of Trieb.

If the Trieb is to remain in that state, unable to re-enter the ego and hence go into action, a permanent anticathexis* must be left in place as a sentinel.

The defence mechanism *par excellence* is repression. At some points in the theory, repression is synonymous with defence, but since *Inhibitions, Symptoms and Anxiety* (1925) it becomes the specific mechanism of conversion hysteria*.

Repression, whose essence is ignorance, consists of two steps. Primary repression is simply anticathexis, the origin of the other ulterior or secondary defence mechanisms*. In the latter, cathexis is also removed from the preconscious word, which consequently cannot be verbalized by the ego but returns to the unconscious id*. This withdrawn cathexis is placed into another word or substitute formation*, a compromise between the ego and Trieb which acts as an anticathexis. The anticathexis is also established in the perceptual apparatus (Pcpt.-Cs.) to avoid perceiving anything in reality* referring to the conflict, or may be displaced onto other unimportant presentations which may become obsessional, for example.

The primarily repressed also attracts to the unconscious anything that may refer to this conflict.

Other defence mechanisms classically described are undoing (what has been done)*, isolation*, reaction formation*, identification* (hysterical and melancholic)*, disavowal* of sexual difference and of object loss, denial*, splitting of the ego*, and others. The factor common to all is that they make the Trieb impulse unconscious in order to avoid the anxiety signal the ego would otherwise experience. If the defence mechanism fails, the quantity of excitation* may destroy ego presentations and lead to automatic anxiety which lacks presentation, a situation similar to the birth trauma*.

The latter is one of the reasons for which, though defence mechanisms produce pathological alterations, they are sometimes a necessary evil to avoid a greater evil (automatic anxiety). We must also recall that the ego forms an unconscious infrastructure from unconscious defence mechanisms upon which the preconscious structure is established, which may then function without harassment from Trieb about which it knows nothing.

When the ego leans too heavily on its defence mechanisms to the extent that they govern its secondary process*, a more or less severe alteration of the ego* may ensue which forms a strong obstacle to the cure and participates in the formation of character disorders; the type of disorder often depends on the most frequently used defence mechanism, which is in turn related to fixation* points.

In Freud's *Project for a Scientific Psychology* (1950), he describes the formation of the ego through side-cathexes, chains of thoughts* that help it to grow and learn from experience as it accumulates presentations with increasingly complex interrelations in order to compare them to new perceptions which then become new presentations, and so on.

When quantities of excitation surpass a certain limit, the side-cathexis is insufficient to conduct them; it must then resort to primary defence which consists of anticathexis that now prevents the entry of Trieb cathexis into new presentations. These are rejected by the ego and accumulate, repressed, in the unconscious.

The side-cathexis enriches the ego (the ego of thought) and moderates Trieb, appropriating it. However, the anticathexis expels Trieb stimulus (its presentations and presentational derivatives) to the unconscious; therefore, it impoverishes the ego or gives it unconscious characteristics (primary process*, pleasure principle*). In this way, both factors gradually shape different parts within the ego, dynamically and not without a struggle: (a) secondary process, thought, the ego with its synthetic function and its reality principle*; (b) a part remaining unconscious functions automatically beyond the preconscious ego's will*; this is the ego of defence or ego defence mechanisms, the unconscious ego.

In the psychoanalytic cure, defence mechanisms become manifest when they express ego resistance. We must then deal with them in order to gain knowledge of repressed wishes*; the ego thereby benefits from this knowledge and the possibility that the previously repressed wish might lead to action (or not) when it is given side-cathexes. In this way, it participates in the associative commerce that integrates the ego of thought or secondary process with the preconscious ego.

DEFERRED REACTION TO EXPERIENCE

Ger.: Nachträglich. – Sp.: a posteriori. – Fr.: après-coup. – It.: posteriore, posteriormente. – Port.: a posteriori.

Freud gives this term, translated by James Strachey from the German *Nachträglich*, to a particular characteristic of sexual Trieb*: a quantity of excitation, usually traumatic, is carried through time (a quantity of excitation* occurring at the wrong time or rather before its time and therefore corresponding to a different predominant erotogenic zone whose history has a different complexity and category: at the moment of its perception no psychical binding was possible, especially with words) by virtue of which this sensation (or an anticathexis* defence* against it) becomes actual. This concept reflects the necessary condition of previous cathexis* of all the subject's organs of perception, including the subject's erotogenic zones*, in order to grasp sensations produced by stimuli (objects), relate them subsequently to presentations* of similar, previous situations, and find some degree of identity – at least concerning the sensation – with which to form thought* bindings by which to understand personal experiences*. When for different causes, and in the absence of previous cathexis, trauma* was produced at some time during infantile sexuality*, this trauma becomes actual in a deferred manner. Because of the necessary condition of perceptual cathexis previous to the stimulus, stimulation of an erotogenic zone becomes traumatic when for some reason it was not previously cathected. For example, in the case of genital stimulation of a boy in whom anal erotism* or oral erotism* still predominates, the child has insufficient phallic cathexes at the moment of the traumatic event (although it leaves a fixation* point due to defensive anticathexis) which becomes traumatic only when the subject enters the corresponding erotogenic phase or its re-edition in puberty. Only at this time is he able to cathect the organ with presentations bound to experiences produced through it. These experiences then return from the repressed* and become traumatic at a deferred time, possibly generating neurotic symptoms*.

Freud elaborated this concept in his *Project for a Scientific Psychology* (1950 [1887–1902]) and returned to it with most genial brilliance in the case history of the "Wolf Man", revitalizing and adding complexity to his theory of sexual trauma*.

The concept of deferred reaction also involves thought that takes place following experience: the traces it has left are necessary for the formation of presentations of these traces and for thinking about them in a deferred and progressively more complete manner in relation to new experiences and changes in the individual. The "deferred" refers to the content of experience and its presentation, including its interpretation or historical truth*. For this reason, history is central in Freudian thought. Thought is deferred in relation to facts and therefore also to their interpretation, even when their theme is the future, since each experience is thought about in terms of the individual's previous experience through the secondary process* of the preconscious, including distortions introduced by repression* (distortions that psychoanalysis aims to repair). But this is not all, nor does it mean that Freud does not contemplate unconscious materials deferred in relation to experience which are "preparations for understanding"* or categories inherited from the experience of our species which Freud calls phylogenetic phantasies*.

Freud takes up this Kantian concept indirectly (not mentioning the concept itself, but utilizing concepts derived from it) and develops it in a different way, giving it new specificity. Although he does not utilize it with a specific term as a concept in his works, he agrees with the philosopher from Königsberg when he considers that the deferred carries a "form" of thought that will serve its "content"; this content is what subsequently fills the presentation* formed by individual experience. In this sense Kant speaks of the notions of time and space as *a prioris* of experience: categories or forms with which to think about its contents. Thus, in his theoretical scheme, Freud considers primary process* thought inherent to the unconscious* and calls it primal phantasies* or *a prioris*. These *a prioris* are deferred in relation to the individual's experience, belonging to experience of the species; they are therefore universal, markedly analogous to "the instinctive knowledge of animals" (*From the History of an Infantile Neurosis*, 1918, p. 120). This means that Freudian *a prioris* are *a prioris* in relation to the subject's experience but are also deferred in relation to experiences of the human species. This conceptualization exemplifies the dynamic character of Freudian thought in which history becomes psyche and conditions biology (in *Moses and Monotheism: Three Essays*, he even considers that mankind likely descends from a primate that concluded its sexual development at the age of five and that, as a product of the history of oedipal repression, a period of latency* was introduced into human sexual development), and elsewhere, that biology may determine history (*Some Psychical Consequences of the Anatomical Distinction between the Sexes*, 1925). Thus, primal phantasies act in unconscious thought as "preparations for understanding" experience by referring it to them. An example is the "Wolf Man" who explains that he somehow understood the primal scene* between his parents since it was not indifferent to him considering that he had a diarrhoeal bowel movement that could very well have been a "preparation to understand" it *a priori*; when he entered the phallic stage, the corresponding erotogenic zones were already cathected and had some experience concerning links with objects, along with their history of pleasures and problems. In psychoanalytic treatment, a new level of understanding* is reached, more connected with words and thought when repression, engaged in anticathecting the contents of this experience, is lifted. Despite infantile *a prioris* and the deferred, this experience becomes traumatic, and only then is the adolescent or adult enabled to work it through with words and their logical relations.

DEFINITIVE REALITY EGO

Ger.: bestimmt Real-Ich. – Sp.: yo realidad definitivo. – Fr.: moi-réalité définitif. – It.: io realtà definitivo. – Port.: ego de realidade definitive.

This type of ego functioning predominates in adults, and also in children following the end of the period of the Oedipus complex*, having established a superego* that watches the ego* to ensure it is attentive to the danger of return of Triebe from the id*.

Since the ego is protected from Trieb danger, it may function more easily with the reality principle*: Trieb is no longer constantly and heavily pressuring it, producing anxiety.

Therefore, secondary process* is established definitively (or rather at last, since primary process* may return at any moment), with its notion that a thing is one thing and not another thing: negation*, notions of space and time, the search for synthesis in thought* activity; everything that predominates in the diverse activities that will be its products.

Thought is produced mainly through words, utilized to seek thought identity* with what is wished for in perceptions*. The wish is to "refind" the object*, "to convince oneself that it is still there" (*Negation*, 1925, pp. 237–8).

Thought functions by studying differences and similarities between the percept and what is wished for. It tries to find similarities; however, it is not enslaved by the wish* to find them but is ruled by reality* which in this case is synonymous with truth*.

The definitive reality ego concludes its formation in the phallic phase when all the erotogenic zones* are bodily united under phallic supremacy, definitively giving all of this unified body the name of ego.

All this coincides with recognition, also definitive, of the object as the most important source of pleasure*. When the object is recognized in this way, love* for the ego or narcissism* is also recognized.

The definitive reality ego slowly grows, buttressed by the initial reality ego* and the purified pleasure ego*; it is a synthesis of the two. Once it develops, it continues to add members to its flock, and therefore the preconscious ego also grows, together with thought and abilities to tame Trieb and lead it to a good end, whether to Trieb specific action* or to its cultural derivatives such as sublimation*.

The concept of health is also associated with predominance in the psychical apparatus* of the functioning of this ego modality.

DELUSION

Ger.: Wahnsinn. – Sp.: delirio. – Fr.: délire. – It.: delirio. – Port.: delírio.

Phenomenologically and in general, these disorders of thought* content remove subjects from reality* or from their integrated interpretation of it by creating a new, imaginary reality* of their own. This occurs when the ego* is severely alienated or has suffered a very deep alteration of the ego (cf. alteration of the ego*). Freud extends this term to some obsessional ideas or actions – some ceremonials*, doubting mania – even products of omnipotent thought* (the obsessional neurotic's magic* and superstition), perhaps to underscore how far from reality obsessional neurotics* are drawn by their symptoms*; in some, their ego's character* is affected, but only in those in whom alteration of the ego is less significant. Various types of delusion are observed in different types of affections. Freud describes a hysterical delusion in Norbert Hanold, the character in Jensen's *Gradiva* (*Delusions and Dreams in Jensen's Gradiva*, 1907). In Hanold's delusions – gratifications of daytime wishes in the manner of dreams* and more credible than fantasies* or daydreams – his infantile memories* are reactivated by and intermingle with the present through sublimations*: he believes he sees a character connected to his studies of archaeology in the figure of a young woman with whom he had had an affectionate relationship in his childhood, reactivated in the present. Repression* appears in the masking of the loved character (which refers to his infantile sexuality*) through a hallucination* which he believes* and which transports him, in his amorous rapture, back to a historical period corresponding to his archaeological studies; this movement is assisted by the surroundings he is visiting: the ruins of Pompeii.

Freud also describes a different type of delusion: acute hallucinatory confusion or Meynert's amentia*. In it, the loss in reality of a loved object* is so unbearable for the subject's ego that it is disavowed: these persons believe they see the object or feel it will return, or that it is in a nearby room and so on. In this case, the perception-consciousness system (Pcpt.-Cs.) is decathected. When perception* of reality is thereby blocked in relation to loss, it may be filled in by topical regression through reactivation of perception of the wished-for object in its crude state, as in a dream. Therefore, the hallucination is perceived. If it is believed, the delusion of the existence of the lost object is elaborated. The ego avoids reality testing* and sometimes even uses elements of reality to prove the existence of what is wished for, a wish that is conscious and not repressed, unlike hysterical psychosis which is quite similar but involves repressed wishes. In amentia, alteration of the ego seems to be deeper than in hysterical psychosis; in both, the wish for the object persists, unlike narcissistic psychoses. This may help, or may be the reason these acute clinical pictures remit *ad integrum*, a prognosis different from that of schizophrenia, for example. They may, however, lead to other, more persistent disorders that alter the ego more severely. We turn now to the main types of chronic delusion: paranoiac delusion which is the classical delusion and the delusion corresponding to paranoid schizophrenia*.

There are also different types of these which usually develop in the following way: first the unconscious cathexis* is withdrawn from the thing- or object presentation* and therefore from the object itself; when libido is withdrawn (cf. libidinal withdrawal*), object libido becomes narcissistic libido: from the unconscious*, the wish* for the object world disappears. This is the end of the world experience, an expression of automatic anxiety produced in this case by presentational decathectization when it becomes mainly energetic, free of presentations, and floods the psychical apparatus as the affect of anxiety.

As we said, the other part of object libido becomes narcissistic when it is withdrawn from the ego, and is expressed clinically as a delusion of grandeur. When it is withdrawn into the body, it is called hypochondria*.

Of the cathexes remaining in the psychical apparatus, those that cathect word-presentations* (preconscious) attempt to reconstruct the object world. These words no longer mean thing-presentations*, since the latter are decathected as if they did not exist. Therefore, they take the place of thing-presentations on the psychical path; they are treated like things rather than words representing things. This means that they may function in primary process* by utilizing associations* by contiguity*, analogy*, or opposition*, and even universal symbols* with which to form condensations* and displacements* which with good secondary elaboration* may take on a certain logical appearance.

Delusions are formed in this way, with specific differences in regard to their different clinical forms. Paranoid delusion is composed of homosexual libido, does not recognize sexual difference, and rides astride both narcissistic and object libido. This libido loses its possibility of sublimation* (socialization), and aim inhibition since it is eroticized homosexual libido. This is a new, unbearable problem for the ego from which it defends itself, since it is unable to sublimate eroticized libido. Then, it relieves love* by transforming it into the opposite: hate* – in the persecutory delusion that is, however, at the base of the others: the erotomaniac, jealous*, and grandiose delusions – and projects the unconscious wish. The paranoiac now feels that what was his own unknown homosexual wish comes from the object's unconscious and is aimed at him though relieved by hate.

All the types of delusion mentioned above contradict the statement: "I love him" in the case of men, of course. It is a very painful "reconstruction of the world" indeed, until the delusion is able, through primary process, to fashion a disguise acceptable enough to the ego to enable the ego to tolerate the homosexual wish. In Schreber's delusion, he comes to the conclusion that he has been chosen by God to give him children. This conclusion is ultimately justified by the delusion (whose richness and complexity reflect his previous intellectual wealth and intelligence), and permits some satisfaction of homosexual Trieb. Thus, a weak but relatively lasting peace is found, and in some cases the ego, through its unaltered parts, is able to re-accommodate itself to some extent with reality.

Other types of delusions are also typical of paranoia* and paranoid schizophrenia, such as the delusion of being watched, accompanied by auditory hallucinations that signal all the subject's acts (thought given sound), or feelings of being looked at which may sometimes be connected to persecution or to erotomania. The self-observing auditory hallucination is produced by regression* to perception*. The parents' observation of the subject in infancy, which later became superego* by identification*, returns now by regression to perception, thus revealing its origin.

In the delusion of influence, regression is even more severe. The entire ego is projected outwards. These patients feel that machines (universal symbols of the body, the ego's place of origin) are influencing their actions and determining their thoughts. These machines are driven in turn by persons, and the relation to persecution gradually becomes clear.

Delusions in paranoid schizophrenia and paranoia show the noisy part of the illness; however, it is in reality the patient's attempted cure (in the sense of reattempting the relation with the object that was lost during the "end of the world" experience). This achievement is more or less peaceful depending partly on the manner in which the previous father complex* was carried through.

Delusions fashioned from words and utilizing primary process are based on historical truth* at the bottom of all delusion which makes it accessible to some construction* or interpretation* in the manner of a dream* or a neurotic symptom*. This does not mean that it is the road to the cure, at least not as in neurotic cases; Freud practises it mainly in his study of Schreber's autobiography. He also attempts it with some patients at the beginning of his career, as for example in *Further Remarks on the Neuro-Psychoses of Defence* (1896). At the acute moment of the illness, this is impossible given the magnitude of automatic anxiety; also because the only possible transference is negative or predominantly negative due to the difficulty of desexualization (sublimation) of homosexual libido. We recall that the possibility of treatment (as in all social links) is based on sublimated homosexual libido.

Perhaps erotomaniac delusions or delusions of jealousy are better examples for reconstructing the past: the delusion itself contains themes involving a predominance of love over hate; thus, the therapeutic relation might be more manageable.

In the case of the "Rat Man", Freud also mentions "a sort of delusion or delusional formation"; in it, the patient as a child felt that his parents knew his thoughts because he had declared them without hearing them himself. "I declare my thoughts without hearing them". Freud explains this phenomenon as a projection of the fact that the patient has thoughts unknown to himself, an endopsychical perception of the repressed.

Freud also gives the term "delusion" to a certain type of obsessional formation, such as the series of thoughts that occupied the patient on his journey when he returned from military manoeuvres; or the absurd action (in the manner of a ceremonial) in which, working until very late at night, he opened the doors to his father's "spectre", then looked at his own genitals in the mirror and tried to correct himself with the admonition: "What would father say if he were really still alive?" This phantasmagoria ceased after he had put it in the form of a "delusional threat": if he repeated this foolishness, something bad would happen to his father in the after-life. This type of "obsessional delusion" is inscribed as forming part of "omnipotence of thought" with its accompanying magic and superstition typical of obsessional neurosis.

DEPRESSION

Ger.: Depression. – Sp.: depresión. – Fr.: dépression – It.: depressione. – Port.: depressão.

A painful, unpleasurable affective state in the order of sadness, provoked sometimes by object loss*, frustration*, failure, or other factors. In all these circumstances, the preconscious ego* is doing the work of mourning* during which anything that in any way recalls the lost object reactivates longing* for it. This increases cathexes of longing (cathexes of the wish for the presentation of the lost object due to which its definitive loss has already been recognized), while reality also shows that satisfaction is impossible, producing psychical pain*. This pain is repeated in every situation that recalls the lost object, each place the subject shared with the object, each moment similar to moments experienced with the object. The mood is sadness, and the ego is enveloped in the task of decathecting* memories* of the lost object or illusion, one by one. Throughout the period in which the ego is occupied with this painful work, it introverts* the libido*, separating it from preconscious wishes* and from any object other than the one that was lost. The ego may in this way gradually accept reality, which it will do eventually, when the libido cathects another object and a new wish appears.

This describes normal depression as a response to external loss, which justifies it, so to speak.

It is quite different when no causes in real life account for the depression, or when these causes do not explain its magnitude or duration. Then the loss is said to be unconscious*. Making it unconscious consists in identification* with the object in the ego. It is in reality hate* (we recall that hate is initially confused with love*) for the object, unknown to the ego since it appears clinically as self-reproaches*. However, in psychoanalytic treatment self-reproaches are revealed as reproaches to the object that is now inside the ego. The superego* is quick to take advantage of this turn of events, adding to these reproaches and applying severe punishments to the ego for "everything it deserves" for not being like the ideal. More libido is withdrawn*, and the subject breaks off from the world of objects; all of which began with unacceptable hate towards the object displaced onto the ego that identified with it. This description corresponds to the clinical picture of melancholia*.

Between mourning and melancholia, we find neurotic depressive pictures with their feelings of inferiority, the sense of guilt* inherent to the formation of their psychical apparatus*, in which the ego can hardly satisfy a superego that demands it be the ideal. Therefore, guilt feelings are nearly constant and therefore the depressive state is basic.

The depressive state deepens with each new failure before the ideal, just as it improves when successes bring it near to the demands of the superego. Everything that decreases self-esteem* leads the ego in the direction of depression.

Unlike mourning, when psychical pain is produced by the impossibility of discharge of object libido, the other types of depression result from a vicissitude of narcissistic libido.

In melancholia it leads to narcissistic psychosis*, and in other depressions to disorders of narcissism* or of self-esteem produced essentially because the ego does not satisfy the superego. These disorders are not severe enough to separate the subject from reality or to withdraw libido from unconscious presentations of objects and wishes for them. However, this does occur in melancholia.

DESEXUALIZATION

Ger.: Desexualisierung. – Sp.: desexualización. – Fr.: désexualisation. – It.: disessualizzazione. – Port.: desexualização.

Desexualization is inhibition* of the aim of sexual Trieb*. Desexualized libido* unites the cultural group*, and forms the base of culture* itself which it inaugurates. It is what is left of the child's link with parents and siblings following repression* and dissolution* of the Oedipus complex*. It is homosexual libido, since its inhibited sexual aim does not recognize sexual difference. Desexualized libido forms links of tenderness and friendship: sublimation*. Since complete discharge is inhibited, it preserves the most lasting links.

Normally, the ego* functions with desexualized libido. This libido has lost some of its peremptory character (*Drang*) when its aim presentation was displaced* (sublimated) from its original objective; by virtue of this operation it is more manageable for the ego; it is thinkable and may enter associative commerce without the urgencies of action or anxiety. When ego libido is resexualized, narcissistic perversions* such as homosexuality* result; alternatively, different types of defence against it may be generated, as in paranoia.

In narcissistic pathologies, libido is sexualized or homosexual. The latter may be repressed and lead to neurosis* ("Dora", 1905; the "Wolf Man", 1918).

The neuroses are, among other things, disorders resulting from desexualization of object libido, which forces their repression. Conversely, it is because of this repression that object libido is not desexualized but "grows in the shadows" in the unconscious.

Since all sublimation assumes desexualization, it involves defusion of life Triebe* from death Triebe*; consequently, although desexualization is necessary for access to culture, it paradoxically liberates death Trieb. Desexualized links, based on inhibition of the sexual aim, may be resexualized as a result of different causal factors, and may also become loving. In the latter case, they again become asocial, since the couple in love seeks exclusivity, is jealous of the loved one, and does not wish to share its love*.

DESPERATION

Ger.: Versweiflung. – Sp.: desesperación. – Fr.: désespoir. – It.: disperazione. – Port.: desespero.
The cathexis of longing* to which fear of object loss* refers or vice versa; the affect* corresponding to mourning* for object loss and also anxiety for the possibility of losing it. Freud considers that this affect is probably felt by infants (*Inhibitions, Symptoms and Anxiety*, 1925) when they begin to notice their mother's absence and to distinguish her as an object before they have differentiated whether her absence is transitory or definitive. If it is transitory, the danger is that she may not return when they feel the tension of necessity (anxiety). If it is definitive, it produces mourning and longing*. Experience gradually separates pain* from anxiety*, although in certain circumstances (for example, when the body of a person who has disappeared cannot be found, and reality is unable to prove the person's definitive absence) they come together and desperation returns when mourning and its longing are joined to fear of object loss.

DESTRUCTIVE TRIEB

Ger.: Destruktionstrieb. – Sp.: pulsión de destrucción. – Fr.: pulsion de destruction. – It.: istinto o pulsione di distruzione. – Port.: pulsão de destruição.
This Trieb results from deflection of death Trieb* onto the external world.

It is fused with Eros* by virtue of action of the muscular system, which produces aggression*, sadism, and Trieb for mastery*, which are complementary and participate in fusion with other, different qualities and proportions of sexual Trieb*. In reality, aggression itself is never pure but may always be seen as an expression of fusion (however small it may be) with Eros.

Death Trieb is mute; that is to say, it has no unconscious presentation* of its own; however, it is no longer mute when it is transformed into destructive Trieb; at that time it is fused with life Triebe (sexual, narcissistic, or object Triebe, and self-preservative Triebe).

Death Trieb seeks to return to the subject's inorganic state; it is a tendency, a *Drang*. Destructive Trieb is fusion of the former with life Triebe which attempts to place the tendency to return to the inorganic in the object* (ambivalence*) or the rival that appears on the phallic-oedipal level; on the previous (pre-oedipal) levels, love* and hate* are mixed in different proportions.

The endeavour to destroy may extend to the entire external world, even the inanimate. Destructive or aggressive Trieb is reintrojected into the psychical apparatus by virtue of secondary identification*, the origin of the superego*, by which incestuous sexual and aggressive parricidal wishes are dissolved or repressed. Here, aggression returns to its starting point, turning round against the ego*, and is not mute, having the words of the superego* (cf. guilt*, masochism*). However, it is no longer death Trieb, or at least only death Trieb, but its deflection (destructive or aggressive Trieb) which re-enters the psychical apparatus as a way to ensure culture* that the ego is taming Trieb. Therefore, it is also a product of fusion with Eros; although sometimes, as in melancholia*, it may fuse with death Trieb remaining as a residue of deflection with the psychical apparatus (but also fused with life Trieb as primary erotogenic masochism*), break its chains, and become a "pure culture of death Trieb".

> Every renunciation of instinct now becomes a dynamic source of conscience and every fresh renunciation increases the latter's severity and intolerance … conscience is the result of instinctual renunciation, or that instinctual renunciation (imposed on us from without) creates conscience, which then demands further instinctual renunciation.
>
> (*Civilization and Its Discontents*, 1930, pp. 128–9)

In this text, Freud presents a very interesting description of the vicissitudes of life and death Triebe in the psychical apparatus in response to culture: "When an instinctual trend undergoes repression, its libidinal elements are turned into symptoms, and its aggressive components into a sense of guilt" (Ibid., p. 139).

DETERMINISM

Ger.: Determinismus. – Sp.: determinismo. – Fr.: déterminisme. – Ital.: determinismo. – Port.: determinismo.

Freud in general adhered to nineteenth-century scientific determinism, though with some exceptions.

In the debate between determinism and free will, he maintains a deterministic position to explain facts, although psychoanalytic treatment aims to disengage individuals from fixations formed in the course of their history, which gives them greater freedom and a freer will.

In the debate between determinism and chance, he does not discard chance (traumatic facts occur to individuals by chance but determine them henceforth). Freud considers that chance* still exists in reality* beyond previous intrapsychical determinism. In regard to complexity, we could say that psychoanalysis itself was born as a complex theory, that it enters other fields of knowledge and makes them more complex; it also utilizes them in order to make itself more complex. In this sense it breaks through limits imposed on scientific disciplines by modernity. Its theory of the unconscious also makes culture more complex and problematic (apart from criticizing it profoundly); it does the same for the human beings in this culture, especially modern culture. Therefore, it is both a product of this modernity and also its critic.

We should therefore say that Freud's determinism is relative. What is its essence? One type of determinism is produced by the inheritance of our species, transmitted as primal phantasies* ("preparations for understanding"). Another is social determinism that enters the subject through language*, and is established in the psychical apparatus, especially in the superego*. More basically, unconscious determinism is the product of individuals' own prehistory, their infantile sexuality* which directs adults' actions even though they know nothing of the histories related to them. Psychoanalysis seeks to break this determinism by making it conscious, thereby interrupting repetition compulsion resulting from repetitive tendencies of Triebe. How does it do this? Through knowledge of these unconscious determinants, made conscious by its action of recovering words that label and interrelate them. Once these words have been recovered, they circulate in thought* activity and seek logical connections that gradually bind them. In this way they reach the deep meaning of symptomatic signifiers or fixation* points, symptoms and fixation points generated in individuals' infantile prehistory, a prehistory unknown since the establishment of repression* or even by their return* from the repressed in disguise.

DISAVOWAL

Ger.: Verleugnen. – Sp.: desmentida. – Fr.: déni. – It.: diniego. – Port.: desmentida (recusa).

This mechanism is utilized by the ego* when confronted by an unbearable reality*. It is able to not perceive this intolerable aspect of reality or to not notify reception of its perception* by withdrawing cathexes* from the perceptual-conscious system (Pcpt.-Cs.). As Freud says, the ego flatly denies it.

Disavowal is never absolute, since reality, even what is meant to be disavowed, is partly perceived. This involves the formation of a splitting of the preconscious ego*. The same aspect of reality is simultaneously accepted and not accepted. In this way a contradiction is authorized that does not, however, disturb its secondary process*. If disavowal clearly predominates over recognition of reality, hallucinatory confusion or Meynert's amentia* ensue. Following topical regression (from word to image), the Pcpt.-Cs. hallucinatorily registers the presence of the wished-for and unrepressed (undisguised) object in the place left by the withdrawn cathexis. In reality, this object was lost. The result is a defence* producing psychosis* as a response to mourning*, a short-lived defence to which non-psychotic persons sometimes resort with little or no alteration of the ego* when the quantity of excitation* is excessively intense.

When disavowal of reality is equal to recognition of reality, a split ego may be clearly observed: an ego whose conscious thought* activity accepts contradictions. For example, fetishism* is a type of sexual perversion* that avoids effective homosexuality* in the individual. It is homosexual libido* that links the fetishist to the object; that is to say, it is libido that disavows sexual difference but is not desexualized. However, heterosexuality is achieved in action by virtue of the fetish; through it, reality is reinforced, which is necessary to sustain the flat "denial" opposing recognition of sexual difference.

In both acute hallucinatory psychosis* and fetishism, disavowal takes place in two steps: (1) nonacceptance of reality (object loss and acceptance of castration, respectively) and (2) active replacement of reality (hallucination* and the presence of the fetish in the woman, respectively).

Splitting of the ego in fetishism is observed clinically in the fact that, even though erection is achieved in the sexual act if the woman possesses a fetish (a fetish shaped by presentations* extracted from experiences of infantile sexuality* and generally displaced, by contiguity* or by symbolism*, from the female penis), castration anxiety* is experienced at other times, which reveals that the ego partly disavowed castration* and partly accepted it (since the man is anxious in relation to an association* referring to castration). The splitting of the ego in this case is intrasystemic, produced in the preconscious ego; it is a failure of its synthetic power by which the ego permits contradictions in secondary process and does not consider them erroneous.

DISGUST

Ger.: Ekel. – Sp.: asco. – Fr.: dégout. – It.: schifo. – Port.: nojo.

A special form of anxiety* that functions as a repressive dam (fixation*) against Trieb* corresponding to a given erotogenic zone* predominant at some period; this predominance passes into another, more developed zone whose problems are more complex.

It is a product of normal primary repression* and constitutes the front line of ego defence (cf. ego), thereby contributing in part to the creation of the ego's unconscious infrastructure. The metapsychological mechanism that constitutes disgust is anticathexis*; it generates a fixation point and changes the affect in response to the possibility of satisfaction of a certain sexual Trieb (what was pleasurable becomes disgusting). Ulterior Trieb regression* returns to this fixation point (with its concomitant presentations, histories, and modalities of ties with the corresponding objects, as well as its modalities of pleasure and now of disgust).

When the oral period passes into the anal, children commonly feel disgust for milk, the breast, and later, in latency following the Oedipus and therefore deferred from it, for cream (symbolic presentation of the nipple). Once the period of anal satisfaction in this predominant erotogenic zone has been overcome, disgust for faeces remains, mainly those of others, as well as anything connected with them.

In the phallic period, some disgust for the sexual may remain if the individual is fixated to this erotogenic zone; for this reason objects* unconsciously desired are predominantly incestuous or derive from incest, a typical phenomenon in hysteria.

Many degrees of fixation are produced by disgust, which depend on the quantities of excitation experienced in each period. Hence, they also depend on traumatic events at those times, which forced the weak ego to increase anticathexis (the only mechanism of primary repression) in order to block Trieb by changing the affect; in this case it does not actually become anxiety although it is one of its specialized forms; the heavier the anticathexis, the stronger the fixation and more intense the disgust.

The ego feels disgust in response to the danger that Trieb might succeed in reaching its objective of discharge. Therefore, the ego utilizes its defence mechanisms* which disgust triggers, providing a signal for the others to unfold (generating hysterical conversions, for example). Placed at the very front line of battle, it may continue to be felt in a conscious and egosyntonic way (and also form certain character traits*). Within certain limits and when controlled by the ego, it is part of normality.

DISPLACEMENT

Ger.: Verschiebung. – Sp.: desplazamiento. – Fr.: déplacement. – It.: spostamento. – Port.: deslocamento.

In this type of mechanism, characteristic of primary process*, psychical energy* (quantum of affect*) passes freely from one presentation* to another, decathecting* one and cathecting* another, according to laws of association*. To achieve perceptual identity*, it is enough for a presentation to be contiguous, analogous, or opposite to another. One presentation can also be the other one because they share superficial attributes. The task of secondary process* is precisely to inhibit* this mechanism (which the Freudian hypothesis considers the first one). This is the only way to distinguish one presentation from another. Then, the cathexis is strong and its displacement weak.

These characteristics of secondary thought* process are operated by the preconscious ego.

However, the unconscious ego may utilize displacement for defensive purposes through free displacement of the cathexis among presentations following laws of association, thereby succeeding in disguising Trieb* or a repressed wish*. Thus, displacement to the trivial is observed in obsessional neurosis*, and may become an ego character trait* (punctilious attention to detail). It is also the typical mechanism in phobias*: the ego displaces fear of the castrating father onto an animal, or the fear of erotic concupiscence onto a phobia of open or closed spaces. Even transference* is an intersystemic form of displacement from the unconscious to the preconscious. The most complex dreams*, those most difficult to understand, are those resulting from more displacement and more resulting disguises.

DISPOSITION

Ger.: Anlage. – Sp.: predisposición. – Fr.: prédisposition. – It.: predisposizione. – Port.: predisposição.

The first factor in the complemental series*, it refers to the propensity of the child who has left behind the period of the Oedipus complex*, now replaced by the superego*, and is therefore taking initial steps in human culture*, beginning in the latency* period and continuing throughout adolescence and adulthood.

The infantile period leaves an indelible impression on this disposition: the subject goes through life with it. When a precipitating factor is added (frustration*), a neurosis* or other psychical affection develops.

Disposition is first composed of all that is inherited phylogenetically: inherited from the parents, grandparents, and even from the entire human species (for example, the Oedipus complex); second, of fixation* points of infantile sexuality* formed by the sum of inherited or constitutional and infantile traumas*. These infantile traumas originate in links with the parents in which excessive amounts of excitation of erotogenic zones* have led to fixations: anticathexes* against Trieb or its hyper-cathexis. Fixations also originate in links with siblings or with the birth of younger siblings, even in relations with caregivers or other persons in their surroundings.

When the inherited predominates over the traumatic, it is more difficult to work through* fixation points* and subsequent concomitant illnesses as well.

Freud describes phylogenetic categories – that is to say, a hereditary tendency to interpret actual events (constitutional subjectivity, so to speak) – according to a line of inherited and universal (corresponding to the species and the history of humanity) primal phantasies*: (a) of the primal scene* (the view of a sexual scene between the parents); (b) of the child's seduction* by an adult; (c) of the threat of castration*. Later, he adds: (d) of the family romance* (the adolescent phantasy of being the child of another family, generally rich, powerful, or having higher social status than the child's own; and (e) the wish to return to the womb.

Some of these inherited phantasies coincide with those most commonly described as traumatic events, which opens a debate regarding the subject of traumatic situations* and historical truth*, as in Freud's discussion of it in the case history of the "Wolf Man".

There is no doubt that there must have been stimulation of the erotogenic zone. Whether it was really excessive or was interpreted in this way by the child based on inherited phantasies must be revealed, or an attempt be made to reveal, by means of reconstruction of the facts through remaining indirect indicators which appear in some dreams*, symptoms*, and other phenomena.

DISSOLUTION (OF THE OEDIPUS COMPLEX)

Ger.: Untergang. – Sp. sepultamiento (del complejo de Edipo). – Fr.: dissolution (du complexe d'Oedipe). – It.: dissoluzione (del complesso di Edipo). – Port.: sepultamento (do complexo de Édipo).

This term is also translated as destruction or mastering of the Oedipus complex, indicating a larger effect than repression*; at least it refers to successful repression which may not return from the repressed (cf. return of the repressed*). Freud apparently refers to the incestuous wishes* of infantile sexuality* which as such are dissolved when the object* cathexis* becomes secondary identification*: transformation of what was a wish into a character trait* belonging to the ego* and therefore desexualized* (we could also say that it partly belongs to the superego), and is able to return only through its unconscious derivatives, never with its original presentations*, unimaginable for the subject's consciousness* (especially the boy's in relation to his mother, but less so for girls in relation to their father).

Therefore, the most thoroughly dissolved is the incestuous presentation in boys, their parricidal presentation is less so, and may even act as an anticathexis* against the former (quite clear in the case of Little Hans).

In girls, repression predominates over dissolution, probably because of the difference in their processing of the Oedipus complex* and also different constitution of the superego*. We are justified in supposing that castration anxiety* in boys must influence successful repression or dissolution. Fear of loss of love would either produce less pressure or this pressure would be less urgent.

DREAM

Ger.: Traum. – Sp.: sueño. – Fr.: rêve. – It.: sogno. – Port.: sonho.

This psychical act is produced during sleep. In it, presentations* of thought* are perceived as images (mainly visual), displaced* and condensed* in time and space, which the sleeping subject believes* at the moment of the dream as if they were perceptions of real experiences.

Sleeping involves libidinal withdrawal* from presentations of objects* of the external world, libido taking refuge in the ego*, or in its representations, which implies regression* to narcissism*. All systems are also decathected* and the total level of cathexis* is lowered; cathexis of the perceptual apparatus is lower, since the ego must leave aside stimuli which might interrupt sleep.

The act of sleeping satisfies a wish of self-preservative Triebe*: the wish to sleep. This preconscious wish is also libidinal, since withdrawal of object cathexes stops in the ego and produces regression to narcissism. This process participates in the general mechanism of dreams. Although this fact is perhaps obvious, it is always advisable to emphasize the end point and the meeting point. In any case, this regression to narcissism inherent to the state of sleep influences the content of dreams, for example, in the sense that they are essentially egoistic and that "the person who plays the chief part in their scenes is always to be recognized as the dreamer" (*A Metapsychological Supplement to the Theory of Dreams*, 1917, p. 223). Freud also observes more sensitivity to bodily alterations in the dreamer due to libidinal withdrawal which, so long as libido is placed in the body, the origin of the ego, it is hypochondriac.

Even so, the ego does not succeed completely in this regression to narcissism in the state of sleep, since repressed unconscious thing-presentations* of object wishes* (therefore object libido) are extracted from the general withdrawal of cathexes, and their functioning is separated from the ego's.

On account of this, withdrawal of cathexes is not total, and therefore the ego must maintain a certain level of censorship*, overseen by the superego*.

Since motility is annulled in the sleeper's ego, unconscious wishes that manage to return from the repressed do not reach specific action*.

The ego generally knows this, although withdrawal of cathexes takes place anyway, but not usually to the extent of making dream images unbelievable; however, at some point in dreaming the ego may resort to "this is only a dream" in order to go on sleeping if its content produces anxiety, for example.

Nonetheless, the ego may wake up as a last resort, since it wants to sleep. If it wakes up, the function of dreaming has failed as the guardian of sleep against the influx of mainly internal stimuli proceeding from repressed Trieb wishes which are always awake and try to attack during the night.

A dream is the result of work done by the ego with its Triebe and repressed wishes, which struggle to return from the state of repression whenever they find an opportunity. The state of sleep is one of these occasions, since the ego is resting and its defences are lower, making it easier to enter.

The mechanism by which the dream is produced is more or less the following: at some point, the cathexis of thing-presentations of repressed object wishes accesses (before or simultaneously) their representation in words, which belongs to the preconscious ego, then transfer their cathexis to mnemic residues of experiences during the day which for some reason retained some cathexis or simply serve as figures for repressed wishes.

In the *Interpretation of Dreams* (1900) Freud calls the repressed unconscious wish* the "capitalist partner" and the day's residue the "industrial partner". The "society" may be composed in different ways.

Once cathexes of repressed wishes have been transferred* to the day's residues, the "wish-fulfilling phantasy" is constituted; its road to action is blocked since motility is cancelled by the state of sleep. This leads to formal regression to cathexis of the thing-presentation (mainly visual); regression is both topical regression, since cathexis regresses to the perceptual end*, its origin, and also ego regression, since the ego regresses to the stage of "hallucinatory satisfaction of wishes"*.

When this regression is produced, thoughts are perceived as images possessing characteristics of primary process* of mental functioning; therefore, presentations are condensed in diverse ways. Cathexes of these presentations are displaced easily from one to another according to the laws of association* which accept neither contradiction, space, nor time and achieve perceptual identity*, decentring the value from the content of ideas belonging to the dream.

Presentations regress from the preconscious to the repressed unconscious; therefore, they become part of the id* and its laws, but also have the additional facility of reaching the perceptual apparatus (the unconscious ego intervenes in these "negotiations"). This complex process is called dream work*.

This primary process functioning of hallucinations* of the dream also acts as censorship for the ego. Its unconscious censorship, which Freud refers to as "the dream censor", utilizes it because it serves as a disguise or substitute formation*.

When awake, the preconscious ego does not usually understand contents of this type, so far removed from its logic (belonging to secondary process*), and tries to repress what was dreamed. For this reason, the dream is forgotten, remembered only partially, or is remembered ego-dystonically, the ego not feeling it is a psychical production of its own.

However, as it does with any other perception, before, during, and after perception of the manifest content* of the dream, the ego tries to procure a formal structure for it with some intelligibility which accounts, for example, for formal alterations in time and space corresponding to images of memories (they are ultimately memories) participating in the dream's contents.

This action achieves the opposite effect, since it unmasks the repressed wish satisfied by the dream's content even more clearly to the preconscious ego.

All of the dream's representational content is composed as if figurability were carefully considered in the selection of presentations.

Some mechanisms inherent to the unconscious are also found among the presentations, such as universal symbols*, remnants of humanity's experience before the creation of speech*, later forgotten but remaining in the unconscious psyche as relics that may be used again to figure unconscious wishes, since the preconscious ego does not understand their meaning.

Clinically, universal symbols tend to produce no associations because they do not belong to the dreamer's individual experience, but their placement in the dream guides the analyst to the global meaning of the content of a complex dream, also including associations for closer analysis. Consideration for figurability, working through, universal symbols, and, of course, condensation and displacement all participate in dream work.

The dream's manifest content is thus an attempt to satisfy repressed unconscious wishes and also a way to honour the ego's wish to sleep. For numerous causes, wishes emerge that were repressed successfully during the day and attempt to return during sleep.

In some cases it is quite difficult to discover the type of satisfaction of wishes, since it has been very effectively disguised.

In other cases, the affect* it produces makes it doubtful, for example, although this is precisely one of the signs of repression*: satisfaction of a repressed wish produces anxiety in the ego.

In other cases, wishes to be punished by the superego are satisfied, resulting in punishment* dreams. They are perhaps reaction formations* in the dream's content in which the need for punishment*, unconscious by definition, predominates in relation to fear of satisfaction of wishes (as in anxiety* dreams*) and Trieb satisfaction (as in more or less indifferent or pleasurable dreams).

Some dreams contradict the theory of satisfaction of wishes: the dreams of traumatic* neurosis. The previous traumatic situation* overwhelms the protective shield* against stimuli whose last resort is preparedness anxiety*. These dreams repeat the traumatic situation, partly due to the repetition compulsion* typical of all Trieb behaviour, especially behaviour corresponding to death Trieb*, by which the pleasure principle* is abandoned. There is also an attempt to return to the pleasure principle by restoring the overwhelmed protective shield. Then, the preparedness anxiety that could not be felt during the traumatic situation may be felt and therefore transformed into a danger-situation*, which may then be referred to other previous danger-situations (castration, for example) close to pleasurable but forbidden or dangerous situations (incestuous or derivatives of incest).

When this is possible, it becomes an anxiety dream* which may then be explained as a satisfaction of wishes. When this is not possible, it remains part of repetition compulsions functioning beyond the pleasure principle, the traumatic quantitative predominating and being repeated in a "demonic" way.

The dream's manifest content has a latent content*. This is the result of the dreamer's associations. From the latent content we arrive at the meaning of the dream, which results from a retranslation of dream work into wish thoughts in preconscious word-presentations corresponding to the wish-fulfilling phantasy that contained them before their regression to thing-presentations.

Thus, repressed wishes are recovered which enter the formal contents of secondary process.

Word-presentations once decathected and therefore remaining in a state of repression are recovered and now form part of the ego, enriching it, mainly its ability to think* or "associative commerce". Because of their potential to provide such direct perception of primary process mechanisms, Freud referred to dreams as the *via regia* to access the unconscious. The meaning of dreams may therefore be interpreted; that is to say, re-translated into secondary process, which allows the ego to understand it. Psychoanalytic technique includes various approaches to dreams. The classical approach and quite probably the most rigorous, although not necessarily the most effective, is to decompose the dream's manifest content into its diverse elements and to ask the patient for associations. In this way, we find a new level of elements that were latent, in which new associative paths appear and from which new and increasingly deeper levels of meaning are derived; their quantity depends on the degree of previous condensation which is initially impossible to determine. Another path is to ask for associations based on day's residues which may also lead to unexpected paths. A certain element is chosen because it stands out or reminds us of something previous in the patient's problems, and therefore we ask for associations with it. Other analysts, or the same analyst on a different occasion, may wait for the patient to choose the place from which to begin to associate; or their interpretive approach may be based on a universal symbol and a request for associations, in search of new meanings. All these interpretive techniques are alternatives, and the analysis does not necessarily complete the analysis of a dream but only finds levels of meaning of the wish or different unconscious wishes expressed in it. It is even possible to analyse the meanings of a certain dream chapter by chapter, connecting them in the representational interweave with other presentations apparently referring to other things, events, or facts. The analysis of dreams is therefore one of the most valuable and exciting aspects of analytic work, leading to knowledge of the unconscious.

DREAMS FROM ABOVE AND BELOW

Ger.: Traum von oben / Traum von unter. – Sp.: sueños desde arriba y abajo. – Fr.: rêves d'en haut et d'en bas. – It.: sogni di su e di giù. – Port.: sonhos de cima e de baixo.

Freud applies these terms to differentiate dreams according to the predominance of the "capitalist partner" or the "industrial partner", at least in relation to the manifest content* of the dream; a distinction, however, to be taken with a grain of salt. "Dreams from below" are created by a repressed unconscious wish* that has managed to get a day's residue* to represent it. It is similar to irruption of the repressed in everyday life (in jokes*, parapraxes*, and other phenomena).

In "dreams from above", however, the thought* content or day's aim predominates; during the night it succeeds in being reinforced by the repressed and remaining separate from the ego*.

In any case, the meaning of the dream, which is the capitalist partner, is still the fulfilment of repressed unconscious wishes in spite of the importance of these dreams provided by the content of the day's residue. They do not in any way modify the theory of fulfilment of repressed wishes in dreams.

DREAM'S NAVEL, THE

Ger.: Traum Nabel / Nabel des traumes. – Sp.: ombligo del sueño. – Fr.: nombril du rêve. – It.: ombelico del sogno. – Port.: umbigo do sonho.

This place remains in the shadows after the analysis of a dream*. Freud infers that it is the origin of a tangle of dream thoughts* which cannot be disentangled, and has not made other contributions to the dream's content. It is the place in the dream where the unknown resides; it is what is unknowable about the history of the unconscious* wish*.

An interpretation* of all dreams is not possible. "It is thus a question of relative strength whether our intellectual interest, our capacity for self-discipline, our psychological knowledge and our practice in interpreting dreams enable us to master our internal resistances" (*The Interpretation of Dreams*, 1900, p. 525).

It is always possible to go a step further until we understand the meaning of a dream. Or to glimpse it through analysis of another dream which confirms or completes the interpretations of the first one. However, we may also reach a point impossible to untangle: "This is the dream's navel, the spot where it reaches down into the unknown" (Ibid.). In this place, cathexis* can no longer be returned to the presentation* from which it was originally displaced, and therefore we are now unable to separate the different condensed presentations (cf. condensation*). Here, multidetermination leaves different roads intermixed and not entirely distinguishable, as they were at the beginning of the functioning of the psychical apparatus.

DREAM WORK

Ger.: Traumarbeit. – Sp.: trabajo del sueño. – Fr.: travail du rêve. – It.: lavoro del sogno. – Port.: trabalho do sonho.

Dreams* disguise their thought* presentations* proceeding from their preconscious wish-fulfilling phantasy to enable their perception by the perceptual apparatus as images constituting the dream's manifest content*, a process produced during the act of sleeping: "the work which transforms the latent dream into the manifest one is called the dream work" (*Introductory Lectures on Psychoanalysis*, 1916–17, p. 170).

This dream work is accomplished by the entire psychical apparatus although essentially by the ego*. It includes several phases. The first is probably regression* of word-presentations* belonging to the preconscious ego to thing-presentations*, and the registration of the latter by the perceptual-consciousness system. Together with this, the laws of functioning or the ties between them regress to primary process* whose condensation*, displacement*, and universal symbolism* are the pillars of dream work.

Perceptions* by the perceptual end* of condensed, displaced thing-presentations symbolizing body parts and sexuality*, death, and other elements are processed by this perceptual-consciousness system and given some consistency from the viewpoint of the preconscious ego, though at the cost of a heavier disguise.

Dream work is accomplished before, during, and even after the dream* depending on the sequences or "parts" composing them and those to which the subject is referring. They are regressions of what already constituted a wish-fulfilling phantasy (had already obtained a word-presentation) in the preconscious by virtue of the transference* of cathexes* of repressed unconscious wishes* on to day's residues* of words, unimportant or rejected during the day, to figure as representations of images of things, since access to motility is cancelled by the state of sleep. They are figured in the perceptual-consciousness system and, like any other perception, are believed*. Because of topical regression, these thing-presentations are handled according to the laws of primary process; therefore they may be condensed in diverse ways according to the laws of contiguity*, analogy*, or opposition*. The *quantum* of energy circulating among them may also be displaced freely, thereby modifying the centre of the scene. Finally, images of universal symbolism may be utilized in order to represent images that would otherwise be repressed. Also before, during, and after production of the manifest content of the dream, the preconscious ego tries to make it intelligible, as it does any other thought or different perceptions considered absurd, giving them for example a certain chronological or spatial order or some rationalization* to explain different elements of the dream whose logic might seem strange, this being the secondary revision* of dream work.

E

EARLY PSYCHE

Ger.: frühe Psyche. – Sp.: psiquismo temprano. – Fr.: psychisme précoce. – It.: psiquismo precoce. – Port.: psiquismo precoce.

We consider the early psyche is the infant's psyche. In practice, it extends from birth to the appearance of spoken language*. This definition does not exclude the foetal psyche, but the latter is necessarily different. Although Freud did not specifically discuss the early psyche, he referred to it indirectly when theorizing on other subjects based on observation of the adult psyche, especially some phenomena such as dreams*. His theorization is therefore basically deferred* and theoretical, and hence he never tried to observe children's behaviour to draw conclusions, although he did observe his own grandson in *Beyond the Pleasure Principle* (1920) and participated in the famous case of Little Hans, a period in which he warmly recommended that infantile material be sent to him for the development of his texts on infantile sexuality*. We could start by taking three lines of discussion to describe this subject: one previous to and two following individual experience. The first refers to primal phantasies*, "preparations to understand", products of the experience of the species, which lead the child to grasp diverse situation in the sense of seduction* and the primal scene*, for example. To these universals must be added the so-called universal symbols* and the individual aspect corresponding to the subject's own experiences* of satisfaction* and pain*, experienced with the object*, in which the object's actions are determinant considering the initial helplessness of human being and their absolute dependency on the mother (or her substitute) to reduce all types of tensions; also because the object's actions constitute presentations (object presentations of what was done with and by the object and what was felt in this experience, a complex subsequently desired) which when cathected* form the subject's wishes*, part of the subject's subjectivity, and part of the subject's protective shield*. The concept of the experience of satisfaction (not one, but their predominance during this stage of life) therefore acquires such importance that it is practically the founder of the entire psychical apparatus. When these experiences are produced, the psychical presentational is inaugurated strictly, the traces gradually left by experiences becoming presentations* or presentational contents. Once these are outlined, what was *biological* becomes *psychical* by means of the *social* (contact with the object, its language, and its actions). That is to say, this experience becomes the trace left by it in the apparatus which, when it re-emerges, cathected by the bodily, constitutes the wish, which is already psychical, whose content is the former pleasurable experience desired to be repeated. However, this description is not as simple as it seems; it becomes complex even on these initial levels. As a result of his study of dreams in adults, Freud hypothesized on a tendency to hallucinatory wish fulfilment*; he thought about the existence of a process of psychical functioning (primary process*) by which the wish appeared at first as hallucination; that is to say utilizing perceptual identity*, which means that, rather than being wished for, it was perceived in hallucinatory fashion as already being fulfilled. In this way, frustration or pain was obtained (depending on which scene was hallucinated: the experience of frustration or of pain) which created a need for a different type of psychical functioning to inhibit this hallucinatory tendency. This second process is secondary process*, an ego* function. The ego functions by placing presentations in the path leading to the hallucination, representations which lead to others, association, and thought. In this way a psychical space is achieved in the path from stimulus to action which may be guided by thought in the search for thought identities*, first with thing-presentations* (reproductive thought and primary judging* through actions) and then with word-presentations*. With the latter, thought may reach a very high level. Later, conflicts corresponding to these wishes arise with the erotogenic zones, and primary* and secondary* repression develop, causing difficulties in this thought; however, this is another aspect.

We return to what is early. A line of analysis simultaneous with the former is development of the ego. Freud first describes two conflicting and simultaneous types of ego which function from the outset, one more bound to body limits, called the initial reality ego*, in dialectic process with the purified pleasure ego* which only recognizes as ego what is pleasurable and as non-ego what is unpleasurable (pain is included in unpleasure) and what is indifferent. The synthesis of these egos which negate each other is the definitive reality ego* which encompasses and surpasses the other previous egos. This definitive ego is constituted when one erotogenic zone gains primacy and unifies the rest; this occurs when phallic-urethral eroticism* predominates. The egos previous to the definitive ego apparently involve contradictory situations; for example, the object is partly recognized at the outset (in reality, only the object's body is recognized as foreign to the subject's own body). At the same time, so long as the criterion of *being** predominates over that of *having**, the object is ego, in direct (unmediated) identification*, which is "the first form of love" (*Group Psychology and the Analysis of the Ego*, 1921). The latter is the first type of identification (primary identification*) with the mother, to which is added in boys their primary identification with the father, already recognized as an object of desire but previous to recognition of sexual difference and therefore lacking the hostile aspect it acquires when he becomes the rival for the mother's desire (the boy wants to be like the father without yet recognizing his essential difference from the mother, which on the phallic psychical level resides in castration). Later, this identification is reinforced by secondary identification*, constituting the superego*.

Therefore we have two supreme elements of this early psyche: the formation of psychical presentations as traces of experiences with the object and identifications with the same object, thing-presentations, and primary identifications which are initially barely distinguishable from each other, as are ego and object. Reality must gradually impose itself (though never totally), depending on the quality of experiences with objects and conflicts which inevitably arise on the road (especially the Oedipus complex* which as such is universal. The individual is the presentational content of each subject's experience).

EGO

Ger.: Ich. – Sp.: yo. – Fr.: moi. – It.: io. – Port.: ego.

Freud describes this agency, institution, and psychical structure, which unifies and localizes the psychical apparatus, in different ways in the course of his works, addressing its many aspects and the diverse perspectives from which it may be examined.

We may, for example, mention an ego constructed from presentations* formed gradually as experiences* occur, leaving their memory traces* which later become presentations (first, thing-presentations* and then, when language* is acquired, word-presentations* which become the ego's marrow). The major experiences are those of satisfaction* and pain*, the two main forms of link with the object*.

In this way the ego grows and is even formed out of experience (in other ways, the ego is also being formed throughout life, although its main characteristics are acquired in the first years of life).

This presentational ego arises, moderating movements of cathecting libidinal energy among presentations, thereby preventing perceptual identity* (which is hallucinatory and therefore frustrating) inherent to primary process* ruled by the pleasure principle* that sought perceptual identity at the beginning of life. It accomplishes this by setting up an inhibitory side barrier composed of cathected presentations that attract libido* to themselves, having strong cathexis* and weak displacement*, and ruled by the reality principle*. Thus, these presentations acquire new attributes that even enable them to change category. As we said, presentational cathexis is strong and displacement of energy among presentations is weak. Identity with what is wished for is still sought, but through thought*; therefore, thought identity* is sought. Thought activity then becomes a highly important function of the ego.

This first type of ego that inhibits hallucination* begins to work in this way following the first frustrating hallucinatory experiences when it learns that the pathway of hallucination, at least concerning self-preservative Trieb*, leads nowhere or, worse yet, leads to the opposite of what it wishes for.

The ego must prevent this by inhibiting (cf. inhibition*) hallucination. How? As we said, by side-cathecting other presentations with which to compare and differentiate it; thing-presentations are essentially images of wished-for objects in which presentations are not condensed (cf. condensation*) and energy is not so freely displaced among them.

Reproductive thought, previous to acquisition of words, is one of the first forms of thought which distinguishes between memory* and perception*, a primitive level of secondary process*.

This first level of thought in images gradually makes more room for memory and psychical activity in the psychical apparatus (*Project for a Scientific Psychology*, 1895–1950); the incipient reality ego thinks and also distinguishes its thought as an expression of a wish*; at the same time, the presence of this wish is not enough for this ego to consider it fulfilled. Reproductive thought is useful at most for recognizing differences between what is wished for and what is perceived, and between the different perceptions as compared to memories.

All these functions, even the smallest, need this primitive ego and some secondary process. In this way, the reality ego is slowly formed, later becoming the definitive reality ego*.

Together with development of reproductive thought based on images, a type of thought is formed, also previous to definitive thought in words. Freud calls it primary judging*, judgement made with bodily movements. Freud's example in the *Project* ... is the baby when it remembers the breast as seen from the front. When the breast is presented in profile, a slight movement of the neck reveals that it is essentially the wished-for breast, which is the same whether it is seen from the front or in profile, since the sensation obtained in the link with it is repeated and a *Gestalt* of the image of the breast is also achieved. Thought through movements and reproductive thought (produced with images) also draw the first outlines of a growing secondary process and therefore of the definitive reality ego.

As the subject acquires language, another type of presentation appears: word-presentations which add complexity to the thought system and inhibition of hallucination. Inhibitory side chains are made more complex by words, which weave an extremely sophisticated presentational fabric. This fabric of word-presentations constitutes the preconscious, perhaps the major part of the ego. The preconscious and the ego are formed in relation with vicissitudes of infantile sexuality*, the main one being the Oedipus complex.

Presentations are ultimately mnemic residues of experiences with objects, experienced through one or another erotogenic zone* predominant in a given moment of infantile sexuality; these experiences with the object left behind fixation* points on the one hand and modalities of satisfaction or pleasure* on the other.

Object wish presentations are constituted from something corresponding to characteristics of images belonging to objects and sensations produced in relation with them. Everything corresponding to presentational complexes related with movements by objects and with objects at moments of experiences of satisfaction and pain are transformed into modalities of ego behaviour, identifications*, and/or ego representations; this ego wishes, and knows what it wishes for: the object.

What does it mean to wish for the object? For self-preservative Triebe, the object is firmly fixed. For sexual Triebe* it is variable. What they seek in reality is pleasure, for which the object is necessary. For this reason, the anaclisis of object choice is formed by objects and their attributes that first satisfied self-preservative Triebe.

Traumatic* situations of infantile sexuality originate fixations with respect to characteristics of objects the ego will choose when it is ready to do so.

Now we consider ego development from a viewpoint more connected with the problem of ego-object differentiation. At first, there is an ego that recognizes differences between the ego and the outside world in terms of a realistic criterion. It is the initial reality ego*. If a small movement (closing the eyes, for example) is enough to stop feeling a sensation in response to a certain stimulus, then this stimulus is not-ego; if the sensation stops without any movement, it belongs to us: it is ego; it is even more: it is the nucleus of the ego (Triebe*).

But it is not all so easy; there are other criteria; the object is not so easily accepted as belonging to the external world, especially if it is the source of pleasure, the object may come to be considered the ego or part of it. Also, anything that produces unpleasure* or is neutral is considered the outside world.

In this way, the purified pleasure ego* is constituted and rules during the period of primary narcissism*. In reality, one corresponds to the other: if pleasure and what produces it (the object) is ego, then the ego is the object or, equally, everything is narcissism, everything is ego, except what is unpleasurable.

From another viewpoint, we may call this process primary identification*, in which the object's attributes become characteristics of the ego.

This type of ego is perhaps indispensable at the beginning of life given the extreme helplessness of human young which involves absolute dependence on the object and its love*.

"Being" the object leaves no room to feel its absence or any wish for it. When some control over the muscular apparatus is gained and certain levels of specific action* are possible, the source of pleasure is gradually accepted as not being the ego; at the same time the object begins to be recognized as such and related anxieties* are felt: first, anxiety for fear of its loss, which becomes more complex as progress is made in the relative predominance of the different erotogenic zones.

This presentational ego is therefore at first a modality of links among presentations, which slowly establishes secondary process.

Not all presentations constitute the ego. Some, for example those of certain wishes, belong to the ego without being the ego. They are presentations of ego wishes.

Presentations of the subject's own body*, those of sensations of pleasure (autoerotic or originating in the relation with the object through the erotogenic zones) and of pain*, originating in the depth of sensations of organs and on the body surface, in images produced through the sensory organs such as sight and its voyeuristic pleasure; perception of the subject's own features and its understanding as an image of the ego requires the mirror image, as well as acquisition of language and thought activity; all these elements constitute presentations belonging to the ego.

An image of the subject's own body is thereby obtained, unifying all the previous autoerotic (cf. autoerotism) experiences* and object experiences as belonging to an ego: a body essence containing a history and the marks of this history.

The formation of this ego notion culminates in the phallic period. In it, all the previously dominant erotogenic zones are united as belonging to one unity that now seeks a type of pleasure which also unifies them and to which they now belong.

This period is contemporary with the Oedipus complex, when formation of the definitive reality ego* is completed and the object is finally recognized as the principal source of pleasure. Therefore, the problem presented by reality for satisfaction of sexual Triebe* must also be accepted, since the object is its major part.

The period of primary narcissism also culminates, although from another viewpoint it is also, paradoxically, recognized as such, together with the object. All the erotogenic zones which were as separate as islands are unified into one continent called the ego, a desiring ego whose type of wish unifies all the previous tendencies; this ego now possesses language and speaks, speaks about what is wished for; what it essentially desires is the object.

As we know, complex problems arise in this wishing for the object which this ego must face as best it can in order to perform the specific actions demanded by Trieb wishes.

The ego is also the seat of anxiety. When the psychical apparatus is invaded by quantity of excitation* coming in from the external world or from Triebe inside the body, the ego suffers traumatic anxiety or automatic anxiety* (when quantity of excitation surpasses the ego's ability to bind it with presentations, it automatically becomes anxiety). In infancy, this invasion was produced when certain erotogenic zones were hyper-stimulated by the object in detriment of others. An invasion may also occur in the present.

As it grows, the ego establishes a certain order of defences to fend off the reappearance of the first form of automatic anxiety aimed against it in infancy.

The first defence, *primal repression**, is composed of anticathexis* of the erotogenic zone that was traumatic in the period of infantile sexuality. This generates *fixation** of this anticathexis to the presentation of the satisfaction of this erotogenic zone and also fixation to the presentation of the object and its attributes.

Although this first ego defence is unconscious and also generates repressed unconscious, when it represses the word-presentation of the object corresponding to the satisfaction of sexual Trieb through a certain erotogenic zone, it also marks the limits of the ego. With each repression*, the ego loses ground and loses wealth, but also inhibits Trieb.

Primal repression therefore limits the ego. It generates character traits*, forms of being or doing or of not doing (ego inhibitions, produced by shame*, disgust*, or moral conscience*, dams originating in primal repression), which may be more or less pathological, more or less normal, rooted within the ego. The formation of primal repression is completed in the period of the Oedipus complex. At that point, the psychical apparatus is split into an unconscious id* including the unconscious that was repressed by this primal repression, an ego that is partly unconscious (essentially, the repressing part) and partly preconscious* and conscious, and the superego* which opposes the ego, forcing it to repress Triebe and punishing it with the sense of guilt* (conscious or unconscious) when it is unsuccessful.

Previous repressions are re-signified in a deferred* manner by making them oedipal, thereby giving previously recorded histories an oedipal tinge.

Thenceforward the ego unfolds another, secondary level of defence; it is also unconscious and not entirely new since it was already functioning when it was recognizing the object as the main source of pleasure.

It no longer defends itself from automatic anxiety directly but instead through anxiety signals* related with dangers of fear of object loss* and castration anxiety*; even tertiary levels of defence are constituted from that point on; one example is phobic inhibition, part of the rampart to avoid reactivation of ego conflicts with id Trieb and the superego (this level is preconscious in the form of rationalization* and conscious censorship*); this defence thereby acquires greater complexity and increasingly distances itself from automatic anxiety, though at the expense of growing impoverishment of the ego and the limitation of its abilities.

The ego's second level of defence, also unconscious, develops *secondary repression or repression proper*; that is to say, most of the *defence mechanisms** in response to anxiety signals, which sometimes create substitutive formations called symptoms*, the ego's compromises with Triebe not accepted by the ego as its own; however, if they become chronic, the ego tries to encompass them within it.

The ego cultivates the anxiety signal with the memory of traumatic birth anxiety and subsequent traumas; it takes a small sample of trauma which it displays as an alarm flag in response to any danger situation* in order to protect the previous level.

The ego as the psychical structure described by Freud in *The Ego and the Id* (1923) complements what we describe above. It develops from the surface inwards, from reality towards Trieb, from identification towards the nucleus of our being, from identification towards wishes, from outside towards the inside.

For this reason, it is also an alienated ego, the "shadow of the object" on the surface of the psychical apparatus, a stranger that entered the house and took possession of it in order to tame Trieb proceeding from the inside, from the very "nucleus of being".

However, the ego also has other functions. It is the seat of language* and therefore of thought, through which it must reach the specific action (while in the service of Trieb, for which it governs action). It is composed, at least its preconscious part, principally of word-presentations signifying thing-presentations. The ego's preconscious part (the official ego that can be seen and is accepted as such by the subject) develops as a superstructure which is in reality edified upon an infrastructure prepared by the unconscious defensive part, which it does not recognize as its own but exists by virtue of it; its "existence" may depend so heavily on it that its influence may alter the ego (cf. alteration of the ego*).

In a different way the ego is also composed of desexualized libido* which appears to itself as a sublimation*. However, sublimation is not a sudden, isolated act but instead a process. The ego undertakes to sublimate Triebe in order to adapt them to culture*, a human creation producing sublimations and also a product of another sublimation: language.

Language with its preconscious word-presentations gives the ego an opportunity to think and also to be the object of thought. The ability to think involves its accessory: responsibility for decisions involving action, for which thought may provide, among other things, a kind of preview.

However, the preconscious ego is subjected to diverse dependencies before reaching action. It is buffeted by the id and its Triebe, which demand satisfaction; by the superego which demands "what you must be" and "what you must not be"; reality also tugs at it.

It must try to impose a criterion of reality and find a synthesis with these other extremely diverse criteria. It must impose the reality principle and secondary process, for which it is important to examine reality by reality testing* using cognitive thought.

The ego is often unsuccessful, since a whole part of itself, its unconscious part, escapes its own control. This part makes compromises with the id, libidinal Triebe, and wishes that strive to return from the repressed*, generating neurotic symptoms. If we take this reasoning to its extreme, we could even say that the ego itself is configured as a compromise established between id Triebe and reality, between the id and the superego, the best agreement these different forces can reach.

When the ego is unable to find pathways to unite all these diverse tendencies, its preconscious part may split (cf. splitting of the ego*); then contradictions arise in its thinking which it does not recognize as such, as if there were two separate egos. This is characteristic of sexual perversions* which accept and also do not accept the existence of two sexes, or rather, the existence of castration.

However, the preconscious ego is the part of the psychical apparatus most worked over in psychoanalytic treatments. Id Triebe, "the nucleus of the ego" early in the theory and also in the origins of each psychical apparatus, are again recognized by the ego as its own, enriching it when interrelations between presentations, their "associative commerce", increase. It no longer needs to defend itself so fiercely from them, since they have lost the danger they represented in childhood when castration anxiety was realistic. Psychoanalysis also endeavours to help the ego to recognize its own unconscious defensive parts in order to diminish the demand for defensive energy and thereby make libidinal energy available for specific action.

Psychoanalytic treatment also aims to help the ego to recognize its superego and to differentiate itself from it, which relieves its sense of guilt and leaves it freer to undertake the type of specific action it finds most enjoyable, including sublimation, which also involves the criterion of reality, an ego principle.

Finally, the ego is the seat of narcissism*. Or rather, libido in the ego constitutes narcissism.

In adults, narcissism is nourished by appreciation the ego carries forward from infancy, by success achieved through obeying the ideal ego*, and by the love of its objects*.

When narcissism is wounded, libido may be withdrawn from objects (from their presentations) and sent to cathect the ego, thereby generating narcissistic pathology whose most regressive form is schizophrenia*.

In the latter, the object is apparently not desired. This loss of desire for the object befalls the ego when it utilizes its last bastion in response to automatic anxiety arising in a poorly defended ego which rapidly succumbs to this type of anxiety in response to frustrations the object may produce in relation to their link or to the ego's intentions towards it, instead of defending itself or facing anxiety signals for object loss* or loss of the object's love*, threat of castration* or loss of the superego's* love (as occurs in transference neuroses*).

The last bastion is therefore withdrawal of libidinal cathexis from unconscious object presentations. They are no longer desired on a deep level (the subject does not say they are not desired; they are no longer desired without saying so); the ego thereby sinks into this state of affairs in which the object is no longer desired, paradoxically, in order to support the ego which is no longer receiving libido from the object, but instead recathects it with libido now coming from the id. Word-presentations of an ego in these conditions are not based on thing-presentations. They are signifiers without signified: word-presentations mistaken for thing-presentations and treated as such; that is to say, by primary process.

Thus, a small circuit or an extremely shaky defensive bunker is thus established, utilizing libido that was object libido but secondarily became narcissistic again, now at the mercy of automatic anxiety and repetition compulsion* which originate all libidinal presentational decathexes*.

EGO IDEAL

Ger.: Ichideal. – Sp.: ideal del yo. – Fr.: idéal du moi. – It.: ideale dell'io. – Port.: ideal do ego.

This is a split-off part of the ego*. Until 1921 Freud describes it in an isolated way, separate from other concepts, more as a function than as having a place in any topic (*On Narcissism: An Introduction*, 1914; *Group Psychology and the Analysis of the Ego*, 1921). After conceptualizing it as synonymous with the superego* (*The Ego and the Id*, 1923), he finally identifies it as a substructure within the superego, with its components and/or functions, together with conscience* and self-regarding (*An Outline of Psycho-Analysis*, 1940).

The ego ideal is the origin of one of the largest components of the superego: "You ought to be like this (like your father)" (*The Ego and the Id*, p. 34).

It is the heir of the perfection and delusions of grandeur of original narcissism* constituting the ideal ego* and infantile sexuality*, which is predominantly autoerotic* and later recognized as being narcissistic by the reality ego*.

The purified pleasure ego* possessed pleasure* as a condition of its being*. No object* was not-ego if it produced pleasure. What produced unpleasure* was considered not-ego.

This is the ideal situation. If the ego is pleasure, there is no chink through which unpleasure, the imperfect, or the impure might enter; the ego is thus "purified" of anything unpleasurable.

As the reality principle* is gradually imposed on the ego and a reality ego* forms, gradual recognition of objects as not-ego and also as potential sources of pleasure becomes possible. The ego accepts that it is not the object but at most may have them (cf. having*), and that they are foreign to it.

The first pleasure object (the mother) is one of the first ways to recognize the object* as such and mainly as a source of pleasure whose loss is feared (fear of object loss*). Then, there is an attempt to master it by Trieb of mastery* (especially in the anal-sadistic phase). However, especially in boys, another type of link continues: the former model of being; the link with the father, which the boy masters by "identifying* himself with him" (*The Ego and the Id*, p. 31).

We repeat: there are two ways to understand the link through the category of being (the purified pleasure ego's link with the mother, the mother being the measure of pleasure; and the link with the father, considered omnipotent or capable of executing specific actions* wished for by the boy, for which he longs to be like him), without any implication of sexual differentiation. These two forms constitute the child's primary identifications*, the base on which secondary identifications will be established, thereby reinforcing the former, and later constituting the ego ideal.

The ego ideal is the heir of original narcissism and of identification* with the ideal father of infancy. Secondary identification*, built on this primary identification* involves a hostile, ambivalent aspect that eventually constitutes the definitive superego. We could summarize by saying that the ego ideal is constituted, together with the ego, from primary identifications with the pleasure object, adding in boys a longing to be like the father of early infancy (also primary identifications, sometimes paradoxically conscious copies*, since the father is recognized as an object that is neither a source of pleasure nor a rival). Primary identification is reinforced by secondary superego identification (with the figure of the oedipal parents: objects desired positively or negatively and a castrating rival) which anticathects (cf. anticathexis*) infantile sexuality, covering it with a mantle of forgetting*. In boys, it also reinforces masculinity; we could even say that it founds it.

In any case, with constitution of the ego ideal, narcissism undergoes changes, since the ego seeks to be like the ideal in its actions. It feels either esteemed by it or guilty* depending on whether it succeeds or not.

Through self-regarding, the superego commands the ego to be like the ideal, punishing it when it falls short of achieving it by means of the conscience.

The ego ideal is therefore formed out of narcissistic libido* (pleasure ego) and homosexual libido (the link of being with the parents); that is to say, sexually undifferentiated libido. Following establishment of the superego, new characteristics are added to the ideal when it acquires the ideals of a community, a group, and other social influences. Human groups are formed by identification links between the egos of the individual members. One of them is chosen as the ideal ego to be the leader in the manner of the father of infancy. For this reason the link is as ambivalent* as the father complex*.

What occurs in hypnosis and being in love? The hypnotized person and the lover place the object (the hypnotizer and the inspirer of love, respectively) in the place of the ego ideal. This object then possesses the virtues and powers of the ideal, whereas the subject's ego is emptied.

The ideal required of the ego by the ego ideal refers to the future, though also to the past (as in the family romance* in which adolescents cannot tolerate the fact that their parents are not ideal as they believed them to be in infancy). The future is a future called upon to be the splendid past once experienced in infantile megalomaniacal delusion: a race towards the future in search of the past, an impossible race. Past and present are thus intertwined in a very particular way in this part of the superego, causing suffering to an ego never or only quite sporadically able to satisfy it. Then, the superego and the ego relate to each other in a way that begins to resemble the relation between their Triebe*. The ego even tries to repress* or suppress* demands of the ideal, almost as if these demands had the features of Trieb demands. In fact, the superego acquires the force of its "categorical imperative" from its roots in Triebe and its phylogenetic roots in the id*. This force is so strong in adults that it is sometimes difficult to differentiate between a Trieb demand and a demand of the ideal (as in some obsessional symptoms, for example), if not for the presumption of sublimation. The latter is not in any case absolutely necessary.

Although sublimation* is a demand of the ego ideal, it is the ego that acts on it: the ideal cannot obligate the ego; it may demand it, but the ego will do what is possible or will rebel.

The origin of the female ego ideal is not fully clarified. Assuming a phallic fixation*, we might think that her castration complex* is formed in the same way as in men: with the longing* of infantile narcissism lacking sexual difference, from which the ego ideal is formed with phallic characteristics, the paternal figure therefore established as the unreachable ideal. "You ought to be like this (like your father)" (generating the longing, so frequent and strong in women, for the penis-child, often constituted as bedrock*, and impenetrable by psychoanalysis). However, we may also think that the girl's pre-oedipal maternal-filial link is far more extensive than the boy's; that the girl's detachment from her mother is more gradual, inevitably culminating in a fight (since girls must change object, they are assisted by their castration complex, castration they blame on their mother in order to proceed to make a paternal object choice). Taking the latter line of thought, we could think about the formation of more purely feminine ideals connected, for example, with maternity (wanting to be like mother), even though this infantile mother is also phallic in infantile sexual theories*. The definitively predominant form arises from fixation points and the complemental series. It is also probable that both forms develop to some extent, one prevailing over the other. This does not mean that the form that has apparently been overcome may, at a different moment in life, again dominate. If the predominant form is the phallic, the female superego is left with a phallic ego ideal which may be more or less unconscious and originate neurosis* or difficulties in the link with men or even more serious pathologies such as paranoia* or homosexuality*, for example.

The second path will probably lead to better feminine identity, although it may also generate problems such as fixations in the maternal link and therefore problems with women in general, not easily reduced. As we see, both roads start with a phallic mother*, and perhaps they are not roads but rather phases in the formation of the ideal. The female ego ideal, like the superego, gradually acquires its definitive form towards puberty; in this sense, the preconscious* part of the ego ideal collaborates more in the labour of working through thought* and female sexuality*. The preconscious bases of the ego ideal are established on its unconscious bases, very important in women, formed in latency* and puberty by virtue of secondary identifications and conscious copies, essentially feminine, more or less facilitated* by those previous infantile experiences.

END OF THE WORLD PHANTASY OR DELUSION

Ger.: Weltuntergang. – Sp.: vivencia del fin del mundo (sepultamiento del mundo). Fr.: expérience de fin du monde. – It.: esperienza di fine del mondo. – Port.: vivência de fim do mundo.

This experience* is produced at the outset of schizophrenic narcissistic psychosis* when libidinal cathexis is withdrawn from thing-presentations* or object presentations*, and the wish* for them is consequently lost.

A clinical result of the phenomenon for which we have given this metapsychological explanation is the subject's growing distance from relationships with objects as if they or the possibility of the link with them were lost forever. For this reason, the subject re-experiences the same feeling of helplessness* that was felt in the birth trauma*. The individual is invaded by tension of need or quantity of excitation*, which is perceived as brutal automatic anxiety*.

Therefore, the subject loses the ability to reach the highest level of binding* of anxiety* (binding with presentations*) such as fear of object loss* or castration anxiety*: signals for the ego* to marshal its defence mechanisms*.

However, the experience of the end of the world is itself a product of a defence mechanism (the unconscious object wish is decathected when the ego is no longer able to bear frustrations* caused by objects previously and actually, resulting from previous narcissistic cathexes stemming from objects and fixations* established very early in life which make self-esteem* very labile): withdrawal of cathexis, common to all repression* (*Repression*, 1915).

Although this repression or defence mechanism is extreme, it fails in this case, since the invasion of automatic anxiety is brutally massive. It results in the loss of psychical organizations because of trouble with them, and therefore the problem grows dramatically.

After the experience of the end of the world, an attempt is made to reconstruct the representational world by creating one more palatable for narcissism (delusions* and other phenomena). Since cathexis was withdrawn from unconscious wish-presentations, the only materials available for this reconstruction are word-presentations* that are cathected (but have lost their unconscious meaning) and are now treated as unconscious thing-presentations were treated before (in primary process*). Then, symptoms* of restitution* appear: hallucinations*, delusions*, and organ speech*.

EPHEMERAL GROUP

Ger.: Glüchtige masse. – Sp. masa efímera. – Fr.: masse ephémére. – It.: massa effimera. – Port.: massa efêmera.

These human groups are formed by an agglomeration of diverse types of individuals sharing a common but generally transitory interest. Freud refers to Le Bon's *The Crowd: A Study of the Popular Mind*, which perhaps considers revolutionary groups, in particular those of the French Revolution. In any case, in our time, we would be inclined to think in terms of social conflicts, sporting events, popular music concerts, and any human group generated spontaneously for a certain reason. Le Bon's view denigrates the acts of groups, attributing to them a tendency to liberation of unconscious* repressed inclinations (cf. repression*), thought* in images, a tendency to action, contagiousness, and loss of intellectual capacity.

Freud shares a good part of Le Bon's view but also recognizes the importance of groups in creations such as language*, folklore, and others. He underscores the importance of the leader and of the link between the leader and each member of the group, which functions through idealization*. The leader occupies the place of the ideal, lifts repressions, and establishes perversions, as does the ideal object*: lovers or hypnotizers in their subjects.

The link between group members functions by identification*; all possess the same ideal: this makes them equals and "brothers" without differences between them. This indiscrimination generates suggestibility and contagion in groups.

EPILEPSY

Ger.: Epilepsie. – Sp.: epilepsia. Fr.: Épilepsie. – It.: epilessia. – Port.: epilepsia.

In *Dostoevsky and Parricide* (1928) Freud mentions hysterical epilepsy and its difference with respect to conversion hysteria*, consisting in a greater degree of ambivalence (referring to love–hate), perhaps with predominance of hate. The repressed in this case is the parricidal wish more than the incestuous wish, although it is still a type of hysteria. The "grand mal", in this perspective, is similar to a hysterical attack; beyond clinical differences, epilepsy presents a predominantly higher degree of masochism and sadism and auto- and hetero-aggression. Freud explains epileptic absences as a realization in the ego of murderous phantasies in relation to the father figure. In this sense it is similar to melancholia, except for a certain degree of conversion* instead of the psychical suffering in melancholia. In any case, Freud's explanation does not refer to essential epilepsy, nor does he elsewhere in his works; however, in some cases it may be highly important to consider this interesting Freudian observation concerning the parricidal phantasy in the "grand mal".

EROS

Ger.: Eros. – Sp.: Eros. – Fr.: Eros. – It.: Eros. – Port.: Eros.

This is the name of the Greek god of love* which Freud utilizes in his second Trieb theory to give a name to life Triebe*: that is to say, sexual Triebe* (in the broad sense given by Freud to sexuality). Life Trieb includes the ego's* self-preservative Trieb*.

Life Triebe or Eros are governed by two principles: the pleasure principle* and its derivative, the reality principle*. Like all Triebe*, they are conservative and tend to re-establish a previous state. Eros endeavours to return to the state of life previous to the stimulus, to return to the quiescence previous to excitation. Since it is impossible to succeed by taking this path, it creates others, more complex convolutions of what it seeks. Other Triebe endeavour to re-establish a state previous to life: to return to the inorganic; Freud calls them death Triebe*. Both types of Trieb endeavour to return to a previous state, the difference being the previous state each seeks, and because of this difference they oppose each other.

Eros tends to unite, to create new and more complex units. In psychical life, it tends to tie quantity of excitation* to presentations*, thereby giving mere quantity presentational quality*, a path aiming towards perceptual quality.

Desire*, an expression of life Trieb, is energy unified with a presentation. Any process tending to interrupt this union – mainly by utilizing unconscious thing-presentations* – seeks to return to mere quantity, the world of the inorganic.

Therefore, Eros enters the second Trieb theory in a complex way, in opposition to death and destructive Trieb. It makes the inorganic more complex, generating what is doubtless the most important complication to emerge from it: life.

EROTOGENIC ZONE

Ger.: erogene Zone. – Sp.: zona erógena. – Fr.: zone érogène. – It.: zona erogena. – Port.: zona erógena.

Any bodily zone may send sexual stimuli to psychical life, and in this sense the whole body is erotogenic, although some zones are more so than others. In the traditional, classical version of these zones, to which Freud contributed evolutionary support, K. Abraham is frankly "evolutionist". For this reason he describes periods (oral, anal, and phallic).

Each erotogenic zone involves a certain type of object* link (for example, whether it is recognized as such or not and to what extent) and a type of pleasure*; its traumatic events (untimely hyper-stimulation of certain zones only apt for stimulation in a deferred* manner becomes traumatic later, when the zone predominates), originating fixation* points with defensive anticathexes* that tend to be utilized in these circumstances. The type of relation established with the object through the erotogenic zones at the beginning of life marks the pathway of subsequent searches; it even in some way determines the predominant type of libido in the subject and therefore also the ulterior type of pathology (whether it involves object or narcissistic libido, for example).

The erotogenicity of the entire body also appears in hypochondria*, which manifests libidinal withdrawal* of cathexis from object* presentations, libido now invested in the body and its organs, felt by the ego* as anxiety* in response to disorders produced by imaginary bodily illnesses.

The magnitude of anxiety in these cases and the irrefutable character of preconscious reasons used to arrest it reveal the proximity of automatic anxiety*, since when the libidinal cathexis is withdrawn from object wishes, anxiety signals* for object* loss, castration*, and fear of the superego* are no longer felt.

The ego is also gradually formed by stimuli sent by erotogenic zones to the psychical apparatus, stimuli at first sent dispersedly (perverse-polymorphously, in Freud's words), the phallic erotogenic zone slowly taking supremacy and unifying them later, whereby they take a decisive step in ego formation. This step coincides with the unfolding of the oedipal period, the culmination of infantile sexuality*.

The erotogenic zone is on the body surface. The pleasurable object link is produced through it, as well as autoerotism*, which mix, since it is very difficult for the ego to recognize the object as foreign to itself. However, they are differentiated first by the initial reality ego* until the definitive reality ego* culminates its formation in the phallic* period.

This formation is strictly concluded after the latency* period in the genital* period during adolescence when events of the infantile period tend to be repeated, sometimes with greater intensity, on account of the possibility of action and the probability of its transformation into real events. These repetitions also leave their traces later in the adult.

ETHICS

Ger.: Ethik. – Sp.: ética. – Fr.: éthique. – It.: etica. – Port.: ética.

Freud did not specifically or theoretically discuss the theme of ethics; at least, this intention was not manifest. However, he did investigate the origins of morals in humanity and in each human being; he considered morals to descend from events that gave birth to humanity in his hypothesis, described in *Totem and Taboo* (1913); that is to say, the prohibition of incest and parricide; individually, the superego's repressive anticathexis*.

However, he was concerned that psychoanalysis as psychotherapy should not lapse into ethical disorderliness given the affective proximity (he called it positive transference*) between therapist and patient, required by the treatment to enable the work of construction to produce psychical change in the patient. In general, ethical failings in the treatment are also technical errors, which is proof of the ethical character of psychoanalytic technique. However, some technical errors are not ethical failings. For this reason and because of the ideal of truth in all psychoanalytic treatment, we consider that this fact in itself is intimately related to an implicit ethical attitude.

What we may unequivocally say is that the growth of their knowledge of their Triebe and unconscious wishes as well as their unconscious need for punishment provide analysands with more weapons with which to make decisions concerning their ethics and to base them on reason. The latter is an ego function. The lifting of repressions does not necessarily produce anti-ethical effects in the patient who, now possessing cathected words, is able to think what was previously repressed, and therefore to decide whether or not to take action by means of thought*, the secondary process. This process takes time, thought involves comings and goings, departures and steps back: a process of working through* which gradually desexualizes the original presentation, thereby diminishing Trieb urgency, thereby enabling the ego to decide more freely. What was sexualized is desexualized (sublimated) and may thus become part of the ego which is then able to tame it and to lead it as a rider does his horse, guiding it to the wished-for destination. Thought is therefore the means by which a wish may access reality through action, a pre-resolved action that will change reality. Therefore, ethics in Freud may be defined on the one hand as eudemonic ethics (those guided by wishes in pursuit of happiness) but also as deontological ethics (those guided by duty), since the happiness sought includes reality on the other hand (with its laws, susceptible to change, susceptible to struggle) and also the categorical imperative of duty towards others. The ego must find a synthesis of these ethical, basically intrapsychical struggles; but to accomplish this, it must know them. This is what psychoanalysis offers.

When individuals expand self-knowledge including their contradictions, when they bring unconscious presentations into the preconscious* and into consciousness*, Freudian psychoanalysis broadens the space of Cartesian and Kantian reasoning, describes a new logic (primary process* logic), and offers a method to transform this logic into reason; the result is that this reason is no longer the same, but now diminishes intrapsychic conflicts (and also conflicts with fellow beings produced by the predominance of projection), thereby improving contact with reality. The place of ethics is in reality (in action with the reality of fellow beings and nature).

EVENLY SUSPENDED ATTENTION

Ger.: Gleichschwebende Aufmerksamkeit. – Sp.: atención libremente flotante. – Fr.: attention (également) flottante. – It.: attenzione (ugualmente) fluttuante. – Port.: atenção equiflutuante.
This is an attitude that Freud advises analysts to take during psychoanalytic sessions, at least at the beginning. Analysts should try to inhibit their aim presentations* and to be equally disposed to register all perceptions* without seeking any in particular; this disposition provides more possibilities to follow the direction of the patient's meanings while leaving aside their own.

This is the technical application of the first level of attention* whose weak cathexis and free displacement leave the way as open as possible to new perceptions, since the wish (in this case the meaning, or perhaps a more repressed level of meaning, of the dream, symptom, or parapraxis) looked for in the patient's associations may be found among them.

Situations analysts seek (which require that they inhibit any active search for their own wish and aim their attention towards everything associated by their patient) indicate meaningful situations brought up by the patient: associations (memories*), dreams*, parapraxes*; all are paths leading to the unconscious. When free association reveals indicators possibly more significant to the patient, the analyst shifts to the second level of attention, which is clearer and more closely focused. Then, attention is copious and its binding is stronger, no longer "free"; expectancy rises, and thought activity utilizes it for its own purposes.

EXCEPTION, CLAIM TO BE AN

Ger.: Ausnahmen. – Sp.: las excepciones. – Fr.: les exceptions. – It.: l'eccezioni. – Port.: as exceções.
Freud described this type of character* trait in 1916, noting that some individuals act as if nature or someone, sometimes undefined and specified in other cases, had done them deep injustice which they must avenge. Others must consequently indemnify them. They expect benefits, privileges, or exceptions. They are usually predominantly narcissistic personalities.

Richard III, Shakespeare's character, in compensation for his ugliness and physical defects, claims the right to commit all kinds of immoral acts to satisfy his ambitious wishes – as if all human beings were indebted to him and he therefore had the right to claim it from them. The narcissistic wound generated by the feminine castration complex* is also fertile ground for cultivation of this type of personality.

Freud explains that

> the claim of women to privileges and to exemption from so many of the importunities of life rests upon the same foundations. As we learn from psycho-analytic work, women regard themselves as having been damaged in infancy, as having been undeservedly cut short of something and unfairly treated; and the embitterment of so many daughters against their mother derives, ultimately, from the reproach against her of having brought them into the world as women instead of as men.
>
> (1916, *Some Character-Types Met with in Psycho-Analytic Work*, p. 315)

In these cases, it is a question of fixations* in the phase when phallic erotism* predominates, in which incipient sexual differentiation depended on the presence or lack of a phallus; at that stage, the feminine was synonymous with castrated. For this castration these women demand compensation from others, especially from their mother.

EXIGENCIES OF LIFE (ANANKÉ)

Ger.: Not des Lebens. Sp.: apremios de la vida. – Fr.: contrainte de la vie. – It.: costrizione della vita. – Port.: premencia da vida.
Also called need. It refers to the breaking of the principle of inertia* to which complex organisms are subject when they receive stimuli from the bodily element: endogenous stimuli that become psychical and are then called

Trieb* which must be discharged since they fight to do so.

The principle of inertia is broken by disequality between the quantity of stimulus provided by need and the quantity of necessary energy the organism possesses in order to satisfy it. Since the latter is lower, a passage to a new level is needed in order to that save energy for carrying out the specific action* at the appropriate time. Therefore, the organism needs to maintain a constant level of energy (principle of constancy*). This quantity of constant energy remains bound to presentations*, giving birth to the psychical apparatus in general and to the ego* in particular.

Energy coming from the body which demands action adequate to an aim probably corresponds to what Freud in *Instincts and Their Vicissitudes* (1915) called the pressure (*Drang*) of Trieb. That is to say, "its motor factor, the amount of force or the measure of the demand for work which it represents. The character of exercising pressure is common to all instincts; it is in fact their very essence" (p. 122).

EXOGAMY

Ger.: Exogamie. – Sp.: exogamia. – Fr.: exogamie. – It.: exogamia. – Port.: exogamia.

Exogamy refers to a social rule or practice by which the sexual object must be chosen from a different clan, tribe, or ascendance, or a different family group. For males, it is

> renunciation of the passionately desired mothers and sisters in the horde – the granting of equal rights to all the members of the fraternal alliance – that is, restricting the inclination to violent rivalry among them.
>
> (*Moses and Monotheism: Three Essays*, 1939, p. 119)

Exogamy, according to Freud, arises as the basic law of human culture* through the prohibition of incest. This prohibition is established when the band of brothers*, having committed parricide and devoured the father of the primal horde*, longs for the father and blames themselves for the crime they have committed. Thenceforward, everything monopolized by the father and forbidden to his sons is prohibited, even repressed and dissolved in each son's psyche: possession of the mother and sisters as sexual objects.

Therefore, exogamy, which in the best of cases had been a punishment for the sons of the primal horde (if they escaped death or castration by their father's hand), is transformed into an inner need following the establishment of the superego*; it is therefore a decisive step, to the extent that we could consider it one of the foundations upon which our present culture was built. The command in favour of exogamy, of which the horror of incest is the negative expression, was a product of the will of the father and carried this will on after he had been removed. Hence come the strength of its emotional tone and the impossibility of finding a rational basis for it – that is, its sacredness (Ibid., p. 121).

EXPECTATION, STATE OF

Ger.: Enwartungs situation. – Sp.: expectación, estado de. – Fr.: expectation, état d'. – It.: aspettazione, stato di. – Port.: expectação, estado de.

This state of hyper-cathexis* of attention* of the ego's perception*-consciousness system (Pcpt.-Cs.) is also heavily cathected with desire* and has the material possibility to put it into action. Expectation may also be described with respect to the situation of danger*. In it, attention is hyper-cathected as indicated by the wish (at the onset), although it is more than attention: it is expectation. An imperious desire (or fear) intensely directs the search for perceptions. That is to say, this wishful hyper-cathexis exists, but in the presence of an ego that inhibits hallucination*; it is hyper-cathected attention in search of signs of quality*. In the state of expectation, the ego searches intensely for something highly wished for and does so while discriminating between phantasy* and reality*, memory* and perception, internal and external worlds. Only real perceptions satisfy it (narcissism* is a refuge when real objects fail), and it proceeds with urgency. It not only discriminates the internal from the external, which is already quality, but also detects signs of quality in relation to things known (remembered) to produce satisfaction, which is discharge*: pleasure*. The ego in a state of expectation is not innocent, simply knowing, but has intentions and takes a precise direction; it does not beat about the bush; it knows what it wants and is on the lookout to "refind" it. It does not hallucinate, nor does it mistake this object for a memory; its perception is ready to effect the specific action* at the right moment.

EXPERIENCE

Ger.: Erlebnis. – Sp.: vivencia. – Fr.: expérience. – It.: esperienza. – Port.: vivência.

Freud does not discuss the term "experience" in isolation, nor does he develop it as a concept in itself; he only describes certain experiences: satisfaction and pain. Since it is implicit in his exposition, we attempt to extract from it what seems important to us in relation to the formation of the psyche.

An experience is lived through, passing through the perception of the senses, through the erotogenic zones. The act of life centres on sensations which are simultaneously registered in connection with whom or what produced them (the object); the object forms psychical presentations* and with them wishes*: wishes that these experiences (satisfaction) may be produced again and others not (pain), wishes represented in the psyche by presentations of objects with which and by which these experiences were produced. This process becomes growingly complex, a multiplicity of concepts coming into consideration; therefore, at some point this basic notion may be forgotten: the notion that the presentation is ultimately the memory* of an experience, mediated and made still more complex by language*.

Although living is a continuum, we arbitrarily separate it into experiences that leave traces in our memory. This arbitrariness is related with the nature of each experience which is specific to each of them but refers to the two major experiences, satisfaction* and pain*. The most intense of these experiences leave the largest trace and induce us to wish for them or to flee from their memory.

The magnitude of an experience is therefore what defines it and its value. At first, this magnitude is purely quantitative, but as complexity increases, experiences are also determined by the qualitative (which results from their comparison with the magnitudes of other experiences) which is ultimately a sophisticated memory of that first quantity, against which it is also a defence.

Since the experience belongs to perception, it also belongs to the present; the perceptual apparatus qualifies the quantities of the external world, perceiving them as certain experiences and not as what they are: "masses in motion and nothing else" (*Project for a Scientific Psychology*, 1895–1950, p. 308). Of course, the object and its action intervene in this qualification (or subjectivation) of the *perceptum*. However, the presentation belongs to the past, to what was experienced, and is wished to return to the present, for which thought* is necessary to determine the relative differences and similarities between the wish, expressed in presentations of the past, and the experience, which is what is perceived in the present. This may succumb to different types of disorders in which the affect gains primacy over this differentiation required of thought, as in the case of transference*, parapraxes*, dreams*, and other phenomena; primary process* infiltrates thought when secondary process* should dominate. At this point we are in the field of psychoanalysis as therapy.

EXPERIENCE OF PAIN

Ger.: Schmerzerlebnis. – Sp.: vivencia de dolor. – Fr.: expérience de douleur. – It.: esperienza di dolore. – Port.: vivência dolorosa.

This type of experience is described by Freud in the *Project for a Scientific Psychology* (1895–1950) and *The Interpretation of Dreams* (1900); it is produced by the invasion of large quantities of excitation* into the psychical apparatus, breaking through the "nerve-ending screens" (1895, p. 306), in 1920 called the protective shield*.

This experience produces in the psychical apparatus: (1) a huge increase in the level of excitation, felt as unpleasure* by consciousness* or the preconscious-conscious system; (2) a tendency to discharge; (3) a facilitation* between the latter and a memory image of the object* that excited this pain*.

Pain possesses a singular quality which places it alongside unpleasure. The image of the object originating the pain persists as the mnemic image of a hostile object. Its memory activates the sensation of pain in an attenuated form as anxiety*. If anxiety is mitigated by presentations binding it, it constitutes the anxiety signal* essential for defence of the ego in response to external danger and the origin of unconscious defence mechanisms in response to Triebe* proceeding from within the body* when the satisfaction of some of these Triebe may produce its anxiety. In general, within the pleasure principle*, an attempt is made to flee from the memory* of the painful experience*.

If this experience is remembered, it may be in order to bind it by relating it with previous presentations* and putting it through the process of thought* with word-presentations* in secondary process*. This attempt to bind is in order to forget afterwards.

The exception is masochism*, especially erotogenic or primary masochism and moral masochism, which have no extra reward of sexual excitation as in feminine masochism.

In the latter, repetition of the experience of pain may involve seeking sexual pleasure.

In moral masochism, pain itself is desired in order to relieve the sense of guilt*.

Therefore, in these cases, the "guardian of life", the pleasure principle, is deadened, resulting in Trieb fusion* and its emerging defusion*.

EXPERIENCE OF SATISFACTION

Ger.: Befriedigungserlebnis. – Sp.: vivencia de satisfacción. – Fr.: expérience de satisfaction. – It.: esperienza di soddisfacimento. – Port.: vivência de satisfação.

Since this is the first type of pleasurable experience*, its main figure an object*, it is paradigmatic; it is subsequently desired, and is experienced in different forms and with different objects in more or less similar ways, at least in terms of sensations sought, for the rest of the subject's life.

Freud discusses it exhaustively in his *Project for a Scientific Psychology* (1895–1950, pp. 317–19) and in *The Interpretation of Dreams* (1900, pp. 565–6). It occurs at a logical moment following the birth trauma* (1925) and internal change* (expression of emotions, screaming, vascular innervation). The object involved performs a certain action that abruptly lowers quantity of excitation* in the nucleus of the ego*, produced by the invasion of Trieb (at first, self-preservative Triebe* which gradually form the anaclisis for sexual Triebe).

This action is provided almost entirely by the object (the baby only needs to suck) given the subject's initial helplessness. "Specific" is the adjective describing this action. It very gradually comes to be carried out by the subject, becoming progressively more complex in the course of life, in correspondence with the different vicissitudes of Trieb*.

The baby's initial helplessness is the cause of all social motivations, since Trieb satisfaction depends from the outset on the object: the subject needs the object, and therefore needs object wishes which it never renounces (1925).

As a result of this experience, a presentation* corresponding to an object together with that of reflex movements effected with this object and those exerted by the object remain on the periphery of the nucleus, in a "place" that Freudian anatomical reminiscences call the *pallium*. The sudden decrease of tension in the nucleus, along with the presentation of the object and these movements, remain mutually facilitated*, constituting a representational complex: the first thing-presentation*. We add: this is a presentation of the thing* that was felt in the experience with the object.

From this moment on, whenever tension arises in the nucleus, it unites with these representations of the object and of movements, thereby originating wishes* for satisfaction or pleasures* that may be obtained with the object. They set psychical functioning into motion.

In his explanation of this experience, Freud succeeds in presenting a simple clarification of the way the *biological* (quantity of excitation proceeding from the body and, we add, inherited representations, for example those of sucking) intertwines with the *social* (extraneous help*: the object), leaving in the apparatus the trace that becomes the *psychical* (the representation* of the object, origin of the wish for it), which interrelate dynamically, giving birth to wishes and to the entire psyche.

Representations remaining from what were perceptions* of objects awaken wishes for them. Representations of the subject's own movements and those of the object in the experience of satisfaction gradually form models of functioning acquired by the ego, thereby generating precursors of the definitive ego that constitute its representations and, later, modalities of its character*.

The actions leading to the experience of satisfaction or pleasure are specific actions* that the ego must gradually learn throughout life.

EXTRANEOUS HELP

Ger.: fremde Hilfe. – Sp.: asistente ajeno. – Fr.: assitant étranger. – It.: assistente altrui. – Port.: assistente alheio.

A term utilized by Freud in the *Project for a Scientific Psychology* (1950 [1895]) to indicate the other, the fellow human being, the mother, whose presence is vital for the helpless child when he shows us how important the presence of the object* is for the structuring of the psychical apparatus.

He also mentions it in *The Interpretation of Dreams* (1900), in *Inhibitions, Symptoms and Anxiety* (1925), and elsewhere.

At the moment of birth, babies enter a state of helplessness* in relation to the quantity of stimuli coming from their own body, their Triebe, and external reality. Quantity of Trieb moves the most primitive process of discharge: internal change* (expression of emotions, screaming, vascular innervation).

This complex, centred on the invasion of quantity of excitation*, in a psychical apparatus too new to bind it owing to lack of life experience, and consequently lacking presentations with which to relate it, is also called the "birth trauma"*.

In babies, internal change is a safety valve. For babies to survive, and for the constitution of the bases of their psychical apparatus, internal change must be transformed into a scream that must be understood by "extraneous help" (that is to say, the attention of no less than the mother or someone carrying out her functions) to cover different kinds of primitive needs, thereby decreasing quantities of excitation: feeding, cleaning, giving warmth and tenderness, and so on. This involves an experience of satisfaction* that leaves deep traces which are foundations of a psyche that becomes growingly complex. The main traces are those of the object: its movements and the feeling of discharge produced in contact with it.

From that time forward, when quantity of excitation reappears in the psychical apparatus already in the process of formation, binding with the memory traces* of previous experience is facilitated. In this way it becomes a psychical wish*-presentation* (a presentation of the wish for the object's presence and the movements to be effected towards the object and with the object in order to obtain the wished-for feeling) of what was quantity of somatic excitation.

Freud's reasoning, which seems biological, is essentially social, or rather an excellent dynamic assemblage of the biological, the social, and the psychological.

This presentation of the object (the extraneous help leading to the experience of satisfaction) is what inaugurates the psyche.

The wish arises when tension due to somatic need reappears, at which time it becomes a wish for the object, partly independent of or parallel to recognition of the object as such by narcissism* then reining in the pleasure ego*.

The thing-presentation* thus founded is principally an object presentation of everything felt with the object. Its presence founds the psyche of the helpless human creature.

F

FACILITATION

Ger.: Bähnung. – Sp.: facilitación. – Fr.: frayage. – It.: facilitatione. – Port.: facilitação.

This concept is utilized by Freud in his *Project for a Scientific Psychology* (1950) to refer to neuronal excitation. In this work, neurones* are classified basically into two types depending on whether they are altered or not when a stimulus passes through them; those that are not altered serve for perception*. Those that do undergo alteration have memory, and are therefore the seat of the psyche. The latter are those destined to be facilitated in different ways, since the passage of a quantity of excitation* has left a trace in them, a trace by virtue of which the next excitation passes more easily, also a trace that attracts other excitations.

If we think about the neurones described by Freud in the *Project* ... as if they were presentations*, the facilitation is at the root of their interrelations, therefore also of memory, and with it, the entire psyche. The concept of facilitation extends, in this line of thought, to psychical associations* and also helps us to understand the Freudian explanation of the conservative tendency (repetition compulsion*) of Triebe* in general, including those ruled by the pleasure principle*. Facilitation therefore consists of what is generated in presentations that is left after the experience of satisfaction* as a desire* to repeat it. It is an expression of the principle of inertia* as the general law of movement, and of the pleasure principle and the reality principle* as the expression of the psyche. It is at the root of repetition compulsion and of the resistance* to change of the unconscious*, attracted by its facilitated archetypes which aim to be repeated beyond the cure.

The experience of pain*, in Freud, leaves an extreme facilitation, perhaps in the sense that one tends to feel pain in response to an experience sharing important points of analogy* or contact with the painful experience, which may provide a base for defence against it.

However, if pain causes such an extreme facilitation, would it not also be connected to the repetition compulsion beyond the pleasure principle, which attracts towards the inorganic, towards quantity, and separates from quality*? In other words: who is guiding repetition? Does repetition take place only through the pleasure principle (repetition of the experience of satisfaction)? Or does the psychical apparatus tend to repeat simply because of facilitation, whether or not it is pleasurable? Or does an attraction to pain and suffering even exist? Freud attempts to give new answers to these questions in 1920 with his hypothesis of death Trieb* and fusions and defusions of Trieb*.

FALSE CONNECTION

Ger.: falsche Verknüpfung. – Sp.: enlace falso. – Fr.: fausse liaison. – It.: allacciamento falso. – Port.: enlace falso.

This type of relation between presentations*, established by superficial associations* (contiguity, analogy*) between their attributes and governed by primary process*, searches for identity between them without subjecting them to examination by reality*.

False connections were described by Freud early in his works, and were replaced by other, slightly different concepts such as displacement*.

False connections are made between unconscious presentations* (for example, displacement in dreams), and consequently some presentations are more highly cathected than others due to an "inversion of psychical values" following lines indicated by censorship*.

False connections are also utilized in defence mechanisms* by the ego* in order to defend itself from the anxiety signal*; for example, displacement to the trivial in obsessional neurosis* or displacement of the original phobia-generating object onto an animal in infantile phobias*.

Once the psychical apparatus is structured, a repressed presentation sometimes manages to transfer its affect* to a preconscious word-presentation* that does not signify it but secretly, by a law of association, refers to it. Then we say that there is transference* from one wished-for presentation to a perception of an actual object, a transference unknown to the ego* and its consciousness*. If they noticed it, they would repress it immediately. Transference is inevitable in psychoanalytic treatment and is sometimes a serious obstacle to its progress. However, it is also the most effective weapon of the cure when it brings the patient to experience, by virtue of an affect perceived in the present, what was felt in the past, which enables the ego to know about it and subsequently tame it.

A false connection is therefore a type of relation between presentations generated by means of codes (laws of association: contiguity, analogy, opposition*). It is the means chosen by primary process to penetrate into secondary process* for the simple purpose of disguising associations as identities. These forms differ from those known by the preconscious ego (thought* activity, secondary process*), with the result that this connection, beyond the knowledge of the ego, is therefore considered "false".

FAMILY ROMANCE

Ger.: Familienroman. – Sp.: novela familiar. – Fr.: roman familial. – It.: romanzo familiare. – Port.: romance familiar.

This group of generally unconscious phantasies* concerning the identity of the individual's real parents is produced in neurotics and also in "normal" persons. Children also have them as soon as they discover their parents' real limitations, for instance that they are not omnipotent as they had believed when they wanted to be adults like their progenitors.

This process develops mainly from prepuberty through late adolescence.

These phantasies are generated when children have experience or knowledge of persons whose attitudes or social positions are superior to those of the children's own parents. An idea forms of being the child of other parents, usually superior in many ways to their own.

In boys, this leads to the development of hostility, more towards their father than their mother. Therefore, they wish to get rid of these depreciated fathers and to replace them with others, thereby also satisfying their envy by the idea of being part of a better family history.

At first, this phantasy is played out on an asexual terrain, but is subsequently sexualized, and since *pater semper incertus est, mater certissima*, the boy accepts being his mother's but not his father's child, thereby triumphing more intensely over the latter in oedipal rivalry.

Then he unconsciously imagines his mother's infidelity and often invents as many amorous adventures as there are rivals (siblings). Being the offspring of different fathers even enables phantasy or sexual games with a sister, resultingly exempt from incestuous barriers.

This phantasy is totally or partially unconscious, since it is expressed towards displaced or disguised figures; however, it always includes denigration of the parents, especially in children at this period of life.

Freud explains that in paranoia*, the family romance becomes absolutely conscious: in this affection, words are not derivatives of unconscious repressed phantasy but are instead preconscious attempts to reconstruct the world through word-presentations* felt to be thing-presentations*. Consequently, the family romance takes on the form of a delusion*, as in the case of Schreber (*Family Romances*, 1909, *Psycho-Analytic Notes on an Autobiographical Account of a Case of Paranoia (Dementia Paranoides)*, 1911), in which the head of the new family is no less than God himself.

FATHER-COMPLEX

Ger.: Vater Komplex. – Sp.: complejo paterno. – Fr.: complexe paternel. – It.: complesso paterno. – Port.: complexo paterno.

The type of relation the son establishes with his father in which feelings of love* and hate* coincide greatly (ambivalence*), this link originates during the positive and negative Oedipus complex* since in both aspects the son feels that danger of castration is presented by the father.

In adults, it is unconscious*, strongly supported by the "bedrock" and the return of the repressed* due to links established with figures corresponding to the paternal line (teachers, leaders, God). Even with the psychoanalyst. In the last case, it may become one of the sturdiest resistances* to the cure.

Products of fixation* to this type of ambivalent link with the original paternal figure appear in transference as fear, defiance, and distrust of any later substitute paternal figure.

The father-complex also plays an important part as the base of the constitution of groups* which involves repetition compulsion* of the history described in Freud's hypothesis: the brothers of the primal horde* murdered their father (parricide) and later established the fraternal alliance*, the genesis of culture*.

The group creates the leader to whom it submits, and at the same time begins to attack the leader, attempting to take over this position.

The father-complex may also be at the base of paranoiac persecution delusion*. It is most clearly observed in obsessional compulsion in which the ego* has an ambivalent relation with the superego* just as the boy had with his father in childhood.

In *The Future Prospects of Psycho-Analytic Therapy* (1910), Freud explains: "in male patients the most important resistances in the treatment seem to be derived from the father-complex and to express themselves in fear of the father, in defiance of the father and in disbelief of the father" (p. 144).

FATHER'S NAME

Ger.: Vatersname. – Sp.: nombre del padre. – Fr.: nom du père. – It.: nome del padre. – Port.: nome do pai.

This is one of the aftermaths of language development, by which the son must carry the father's name* (we now call it the family name), inheriting it in a patrilinear fashion.

It reveals the pride of humanity, expressed in omnipotence of thought*, a product of language development by which the terrain of spirituality was inaugurated, in which presentations*, memories*, and reasoning processes became decisive through opposition to psychical activity limited to immediate perceptions* of sensory organs.

A matriarchal period (cf. matriarchy*) existed after parricide and before the fraternal alliance*. The patriarchal system took over because it meant the triumph of spirituality over sensuality; that is to say, the progress of culture*: "maternity is proved by the evidence of the senses while paternity is a hypothesis, based on an inference and a premiss" (*Moses and Monotheism: Three Essays*, 1939, p. 114).

The feeling of superiority of the spiritual over the sensual is based on narcissistic pride (implicit in culture because the superego's* love for the ego* is greater in narcissistic pride when Trieb is renounced).

> An advance in intellectuality consists in deciding against direct sense-perception in favour of what are known as the higher intellectual processes – that is, memories, reflections and inferences. It consists, for instance, in deciding that paternity is more important than maternity, although it cannot, like the latter, be

> established by the evidence of the senses, and that for that reason the child should bear his father's name and be his heir
>
> (Ibid., pp. 117–18)

If we add to this the importance of the name in the child's and the primitive's thought* and the valence of its thing-meaning, we see how the father's name becomes a source of identification* and paternal inheritance which sometimes generates problems that are ultimately foreign to the subject's own experience and are produced beyond it, as if they were "borrowed" (*The Ego and the Id*, 1923, p. 50, Note). A clinical example is the compulsion* to pay the debt for the eyeglasses that harried the "Rat Man", which was related to a debt of his father's. The father's name the son is to carry forward includes all the meaning this name implies, including its repressed and therefore unconscious histories.

FEAR OF DEATH

Ger.: Todes Angst. – Sp.: angustia de muerte. – Fr.: angoisse de mort. – It.: angoscia di morte. – Port.: angústia de morte.

This is a type of preconscious* realistic anxiety* produced in response to recognition of the existence of the end of individual life, and therefore in response to the near or distant possibility of the subject's own death. It is a form of secondary working through* of fear of the superego*, unconscious* (for example, as fear of fate), and sometimes of fear of castration*, also unconscious (for example, fear of accidents, venereal diseases, and much more).

There is no unconscious thing-presentation* of one's own death, since it could never have been experienced. Presentations* arise from experiences and are ultimately traces of them.

In order to have a notion of one's own death and even of another's, it is necessary to possess word-presentations* that enable preconscious or conscious thought about it.

On this basis, therefore, another's death may be related to one's own, but no more is gained than theories, myths, phantasies, and external presentations created basically by words ("the chill of graves") speaking of death rather than a complete, vivid presentation of what death is that has gone through personal "bodily cathexis" (these are thing-presentations of the unconscious).

Therefore, fear of death is preconscious working through of anxiety.

The anxiety signal* is produced in response to danger. The real danger during the Oedipus complex is castration; before this phase, it had been object loss, and afterwards punishment from the superego; all are consecutive levels of mediation in response to defencelessness* against quantity of excitation* or tension due to need whose prototype is the birth trauma*.

FEAR OF THE SUPEREGO

Ger.: Angst vor den Über-Ich. – Sp.: angustia ante el superyó. – Fr.: angoisse face au surmoi. – It.: angoscia di fronte al super-io. – Port.: angústia frente ao superego.

This is a type of anxiety signal* felt by the ego* when the latter produces defence mechanisms against the Trieb impulse, or rather, against threat of punishment received from the superego* when there is danger of an advance of Trieb coming from the id*. It implies formation of the superego, produced through introjection of parental figures (especially the father) as secondary identifications* prohibiting and punishing Trieb satisfaction. This is the subject's experience of them in infancy. After the dissolution of the Oedipus complex* they become identifications*.

The sole presence of an unconscious wish* (presentation of the cathected object) merits sanctions by the superego. On the one hand, it reinforces the need to ignore it by utilizing the ego's defence mechanisms which are able to bring about ignorance of this wish, which is, however, insufficient for the ego, since the superego's unconscious* aspect grasps the unconscious Trieb wish *in statu nascendi*, with which the ego produces the anxiety signal which thereafter takes on the tone of a sense of guilt*.

Fear of the superego* refers to castration anxiety* in men and anxiety for loss of the object's love* in women, the most feared of all real anxieties* during the period of the Oedipus complex whose dissolution* and repression* originated the superego.

In order to avoid fear of the superego, other defence mechanisms such as judgement of condemnation, isolation, inhibition, even repression, and others may arise.

This type of anxiety signal predominates in obsessional neurosis* in which isolation* and undoing (what has been done) predominate.

In the latest phases of obsessional neurosis, anxiety coincides with the sense of guilt, the ego's guilt before the superego, independent of the facts of reality* (for example, the law). Obviously, fear of the superego also seems to be typical of melancholia*, although in this affection the superego has overpowered the ego and punishes it mercilessly.

Fear of the superego may appear in psychoanalytic treatments in the form of fear of death* or fear of fate, which in reality represent superego punishment.

FEMININE

Ger.: Frauen / weiblich. – Sp.: femenino. – Fr.: féminin. – It.: femmineo. – Port.: feminino.

"Feminine" describes attributes referring to characteristics of women. This does not mean that the feminine is limited to women; all men, even the most masculine, possess feminine characteristics. The adjective "feminine" therefore describes secondary (social) sexual traits and modalities of functioning and relating with others to define gender rather than biological characteristics. This term also refers to cultural and historical characteristics of women, women's ways of acting over long periods of time; for this reason it is sometimes a difficult concept to grasp, since it varies with cultural customs in part, while at the same time retaining an unchanging base.

In the individual, feminine and masculine characteristics are acquired in the course of each person's history; this process involves all the developmental vicissitudes of infantile sexuality, traumatic events experienced in it and fixation points produced in consequence, events of the Oedipus complex, identifications primary to this period of life, and identifications secondary to it. Most commonly, the positive Oedipus complex predominates, and consequently, the masculine predominates in boys and the feminine in girls. However, as experience shows, this does not necessarily occur. Considering the social character of this term, its meaning and value probably change depending on social determinants. The feminine at the dawn of the twentieth century is not the same as at the end of it, although this does not mean that its explanation differs greatly.

When Freud refers to the feminine, he generally considers that it emerges from Triebe with passive aims. This does not exclude the requirement of activity in order to achieve them. For example, it is feminine to seek the object in order to be loved by it (which in reality applies to every human being, feminine or masculine; Freud is referring specifically to the predominant aim in this search); in this sense, needing the object to balance her narcissism* (we could instead say her "self-esteem"*). On the other hand, what characterizes the masculine* starts from an established narcissism and directs an active aim towards the object in order to love it; therefore, his narcissism (we would instead say his self-esteem*) depends less on the object, or at least its love, or its manifestation of love. In this sense, in reference to the Trieb aim, Freud considers that feminine love is narcissistic and depends more on praise from the object to help her overcome the narcissistic wound involved in castration in a previous period of life which, from the repressed unconscious, is endeavouring to transfer into the present.

The feminine may be a characteristic of behaviour, of speech, even a way of thinking, we could even say of an "ideology", but it may also be part of elements emerging from the unconscious such as symptoms. In the "Wolf Man" case, when Freud mentions the three lines of confrontation with castration, he observes:

> In the end there were to be found in him two contrary currents side by side, of which one abominated the idea of castration, while the other was prepared to accept it and console itself with femininity as a compensation.
>
> (*From the History of an Infantile Neurosis*, 1918, p. 85)

Therefore, if we detach ourselves from this case concerning a man, we think that in women the feminine has points of contact with the castrated, even though she overcomes it in the sense of accepting not having a penis; and yet femininity, with all its implications and possibilities (including nothing less than to have children, a real possibility for women, but actually a feminine phantasy which may therefore even become a man's feminine phantasy), involves a greater degree of complexity that women must attain in adolescence when their sexual path leads them to genitality.

The subject of femininity in men is different, as mentioned above. It is generally complementary in male homosexuality, but is not the same, since there are absolutely masculine homosexual men. Of course, heterosexual men have feminine aspects. But we know that the complete Oedipus complex* always exists and with it the possibility that the feminine may correspond to repressed homosexual elements. We could say that feminine elements in men originate in identifications with women in his life or at least with their feminine aspects (the major figure being the mother, although the father may also have feminine aspects). What changes with the times is the degree of social acceptance, in this case of the feminine in men; we could say the same in reference to the feminine in general, with exception of the metapsychological explanation, which remains complex and problematic.

Just a few words about feminine masochism*: it is produced by masochistic perversion. In both men and women, it is described as feminine because of the content of its erotic phantasies (being castrated, being possessed, giving birth, suffering in general, suffering that produces pleasure).

FETISHISM

Ger.: Fetichismus. – Sp.: fetichismo. – Fr.: fétichisme. – It.: feticismo. – Port.: fetichismo.

A certain type of sexual perversion* in men whose female object choice* is governed by the presence of a fetish.

Fetishism is not felt as a discomfort or anything abnormal, not even as a symptom* that might potentially provoke the subject's suffering. It is instead a condition for achieving an erection and, with it, access to pleasure in sexual relations with women. It is therefore appreciated for its contributions to love life.

The fetishist thereby enjoys sexual relations with a female object that must possess a fetish. There are many fetishes, generally consisting in a body part (the foot, nose, braids, and others), clothes (stockings, underwear, furs, shoes, or hats). This feature in the woman provokes his erection. If these details are missing, the symptom of impotence appears.

Analytic treatment reveals that the fetish is a substitute for the woman's phallus. The boy always believed his mother had one, and has not wanted to give up this belief, since this involves the possible existence of castration and the consequent danger to his narcissism*.

It is not an alteration of perception*. Although the fetishist maintains some degree of alienation with respect to knowledge of female genitals, he perceives them. He must take very energetic action in order to support his disavowal*. That is to say, he partly believes in reality* (castration, in the period to which he is still fixated) and partly disavows it. A compromise has formed, following the laws of primary process*: psychically, women have a penis, though not the original one. This substitute inherits the interest once directed towards the original one.

The fetish "remains a token of triumph over the threat of castration and a protection against it. It also saves the fetishist from becoming a homosexual" (*Fetishism*, 1927, p. 154) since his prevailing libido* is homosexual*: object libido not cognizant of sexual difference or an intermediate form between narcissistic and object libido.

The fetish may rarely be chosen in a symbolic way; it usually retrogresses, in the manner of traumatic amnesia, to the moment previous to discovery of the female genital or to what was nearby. This leads to shoes (infantile spying from the floor upwards) or underwear, furs (analogous to pubic hair), and so on.

The fetishist's disavowal produces splitting of the ego*. A split ego accesses exigencies of both the id* and the superego*, and then contradictions are created in secondary process* although they are more limited in the ego than in homosexuality*. Participation in culture avoids social anxiety* involved in the homosexual's participation, although he cannot avoid fear of the superego* or the sense of guilt*, and even castration anxiety*.

In any case, his sexual pleasure* is limited by his dependence on the fetish and so long as this fact is hegemonic, since his libido is predominantly homosexual, it is at risk of narcissistic withdrawal* in response to frustration*. His "health" is precarious, and his need for the fetish may become rigid and acquire characteristics of a ritual or ceremonial, in this sense resembling an obsessional character*.

All this process starts with disavowal and depends on the extent of its use as a defence mechanism* of the ego, whose structure it alters. The more disavowal there is, the more repression* or dissolution* there will be (another solution, of course, is sublimation*), in this case still within the clinical picture of the neuroses or normality.

Fetishism may be combined with debasement of love life* and with sadism*. The subject at this point clearly leads two separate lives concordant with his egos: one life with his phallic and asexual beloved who corresponds to the phallic mother* of infancy, and the other, strictly sexual and also phallic (the fetish), with debasement of the erotic object and sadism or masochism* depending on the amount of homosexuality present.

FIXATION

Ger.: Fixierung. – Sp.: fijación. – Fr.: fixation. – It.: fissazione. – Port.: fixação.

Fixation occurs when development of libido* is arrested by one of the partial aspirations of sexual Trieb*.

Libidinal fixation established in the ego* concerns everything related to the form of satisfaction of an erotogenic zone* to which the libido is fixated (for example, anal-sadistic fixation); fixation is also to certain infantile object* presentations* (for example, incestuous objects in hysteria). Libidinal fixation points are weak points in development, zones that, in a hereditary way or as a result of traumatic experiences, or both at the same time, again dominate a person's psychical panorama when the ego, in response to a frustration*, resorts to regression* as defence against anxiety* re-experienced in the actual phenomenon.

Libidinal regression immediately seeks fixation points. Therefore, libidinal fixation and regression are always two interrelated concepts: the fixation point attracts regression, and regression seeks the fixation point, returning to it. Then, subjects act, feel, and experience object links, their lack, anxieties, or satisfactions, in the same way as in the period of life when the erotogenic zone to which they are fixated was predominant; for example, anal-sadistic regression in obsessional neurosis*.

Traumatic events producing fixations in the different libidinal phases* are generally premature hyper-stimulation of the corresponding erotogenic zones; they may also originate from lack of stimulation, mainly in the earliest stages (deficiencies in the awakening of erotogenic zones by extraneous help*).

We are referring to fixations motivated by untimely hyper-stimulation of the erotogenic zone, when the child's incipient psychical apparatus has not yet acquired thing-presentations* and word-presentations* (the infant acquires them with the traumatic situation*, but they are traumatic, their quantity of excitation carried through time; later, in a deferred reaction to experience*, the corresponding word-presentations are repressed, thing-presentations remaining in the repressed unconscious*) with which to give some binding to the quantity of excitation provoked by the stimulus and some working through of sensations. To the extent that they are not worked through, they become traumatic, reappearing at the corresponding stage with the quantity of excitation* pertaining to the traumatic event.

When fixation may be attributed to traumatic events, the ego resorts to extreme defences* such as anticathexis* (primary repression*), the major mechanism in the formation of fixation.

By virtue of anticathexis, part Trieb* is expelled to the unconscious*, cathecting an opposite presentation (the classical example is reaction formation*, the origin of ego character traits*). With the libido fixated to it and its anticathexis, the repressed presentation remains unconscious. It then pressures to return from the unconscious.

These cases originate neurosis* or character traits. The most intense fixations are the most regressive (to the phase of oral erotism*, autoerotism*, and narcissism*) in which the problem resides more in lack of object stimulus than in hyper-stimulation; the bases for narcissistic regressions are created when the fixation is produced.

Traumatic facts of infantile sexual life have many points of contact with hereditary primal phantasies*. The sexual scene between the parents, seduction by an adult, threat of castration, together with everything related to infantile sexual theories* (the birth of a sibling and discovery of sexual difference) are probably the most common traumatic facts. Depending on the period and the manner in which they occur, they generate fixations to one erotogenic zone or another with its corresponding history.

Fixation is not only the base of transference or defence neuroses* (fixations through anticathexis or primary repression) or narcissistic neuro-psychoses (cases generated more by weakness of object cathexis* due to insufficient stimulus in the subject's history with the object that originated its presentation; we need to recall that the object's love* is the infant's major or perhaps its only defence against helplessness*). It is also the base of perversions* in which anticathexis takes a more complex route, establishing itself on disavowal* of sexual difference instead of on repression* of infantile sexuality*.

FLIESS PAPERS, THE

Ger.: Manuskripte an Fliess. Briefe an Wilhelm Fliess, Abhandlungen und Notizen – Sp.: manuscritos a Fliess. – Fr.: manuscrits à Fliess. – It.: manoscritti a Fliess. – Port.: manuscritos a Fliess.

Fourteen drafts of scientific papers written by Freud between 1893 and 1897 were found in the Freud–Fliess correspondence. They were assigned letters from A to N to identify them.

The first three discuss questions in connection with anxiety* and themes focusing on neurasthenia*, described by Beard, on the basis of which Freud begins to describe a different clinical picture: anxiety neurosis*. The problem of neurasthenia is presented in part by Freud, who generally accepts Beard's description but adds his own attempts to explain its causes. He seeks them in the actual factor of the non-psychical form of sexual discharge. That is to say, Freud considers that somatic sexual tension may not necessarily bind to presentations* or, in any case, produce actual-neurotic consequences, not due to its presentational binding but simply as a mechanical effect of its abnormal discharge or lack of discharge.

In these three drafts, he clearly explains that cathartic therapy does not act on these neuroses but that what produces better effects is prophylaxis of sexual relations. Anxiety neurosis improves only indirectly, through psychotherapy, but not neurasthenia.

Draft D summarizes knowledge of the neuroses and contains theoretical sketches of its aetiology. Some theoretical concepts even appear (such as internal alteration*, specific action*, principle of constancy*) which he discusses more deeply in another draft that is not part of this series: the *Project for a Scientific Psychology* ([1895] 1950).

Draft E is titled "How Anxiety Originates". It is another interesting approach to the problem, with reasoning strongly based on clinical work. On this base, he refutes or deepens theoretical postulates based on observation and varying with it. After various considerations, he comes to a first conclusion: anxiety is engendered by a physical factor of sexual life. But which one? He then discusses all the conditions in which he has observed anxiety for sexual causes: in virgins, in persons with deliberate abstinence or obligatory abstinence, women subjected to interrupted coitus, men who practise interrupted coitus, others who exceed the measure of their desire or strength, and occasionally abstinent men. Since the common factor is abstinence, he concludes that anxiety is caused by an accumulation of physical-sexual tension when its discharge is prevented.

He interpolates in this reasoning a notion of the mechanism of melancholia*. Melancholics tend to suffer from anaesthesia: they feel no need of coitus but do have great longing for love "in its psychical form". Thus subjected to deep psychical erotic tension, when it accumulates and is not satisfied, melancholia develops.

Then, physical-sexual tension leads to anxiety neurosis and accumulation of psychical sexual tension (apparently, the need to be loved without having coitus, a need for tenderness or to be valued, something we could assume to be related with the ego ideal*) generates melancholia.

He then discusses endogenous tension (hunger, thirst, sexual instinct), a term which later acquires theoretical status as Trieb* (self-preservative Trieb* and sexual Trieb*). He anticipates concepts in the *Project* ... when he states that this tension is discharged by specific actions. It is noticed when it accumulates and reaches a certain threshold at which it binds to presentations, working itself over psychically and thereby organizing itself into a specific action. If this action is prevented, physical-psychical tension (sexual* or sensual affect) grows out of proportion. A disturbance is felt then, but not yet anxiety. In anxiety neurosis it is transformed into anxiety.

> The psychical tension increases, reaches the threshold value at which it can arouse psychical affect; but for some reasons the psychical linkage offered to it remains insufficient: a sexual affect cannot be formed, because there is something lacking in the psychical determinants. Accordingly, the physical tension, not being psychically bound, is transformed into – anxiety.
>
> (1892–9 [1950], p. 193)

This explanation is similar to another in *Inhibitions, Symptoms and Anxiety* (1925) regarding automatic anxiety* in response to quantity of excitation* when the latter destroys other types of anxiety (anxiety signals* of castration*, loss of love*, and object* loss) interposed as mediating signals to prevent its entry; when presentational quality* is lost and the psychical apparatus is invaded by quantity of excitation. The draft goes on to state that then, anxiety neurosis exhibits a deficit of sexual affect; that is to say, of psychical libido*, which is observable and is illustrated by several examples.

It concludes with theoretical reasoning stemming from the foregoing; it is followed by an interesting explanation of the way accumulated tension is transformed precisely into anxiety.

> Anxiety is the sensation of the accumulation of another endogenous stimulus, the stimulus to breathing, a stimulus which is incapable of being worked over psychically apart from this; anxiety might therefore be employed for accumulated physical tension in general.
>
> (Ibid., p. 194)

The physical manifestations of anxiety – dyspnoea, palpitations, the feeling of anxiety – are also paths taken normally by physical-sexual tension when it may be and is psychically worked through. Dyspnoea and palpitations are simply concomitants of coitus as subsidiary paths of discharge in it. In our case, they become facilitated paths for discharge of excitation. Something similar to a conversion* is produced, except that it is of physical tension, unlike hysteria, in which it is psychical tension (with presentational cathexis*).

Draft F narrates a clinical case of anxiety neurosis* in which Freud discusses whether or not anxiety is hereditary, and another case of what he refers to as periodical dysthymia or melancholia, which he tries to differentiate from neurasthenia.

Draft G describes melancholia, which Freud again relates with sexual anaesthesia. The specific affect of the melancholic is the same as in mourning* or grieving; that is to say, longing for something lost. What was lost? A part of Trieb life, its Triebe* and desires*. He takes anorexia as clinical grounding: "Loss of appetite: in the sexual, loss of libido". This clinical observation reveals the importance in his theories of infantile sexuality, information officially lacking until

Three Essays on the Theory of Sexuality (1905). He concludes his early reasoning with this statement: "melancholia consists in mourning over loss of libido" (Ibid., p. 201).

He draws the "diagram of sexuality": an initial schema of the psychical apparatus in which limits are clearly marked to differentiate the organic from the psychical (presentational), the external world with the object* as its only figure, the specific action*, ego* boundaries, and sensations. We could think that Freud basically never changed this schema in all his works; in any case, he worked to add complexity (to the nth degree) to what he designates here as a "psychical group"; however, as for the rest, with few exceptions, the relation between the psychical and the organic remains the same to the end.

He also mentions voluptuous feelings, interconnected somato-psychically, which are absent in anaesthesia. "The voluptuous feeling is measured by the amount of unloading" (Ibid., p. 203).

He describes different types of anaesthesia and melancholia. Melancholia is related with absence of somatic excitation, whereas anaesthesia is related with lack of voluptuousness (we recall that voluptuousness originates in the somatic and culminates in the psychical group according to this schema). In any case, anaesthesia is also a forerunner of melancholia. He concludes with this description of melancholia: "psychical inhibition with instinctual impoverishment and pain concerning it" (Ibid., p. 205).

> We can imagine that, if the ps. G. [psychical sexual group] meets with a very great loss in the amount of its excitation, there may come about an in-drawing (as it were) in the psychical sphere, which produces an effect of suction upon the adjoining amounts of excitation.
>
> (Ibid.)

The neurones* (which we consider presentations) give up their excitation, producing pain*. The process of drawing-in (the description is similar to what he later calls narcissistic "withdrawal" and utilizes as an analogy* in *On Narcissism: An Introduction*, 1914: it acts like a wound, attracting cathexes. The opposite process occurs in mania* in which excess excitation extends to all associated neurones.

As we see, this is a basically physiological explanation involving sexuality*, but also a "psychical group" (presentations, phantasies), the object, action, and other elements which increasingly take Freud into psychology.

Draft H. Paranoia. In this essay, in opposition to classical psychiatry, he presents an almost purely psychological theory of paranoid delusion, which he considers on a par with obsessional neurosis*, even hysteria* and acute hallucinatory confusion (Meynert's amentia), in terms of pathological modes of defence*. Paranoid delusional ideas are a consequence of affective disorders whose force is due to previous conflictive psychological processes not tolerated by the subject and from which the subject defends him or herself.

He presents the case of a thirty-year-old woman who, sometime after suffering an attempted traumatic seduction, developed a delusion of observation and persecution. Freud is unable to help her to remember the traumatic event. The patient defends herself, and does not want to remember it; but what is it that distinguishes paranoia* from other neuroses? This woman was avoiding the reproach of being a "bad woman", but this reproach was reaching her ears from outside. Thus, the content remained unchanged, but something in the placement of the whole matter changed: judgement of her was transposed to the outside, from where it could be rejected. The judgement or reproach was kept apart from the ego.

"The purpose of paranoia is thus to fend off an idea that is incompatible with the ego, by projecting its substance into the external world" (Ibid., p. 209).

Strachey points out that in this letter (1895), projection* is mentioned for the first time as a type of defence. Freud states that it is a very common mechanism in normal life, that even a certain observation delusion is normal so long as we remain conscious of our own internal modification.

> If we forget it and if we are left with only the leg of the syllogism that leads outwards, then there we have paranoia, with its overvaluation of what people know about us and of what people have done to us. What do people know about us that we know nothing about, that we cannot admit? It is, therefore, abuse of the mechanism of projection for purposes of defence.
>
> (Ibid.)

He then reviews different types of paranoia and concludes that the delusional idea is supported by the same energy with which another idea, intolerably painful, is expelled from the ego.

"Thus they love their delusions as they love themselves. That is the secret" (Ibid., p. 212). Here we find an interesting list which differentiates pathological entities:

In *hysteria*, the irreconcilable idea is not admitted to association with the ego. It is removed from associative commerce outside of consciousness*. The affect* is displaced (cf. displacement*) by conversion to the somatic sphere.

*Obsessional idea**: the incompatible idea is also refused admission to association (with the ego). The affect is preserved, but its content is substituted.

*Hallucinatory confusion**: the entire incompatible idea – its affect and content – is excluded from the ego and partially detached from the external world. Hallucinations are agreeable to the ego and support the defence.

*Paranoia**: Both content and affect of the incompatible idea are preserved, but are projected into the external world. These hallucinations are hostile to the ego although they support the defence. In *hysterical psychoses** the rejected ideas acquire predominance and may acquire a paroxysmal type: the "second state". These hallucinations are hostile to the ego.

Draft I discusses migraine. Freud observes that it is produced by summation during the period he calls "sexual" (neither in childhood nor in senescence), and is relieved during pregnancy. He explains it as a toxic chemical effect produced by stimulation of sexual substance to which a particular path of conduction is added. The rest of his reasoning is neurophysiological.

Draft J concerns a clinical case of conversion hysteria*. Frau P.J., aged twenty-seven, suddenly feels ill in the abdomen and stomach, and her head swims. The fear of going mad becomes an anguishing obsession.

Freud believes it is an attack of anxiety over sexual longing* for her husband who had gone on a trip. He continues to question her, searching for accessory details of the episode. The patient tells him that she had been singing Carmen's aria entitled: "Près des remparts de Séville". Freud wishes to know the contents of the aria, thinking about a train of ideas awakened by the song's lyrics. He forces association* by the method of pressure on the forehead, to which "husband" and "longing" arise. He insists. Freud defines what has happened to the patient as a state of "outpouring of love", longing provoked by the husband's absence. In a second session the patient arrives, reticent and sceptical about the treatment: her "resistance was already stirred up and progress was far more difficult". Finally, the patient tells him that she had had a similar attack before, and slowly brings up memories* from her life before marriage, when she was a singer. Her former companions led a licentious life. Their "touching" and kisses were repugnant to her. At rehearsals, the tenor tried to touch her breast. On one of these occasions (when he probably went further than before, or she was less repulsed), she had an attack two days afterwards.

Freud simply describes the case and does not theorize on it; we see how he reconstructs the history and gradually finds the meaning of the desire hidden behind the symptom*, although it is not entirely clear or explicit.

Draft K (January 1, 1896). *The Neuroses of Defence (A Christmas Fairy Tale)*. This essay was written after *The Neuro-Psychoses of Defence* (1894) and before *Further Remarks on the Neuro-Psychoses of Defence* (1894) which it resembles in regard to its overall structure and themes discussed.

Freud states that neuroses of defence are pathological aberrations of normal psychical states: of conflict (hysteria), self-reproaches* (obsessional neuroses), mortification (paranoia), and mourning (acute hallucinatory amentia). They lead to permanent damage to the ego. They appear in the same circumstances as their affective prototypes, so long as their determination includes two other conditions: that their character is sexual and that they occur before sexual maturity.

The defensive tendency is utilized against presentations or memories of experiences, especially those capable of causing actual unpleasure*. It is therefore aimed basically against sexual presentations, since other types of presentation become diluted in time.

One condition must be met: that between this experience and its repetition in memory, puberty must intervene, a factor that intensifies the effect of remembering. The psychical mechanism does not seem to be prepared to face this "intensified" memory and must resort to an extreme, pathological defence.

Freud wonders about the origin of unpleasure caused by premature sexual experience. He rejects shame and morality as repressing forces, as well as physical proximity between the anus and the genitals (Freud has not yet discovered infantile sexuality), since when libido is sufficiently intense, repugnance is not felt and morality is easily overcome, although he thinks that shame is more intimately connected with sexuality. Finally, he presents the hypothesis that sexual life must involve an independent source if it is to provoke unpleasure.

He outlines the typical course of a neurosis of defence. First there is a premature and traumatic sexual experience which is repressed. Then, another experience, for whatever reason, evokes the memory of the first experience and is therefore also repressed, thereby generating a primary symptom. This is followed by a phase of effective defence which appears as normal health except for the primary symptom. Finally, a phase follows in which the repressed ideas return (cf. return of the repressed*) and new symptoms are formed in the midst of struggles between these and the ego, symptoms which constitute the neurosis proper.

The difference between the various neuroses resides in the way repressed ideas return, symptom formation*, and also the course of the illness. The specific character of these diverse neuroses therefore lies in their dissimilar modes of repression*.

In *obsessional neurosis** the primary experience was accompanied by pleasure*. When it is remembered in a deferred* manner, it provokes unpleasure* in the form of self-reproaches*. The memory and the self-reproach are repressed and in their place an antithetic symptom is formed: conscientiousness.

In the phase of return of the repressed, the self-reproach also returns unchanged, at first in the form of a sense of guilt*; then, in response to the results of the reproached act, its affect is transformed into anxiety*, hypochondria*, or fear of somatic consequences, a persecutory delusion or fear of social effects: shame or fear that others might discover the reproached act.

The conscious ego finds the obsessional idea foreign to itself, disbelieves it, based on previous conscientiousness (an ego characteristic), and subjects it to logical criticism although its compulsive force is immovable.

Then, three types of symptoms are produced: (1) the primary symptom of defence: conscientiousness; (2) compromise symptoms: obsessional ideas or acts; (3) secondary defence symptoms: obsessional brooding, hoarding, dipsomania, ceremonials.

> Obsessional neurosis can be cured if we undo all the substitutions and affective transformations that have taken place, till the primary self-reproach and the experience belonging to it can be laid bare and placed before the conscious ego for judging anew. In doing this we have to work through* [Durcharbeiten] an incredible number of intermediate or compromise ideas which become obsessional ideas temporarily ... resistance during therapeutic work avails itself of every possible motive of defence.
>
> (Ibid., p. 226)

With respect to *paranoia*, he states that the primary experience seems to be similar to the one in obsessional neurosis: repression takes place once the memory of the primary experience leads to a release of unpleasure through an unknown mechanism. This unpleasure is attributed to others by projection*. The primary symptom formed is distrust (sensitiveness to others). There are diverse types of paranoia* depending on whether only the affect of the experience or its content as well have been repressed by projection.

What returns is therefore the painful affect or also the memory. In the latter case, the experience returns as a visual or tactile hallucination. The affect always returns in the form of hallucinations with perception of voices. In all cases, memories return deformed by analogous images from actual life and by chronological displacement rather than by substitute formations*. The voices represent the return of self-reproaches in the form of a compromise symptom, deformed and related to the primary symptom (distrust) instead of the primary experience.

These patients deny the self-reproach, but do not consider it foreign. They are forced to explain it by an assimilation delusion, precipitating an alteration of the ego*: the ego is being dominated. These deformations are gradually believed, forming delusions of protection, until the ego is finally completely remodelled.

Thus, we find four types of symptoms in paranoia: (a) primary defensive symptoms; (b) return of the repressed characterized by compromise; (c) secondary defensive symptoms; and (d) symptoms of the ego's submission.

Hysteria implies an unpleasurable, passive primary experience. "The natural sexual passivity of women explains their being more inclined to hysteria" (Ibid., p. 228).

The primary experience of hysteria must not occur too early, in a period when release of unpleasure would still be too small.

> Hysteria begins with the overwhelming of the ego, which is what paranoia leads to. The raising of tension at the primary experience of unpleasure is so great that the ego does not resist it and forms no psychical symptom but is obliged to allow a manifestation of discharge – usually an excessive expression of excitation. This first stage of hysteria may be described as "fright hysteria"; its primary symptom is the manifestation of fright accompanied by a gap in the psyche.
>
> (Ibid.)

Repression and defensive symptom formations come later, in relation to the memory. The defence and the overwhelming of the ego provoke symptoms and precipitate attacks*. Repression is achieved by reinforcing a "boundary idea" which belongs, on the one hand, to the conscious ego and, on the other hand, to an undistorted part of the traumatic memory. This boundary idea results from a compromise through displacement of attention on to different ideas which are related by their temporal simultaneity.

Draft L. This draft and the following two, M and N, are simply outlines of ideas or small lines of thought on different and apparently only loosely connected subjects.

In "The Architecture of Hysteria", Freud sketches an interesting theory of memory which remains present throughout Freudian thought.

The objective (it is unclear of what, whether of Trieb in the sense of repetition [cf. repetition compulsion*] or, it would seem, of treatment seeking the memory* and working it through) consists in reaching the primal scenes. He is certainly referring to the primary traumatic experiences of the previous drafts whose memory the defence is preventing; he is not discussing the primal scene* as the primal phantasy* of viewing parental coitus, a later concept in his theory, although this primary scene might well be the primal scene. In some cases the memory is attained directly and in others by way of lengthy detours through phantasies*. The latter are psychical façades erected to block access to these memories and also to refine or sublimate them. They are constructed with things heard and applied only subsequently, thereby combining the experienced with the heard, the past (of parents' and forebears' history) with what the subject has witnessed (the subject's own past).

Then he discusses the role of female servants in neurosis. "There is tragic justice in the fact that the action of the head of the family in stooping to a servant-girl is atoned for by his daughter's self-abasement" (Ibid., p. 249).

The father's attitude generates certain problems in his daughter, such as phobias* or fears of prostitution (fear of being alone in the street).

He also mentions examples of explanatory associations of meanings of diverse behaviour. He mentions identification* in relation to multiplicity of psychical persons (multiple personality, now considered "borderline" patients).

Finally, he returns to the subject of phantasies and the way they are constructed:

> It is possible to follow the path, the time and the material of the construction of phantasies. It is then seen closely to resemble the construction of dreams. But there is no regression in the form [of presentation] phantasies are given, only progression.
>
> (Ibid., p. 250)

Draft M. As we said, these notes beginning here on the architecture of hysteria continue to refer to what Freud refers to in these manuscripts as primal experiences; he mentions that some are accessible directly, whereas others may be reached only by going through superimposed phantasies.

> The scenes are arranged in the order of increasing resistance: the more slightly repressed ones come to light first, but only incompletely on account of their association with the severely repressed ones. The path taken by [analytic] work first goes down in loops to the scenes or to their neighbourhood; then from a symptom a little deeper down, and then again from a symptom deeper still. Since most of the scenes converge on the few symptoms, our path makes repeated loops through the background thoughts of the same symptoms.
>
> (Ibid., p. 251)

He returns to this subject later: "Phantasies arise from an unconscious combination, in accordance with certain trends, of things experienced and heard. These trends are towards making inaccessible the memory from which the symptoms have emerged or might emerge" (Ibid., p. 252).

The first type of deformation consists in a process of fragmentation, totally disconnected from chronological relations (these seem to depend on the system of consciousness*).

> A fragment of the visual scene is then joined up with a fragment of the auditory one and made into the phantasy, while the fragment left over is linked up with something else. In this way it is made impossible to trace an earlier connection. As a result of the construction of phantasies like this (in periods of excitation) the mnemic symptoms cease. Instead, unconscious fictions are present which are not subjected to defence. If now the intensity of such a phantasy increases to a point at which it would be bound to force its way into consciousness, it is repressed and a symptom is generated through a backward impetus (*Rückdrängung*) from the phantasy to its constituent memories.
>
> (Ibid.)

Then, he postulates different types of compromise displacement*; by association: hysteria.

By conceptual analogy: obsessional neurosis. By causal relation: paranoia.

He adds: "Further, that repression proceeds backwards from what is recent, and affects the latest events first" (Ibid., p. 253).

He continues: "It is not sufficient to take into account the repression between the preconscious and the unconscious; we must also consider the normal repression within the system of the unconscious itself. Very important, but still very obscure" (Ibid.).

What does Freud mean at this point when he refers to the "unconscious system"? If we consider that he completed the conceptualization of the preconscious* and unconscious* systems in 1915, and understanding the meaning of this statement within the limits of this conceptualization, it is unclear at this moment in his theory where repression is placed within the unconscious system; unless he is referring to repression as a defensive mechanism of the unconscious ego, a problem he resolves in 1925 in *Inhibitions, Symptoms and Anxiety*, or unless he has not yet clearly defined the concept of the unconscious. At this time, it is taking shape, but we are surprised to note that theoretical developments he resolves much later are outlined here.

Draft N. He continues with notes on hostile impulses towards the parents as elements in neurosis. These impulses come to light consciously in obsessional neuroses. In paranoia they are expressed as persecutory delusions; in mourning and melancholia as self-accusations, and in hysteria as self-punishment. In these latter cases, the phenomenon of identification appears. Although aggression* is not missing, the theme is sexual and refers to the sexual rival in general: the boy against his father, the girl against her mother, which announces what is later the Oedipus complex*, the core complex of the neuroses.

Then he discusses beliefs*, a phenomenon belonging to the ego. In neurosis it is displaced to the defence mechanism, in which the ego believes as something of its own, something natural rather than defensive (for example, disgust* or shame*). In contrast, what it defends against remains unknown, or else the ego does not believe it or acquiesce to it.

In this draft, Freud relates phantasy with literary creation, in reference to Goethe and his *Werther*, subjects he develops in later works. He also states that symptoms, like dreams*, are wish fulfilment. He refers to "saintliness" as a form of resignation of sexual perversions*: that incest is antisocial and culture* is strengthened by progressive renouncement of it.

FORECLOSURE OR REPUDIATION

Ger.: Verwerfung. – Sp.: desestimación. – Fr.: forclusion. – It.: reiezione. – Port.: desestimação (rejeição ou repúdio).

This is a mechanism for nonacceptance of a new fact of reality* considered unimportant by the conscious ego* which this ego fails to study sufficiently to exercise judgement, instead retaining previously established judgements*.

This rejection of judgement of existence* is universal and "normal" in childhood. Children are reluctant to recognize sexual difference or castration in the stage of predominance of phallic eroticism*. The cloacal theory* had explained the birth of children in a much less conflictive way. In general, children react to the threat of castration like Little Hans (*Analysis of a Phobia in a Five-Year-Old Boy*, 1909): when threatened with the loss of the "peepee-maker" he was not anxious because he still had the "pooper" (in theoretical terms, the cloacal theory).

Acceptance of the possibility of castration is the next step, a gradual and perhaps forever incomplete acceptance.

The cloacal theory is partly overcome when the existence of castration is recognized, though never absolutely, in the phallic stage; it partially remains in the repressed unconscious* together with everything related to infantile sexuality*. It may return, for example, as an intestinal symptom* with phantasies* of pregnancy (the "Wolf Man") or as any other product of the unconscious.

When children recognize the existence of castration, even partially – which becomes inevitable upon perception of female genitals and understanding* of the difference through the fellow being complex* – they enter the castration complex*. A multitude of excitations and affects* are then connected to loss of the penis; this is the case of castration anxiety* in boys and penis envy* in girls.

The "Wolf Man's" famous dream is one proof that the boy had entered the castration complex, at least at the moment of the dream. Therefore, he had partly overcome its initial foreclosure*, although the cloacal theory on which it was established could return at any time and even coexist with recognition of sexual differences that generated castration anxiety. Thus, in one conversion symptom, recognition of sexual difference (anxiety in regard to dysentery) coexisted with the cloacal theory (the unconscious phantasy of intestinal pregnancy). The latter included recognition of sexual difference since the anus was recognized as if it were a vagina (because of the dysentery, blood issued from his anus as in his mother's menstruations), which generated renewed castration anxiety since the boy understood the vagina as castration, which apparently created contradictions which, as we know, have a place in the unconscious. These contradictory presentations continued to belong to the unconscious and were able, by virtue of these substitute formations* – intestinal pregnancy symbolized by constipation – to access the preconscious in disguise.

Trieb motions are also foreclosed or repudiated whenever they are conscious or have a preconscious cathexis (a word-presentation*, cathected or not with attention*).

In this case the ego may foreclose or repudiate them by emitting judgement condemning them. Judgement of condemnation* is one of the last defences* the ego uses against Trieb* once it has overcome negation* and the ego has accepted this Trieb as its own; it is perhaps the most highly developed defence mechanism and the one most closely related to binding* and mastery of Trieb*.

Freud considers disavowal* the nonacceptance of facts of reality, such as the existence of sexual difference (partial nonacceptance in sexual perversions*) or of facts of a painful reality (such as loss of a loved one in Meynert's amentia*). In both cases, flat denial of certain facts of reality is produced, and they are covered up with a different perception*: the fetish in fetishism*, the penis in homosexuality*, and hallucination of the lost object in amentia.

FORE-PLEASURE

Ger.: Vorlust. – Sp.: placer preliminar. – Fr.: plaisir préliminaire. – It.: piacere preliminare. – Port.: prazer preliminar.

This type of pleasurable discharge is produced by stimulation of erotogenic zones* predominant in the individual's prehistory before genital primacy developing during the period of adolescence but with a precedent in the phallic stage. We are referring to erotism of Trieb for seeing, oral* cannibalistic erotism, anal* sadomasochistic, even phallic-urethral* and other pregenital erotisms.

In childhood, fore-pleasure is part of normal development of erotogenic zones. At first they act in an isolated manner, separate from others, one predominating over the others (the origin of the names of the different phases of infantile sexuality*: oral, anal, and others). In the phallic phase, this erotogenic zone begins to predominate over the former ones, mainly in boys, because of the quantity and quality of feeling originating in it and the type of attraction to the object it creates, together with autoerotic pleasures* experienced. This predominance is so great that it subsumes the other zones, presides over them, and gives them unity, a unity leading to an aim. This predominance permits the union of all these sensations in the same body, thereby definitively forming a reality ego* which has been waiting for this moment to become a reality ego.

By virtue of puberty and adolescent development, aptitude for reproduction, and the voluptuous sensation of genital orgasm, phallic primacy becomes genital primacy. At this point its primacy is absolute. Genital discharge results from the definitive pleasure of sexual Trieb*. Therefore, both the previous period in the object relation or even masturbatory play should be unpleasurable (due to an increase of tension and lack of genital discharge). However, not only is it not unpleasurable, but it is also proof of evolutionary development of sexual Trieb, since each erotogenic zone has its own level of small pleasurable discharge or fore-pleasure, participating in the path leading to final pleasure.

Approach to the sexual object goes through all the steps of infantile sexuality (except those repressed most successfully and therefore unknown to the official ego). It generally begins with sight, the pleasure of seeing, then goes through the different erotogenic zones with their forms of object relation. Stimulation of each zone generates some fore-pleasure, while at the same time unpleasurable tension is created in relation to the genital so long as final discharge has not been reached.

Sometimes, stimulation of the pregenital erotogenic zones may be sufficient (in this case, rather than fore-pleasure it becomes final pleasure, configuring a certain type of sexual perversion*), or this stimulation, instead of pleasure, may cause anxiety* or some other unpleasurable feeling such as disgust* or shame* (neurosis* or "normality").

The origin of different sensations that may be felt upon stimulation of erotogenic zones is partly hereditary, but is mainly related to history experienced through them by the subject in the object relation: fixation* points formed during the development of sexuality* in them (in the erotogenic zones and in presentations* of these objects and their forms of relation with them). These fixations are products of traumatic events occurring in the link with objects of infantile prehistory.

If the quantity of stimulus that penetrates the psychical apparatus exceeds its possibilities of binding*, in traumatic neuroses, a compulsion* to repeat the scene remains, first in dreams*, and may even reach actions, in an effort to force the psychical apparatus, through repetition, to feel the anxiety signal it did not feel when the last barrier was broken through. It may also do this merely to repeat, in a demonic (death Trieb*) manner.

FORGETTING

Ger.: Vergessenheit / Vergeßlichkeit. – Sp.: olvido. – Fr.: oubli. – It.: dimenticanza. – Port.: esquecimento.

This disturbance of conscious memory*, transitory and functional, is not produced by organic causes. It consists in the impossibility to repeat a name or a word, to carry out a required action or a plan. Forgetting is the most common parapraxis* in normal persons, especially of proper names.

We describe this phenomenon clearly. During a conversation we cannot remember a name which we know quite well, which provokes the excitation of unequivocal anger "similar to that of motor aphasics" (Freud, 1901). Energetic efforts of attention* are impotent to retrieve the lost name as long as this endeavour continues. Also, instead of the name being sought, another comes to mind, recognized as being incorrect, but nonetheless persistent. Some letters or a syllable may come to mind, identified as parts of the forgotten name.

> The mechanism of names being forgotten (or, to be more accurate, the mechanism of names escaping the memory, of being temporarily forgotten) consists in the interference with the intended reproduction of the name by an alien train of thought which is not at the time conscious. Between the name interfered with and the interfering complex either a connection exists from the outset, or else such a connection has established itself, often in ways that appear artificial, via superficial (external) associations.
>
> (*The Psychopathology of Everyday Life*, 1901, pp. 39–40).

The most disturbing complexes are those referring to the subject (attacks on narcissism*).

> A name which has more than one meaning and consequently belongs to more than one group of thoughts (complexes) is frequently interfered with in its connection with one train of thought owing to its participation in another, stronger complex. Among the motives for these interferences the purpose of avoiding arousing unpleasure by remembering is conspicuous.
>
> (Ibid., p. 40)

Two causes may be found: the name itself touches on something unpleasant (which produces a secret aversion in the subject, for example) or it is connected with another having the same effect, so that remembering some names may be disturbing in their own right and others due to nearer or more distant associative ties.

The forgetting of proper names is highly contagious, and this contagion may involve identification*.

The example of Signorelli is classical. Freud, travelling by train, converses with his seatmate about Turks living in Bosnia and Herzegovina (places the train was passing through at the time) concerning death, which they accept with total resignation. He associates with an attitude of the Turks in relation to sexuality, absolutely not resigned; he suppresses this thought and decides not to mention it, since he was still affected by an event that occurred a few weeks previously during a brief stay in Traffoi.

A patient he was interested in had committed suicide because of an incurable sexual disturbance. However, Freud did not consciously remember this episode at any time during this journey.

The conversation continues. They turn to the subject of Italian painting, and it is then that Freud tries to remember the name of the painter of the frescoes in the cathedral at Orvieto on "the last things" (Death, Judgement, Heaven, and Hell). Freud pressures his memory, remembers all the details of the day he spent in Orvieto, remembers the paintings with more sensory detail than usual, and in particular the painter's self-portrait – the severe expression, the hands folded together – placed in one of the corners of the paintings, but the artist's name continues to escape him. Then the names of *Botticelli* followed by *Boltraffio* come to mind. This episode lasts for a while until a cultured Italian tells him: *Signorelli* and Freud immediately remembers even his first name, *Luca*, which indicates how familiar it was to him.

It is interesting that he states that remembering the name involved a sudden fading of his hyper-clear memory of the artist's faces painted on the fresco.

Freud utilizes this example to explain quite clearly how the mechanism of repression*, the origin of forgetting, is produced. He shows the associations* between the *Signor* of *Signorelli*, the respectful *Herr* (Sir) of the Turks when addressing their doctors and *Herzegovina*, the subject of the Turks leads to sexuality and death and to the patient who committed suicide for sexual reasons (not remembered at any time). From *B*osnia the association is with *B*otticelli, also because like *Signorelli* it ends in *elli*. Also associated with *B*osnia is *B*oltraffio, also related with *Traffoi* in its last syllable, the place where he had received the tragic news about his dear patient. Through this tangle of superficial linguistic connections, the word *Signorelli*, which carries these multiple connections, and is therefore a derivative of something repressed, is decathected (cf. decathectization*) in order to be cathected (cf. cathexis*), instead, with *Botticelli* and *Boltraffio*, which now act as anticathexes, since so long as they are in place, the repressed is sure not to return, and so long as the attention of the preconscious ego* continues to be directed at them, success of repression is doubly ensured.

Conscious remembering needs words since, despite the hyper-clear memory of the image, the place of the word indicates forgetting. It is also important to point out that in the example of patients who forget having had illnesses, usually not valued socially and causing narcissistic wounds, Freud mentions disavowal* as a generator of forgetting, as not wanting to know, with an energetic refutation concerning wounded narcissism.

FRATERNAL ALLIANCE, BAND OF BROTHERS

Ger.: Brüder Bündnis, Brüderbund. – Sp.: alianza fraterna. – Fr.: alliance fraternelle. – It.: alleanza fraterna. – Port.: aliança fraterna.

In the Freudian hypothesis presented in *Totem and Taboo* (1912–13), this agreement comprises the unifying homosexual ties established between brothers expelled from the primal horde* by the primal father. Thus, by means of the invention of a weapon and these unifying bonds generated in exile, they were able to consummate parricide and devour the cruel, omnipotent father.

Following the father's murder, which discharged their hate* towards him, remorse* and guilt* for what they had done remained as products, including the wish* to preserve these fraternal ties formed during exile.

In this way, the basic laws of prohibition of incest and parricide, laws on which culture* was built, were gradually born from within their own psyche.

The change in social structures generated by the band of brothers and its consequence, parricide, allowed progress to a higher level of culture, our present culture, and also configured a new structure of the human psychical apparatus: the eternal legacy of the superego*.

During this hypothetical period they agreed upon a sort of social contract:

> The first form of a social organization came about with a *renunciation of instinct*, a recognition of mutual *obligations*, the introduction of definite *institutions*, pronounced inviolable (holy) – that is to say, the rudiments of morality and justice. Each individual renounced his ideal of acquiring his father's position for himself and of possessing his mother and sisters. Thus the *taboo on incest* and the injunction to *exogamy* came about. A fair amount of the absolute power liberated by the removal of the father passed over to the women, resulting in a period of *matriarchy*. Recollection of their father persisted in this period of the "fraternal alliance". A powerful animal – at first, perhaps, always one that was feared as well – was chosen as a substitute for the father. A choice of this kind may seem strange, but the gulf established later by men between themselves and animals did not exist for primitive peoples: nor does it exist for our children, whose animal phobias we have been able to understand as fear of their father. In relation to the totem animal the original dichotomy in the emotional relation with the father (ambivalence) was wholly retained. On the one hand the totem was regarded as the clan's blood ancestor and protective spirit, who had to be worshipped and protected, and on the other hand, a festival was designated for which the primal father's fate was prepared for this animal. He was killed and devoured by all the tribesmen in common. (The totem meal, according to Robertson Smith [1894].) This great festival was in fact a triumphant celebration of the united sons' victory over their father.
>
> (1939*a*, pp. 82–3)

This passage from *Moses and Monotheism: Three Essays* provides the best definition, and underscores the importance Freud gave to his hypotheses presented in 1913, even to the end of his works; in them he develops the concept of the fraternal alliance, the band of brothers united to commit parricide whose eventual consequence forms the substantial seed of human culture.

FREE ASSOCIATION

Ger.: freie Assoziation. – Sp.: asociación libre. – Fr.: méthode o règle de libre association. – It.: libera associazione. – Por.: associação livre.

The fundamental technical rule of psychoanalytic technique. Patients are asked to voice all their occurrences, to suppress their conscious censorship*, and to cathect with attention the word-presentations linked by associative laws with a weak level of binding and a certain freedom of displacement*. In other words, patients are actively invited to express aloud their free fantasy and daydreaming, usually censured by conscious censorship.

Not all patients are able to associate to the same extent. Association* is freer when positive transference* predominates, resistance* is low, rigid, defensive character traits are not predominant, and so on. Among these words, which in a different context would seem senseless or absurd, indicators or traces are left behind on departure from the unconscious by the repressed unconscious wish* hidden behind the symptom*. They enable the analyst to assemble interpretation-constructions* to gradually make conscious the unconscious.

Free association is in reality a gradual pathway leading to the unconscious. On this path, precisely in the vicinity of the repressed nucleus, ego* resistances arise. Their analysis occupies a large part of the analytic task. They are not only resistances to learn about the repressed but also about the repressor, also unconscious, but pertaining to the ego*. Analysis of resistance helps analysands to gain knowledge of the repressed unconscious on the one hand and, on the other hand, of the unconscious part of the ego (its defence mechanisms*); therefore, also of their characteristics and the extent of alteration of the ego* produced by these mechanisms. The overcoming of resistance, besides enabling access to knowledge of unconscious mechanisms, also clears the way for progress to new levels of association accompanying the reconstruction of forgotten childhood history and prehistory and the historical origin of these defence mechanisms, in a dynamic spiral of meaning.

FREE ENERGY

Ger.: freie Energie. – Sp.: energía libremente móvil. – Fr.: énergie libre. – It.: energia libera. – Port.: energia libremente móvel.

This is the state of energy in the id* and in what we understand globally as the unconscious*, governed by the pleasure principle*; from the id or the unconscious it seeks perceptual identity* through which it hallucinates conditions of satisfaction or finds identities with the wished-for object* in small attributes of perceptions. The unconscious ego's defence mechanisms*, also ruled by the pleasure principle, work with this energy, forming the unconscious ego structure upon which the preconscious is edified.

This energy moves freely among thing-presentations*, constantly generating displacements* and condensations*. In this state, energy is ineffective and needs to be tamed, at least partly, in order for it to advance towards discharge.

When free energy is suffocated*, it gains some effectiveness if it returns from the repressed* through symptoms*, parapraxes*, compulsions*, and so on.

When it is bound by word-presentations* and/or thought* activity of the preconscious ego*, it becomes bound energy*, less free but with greater probability of completing a specific action*.

FRUSTRATION

Ger.: Versagung. – Sp.: frustración. – Fr.: frustration. – It.: frustrazione. – Port.: frustração.

An alteration of reality* by which the subject is denied satisfaction of certain sexual Triebe* or their sublimations, including aim-inhibited love relationships. Sometimes a failure to reach a proposed objective is also involved, an amorous disappointment, for example.

It is the precipitating cause (the second in the complemental series*) which, added to predisposition (the first of the complemental series), sparks neurosis* (return of the repressed*). In other words, the external factor was all that was missing from the internal factor to cause the looming neurosis to emerge (or a psychosis, as well as a normal process such as mourning*).

The specificity of frustration is that it produces libidinal stasis. Since the cause originates in the exterior, if the psychical apparatus is prepared to bear it, apparently nothing would happen. If not, equilibrium reached up that that instant would be upset.

FUNDAMENTAL RULE

Ger.: Grundregel. – Sp.: regla fundamental. – Fr.: règle fondamentale. – It.: regola fondamentale. – Port.: regra fundamental.

At the beginning of a psychoanalytic treatment, the analyst asks the patient to eliminate conscious censorship* of preconscious associations* and to allow them to take the lead; that is to say, whatever comes to mind, lending them a cathexis* of attention*.

Thus, latent ideas emerging by association, following laws of contiguity*, analogy*, or opposition*, some of which are phantasies* or daydreams, ruled mainly by the pleasure principle*, access the spoken word and their perception* by the analyst; in this way, by retracing their path, they may become one of the access roads to knowledge of the unconscious*.

It is not always easy to associate freely and it may even be said that neurosis consists in short-circuits of associations. For this reason, it is a rule whose compliance is requested, although it is difficult for the patient to comply constantly, since defensive ego anticathexes* are blocking precisely the passage of any wish* presentation* that might cause the ego* anxiety* or, in another area, any external perception that might evoke its memory*. The analysand brings up associations and finds other new ones by virtue of eagerness to investigate and the desire for a cure, supported by confidence in the analyst (positive transference). What comes to mind tends to get stuck when it leads to perceptions or presentations that might develop transference affects* (erotic* or hostile transference); also when they touch a core resisted by the ego.

We therefore tell him that the success of the psycho-analysis depends on his noticing and reporting whatever comes into his head and not being misled, for instance, into suppressing an idea because it strikes him as unimportant or irrelevant or because it seems to him meaningless.

(*The Interpretation of Dreams*, 1900, p. 101)

However, if the patient is invited – and not threatened – to associate freely, it is because part of censorship is conscious.

This conscious censorship is based on the existence of a previous unconscious censorship, the real cause of the neurosis, the latter (repression) being what the treatment actually aims to lift.

G

GENITAL

Ger.: Genitale. – Sp.: genital. – Fr.: génital. – It.: genitale. – Port.: genital.

Genital refers to the genitals. Therefore, genitality develops in human beings when a person's genitals develop and become capable of reproduction. Psychoanalysis (and culture*) is interested in its psycho-socio-cultural consequences.

Human beings are the only animals that develop sexuality* in two steps with a period of latency* between two libidinal surges. The genital is connected with the second surge. It is a problematic feature of puberty, adolescence, and adulthood.

Libido* conquers evolution in a figurative journey through the erotogenic zones, each with its individual history and type of object relation (the oral zone, the anal zone, skin, muscles, sight, the phallic-urethral). Upon arrival to the phallic zone, the pleasures* inherent to the other zones submit to its supremacy, a unification that enables maximum pleasure. This coincides with other facts: for example, with the consolidation of a highly important stage in the formation of an ego* which, although it continues to grow and change with future experiences, has a first and basic configuration of its own. This is an initial reality ego*. When the ego is configured, autoerotism*, until then predominant in satisfaction of sexual Triebe*, becomes more complex when it becomes narcissism*. The libido cathecting (cf. cathexis*) this ego is narcissistic libido. The ego is an abstract entity that originates in the subject's own body and carries its attributes and its history; this history is present in presentations* of this individual's wishes* and identifications*.

To recognize the ego involves recognition of not-ego: the object*. Thus, the latter becomes the main source of pleasure, its choice supported by self-preservative Triebe*. For this reason, the first object choice*, which was already being configured with the first erotogenic zones (though partially), falls upon the mother.

At the phallic level, the choice of the mother object acquires incestuous characteristics. This inaugurates the period of the Oedipus complex*, associated with castration anxiety* in boys and the castration complex in girls: everything intimately related to dawning recognition of sexual differences. This phallic level is not, however, genital, although it prepares the way for it. In this phase, the "masculine" genital, the phallus, is considered the only genital. Girls feel they have been deprived of it, castrated, whereas boys feel they are in danger of being castrated. The accepted sexual difference is phallic–castrated. Castration anxiety in boys leads the ego to complete primary repression* of all infantile sexuality* by virtue of an immense anticathexis* and secondary identification* with the parental figures which is then referred to as the superego*.

Once the superego is definitively established, the period of latency begins, and the first surge of libidinal evolution comes to an end.

This phenomenon in girls is more complex. Their recognition of sexual difference involves the castration complex, phallic envy*, confrontation with the mother who they are gradually forced to recognize as being castrated, and a desire to possess a child to replace the longed-for penis. When they recognize their mother as being castrated, and because of their consequent separation from her, they enter the positive Oedipus complex; at this point, the desire to get a child from their father arises, followed by the desire to give him a child. Therefore, configuration of the girl's superego involves nothing that would hurry it. Incestuous wishes do not involve renewed anxiety except the fear of not being loved by the object (at this time the father, but also the mother), anxiety that is the counterpart in girls of castration anxiety in boys, though lacking the dramatic, urgent quality of the latter. In women, latency is less perceptible and the superego is established more progressively and consciously.

Oedipal issues in both girls and boys are re-experienced at puberty with the definitive re-emergence of libido, and they inherit the dramatic quality and even the script, engraved on the unconscious during that forgotten period of life.

In boys, the types of affect* towards women that arose in the latency period are kept separate at first: that is to say, tenderness towards the mother and its derivatives; sensuality towards objects without any type of association with representatives of the maternal line. Boys gradually need to overcome debasement of the erotic object*, and at the same time to recognize the female genital as different from their own and all women as different beings, not as phallically castrated beings, in order to reach a definitive object choice*. This process is slow and tortuous, with progressions and regressions*. In this period we say that the individual enters a true genital phase.

Girls need to recognize:

Their female genital, which is not the lack of the male genital (literally or symbolically); that her ego may be configured as a subject, with Triebe* whose aims are both active and passive and not necessarily be only an object; as a consequence of previous recognition, her phallic envy decreases, and she is able to accept males as the predominant objects of her pleasure. She also needs to integrate tenderness and sensuality.

In any case, certain psychoanalytical theorizations on genitality sometimes acquire abstract or ideal connotations that would aspire to include it in the concept of health. Freud never spoke of considering genitality in this sense, although a relation exists. We consider that the genital, psychoanalytically speaking, is a dynamic concept and a state sometimes achieved by individuals, from which they may regress due to the inevitable frustrations* of life. The genital aim is the supreme aim of sexual Trieb in which the greatest fusion of life Trieb* and death Trieb* is produced, the former managing to neutralize the latter to a great extent (achieving a good synthesis of love*, hate*, and aggression*). When libido is inhibited* in its aim, it is also inhibited in its genital aim. When the genital aim is inhibited, the portion of death Trieb neutralized by fusion is defused (fusion and defusion of Trieb), and a portion of death Trieb is freed. This defused death Trieb is liberated as aggression and is turned against the ego as self-aggression, bound in this case by the superego. This occurs in sublimation* and in cultural facts in general. It is part of the price human beings pay to access culture. Also, if the subject's only genital aim is sexual discharge, when this aim is not inhibited, difficulties generated in sublimations and social links lead to other sources of discontent.

GREAT MAN

Ger.: großen Mannes. – Sp.: gran hombre. – Fr.: grand homme. – It.: grande uomo. – Port.: grande homen.

This paternal archetype is described mythically or historically in the origins of peoples:

"a great man influences his fellow-men in two ways: by his personality and by the idea which he puts forward" (1939, p. 109).

The human community tends to produce great men. Individuals are animals of the horde, grouped around a leader, and in this sense are products of history and also its generators.

Freud writes in *Moses and Monotheism* (1939):

> We know that in the mass of mankind there is a powerful need for an authority who can be admired, before whom someone bows down, by whom one is ruled and perhaps even ill-treated. We have learnt from the psychology of individual men what the origin is of this need of the masses. It is a longing for the father felt by everyone from his childhood onwards, for the same father whom the hero of legend boasts he has overcome.
>
> (Ibid.)

The great man is given paternal traits: clearness of thought*, a strong will, forcefulness in action, and, especially, autonomy and independence, a divine heedlessness that may go so far as recklessness. "One must admire him, one may trust him but one cannot avoid being afraid of him too" (1939, p. 110).

The "great man" becomes the mythical, historical or actual leader of human masses, more a representative of the father of the primal horde* and of the childhood of each human being. On the other hand, the hero, a creation of poets, represents the fraternal alliance*, the pact between the brothers that led to parricide. That is to say, to killing and devouring the father, as well as longing* for the father who, now devoured, is inside the son. This was the origin of the superego and with it the advent of culture*: a culture that bears the traces of its origin.

The great man also becomes a god when religions are formed (paternal deities following totemism and maternal deities that emerged in the period of matriarchal* society immediately after the original parricide.). These deities are polytheistic at first, and later monotheistic.

GROUP IDENTIFICATION

Ger.: Identifizierung in der Masse. – Sp.: identificación en la masa. – Fr.: identification dans la masse. – It.: identificazione nella massa. – Port.: identificação na massa.

In this type of secondary identification*, the ego* loses its boundaries in favour of common objectives, and group* members become part of a whole directed by a leader who is put into the place of the ideal. In groups, identification is secondary but also narcissistic* since it is produced in the ego, though fleetingly, since it does not necessarily become a lasting ego trait. It may perhaps become relatively lasting in artificial groups*, not because identification is lasting but because this type of group is.

It generally lasts as long as the group does, although sometimes, long-term membership in a certain artificial group may leave a characteristic in the ego as a "souvenir".

Freud referred to it as "psychical infection" (*Group Psychology and the Analysis of the Ego*, 1921) and compared it to a type of hysterical* identification with a community of interests. (Freud offers this example: in a girls' boarding school, a girl faints when she receives a letter from her boyfriend, which leads to generalized fainting of her classmates as an unconscious means of receiving a love letter.)

GROUP PSYCHOLOGY

Ger.: Massenpsychologie. – Sp.: masa, psicología de la. – Fr.: psychologie collective. – It.: massa, psicologia della. – Port.: massa, psi-cologia de.

This concept is Freud's attempt to explain social psychology, the psychology of human groups. For this purpose, he changes his object of study which is no longer the singular, unique, unrepeatable subject, but not his basic theoretical postulates. However, instead of applying psychoanalysis to other sciences, as some of his disciples do, he finds new incentives and ideas in these sciences. We could say that he utilizes them for his own benefit. Thus, several of these postulates are useful to explain some problems generated in human groups and the close relation between individual and social psychology.

The text in which he develops this attempt is principally *Group Psychology and the Analysis of the Ego* (1921). He discusses ideas of authors such as Le Bon and MacDougall. He utilizes Le Bon's conceptualizations on the spontaneous group, with its tendency to action on liberated unconscious* tendencies, suggestion, the primacy of affectivity over intellectual activity, and others.

MacDougall finds that something in common joins the individuals of a group, pointing out increased affectivity, and also examining highly organized groups.

As usual, Freud is enriched by his reading and gives it his own vision. The links which unite the group are libidinal, but aim-inhibited libido* not seeking a genital* aim (in Freudian language, it is homosexual libido, ignoring sexual difference).

Instead of MacDougall's highly organized groups, we have Freud's artificial groups*. A certain external compulsion prevents the dissolution or any alteration in the structure of these groups, whose prototypes are the army and the Church, which he analyses very deeply. The artificial group attains greater libidinal binding than ephemeral groups. He also underscores the importance of the leader and the double type of libidinal tie: between the members and the leader and among the members.

"Group anxiety" is produced when these libidinal links held together by the leader are broken. This is panic.

The link with the leader is like being in love, idealization* as with a hypnotizer. (Le Bon had written that the group acts in a state of hypnosis.)

The leader may be replaced by an idea (Christianity, Communism, Freudism), in which case the group reaches higher levels of binding of libidinal energy. The leader, the idea, or the image replacing the leader has been situated by all the members of the group in the place of the ego ideal*: links among group members are "the earliest expression of an emotional tie with another person" (1921, p. 105), identifications*.

A group is therefore "a number of individuals who have put one and the same object in the place of their ego ideal and have consequently identified themselves with one another in their ego" (1921, p. 116).

He objects to, or rather, organizes Trotter's statement that human beings are gregarious animals, explaining that they are instead horde* animals led by a chief.

Freud considers group psychology the oldest human psychology. Individual psychology (perhaps understanding individual psychology as what leads to action) grows progressively from group psychology, although it was in the leader from the outset, since the leader was in charge of action or of planning for its completion by group members.

He therefore defines leaders as persons who have no need to love (cf. love*), sure of themselves, and autonomous. They have no need to confirm their will with others. Actually, they have the characteristics of the primal father; the leader of the group ultimately remains the primal father; the group wants to be governed by an unlimited power because of its extreme yearning for authority (in Le Bon's expression, "thirst for submission").

Human beings progressed from individual psychology through myths*, heroic myths sung by poets, in which the feat once accomplished by the group of brothers (fraternal alliance*) united against their leader (parricide, one of the events generating culture*) is attributed to an individual. Nature myths doubtless come later. The falsehood of the heroic myth culminates when the hero* is set up as a god: the father god, thereby generating the return of the primal father as a divinity.

Perhaps what is most fascinating about this theoretical discussion is the link Freud describes between individual psychology (the structure of the psychical apparatus and the establishment of its ego ideal*) and social psychology (the human group formed around a leader) plus the social ties (with the leader and among members), two psychologies that may be acting in one individual (individual and group psychology), and the interrelation between all this and the hypothetical origins of culture (the primal horde–primal father). All this is also functioning in a dynamic way, simultaneously, in an individual and a group, in a constantly interrelated manner.

GUILT, SENSE OF

Ger.: Schuldgefühl. – Sp.: culpa, sentimiento de. – Fr.: culpabilité, sentiment de. – It.: colpa, sentimento di. – Port.: culpa, sentimento de.

A special type of anxiety* felt by the ego* before the superego* when the ego's attributes stray from the ego ideal* demanded by the latter; it is also called "moral anxiety" or "fear of the superego"*.

Because this ego anxiety is felt before another internal structure of the psychical apparatus, it is not relieved by repentance, since the superego, which springs in part from the id*, is in itself an anticathexis against its Triebe*, and therefore has direct notice of unconscious* desire*, of sexual Trieb* which, although repressed, continues to exist. Hence, guilt is still felt, in this case, independent of any acts or conscious and preconscious* phantasies, since it originates in unconscious repressed Triebe*. This produces an apparently paradoxical effect: the greater the ego's beatitude – the greater the anticathexis, reaction formation*, or even sublimation* – the greater the sense of guilt (when the defence is stronger, it is because the unconscious wish is also stronger).

We could say that a sense of guilt originating in external authority initiates suppression* of Trieb* in the pre-oedipal child. Then, following oedipal events, the superego is established with its sense of guilt or anxiety before conscience, which thereafter dedicates itself to increasing suppression of Triebe and to punishment of the ego for not doing so.

A sense of guilt is therefore inherent – of course in varying degrees – to the structure of the human psychical apparatus. It is universal. It is observed in all the neuroses, generating frequent feelings of inferiority. It appears especially in obsessional neurosis* and in a narcissistic affection such as melancholia* (mania* is a defence against melancholia). In obsessional neurosis it is expressed in self-reproaches*, scrupulousness, in some symptoms* such as ceremonials* and others produced by defence mechanisms* against this anxiety of conscience which in obsessional neurotics may or may not be known to consciousness.

In melancholia, a sense of guilt occupies the entire clinical picture. It is therefore conscious guilt. What the subject does not know is the cause. The superego vents its cruelty sadistically on the ego, identified with the object*, the ego consequently submitting masochistically to the sadistic superego.

A sense of guilt is, again paradoxically, a cause of crime, as if the ego sought relief in finding a real cause for this unpleasurable feeling. It is an interesting explanation for some cases of asocial personalities (cf. criminals from a sense of guilt*).

A fairly common element in preconscious or conscious fantasies which generate a sense of guilt is masturbation* in puberty and adolescence. It conceals all the repressed infantile sexuality* whose activity is almost solely autoerotic* and from which its second level of masturbation is laden with incestuous and parricidal fantasies: precisely the oedipal fantasies.

The onanistic and masochistic perverse fantasies of some adults (like those in *A Child is Being Beaten*, 1919, or beating fantasies*) carry the sense of guilt interwoven among their motivations; for example, feminine masochism* (found more in men) and even more so, moral masochism, in which the sense of guilt is the principal though unconscious part.

Concerning degrees of fusion of Triebe, Freud presents the following hypothesis: "When an instinctual trend undergoes repression, its libidinal elements, are turned into symptoms, and its aggressive components into a sense of guilt" (*Civilization and Its Discontents*, 1930, p. 139).

GUILT, UNCONSCIOUS SENSE OF (NEED FOR PUNISHMENT)

Ger.: Unbewusstes schuldgefühl. – Sp. culpa, sentimiento inconsciente de (necesidad de castigo). – Fr.: culpabilité, sentiment inconscient de (besoin de punition). – It.: colpa, sentimento inconscio di (necessità di castigo). – Port.: culpa, sentimento inconsciente de (necessidade de castigo).

A special type of resistance* to the cure of illness and to well-being generated by the superego*, the latter strives to penalize the ego* (which it considers guilty) with the constant suffering caused by illness.

It is quite possibly the most difficult resistance* to overcome, tending to manifest in clinical work as a "negative therapeutic reaction; that is to say, when the treatment has advanced, after the conclusion of a construction* which reveals the meaning of a symptom* or of an ego character trait*; instead of disappearance of the symptom or changes in the ego, both worsen as if the patient were unknowingly clinging to illness. Guilt is not felt. It is the debt collected by the superego through the ego's suffering caused by illness.

It is also manifested in a type of person that Freud called "those wrecked by success". Whenever they are about to achieve something intensely desired, they avoid it or endeavour by all means to keep it from happening: they either fall somatically ill or begin to have accidents. In these people, guilt is inferred from behaviour which demonstrates a need for punishment.

The term "unconscious sense of guilt" is therefore incorrect since there is no "sense" in this case. The existence of need for punishment is deduced from this clinging to suffering produced by the continuation of illness, in some cases, or by different types of punishment suffered in others.

The degree of fusion or defusion* between life Trieb* and death Trieb* (with some predominance of the latter) is directly related to this type of phenomenon, always ready to join the list of causal factors whenever possible.

H

HALLUCINATION

Ger.: Halluzination. – Sp.: alucinación. – Fr.: hallucination. – It.: allucinazione. – Port.: alucinação.

This perception of a wish*, thought*, memory*, even a punishment or a threat also springs from memory storage as if these perceptions originated in the external world; they are registered – like any other perception which therefore makes it worthy of belief* as something real – by the perceptual-conscious apparatus (Pcpt.-Cs.).

Hallucinations occur when the ego* is momentarily altered as in dreams* (it is sleeping and is therefore much less cathected) or is experiencing a state of privation due to external causes. In other cases the cause is toxic (hallucinogenic drugs). They may be due to a more or less deep alteration of the ego* as in cases of hallucinations in hysterical psychoses* and in acute hallucinatory psychoses or Meynert's amentia*. In the latter cases, the alteration is that the ego is unable to discriminate between wish fantasies and real perceptions. In the case of hysteria*, rather than fulfilled wishes, they may be hallucinated punishments derived from these or disguised unconscious wishes that generate anxiety* in the manner of anxiety dreams as for example Anna O*'s snake hallucination.

In amentia or acute hallucinatory psychosis, hallucinations are more closely related to processes of disavowal* of mourning* for the loss of a loved object*, a disavowal produced together with regression* of the ego to perception* in images, withdrawing it from cathexis* and placing it into the perceptual apparatus. By virtue of this perception-consciousness system pertaining to the ego, it mistakes the wishful memory of the object for its real perception.

In cases of schizophrenia*, paranoid schizophrenia, and paranoia*, ego regression is deeper, though not formal (without regression to the image; this hallucination consists of words perceived): the individual's own preconscious* thoughts* are perceived as entering from the outside as if the ego were now located in machines (symbols* of the body) or in other persons manipulating the subject (apparatus of influence); also as perception of the critical part of the ego (superego*) that is felt to be a perception by the perceptual apparatus, giving it credence in reality*. A simple personal thought or occurrence is felt to be an external voice, a phenomenon which occurs by virtue of regression to perception, in the manner in which it was perceived originally (the observing and critical voices of the parents). In these latter affections featuring narcissistic libidinal withdrawal*, auditory hallucinations predominate, whereas in hysteria and amentia visual hallucinations predominate.

HALLUCINATORY SATISFACTION OF WISHES

Ger.: Aluzinatrisches wunsch Befriedigung. – Sp.: satisfacción alucinatoria de deseos. – Fr.: satisfaction hallucinatoire du désir. – It.: sodisfazione allucinatoria di desideri. – Port.: satisfação alu-cinatoria de desejos.

This primitive form of infantile mental life was constructed theoretically by Freud based on his study of dreams* in adult life, which consist in part of regression* to this type of functioning of the psychical apparatus in general and of the ego* in particular. As the term indicates, in the origins of mental functioning, wishes* are not perceived as such but as being satisfied in a hallucinatory manner. An ego able to inhibit wishes must develop before a wish may be discerned as such, since so long as it is a wish it is unsatisfied and avid for satisfaction, and when satisfaction is obtained, this particular wish disappears.

Following the experience of satisfaction*, when bodily need returns, it is transformed into a wish by binding with presentations* of things experienced with the object during that experience; first, there is perceptual identity*: wishes are perceived as being satisfied as soon as they are remembered; they are satisfied by hallucination. Since there is no discharge at the source of Trieb*, frustration* ensues. For this reason the psychical apparatus must necessarily inhibit this tendency to hallucinatory satisfaction of wishes; thus, a first level of functioning emerges in an initial reality ego* which in time becomes a definitive reality ego*: an ego that inhibits hallucination*, since it is frustrating; absolutely frustrating in relation to the ego's self-preservative Triebe* which must necessarily recognize reality* practically from the outset, functioning with laws of the initial reality ego. However, in the case of sexual Triebe*, this state or stage of hallucinatory satisfaction of wishes can be sustained longer, though only partially. Recognition of reality is not as urgent, at least the reality of recognition of objects as a source of pleasure*, since at first they are basically autoerotic (this implies that they are not absolutely so).

Hallucinatory satisfaction of wishes corresponds in general to the logic of the purified pleasure ego* ruled by the pleasure principle* which in turn belongs to the first ways of differentiating the internal from the external in relation to sexual Triebe (the pleasurable is ego, the unpleasurable is not). This corresponds to: what I wish for I hallucinate and perceive as being satisfied; if what is pleasurable is I, then I decide.

This illogical logic (as judged by the ego's secondary process*) is worn down by reality, which gradually imposes its formal, real logic. The object* slowly begins to be recognized as what is wished for, separate from the subject; its absence or not being loved by it may therefore produce anxiety*.

These are different aspects of the progress of an ego, inhibitor of hallucination, which enable the ego to differentiate perceptions* from wishes*. Then, by virtue of language*, or rather word-presentations* which are its major instrument, individuals may acquire conscious knowledge of their own wishes. They may then think them, interrelate them, and, with knowledge of reality, put them into action.

This primitive functioning or primary process* ruled by the pleasure principle, a type of thought* with predominantly visual images, which considers wishes satisfied, becomes in adulthood part of the functioning of the unconscious*. The presentation cathexis* regresses topically to this type of psychical functioning and reaches the perceptual end* during dreams*. It is also a regression of the type of ego functioning and is therefore temporal. When the preconscious cathexis regresses topically to unconscious thing-presentations*, it regresses to those that belong to fixation* points in libidinal development; for this reason there is also some libidinal regression, apart from regression corresponding to the narcissism* inherent to the state of sleep.

Phantasies* (or daydreams) partly respond to this logic without reaching the hallucinatory state but considering wishes satisfied, even though they belong topically to the ego's preconscious. The ego may sometimes accept them as its own, subjecting them afterwards to the reality principle*; the ego accepts that it only aspires to this reality and therefore does not possess it.

Phantasies drawing too near the repressed (by analogical*, contiguous*, or opposite* association*) are unconscious derivatives of this. In this case, the ego prevents their progress by repressing them in order to avoid suffering anxiety signals* ordered by castration anxiety*.

When these repression* fail, the repressed* returns through substitutive formations* and originating symptoms* of transference neuroses.

Some acute psychoses may also regress to the stage of "hallucinatory satisfaction of wishes", such as Meynert's amentia* (acute hallucinatory confusion) and hysterical psychoses; but not the narcissistic psychoses, since these lack any unconscious wish to be satisfied (cf. schizophrenia*, paranoia*, melancholia*, and others).

HATE

Ger.: Haß. – Sp.: odio. – Fr.: haine. – It.: odio. – Port.: ódio.

This unpleasurable affect* is felt towards the object when it is the source of unpleasurable sensations. It produces a tendency in the ego* to enlarge the distance between the object and the ego*. The object is repulsive to the ego* and is hated. This hate may grow and become an inclination to attack the object with the aim of annihilating it.

The ego feels hate in response to aggression* or frustration* produced by the object. It is an affect that may or may not lead to aggression; it is a step towards it but does not necessarily include action. Although aggression is committed because of hate, hate may be felt without coming to aggression (it may be unconsciously repressed and return with the forgetting* of a name, a parapraxis* or even a neurotic symptom*; it may also be suppressed* by conscious* judgement of condemnation*).

Freud describes hate as the first type of link with what is recognized as an object by the purified pleasure ego* (by definition, since the purified pleasure ego recognizes everything pleasurable as ego and everything unpleasurable as not-ego, as an object). Therefore, the notion of object is defined in this type of ego as unpleasure; hence, the only possible type of relation with the object or what is recognized as the object is indifference or hate.

Everything becomes more difficult as reality* is gradually imposed, and the object can only be accepted as a source of pleasure*; at this point, fear of object loss* begins to appear, and Trieb for mastery* of the object enters the scene. Trieb for mastery develops in the anal period by virtue of progressive domination of striate muscles. It expresses sadism* in which hate and love* are mixed, a vivid expression of affective ambivalence*.

In these initial stages, hate is not distinguished from love. At the same time, self-preservative Trieb* develops greatly. Trieb for mastery is supported by it in its attempt to dominate the object when it progressively recognizes it as a source of pleasure and its absence as producing fear of object loss.

In the phallic period, hate is clearly separated from love, and they become opposites. Love then seeks closeness to the object as a source of pleasure, and hate begins to predominate in the link with the rival (the father in the boy's case); thus the Oedipus complex* is gradually configured, identification with the father takes on a hostile tone which culminates in establishment of the superego*, a psychic structure in which the latter tone predominates, charged with hate.

In melancholia* the situation is similar: when the unconscious* object wish is broken off, identification with the object ensues in the ego and, due to the previous unconscious hate relation, this relation of hate now exists between the superego and the ego. This is seen in clinical work as self-reproaching*, which may or may not be put into action by self-aggression or even attempted suicide.

Love may become hate and vice versa. In persecutory paranoia*, homosexual love becomes hate as a type of repressive disguise for the unconscious wish now projected (cf. projection*) on to the object; love that is now hate returns from the object, and the subject is persecuted by it.

When a love relation is interrupted, it is not infrequently replaced by hate. However, apparent hate in this case may be produced by regression* from loving to the previous sadistic stage, and consequently this hate acquires an erotic character; consequently, the love relation may continue on this loving level filled with hate, which is once more indistinguishable from love. Hate involves a degree of Trieb fusion since it is a way to relate with the object; therefore, it contains a small amount of libido; however, it is so little that the liberation of destructive* or death Trieb in the phenomenon of hate is nearly obvious.

HAVING

Ger.: Haben. – Sp.: tener. – Fr.: avoir. – It.: avere. – Port.: ter.

This category of functioning of the reality ego* involves acceptance of the object* as the origin of pleasure*. In having, there is no longer any confusion between subject and object, the object is not part of being*, and now the ego wishes to have it. Its recognition as something foreign to the ego is acquired gradually, proceeding by degrees from narcissism*, going through homosexual object choice (in children, previous to recognition of sexual difference) and arriving at heterosexual object libido*.

Recognition that the ego is not the object and that the object may only at most be had produces fear of object loss. Then the ego endeavours to master the object (Trieb for mastery*) in diverse manners, some of which are symbolic forms (play, language*).

Having is more highly evolved (in this line of thought concerning ego categories in relation to the object) than being*, which is the first category inherent to the pleasure ego* when the object is pleasurable. The category of having also involves the characteristic of object wish*, since the ego recognizes that it is not the object and also that it does not have it; therefore, the ego desires the object.

HELPLESSNESS

Ger.: Hiflosigkeit. – Sp.: desvalimiento. – Fr.: état de détresse. – It.: l'essere senza aiuto. – Port.: desvalimento.

This is the state of defencelessness of the infant, invaded by tension of necessity. A great economic disturbance is produced by the increase in quantities of stimulus awaiting handling. This is the genuine nucleus of danger. It corresponds to the birth trauma* when tension of necessity invaded a psychical apparatus without any capacity to bind this quantity of excitation* since it had insufficient or only phylogenetic presentations.

This is henceforth the feared danger-situation*. Experience gradually shows that danger withdraws in the presence of the object*, the first step in all the growingly complex presentations of anxiety*: castration anxiety*; fear of the superego*; and social anxiety*, which become danger signals indicating that the psychical apparatus may enter the situation of helplessness* (nonpresentational automatic anxiety*). The psychical apparatus may be invaded in various ways by tension of necessity: when defence mechanisms* fail (neuro-psychoses of defence*) or when an invasion of quantity of excitation enters from reality (traumatic neuroses*) or due to mechanical reasons that prevent discharge of the quantitative factor of sexual Trieb (actual neuroses*), also due to decathexis* of thing-presentations (narcissistic psychoses*). Then, an attack of automatic anxiety ensues: a state of psychical helplessness in response to the economic invasion, thereby repeating a situation similar to the birth trauma.

When the quantity of force of a real external danger is much greater than the subject's own, it produces a material situation of helplessness, this time not in response to an internal stimulus but to an external stimulus.

HERO

Ger.: Held. – Sp.: héroe. – Fr.: héros. – It.: eroe. – Port.: herói.

This universal mythological being, a creation of peoples in relation to their origins, transforms important historical individuals into heroes. This concept, corresponding to social psychology, is connected with individual psychology through the primal phantasy* of the family romance*.

Both phenomena contrast the value of two families: one is overvalued and the other undervalued; father–son rivalry is also contrasted.

In the myth, the hero is born into a "royal", noble family that abandons him because the father is jealous of the son. The infant is thrown into the water (a universal symbol* of birth) and then saved by persons of low social status. In time, the hero becomes king, and recovers the "grandeur" of his lineage.

The myth* of the birth of the hero, universal and social, is repeated in each individual, mainly in adolescence, when idealization* of the father (an omnipotent, aristocratic ex-king in infantile thought) enters a crisis and the father is devalued. As a compensation, the subject fancies having been born into a different family with better social standing.

This phantasy involves a wish* to be the hero who in the saga, the drama created by the poet, represents the "band of brothers" which in the Freudian hypothesis or "scientific myth" (1915), existed at the dawn of humanity when the brothers killed their father and created the new social order. In this way, the hero (myth*) moves into the place corresponding to all brothers (historical truth*).

The myth of the hero is linked to the oedipal and represents in boys the implicit parricidal and incestuous wish it involves. It is rivalry with the father, the ambivalence* of the father complex*, inspired by the wish, demanding success in this struggle, or alternatively, blocking it if guilt* predominates.

> But no matter whether what we have here is a phantasy or the return of a forgotten reality, in any case the origin of the concept of a hero is to be found at this point – the hero who always rebels against his father and kills him in some shape or other.
>
> (1939, p. 87)

HISTORY

Ger.: Geschichte. – Sp.: historia. – Fr.: histoire. – Ital.: storia. – Port.: história.

To understand Freud, the theme of the subject's history is central. We see this from the outset, since Freud considers that the concept of presentation* (capital in the psyche described by Freud) arises after the trace left by perception through experiences* (satisfaction and pain*) in links with objects*. That is to say, the psyche, the presentation, arises from a union between the biological (the body) and the social (the object); it is what is left of this union in the individual's psychical apparatus. In other terms, the presentation is the trace of past events remaining in the psyche and configuring their history; it is the configuration of their history. This history in reality is formed gradually by relations between presentations separated by the repressive-defensive process. We could say that almost all the psyche, in its diverse forms, is a product of the subject's history with the object. This does not mean that Freud is a historian of the mind or that he is interested in the material truth* of what happened in reality; he is instead interested in learning the historical truth of what remained of it in the individual. Therefore, we may say that ascertaining historical truth is what guides psychoanalytical work, since the meaning of symptoms and other returns of the repressed* from the unconscious* resides in traces they leave, including ways of being or the ego's* character traits*.

However, Freud conceptualizes the psyche not only as being deferred* in relation to experiences, but also as having *a priori* phenomena; these are inherited primal phantasies* which lend a certain universality to some phenomena as "preparations for understanding" (quite similar to instincts*, the nucleus of the unconscious*) originating in experience of the species and therefore historical or rather prehistorical.

This means that individuals are at first *a priori* of their own experience, partly determined in a formal and universal manner by experience of the species, but are to be determined by their own history (which also partly repeats the history of the species) in a deferred manner in relation to their own infantile experience; their personal history determines the content of their wishes*, Triebe*, etc., and also of their defences* against them, satisfying them or not, or even ignoring them (this is the main defence against wishes and Triebe by making them unconscious; it is called repression* in the broad sense and has diverse modes and mechanisms). Therefore, individuals are determined by their unconscious which is essentially the history of their infantile sexuality*, their own prehistory. This does not exclude chance, but it belongs not to their psychical apparatus but rather to external reality. Although it is forgotten, history may reappear in transferences to the actual, unknown to the subject. Psychoanalysis is needed in order to acquire this knowledge, which may sometimes interrupt determination of the historical past. For this reason, Freud presents clinical cases as case histories; it is a matter of revealing the subject's own history (historical truth), disguised in myths* the subject has created regarding this history, in symptoms, dreams, and other phenomena.

This central place occupied by history in Freud (and consequently the value of memory*, remembering*, and construction* in his thought) places him in the movement characteristic of modernity. However, he could also be placed in certain lines of thought of post-modernity considering the criticism implicit in his theory of discontent generated by the cultural phenomenon in each member of culture, in view of the defensive and uncognizant psychical apparatus (struggling against Trieb for knowledge) originated prevalently by this culture, also a product of the history of humanity (although culture's way of "making unconscious" differs from Freud's description).

HOMOSEXUALITY

Ger.: Homosexualität. – Sp.: homosexualidad. – Fr.: homosexualité. – It.: omosessualità. – Port.: homosexualidade.

This sexual "abnormality" is the paradigm of the so-called "perversions"*, in which sexual pleasure* is obtained only or preferentially with a person of the same sex.

It may be absolute, amphigenous (bisexuality), or occasional. The homosexual's attitude towards it also varies. Some homosexuals consider it natural and defend, for example, their equal sexual and social rights in relation to normal persons (this struggle for human rights, rights for homosexuals as for other human groups, among them even women, who have had to and still have to fight constantly). Others rebel against it and feel that it is a pathological compulsion*. Neurotics (or "normals") do not know it in themselves but fear it; it is taboo*; what they fear is contagion. This fear produced in response to tendencies unknown to the ego*, unknown because by virtue of the action of their unconscious defence mechanisms* they remain in the neurotic's unconscious.

Homosexuality includes innate hereditary factors, since all human beings are bisexual, and factors acquired ontogenetically. In the psychoanalytic perspective, we shall refer to the latter.

We may say that the central problem of homosexuality and perversions in general centres on recognition of sexual difference. Object libido* is satisfied, strictly speaking, with a sexual object* different from the subject, possessing a different sex. Of course, we form links with objects of the same sex and/or objects that we do not recognize as belonging to a different sex. But then it is not a question of object libido but rather homosexual libido, which sits astride object and narcissistic libido. It is object libido because it is satisfied by experiences with objects, but is narcissistic because of the type of object choice*, similar to the ego in the sense of characteristics defining its sex; sexual differences are not accepted (but instead disavowed) since acceptance would endanger narcissism*.

The basic mechanism is disavowal* of sexual difference and splitting of the ego* (since disavowal is successful only for part of it).

Sexual difference is not accepted because on the infantile phallic level, where this problem first appears, there are not actually two sexes but simply a being with a penis and a being with nothing (the female genital is analogous [cf. analogy*] to lack of the male genital), which in this theory is phallic–castrated opposition. The danger is castration. Since it seems to have been executed in girls, castration anxiety* is felt. Since it must be avoided, the existence of castration must be disavowed (in this way primary repression is established in homosexuality). This anticathexis* generates a fixation*, and from this point on, the pleasure object must secondarily disavow sexual difference. Pleasure is obtained by confirming the falsehood of existence of castration in each sexual encounter.

Other causes are added to the major mechanism.

In some adult males, maternal identification* leads them to choose as objects adolescents representing themselves, thereby disavowing the mother's castration and preserving in themselves (by identification*) the image of the phallic mother*.

The most common form of pleasure in males is derived from mutual masturbation or fellatio; previous anal fixations may facilitate maternal identification (the anus as a vagina), returning to the cloacal theory*. In this case, they seek active or passive coitus *per anum*. In the latter type of relation, masochistic* and sadistic elements are added.

A contributing factor may be repression* of aggressiveness and rivalry with brothers, "stepping aside"* and leaving women for them; homosexual women utilize the same mechanism in relation to their sisters or their mother, to whom they leave men. Female homosexuality originates as a consequence of phallic envy which forces disavowal of castration, reinforced by paternal identification and acquisition of masculine characteristics in the character*. Forms of pleasure of female homosexuals usually involve oral sexual games, since oral fixations established in the maternal link establish solid bases for recovering the phallic mother or identifying with her. In homosexual women, active and passive roles are more interchangeable.

Some types of homosexuality, the amphigenous and the occasional, especially when considered foreign to the ego or are rejected by it, are "curable" by psychoanalysis; not by reinforcing repression, of course, but by making homosexual wishes conscious through reconstruction of the history of the subject's infantile Trieb formation and its relation to what is actual in transference; leaving patients more freedom to choose between two aspects of themselves, only one of which they accepted or knew of, providing a possibility to add what was repressed and is now desexualized to preconscious ego forces, to be transformed into sublimation, for example. Those in whom the traumatic factor generated fixation points or changes in the Trieb* aim (from active to passive) have a better prognosis than those in whom the hereditary factor predominates.

As in any psychoanalytic treatment, the task is to reconstruct – through analysis of dreams*, parapraxes*, symptoms*, free association*, and so on – facts that gradually generated fixations and to work them through*: to interrupt the tendency to repetition through understanding* of the memory* and construction* of its circumstances; to face sexual differentiation, castration anxiety, and so on. In any case, since resistances* and predominantly negative transference* are common characteristics of homosexual patients given their narcissistic predominance, this reconstructive psychoanalytical work is not easy.

Homosexuality is part of narcissistic pathology. Since social links are formed with sublimated homosexual libido, homosexuals tend to have social difficulties (sometimes corrected by maternal identification as a feminine characteristic) and social anxiety*, mainly when homosexuality is ego-dystonic. Although ego-syntonic homosexuals also have them, they usually appear as defences* in response to narcissistic wounds, as a character trait: for example, arrogance, which generates difficulties in social links.

HUMOUR

Ger.: Humor. – Sp.: humor. – Fr.: humeur. – It.: umore. – Port.: humor.

This intellectual operation accomplished by the preconscious* part of the ego* through a small displacement* of preconscious presentations* creates a joke, transforming a situation of suffering originating in reality* into something pleasurable.

Therefore, humour is a conscious defensive ego attitude in response to a distressing reality by which it succeeds in saving itself painful feelings by converting it into pleasure*.

Unlike the comic* or the joke*, humour does not necessarily require another's presence: it is enough for a subject to laugh at him or herself and reality. In this sense, humour is narcissistic (cf. narcissism*), a type of link between ego and superego* in some people which enables the ego to identify momentarily with the ego ideal* (in this sense it is similar to mania or a manic mechanism, if you wish, but a healthy one), and it smiles at the ego's fear of reality. The ego ideal thereby becomes like a father who tells his son: "Look! Here is the world, which seems so dangerous! It is nothing but a game for children – just worth making a jest about!" (1927, p. 166). "[H]umour would be the contribution made to the comic through the agency of the superego" (Ibid., p. 165).

This form of the comic rejects suffering, triumphantly upholds the pleasure principle*, raises the ego's omnipotence, and achieves all this in the sphere of psychical health, even though it simply rejects reality and serves as an illusion* though momentary. However, while recognizing reality a bit, it is "wise".

"[N]ot everyone is capable of the humorous attitude. It is a rare and precious gift, and many people are even without the capacity to enjoy humorous pleasure that is presented to them" (Ibid., p. 166).

The observer enjoys humorous pleasure by identification*. The man condemned to death on a Monday, who says, "Nice way to start the week", creates this piece of humour for his own consumption, although an occasional observer may also detect the omnipotence or hyper-cathexis* of an ego identified momentarily with the ego ideal. This pleasure is perhaps not as intense as in jokes or the comic, but is "particularly liberating and elevating".

Humour is therefore a form of defence, among the highest, in response to difficulties of reality momentarily defeated affectively while the ego prepares an appropriate specific action through thought* activity, if this action is possible.

HYPER-CATHEXIS

Ger.: Überbesetzung. – Sp.: sobreinvestidura. – Fr.: surinvestissement. – It.: superinvestimento. – Port.: superinvestimento.

Any cathexis placed on a previous one is a hyper-cathexis. This hyper-cathexis may be in the presentation* (thing-presentation* + word-presentation*, for example) or in the *quantum* of affect* or libidinal energy.

During the state of preparedness anxiety* previous to a specific action* or in a danger-situation*, the entire perceptual apparatus is hyper-cathected with attention. Also, quantities of excitation* proceeding from the body are hyper-cathected by thing-presentations*, and the latter are hyper-cathected by libido*, acquiring the term Trieb* or object wish* without leaving the unconscious.

Hyper-cathexis may be produced by energy, and in this case it has an economic, energetic meaning. However, the somatic quantity of energy may also be cathected by the presentation, "clothed" by it. Then, hyper-cathexis acquires meaning possessing representational quality.

Passage from a presentation on one level to another higher one on the psychical scale requires hyper-cathexis. It may occur in different ways. For example, to access the ego's preconscious from the unconscious, a thing-presentation must be cathected by a word, and for this word to reach consciousness, it must receive a hyper-cathexis of attention from the latter.

In a psychical apparatus conceived in a dynamic way, able to move in different directions, hyper-cathexis acquires a progressive direction, opposed to regression* and, in some way, tends towards greater taming* of Trieb and more Trieb fusion, independent of complexities stemming from repression* and the splitting of the psychical apparatus into different parts.

The quantity of excitation hyper-cathected by an unconscious thing-presentation, which finds its word-presentation and thereby becomes preconscious, and may consequently be thought with a hyper-cathexis of attention, which take representational paths with strong cathexis and weak displacement* (characteristics that define secondary process*), reaching conclusions and deeper knowledge of wishes proceeding from Trieb; these wishes may or may not become realities through action in the external world and will be experienced as pleasurable experiences; this original quantity of excitation passes through all these stations, acquiring different and increasingly higher levels of the psychical: hyper-cathexis may reach the perceptual apparatus, in charge of perceiving reality and also of acquiring increasingly intense and perfected levels of Trieb binding and taming.

The diverse ego defence mechanisms* or secondary repression share the anticathexis of presentations not accepted by the ego which does not "acquiesce" to recognize them as its own.

Therefore, the ego possesses different means of subtracting cathexis from presentations whose presence produces anxiety: for example, by withdrawing its hyper-cathexis of attention, a defence for which it finds causes based on rationalizations*, blocking its access to consciousness, although it may have word-presentations in the preconscious, although they are ignored.

It may also subtract hyper-cathexis from the preconscious word-presentation and give it to another which thereby becomes an anticathexis* of the previous one, which enters a state of repression and is sent to the repressed unconscious.

This is produced by classical secondary repression whose return produces the origin of transference neuroses*, forgetting, dreams*, parapraxes*, and other phenomena.

In narcissistic psychoses*, cathexis is withdrawn from the unconscious thing-presentation, the motor of the unconscious object* wish*, whereas presentations corresponding to the ego (definition of narcissism*) are hyper-cathected, causing clinical phenomena such as megalomania* or hypochondria*. In cases of less severe narcissistic pathology, character traits*, such as haughtiness or arrogance, more compatible with the criterion of reality, may be established.

Therefore, in order to defend itself from anxiety provoked by certain Trieb wishes, the ego does not hesitate in response to its loss of degrees of mastery over Trieb, so long as it is able to expel them by cutting off all opportunities for them to reach action.

This is precisely what it obtains with its secondary repression ("pressure to hunt") or unconscious defence mechanisms besides succeeding in suppressing* Triebe and their derivative affects (in the neuroses this tends to fail, except in conversion hysteria*), not because of hyper-cathexes but just the opposite, because of anticathexes which, although they defend the ego at some point, tend to provoke pathology afterwards.

When the preconscious presentation has been decathected, even though the ego's consciousness hyper-cathects the rest of the presentations in the ego, it cannot find them since they have passed into the unconscious.

However, when it was the unconscious thing-presentation that was decathected, libido withdrew from the object world, manifested clinically as diverse degrees of withdrawal from social ties, even the end of the world experience in schizophrenia*.

In these cases, preconscious word-presentations are hyper-cathected without any type of unconscious grounding; they replace it, and paranoiac delusions* or any type of empty discourse not supported by unconscious thing-presentations are generated in this way. Sometimes, different levels of reconnection with the world are achieved, ruled more by the pleasure–unpleasure principle* than by the reality principle*; however, they are reconstructions, based ultimately on this preconscious hyper-cathexis.

The concept of hyper-cathexis is therefore highly complex, since it sometimes participates in health and Trieb mastery, and other times in pathology; it depends on what is hyper-cathected and how, although attempts to hyper-cathect tend to aim to master Trieb.

HYPOCHONDRIA

Ger.: Hypochondrie. – Sp. hipocondría. Fr.: hypocondrie. – It.: ipocondria. – Port.: hipocondria.

This psychical affection corresponds to narcissistic pathology or symptomatology typical of this type of affections: it presents a high degree of anxiety* whose main cause, for the subject's preconscious ego*, is apparent bodily illness. As in organic illness, bodily sensations are distressing and painful, and involve libidinal decathectization* of object presentations* of the external world and of objects themselves, libido being concentrated in fear or worry about the subject's body, health, or a certain organ. Libidinal cathexes* are therefore concentrated on the body itself, the origin of the ego, or on its presentations; it is differentiated from conversion hysteria* by its feature of uncontrollable anxiety, narcissistic withdrawal*, and other characteristics.

It is also differentiated from organic illness precisely by the bodily alteration justifying all the anticathexis* placed in the diseased organ, in order to prompt appropriate action for defence*. In hypochondria, the only alteration is a functional alteration corresponding to the erotogenic burden on the organ. What does exist is deep anxiety concerning an illness felt to be real.

Hypochondria is produced in processes of withdrawal of object libido and its transformation into narcissistic libido, with bodily stasis. The fact that it is unpleasurable, that it is hypochondriacal anxiety, originates in this stasis (quantitative accumulation of excitation, not variable by contact with the object world); it is an actual neurosis with narcissistic libido. It is the correlate, in terms of narcissistic libido, of the anxiety of actual neuroses belonging to object libido.

Processes of narcissistic libidinal withdrawal nearly inevitably go through a hypochondriacal period corresponding to withdrawal of cathexis from the unconscious object presentation and its shift onto the ego, beginning with its body. This situation may become chronic and participate in the constitution of the person's character*.

Another expression of narcissistic libidinal hyper-cathexis* in the ego is the clinical indicator of megalomania*.

In attempted restitution* of the world in narcissistic affections in general and in hebephrenic schizophrenia* in particular, what Freud calls organ speech* may emerge in which words are felt to be things, not as signifiers of thing-presentations* but as themselves, things that are body organs in a concrete sense, with a loss of the metaphor. The word-presentation* is no longer the signifier of the thing-presentation* in consciousness*, but rather takes its place and replaces it. The psychical apparatus therefore treats it as it treated unconscious thing-presentations*; that is to say, with primary process*. Thus, in this organ speech, syntactic alterations are produced referring to body organs; what was previously a metaphorization of organic concreteness takes the opposite road, returning to the concrete from the abstract ("my eyes get twisted", as Tausk's patient says, referring to her eyes rather than to her fiancé who changes her points of view).

Hypochondria may also be a predominant or chronic clinical picture in narcissistic personalities that have placed libido, and with it self-esteem, in the body ego, and may be expressed as anxiety in moments of greater stasis. In this sense, Freud considers it an actual neurosis* with narcissistic libido.

HYSTERICAL ATTACK

Ger.: hysterische Anfalle. – Sp.: ataque histérico. – Fr.: ataque histérique. – It.: attacco isterico. – Port.: ataque histérico.

Acute form of the symptomatology of "major hysteria" which Freud describes as a convulsive attack with an aura and three phases (Charcot postulated four phases including a terminal delirium*).

The aura is produced by a sensation in the hysterogenic zones*: hypersensitive places in the body whose stimulation triggers the attack. The first phase is the epileptoid, similar to a common epileptic attack; the second, with movements, presents very large movements such as "waving movements", the *arc de cercle*, and contortions. These movements are executed with elegance and are well coordinated, unlike the clumsy movements of epileptics.

The third phase is hallucinatory with passionate gestures. It is characterized by postures corresponding to hallucinated scenes of passion. Most frequently, consciousness* is maintained during most of the attack except some moments similar to the climax of sexual excitation.

In some cases, a single phase of the attack may substitute a full attack. Apoplectic attacks called "attacks of sleep" are also important.

The attack is composed of fantasies projected onto motility, represented in pantomime and disfigured in the manner of dreams*. This attack expresses a number of condensed fantasies with several identifications* (representing in this case two or more characters), sometimes with mutually opposing roles. It may also invert the temporal sequence of the fancied facts. The attack may be brought on associatively or organically and as a primary tendency (consolation) or a secondary gain from illness* (for example, when attacks are produced before certain persons).

The attack is a substitute for previously renounced autoerotic satisfaction (masturbation*) which returns but is not registered as such by consciousness.

Loss of consciousness, called an "absence" in hysterical attacks, comes from the transitory but unmistakable loss of consciousness that is registered at the height of all intense sexual satisfaction (even autoerotic). The reflex mechanism of the action of coitus shows repressed libido* the path towards motor discharge in the attack.

HYSTERO-EPILEPSY (CF. EPILEPSY)

HYSTEROGENIC ZONE

Ger.: hysterogene Zone. – Sp.: zona histerógena. – Fr.: zone hystérogène. – It.: zona isterogena. – Port.: zona histerógena.

This is a bodily zone whose stimulation may precipitate a major hysterical* attack or a hysterical symptom*. Some of them are described in typical areas of the body*, zones predisposed to sexual excitation and common to most cases of hysteria.

However, in a person suffering hysteria, any zone in certain circumstances may become a predominant, anomalous erotogenic zone* with its own anticathexis; for example, Elizabeth von R.'s* thigh as a result of placing her father's leg on it during caregiving in the period of his terminal illness (cf. cases of hysteria from the first period*), generating a stimulation point for the subsequent appearance of the hysterical symptom.

Sometimes, stimulation of the hysterogenic zone may encourage the appearance of the symptom or hysterical attack; this stimulation may even be verbal; during psychoanalytic treatment, symptoms may also flare up and thus "participate in the conversation" in the midst of a still incomplete therapeutic process. The hysterogenic zone may also be stimulated in other ways.

Ultimately, hysterogenic zones are erotogenic zones* which, instead of being sensitive to sexual stimulation, are debased to stimulating the emergence of neurotic symptoms.

I

ID

Ger.: Es. – Sp.: ello. – Fr.: ça. – It.: es. – Port.: isso.

One of the psychical structures of the "second topography", it is the seat of Triebe* from which psychical energy* springs.

At the same time it seems to be a dark, inaccessible part of our personality. It is described by opposition to the ego*; in reality, the id could correspond to what Freud calls the "nucleus of the ego" (*Project for a Scientific Psychology*, 1950, p. 328); that is to say, the part of the psychical apparatus that is more in contact with stimuli originating in the body. these stimuli cathect (cf. cathexis*) presentations* and are then referred to as Triebe; he also mentions it in *The Interpretation of Dreams* (1900) as "the core of our being" (p. 603).

The id is "open at its end to somatic influences, and as there taking up into itself instinctual needs which find their psychical expression in it" (*New Introductory Lectures on Psycho-Analysis*, 1933, p. 73).

The id is unconscious* but is not all the unconscious, since parts of the ego and the superego* are also unconscious.

The unconscious of the id is not synonymous with the repressed: the repressed is only a part of it, since other parts do not correspond to the repressed.

The id includes thing-presentations* having larger or smaller cathexes, interconnected by associations* of contiguity*, analogy*, or opposition*. Energy is displaced freely among them (free energy*), governed by the pleasure principle*, seeking perceptual identity*.

> The logical laws of thought do not apply in the id, and this is true above all of the law of contradiction. Contrary impulses exist side by side, without cancelling each other out or diminishing each other.
>
> (Ibid., 1933, p. 75)

These contrary impulses produce condensations*. There is no negation* in the id; nor is there any notion of space or time. Wishful impulses that have never left the id and impressions buried in it by repression* are virtually immortal.

> The id of course knows no judgements of value: no good and evil, no morality. The economic or, if you prefer, the quantitative factor, which is intimately linked to the pleasure principle, dominates all its processes. Instinctual cathexes seeking discharge – that in our view is all there is in the id.
>
> (Ibid., p. 74)

By the way, we recall that "instinctual cathexes" involve quantity cathecting presentations and vice versa (cf. Trieb*; cathexis*).

Primary process* reigns, its characteristic condensation* and displacement* providing links between thing-presentations*.

Freud adopted Groddeck's term, [Es] "id". He chose it mainly because of its meaning as something extraneous to the ego, metaphorically an "alien internal province".

Paradoxically, the id, the most deeply intimate part of our internal life, "the core of our being", is not felt by our ego as anything foreign to it, which shows us the ego's "alienation" within its own formative structure. It feels foreign to the deepest part of itself.

The id includes all the phylogenetic baggage left to us by experiences of former generations, which is summarized in the five primal phantasies* (the primal scene*, seduction*, castration, return to the mother's womb, and the family romance*) which, like the Kantian categories of understanding (time and space) function *a priori* in relation to experience, providing the child's understanding (and later the adult's, also unconsciously) an unconscious orientation concerning phenomena presented to the individual's perception* by placing them into "categories" or primal phantasies (*From the History of an Infantile Neurosis*, 1918). They are like pre-shaped channels to be filled with experience and even with other inherited memory traces (*Moses and Monotheism: Three Essays*, 1939), which thereby guide the way to understanding actual phenomena: a kind of instinctive knowledge akin to that of animals. Another element of this phylogenetic equipment, universal symbolism*, familiar to all (pre-oedipal) children regardless of their linguistic diversity, also belongs to the id.

IDEAL EGO

Ger.: Ideal-Ich. – Sp.: yo ideal. – Fr.: moi-idéal. – It.: io ideale. – Port.: ego ideal.

This part of the ego* is synonymous with the ego ideal* in works such as *On Narcissism: An Introduction* (1914) and *The Ego and the Id* (1923). However, in 1914, Freud mentions aspects that clarify the road to understanding this concept, although they are not enough to give it status as a structure.

"Observation of normal adults shows that their former megalomania has been damped down and that the psychical characteristics from which we inferred their infantile narcissism have been effaced" (*On Narcissism: An Introduction*, 1914, p. 93).

At a certain moment (following the Oedipus complex*), the psychical apparatus sets up an ideal by which it measures its actual ego. "For the ego the formation of an ideal would be the conditioning factor of repression" (Ibid., p. 94).

> This ideal ego is now the target of the self-love which was enjoyed in childhood by the actual ego. The subject's narcissism makes its appearance displaced on to this new ideal ego, which, like the infantile ego, finds itself possessed of every perfection that is of value ... What he projects before him as his ideal is the substitute for the lost narcissism of his childhood in which he was his own ideal.
>
> (Ibid.)

Therefore, the ideal ego is what the ego ideal (part of the superego*) demands of the ego, and consists of memories* of the omnipotence* of thought* of infantile sexuality* and even, farther back, the purified pleasure ego*, since what ego could be more ideal than this one?

This is further proof that the ego ideal is not ruled by the reality principle* but by the pleasure principle*. Ultimately, it is ruled by the superego's pleasure* in its power to punish the ego when it disobeys demands of the ideal.

It is also interesting to emphasize Freud's reasoning: the ego ideal demands that the ego be ideal regarding the future, but also requires it dictatorially to be the ideal it "possessed" in the past, a past now repressed and part of the unconscious, since it belongs to infantile sexuality, which thereby becomes idealized as well as repressed.

IDEALIZATION

Ger.: Idealsierung. – Sp.: idealización. – Fr.: idéalisation. – It.: idealizzazione. – Port.: idealização.

Overvaluation of the object* by the ego*, which has put the object in the place of the ego ideal*.

In relation to the object thereby idealized: "The criticism exercised by that agency is silent; everything that the object does and asks for is right and blameless" (1921, p. 113).

The object possesses all the virtues, beauties, and capacities the ego wishes for. Examples of idealization are being in love and hypnosis. When the subject is in love, object libido* but also a larger measure of narcissistic libido flows into the object. The object replaces the subject's own ego ideal which the subject would like to attain in order to satisfy narcissism* by this roundabout route.

In hypnosis, the hypnotizer is the idealized object, excluding all sexual satisfaction. (The same occurs in groups* in the link with the leader, who synthesizes the ideals of group members.)

> Idealization is a process that concerns the object; by it that object, without any alteration in its nature, is aggrandized and exalted in the subject's mind. Idealization is possible in the sphere of ego libido as well as in that of object libido.
>
> (1914, p. 94)

Children apply this type of valuation when they begin to recognize their objects. They want to possess some and want to copy others, to be* like them. Parents are idealized by their children, since the latter consider them omnipotent because they complete specific actions* children know about and wish for but are beyond their reach or forbidden.

Towards adolescence, paternal figures are deidealized. Idealization is displaced (cf. displacement*) on to others. Then they experience being in love and fascination for idols and heroes* which were once the parents. Gradually, as the ego is enriched, the reality principle* imposes itself and the ego has less need to occupy the place of the ideal with an object, although it often persists, especially when fissures in narcissism need to be filled up.

IDENTIFICATION

Ger.: Identifizierung. – Sp.: identificación. – Fr.: identification. – It.: identificazione. – Port.: identificação.

This primitive form of psychical functioning and object relation (prior even to recognition of the object as such) comprises, in principle, the action of becoming identical: identical to one or many of the object's* attributes. The object's attribute or attributes then constitute characteristics of the ego* which develops in this way.

Identification is an unconscious process, rather than simple imitation; though they share some points of contact), but is an appropriation expressing an "equal to" and referring to something in common that remains in the unconscious*.

"First, identification is the original form of emotional tie" (1921, p. 107).

In this first stage, when the logic of the purified pleasure ego* predominates, when there is no distinction between ego and object (or rather, what is recognized as ego is accepted in the future as an object, especially if the link with it produces pleasure*), we may say that ego and object are identical: the ego has identified with the object. It does not consider it foreign to itself but simply itself. The category of having* does not exist: everything is being*. This is quite likely the predominant type of link between baby and mother (a symbiotic link according to M. Mahler's terminology). This type of identification between baby and mother may be considered primary, since it is previous to recognition of the object as a source of pleasure. The oral erotogenic zone predominates at this time (cf. oral erotism*) and the prevalent link is established by anaclisis* on incorporation of food and the pleasure of sucking: the incorporation model marks the direction to identification. Preponderance of the oral erotogenic zone* lends its model for this to occur. The object's attributes become the ego's, and the ego begins to move and to do things as the object once did for it.

The concept of primary identification* includes the first type of the baby's link with its father: when the "Wolf Man" as a child "was always declaring that he would like to be a gentleman like [his father]" (1918, p. 17). Not yet distinguishing sexual difference and therefore the father's real place in the family, incipient object discrimination exists.

In any case, unlike identification with the preoedipal mother*, this identification with the father is not linked to the latter as the child's pleasure object; at least, not predominantly in what defines his paternal role. This is previous to later oedipal rivalry but after the purified pleasure ego; for this reason it is still primary, although there is some discrimination between ego and pleasure object. The difference is that the father is not yet a rival (positive Oedipus) nor is he a pleasure object (negative Oedipus). In the phallic period (cf. phallic-urethral erotism*), primary identification acquires a hostile tone. Then the father complex* is established, culminating in establishment of the superego* by virtue of secondary identification*, basically with the father. Primary identification is thereby reinforced (*The Ego and the Id*, 1923) and with it, masculinity (in the positive Oedipus complex). From this moment, the unconscious mechanism of identification must be secondary, and now also reinforces in transference previous identifications with the parental figures of infantile sexuality*, since the repressed may also return (cf. return of the repressed*) through secondary identifications.

When the primary link is severely altered, the psychical apparatus in response to new frustrations* may again utilize mechanisms by which presentations* of the ego and the object were differentiated, since it is nearly impossible for the subject to form links in which the desired object is recognized as such. Consequently, the first form of loving is re-established: transformation into the object or "being" the object, as the baby once felt. This is typical of narcissistic affections, especially in borderline patients and in melancholia*; it is also observed as identification with an attribute connected with a repressed erotic wish in conversion hysteria*.

When an ego's characteristics have been successfully established by primary identification and those of the superego by secondary identification, identification may appear as an unconscious mechanism in dreams*, in symptoms*, and as a form of link among members of a group* by virtue of the community of wishes.

In hysterical symptoms, identification is partial, established with only one of the object person's attributes (a loved or hated person; Anna Freud referred to the latter as "identification with the aggressor").

Identification may also dispense with the object relation with the person copied and be done to acquire power or to put the subject's self into the same situation. Freud called this phenomenon "psychical infection", present in group formation and even in empathy towards a work of art*: the subject feels like the artist, "is" the artist.

ILLUSION

Ger.: Illusion. – Sp.: illusion. – Fr.: illusion. – It.: illusione. – Port.: ilusão.

This belief, motivated particularly by wish fulfilment*, sometimes relinquishes its connection with effective reality*.

Freud considers religious presentations* illusions.

> These, which are given out as teachings, are not precipitates of experience or end-results of thinking: they are illusions, fulfillments of the oldest, strongest and most urgent wishes of mankind. The secret of their strength lies in the strength of those wishes.
>
> (*The Future of an Illusion*, 1927, p. 30)

In response to their helplessness before nature, their fellow beings and their own Triebe*, children need first maternal and then paternal protection. Recognition that this helplessness lasts a lifetime sets them in search of a much more powerful father.

> Thus the benevolent rule of a divine Providence allays our fear of the dangers of life, the establishment of a moral world-order ensures the fulfillment of the demands of justice, which have so often remained unfulfilled in human civilization; and the prolongation of earthly existence in a future life provides the local and temporal framework in which these wish-fulfillments shall take place.
>
> (Ibid.)

"An illusion is not the same thing as an error; nor is it necessarily an error" (Ibid.). Its characteristic is that it always derives from human wishes.

Neither is the illusion necessarily false, unrealizable, or contradictory with respect to reality. It is a belief based on wish fulfilment, not demonstrable and irrefutable.

Freud considers that

> the riddles of the universe reveal themselves only slowly to our investigation; there are many questions to which science to-day can give no answer. But scientific work is the only road which can lead us to a knowledge of reality outside ourselves.
>
> (Ibid., p. 31)

"Ignorance is ignorance; no right to believe anything can be derived from it" (Ibid., p. 32).

INFANTILE AMNESIA

Ger.: Infantile Amnesie. – Sp.: amnesia infantil. – Fr.: amnésie infantile. – It.: amnesia infantile. – Port.: amnésia infantil.

A universal process by which the adult human being does not remember all the events that took place in life before five years of age, approximately, despite having had resources, not fully developed, during most of this period, for remembering (language*, thought*, ego*, reality principle*, anxiety for object* loss, recognition of the object as a source of pleasure*).

Amnesia is produced following the dissolution* of the Oedipus complex* and the definitive establishment in the psychical apparatus of the superego*, an agency which acts as an immense anticathexis* that encompasses all previous anticathexes (primary repressions*), thereby producing repression* (primary by antonomasia) and with it the forgetting* of all infantile sexuality*.

The latter may subsequently be reconstructed by psychoanalysis of dreams*, symptoms*, screen memories*, parapraxes*, and so on.

An interesting example of infantile amnesia is Little Hans, the first child patient in the history of psychoanalysis, who was treated between three and five years of age. Later, when he was nineteen, he remembered almost nothing of his analytic process or of events that occurred at that time, when he had manifested brilliant intelligence, precocious capacity to think, and a magnificent memory.

The producer of infantile amnesia is none other than infantile sexuality itself commanded by the phallic erotogenic zone; with the union of all the erotogenic zones* generating a definitive reality ego which definitively recognizes the object* (centre of reality*) as a source of pleasure, now with characteristics different from the ego (its sex is different, although the first difference recognized is only that of possession or not of the phallus); in sum, the entire oedipal problem. This complex problem is "dissolved" or goes into the state of repression* and with it, all the antecedent problems; in this way primary repression, the superego, and the psychical apparatus in general are definitively constituted.

Infantile sexuality is dissolved or repressed and the repressed unconscious* is born – a crucial discovery by Freud – containing all the presentations of that infantile sexuality.

INFANTILE SEXUALITY

Ger.: infantile Sexualität. – Sp.: sexualidad infantil. – Fr.: sexualité infantile. – It.: sessualità infantile. – Port.: sexualidade infantil.

This is the sexuality of children up to five or six years of age, before establishment of the superego* following the Oedipus complex*. Infantile sexuality emerges as extra pleasure* above satisfaction of self-preservative Trieb which is thereafter gradually differentiated from it. It is basically autoerotic (although not absolutely, since the erotogenic zones* awaken in the object* link) and different erotogenic zones predominate in it corresponding to the different phases. Each zone has its own means of pleasure, but these zones do not form a bodily unit; for this reason, Freud describes infantile sexuality as "perverse polymorphous". It is part of the development of sexuality, its aim being pleasure rather than procreation; at the end of its development, its object becomes incestuous (precisely during the Oedipus complex*), and is therefore repressed in order to enable the subject to access culture*. In his treatments of adult patients, Freud observed phenomena which are normal in childhood. Based on his observations, he was able to investigate behaviour in children which derives from the development of their sexuality.

The text presenting the discovery and description of phenomena related to infantile sexuality is *Three Essays on the Theory of Sexuality* (1905), and the first case of psychoanalysis of a child, Little Hans, transcribes the narration of all the events related to the development of his sexuality and the relation between these events and the child's pathological symptoms.

Since that time, the concept of infantile sexuality has become a fundamental pillar of psychoanalytic theory and clinical work.

The unconscious* as a topical seat of the psychical apparatus is essentially populated by presentations* of events experienced with objects through the erotogenic zones which predominated in the different periods of infancy and early childhood. They form thing-presentations* which later refer to subsequent experiences, seeking identity with them, trying to "refind" them or to refind* in reality the object or its attributes which may produce this identity or some degree of it (*Negation*, 1925).

Infantile sexuality has great freedom in regard to the forms of pleasure with objects and the types of choice of these objects, but follows a certain order in its development (an order perhaps originating in phylogeny).

Therefore, it has phases of libido* development in which certain forms of pleasure predominate over others in different periods.

All these phases are predominantly autoerotic. There is pleasure through auto-stimulation of the body and also pleasure produced in the object link, except that at first this object is not recognized as such but only gradually; therefore, the link with it is ultimately also autoerotic even though the object is recognized as a different body by the initial reality ego*; it must await development of the definitive reality ego* in order to be recognized as an object of pleasure external to the ego*; this occurs together with changes in predominance of each erotogenic zone of sexuality*.

The phases classically described are the oral, the anal, and the phallic (cf. oral erotism*, anal erotism*, and phallic-urethral erotism*), each with its different forms of pleasure and specific problems.

However, we may also add to these the erotism of the whole body, the skin, vision, sadism*, masochism*, the vicissitudes of Trieb* previous to repression*, such as reversal into the opposite*, turning round upon the subject's own self*, the disorder of Trieb activity turned into passivity, and other mechanisms.

These events occur partly with Triebe corresponding to those libidinal phases, although they may also be independent or parallel vicissitudes, or may be subject to subsequent transformations, forming diverse pathologies with different complexities.

The type of pleasure of Triebe of infantile sexuality is poorly organized. In spite of periods of predominance of one Trieb over another, they do not form a bodily unit, and for this reason they are part Triebe*. Each one seeks pleasure in a disperse way, isolated from the other erotogenic zones: pleasure produced by its stimulation does not unify the body as it does when the development of sexuality (genital) concludes and the ego is formed definitively.

However, the phallic phase attains a level of pleasure that unites the former phases under its supremacy, and then the objective of sexuality is to produce phallic pleasure, which is associated with growing recognition of the object of its pleasure; also, this union of the erotogenic zones organized under its supremacy, each bearing its own history with the object, contributes greatly, proceeding from the body (the body essence of *The Ego and the Id*, 1923) to the formation of the definitive reality ego, the culmination of the narcissistic period when predominance of object libido over narcissistic libido is achieved.

It is in this phase that the most traumatic period of infantile sexuality arises: the Oedipus complex.

This phase also leads to the greatest consequences, since it re-includes the previous phases and re-signifies their histories from its own viewpoint. It concludes infantile sexuality as well.

The sexual object, chosen by anaclisis* on self-preservative Triebe, has now become incestuous, and consequently, the idea of seeking pleasure provokes castration anxiety*. The child's unconscious (reinforced by phylogeny) believes that castration would be executed by the father, felt to be the rival; this phantasy is accepted as a possible reality* by what is now full understanding* of the meaning of the appearance of the female genital (an analogy, mistaken for identity in this phase, of the feared castration of the male organ, the only genital recognized as such). The result is a first level of recognition of sexual difference between objects: they are either phallic or castrated.

Since this problem has no solution at this time of life, it is repressed and dissolved, and the superego is finally established along with clearer definitions of the limits between the ego and the id. A blanket of forgetting is thrown over all events corresponding to the period of infantile sexuality. Constitution of the psychical apparatus is completed, and the subject accesses culture.

However, infantile sexuality leaves its trace in thing-presentations of the repressed unconscious belonging to the id*; as such, it will no longer have access to the ego, since the ego utilizes the anxiety signal*, especially that of castration, to defend itself from infantile Triebe which are now anticultural since they have become incestuous.

However, taking advantage of the possibilities of sexual Triebe to change their object, their aim may also be inhibited and sublimations* formed to generate culture and social ties. They also participate in the fore-pleasure of courtship and sexual play.

Everything that was repressed struggles to return from the repressed through neurotic decompensations facilitated by a triggering factor or frustration*.

Sexual perversions* may also be generated when fixations* are established by disavowal* of sexual difference, and even the splitting of the ego.

INFANTILE SEXUAL THEORIES

Ger.: infantile Sexualtheorien. – Sp.: teorías sexuales infantiles. – Fr.: théories sexuelles infantiles. – It.: teorie sessuali infantili. – Port.: teorias sexuais infantis.

Freud discovered not only infantile sexuality* but also, dazzling us again with his genius, infantile thinking, children's theories on birth and sexuality*, products of the infant's curiosity and Trieb for knowledge* previous to establishment of the period of phallic supremacy and therefore pre-oedipal* and universal in all children.

Infantile sexual theories involve sexual non-differentiation which implies possession of a penis by all human beings (men and women), and later at least by the mother, which gives her a phallic characteristic (theory of the phallic mother*).

It is followed by the cloacal theory*. According to this theory, babies are born through the anus, and delivery is not limited to women (strictly speaking, the feminine-masculine category does not exist at this age, which does not mean that secondary sexual characteristics are not recognized). Delivery is intimately connected with the idea of a "gift" and with faeces, identified in the unconscious by the equation:

$$\text{child} = \text{penis} = \text{faeces} = \text{gift}.$$

These theories seem to succumb to the reality of sexual differentiation, the first level of which becomes evident in the phallic period.

However, they are left in the unconscious and in some cases are part of the unconscious ego which retains certain contradictions which may lead to splitting: recognition and non-recognition of sexual differentiation in order to defend itself from castration anxiety* involved in the phallic period, to which the subject may continue to be fixated. This persists as each person's own "bedrock"*, a place analysis reaches, or a degree to which a person's ego tolerates castration anxiety.

Infantile sexual theories involve some degree of foreclosure* of reality*, a reality carrying little weight in this period of life (since it is closely mediated by the parents), but which is important and difficult to bear in the phallic period; for this reason, different defence mechanisms* are called upon such as disavowal* of the existence of castration (the base of some narcissistic disorders such as perversions* and of some psychoses* such as acute hallucinatory confusion or Meynert's amentia*) or repression* of Trieb* which succeeds in avoiding castration anxiety (the base of transference neuroses*).

Infantile sexual theories repressed in the period of the Oedipus complex* may return and originate neurotic symptoms*, as in the case of the "Wolf Man" whose hysterical symptom of constipation was based on a homosexual and masochistic phantasy of giving his father a child, involving regression to the cloacal theory.

In general, when the period of the Oedipus complex is reached and following its dissolution*, these theories sink to the bottom of the unconscious together with all infantile sexuality; they have entered a dead end where they are unable to survive attacks by reality, the castration complex*, and the wound to narcissism produced by the castration complex in women and castration anxiety in men.

Then, the ego splits to a greater or lesser extent, forming some kind of "bedrock" (parts of the ego in which castration is not accepted). In these defensive narcissistic bunkers, infantile sexual theories remain standing.

INHIBITION

Ger.: Hemmung. – Sp.: inhibición. – Fr.: inhibition. – It.: inibizione. – Port.: inibição.

The concept of inhibition has two definitions in Freud's works. At first, in the *Project for a Scientific Psychology* (1895), it is action exerted by the ego* on primary process*. More precisely, on the energy of cathexis* displaced* freely from presentation* to presentation (understanding these neurons* as presentations) in search of perceptual identity* with the experience of satisfaction* and even with that of pain*.

If there were no inhibition, the experience of satisfaction could be hallucinated and generate the consequent frustration*; that experience of pain could originate pain in absence of the real object* that once caused it. In order to avoid this, the ego places collateral chains of cathected presentations which form the activity of thought*; this enables passage from free energy to another that is bound*; that is to say, with a strong cathexis and weak displacement.

Inhibition modifies the route of the energy of cathexis by impeding direct hallucination* of the desired image, and allows space for "perhaps" or "afterwards" as well as reality testing*. Comparison between the perceived object and the wish* shows to what extent they are the same, analogous, or different. The ego applies this inhibition through its presentations and its energy stored in a bound state. This ego is constantly growing, receiving presentations that are products of new experiences in life.

In order for the ego to utilize this inhibitory mechanism, quantities of energy must not surpass a certain limit (a situation we refer to as traumatic*), since in this case the ego is unable to bind them and must resort to an extreme defence* such as anticathexis*. The latter fixates the Trieb* (the erotogenic zone*, the object presentation, and the type of satisfaction or pleasure* this erotogenic zone derives from the object) and does not allow its presentations to be part of the ego; they are instead expelled from it.

Inhibited by the ego, primary processes may access secondary process*, which involves a higher level of binding, the reality principle* and the possibility to enter into specific action*.

However, in *Inhibitions, Symptoms and Anxiety* (1925), Freud presents a different, more phenomenological conception of inhibition referring to a process with certain pathological characteristics. In it, inhibition consists of something that occurs to the ego as a functional limitation in relation to a certain activity in order to evade the conflict that it might cause it, which may or may not be pathological. It is differentiated from the symptom* which is something foreign to the ego, the product of a compromise, a substitute formation* between Trieb* and the ego or between the superego* and the ego. By limiting its possibilities, the ego also avoids conflicts by inhibiting confrontation with their possible presence. This is the other concept of inhibition.

Inhibition of the ego may also be one of the consequences of repression* and suppression* of affects*. An ego so busy repressing has no energy for other activities.

INITIAL REALITY EGO

Ger.: Wirklichkeit-Ich. – Sp.: yo realidad inicial. – Fr.: moi-réalité initial. – It.: io realtà iniziale. – Port.: ego de realidade inicial.

The functioning of this ego* predominates at the outset of mental work of human young. A realistic criterion reigns in this type of ego.

It is based on the ability to perform certain movements (at first they are reflexes) such as approaching or drawing away from some sources of stimulus (for example, opening and closing the eyes in response to stimulus by light or kicking in response to a heat stimulus). These movements generally respond in connection with self-preservative Triebe* which rapidly submit to the reality principle*; therefore, internal Trieb stimuli, for example, hunger or thirst, are allowed to be felt as the subject's own.

The initial reality ego enables recognition of bodily limits. In this line, whatever we are able to escape does not belong to our body*; it is not-ego (this ego is synonymous with the body); the stimulus from which we cannot escape except through specific action* is ego.

The initial reality ego is one of the pillars supporting the definitive reality ego* in order to impose the reality principle* upon sexual Triebe*; the background to this is that at the beginning of this type of ego functioning as described above, the reality* of the object* is somehow recognized (partly) from the first moment. In the second step, when something more than satisfaction intervenes, the situation becomes growingly complex, and other types of ego functioning come into play.

INSTINCT

Ger.: Instinkt. – Sp.: instinto. – Fr.: Trieb. – It.: istinto. – Port.: instinto.

A more or less complex action carried out without previous learning, it may also be learning already acquired by forebears, by the species. Instinct is inherited, phylogenetic. Behaviour is predominantly instinctive in animals. In human beings, it is much more unpredictable and differs from one subject to another. The term Trieb utilized by Freud is explained more as a product of the subject's own experience.

Experiences of satisfaction* leave residues: presentations* of wishes* to recover the experience. When these presentations are cathected*, they endeavour to search for satisfaction; in this way Trieb is originated, a concept astride the psychical and the biological, an effort of the somatic that pushes the psychical to reach an action, its aim given by the presentation.

However, aside from being restless seekers, Triebe are conservative. They tend to repeat previous experiences of satisfaction (libidinal or life Triebe*) or to return to the original state before life, the inorganic (death Triebe*). In this repetition, Trieb is similar to animal instinct, beyond the complexity humans may put into their repetitive acts. Therefore, both points of difference and points of contact exist between Trieb and instinct.

In his clinical experience, Freud encounters evidence of behaviour not originating in experience. In the life of the "Wolf Man", castration threats always came from maternal representatives. However, in this patient's unconscious*, fear of castration is felt before the father. Phylogeny defeats ontogeny. This fact forces Freud to the hypothesis of inherited schemas which, like the Kantian categories (time and space), "put order" into vital impressions and "prepare for their understanding". These schemas are called "protophantasies", "primal phantasies", or "phylogenetic presentations". They are inherited schemas that must be filled up with experience.

In *Moses and Monotheism: Three Essays* (1939), he goes even further: "the archaic heritage of human beings comprises not only dispositions but also subject-matter – memory traces of the experience of earlier generations" (p. 99).

"Universal symbols"* are part of this archaic inheritance, original knowledge that the adult has forgotten but which appears in dreams* although they are not understood (for this reason he says, "they have been forgotten").

"[S]ymbolism disregards differences of language" (Ibid., p. 99). "Here, then, we seem to have an assured instance of an archaic heritage dating from the period at which language developed" (Ibid.). Freud also considers that all inherited dispositions for understanding are "the single analogy … of the far-reaching instinctive knowledge of animals" (1918, p. 120).

> This instinctive factor would then be the nucleus of the unconscious, a primitive kind of mental activity, which would later be dethroned and overlaid by human reason, when that faculty came to be acquired, but which in some people, perhaps in every one, would retain the power of drawing down to it the higher mental processes.
>
> (Ibid.)

INTEREST

Ger.: Interesse. – Sp.: interés. – Fr.: intérêt. – It.: interesse. – Port.: interesse.

This energy cathects (cf. cathexis*) presentations* belonging to self-preservative ego* Triebe.

They correspond partly to the initial reality ego*, which recognizes reality* quite soon. Therefore, interest is bound energy* which only becomes conflictive for the ego when it is eroticized; however, in this case, the conflict already belongs to sexual Triebe*. The latter are born with the support of satisfactions of self-preservative Triebe, then slowly differentiate from them and at some point oppose them.

In the second instinctive theory, interest is included in Eros* or life Triebe*, which does not mean that they disappear, since they retain their differences in relation to sexual Triebe.

Although self-preservative Triebe and also interest may conflict with a difficult reality if it blocks their satisfaction, they do not generate intrapsychic conflict.

INTERNAL CHANGE

Ger.: inneren Veranderung. – Sp.: alteración interna – Fr.: altération interne. – It.: alterazione interna. – Port.: alteração interna.

This phenomenon was conceptualized by Freud in direct relation to the form of emotional expression described primarily with respect to the new-born infant, but may be extended to include adults. Freud discussed it in the *Project for a Scientific Psychology* (1950) and *The Interpretation of Dreams* (1900), and mentioned it in other works such as *The Unconscious* (1915) in which he describes: "Affectivity manifests itself essentially in motor (secretory and vaso-motor) discharge resulting in an (internal) alteration of the subject's own body without reference to the external world; motility, in actions designed to effect changes in the external world" (p. 179, Footnote).

He also mentions it in *Inhibitions, Symptoms, and Anxiety* (1926*d*) as part of the neurotic symptom*:

> The substitutive process is prevented, if possible, from finding discharge through motility; and even if this cannot be done, the process is forced to expend itself in making alterations in the subject's own body and is not permitted to impinge upon the external world. It must not be transformed into action.
>
> (p. 95)

In essence, internal change consists in the body's first form of discharge in response to Trieb *Drang* (pressure, force of work) which instead of producing a change in the external world (provision of food, nearness of the sexual object*) produces a change within the body, this change manifested qualitatively as emotion or affect through screaming and vascular innervations.

Internal change is therefore the form of expression of emotions (screaming, vascular innervation) which thus have a very major form of bodily expression.

In *Inhibitions, Symptoms and Anxiety* (1926*d*) he describes three constituent parts of anxiety*: a small bodily discharge, perception* of this discharge and finally perception of a particular unpleasurable feeling. The latter is qualitative perception of quantity by which it becomes a psychical feeling. The form of bodily discharge consists mainly of tachycardia and hyperventilation. He even states that this mode of discharge is acquired during the birth trauma*. At birth this bodily reaction is adequate and specific, given that it is the way to obtain oxygen after the change of respiratory system. However, it would seem that the organism remains fixated to this prototypical situation and therefore responds to any other danger situation* with this type of response, at least as the most immediate response, the affective response. This path then becomes an expression of emotions in general.

Later, when tension due to need in the organism increases, the baby expresses its emotion with screaming and vascular innervation. This "internal change" is then understood by "extraneous help", generally the mother, in charge of bringing about the specific action* at that moment. This causes quantity of stimulation to decrease in the Trieb source, thereby producing an experience of satisfaction*.

Emotional expression, at first a simple bodily discharge, is gradually transformed into an entreaty, in the context of a growing tie between mother and child; this is one of the bases upon which language* is learned.

The concept of internal change is therefore a dynamic concept, since it refers to a process that is transformed (from emotional expression into a call and the call into language) on the one hand, and on the other hand, persists as a form of emotional expression, mainly of anxiety.

A biological response is transformed into social ties with their pertinent feelings and also preserved as a bodily response. It is therefore interesting to again underscore different themes that lead us unexpectedly to others, all deriving from this concept: emotional expression (anxiety), screaming (the maternal tie and with it language), and vascular innervations (psychosomatic pathology).

INTERPRETATION

Ger.: Deutung. – Sp.: interpretación. – Fr.: interprétation. – It.: interpretazione. – Port.: interpretação.

One of the psychoanalyst's major technical weapons, it is a product of the patient's previous associative work, the universal symbolic, symptoms* as memory symbols* or previous knowledge of the case history.

Interpretations may recover an unconscious* level of meaning, and their formulation (when the analyst verbalizes them, speaking them in words) may bring to the analysand's consciousness* the meaning of a dream*, a parapraxis*, character trait*, symptom, repetitive behaviour, transference*, resistance*, or affect* hitherto unknown, at least to the subject's conscious ego*.

Therefore, psychoanalytical interpretation attains the aspiration to make conscious the unconscious.

Presentations* of the unconscious we seek are the repressed and the repressing (resistance * and anticathexes*). When the analyst finds them and communicates them to the patient, they recover words lost in the repressive process and, passing through negation*, may be reinserted in associative commerce, a thought* activity, and thereby become part of the person's preconscious ego. The ego then chooses what to do with them: to put them into action, postpone them for another, more adequate occasion, or condemn them by judgement*; they may be tamed*, placed into secondary process.

An interpretation may be separated into parts, which are then sometimes referred to as "indication". It is sometimes put together with questions, also based on other interpretations; or simply connecting the patient's current words with others spoken at another moment, in the same session or a previous one. This formulation opens new meanings or novel associations*, or brings up fresh memories* or dreams. In sum, to interpret is an attempt to take apart by unravelling the hardened and repetitive skein of phantasies* in which the patient is enveloped until new meanings are found for the ego and old ones for the patient's history (the basic ones from infantile sexuality*).

Different levels of depth in the unconscious are reached by virtue of interpretation. The deeper it goes, the more change it generates, and the more lasting this change may be. Each patient has a unique "bedrock", a metaphor utilized by Freud to indicate the limits of the treatment.

There are different kinds of interpretation.

Transference interpretation is indicated when transference emerges as an obstacle to knowledge of the unconscious; however, the history the repressive ego aims to ignore and repeat tends to be inserted precisely in the characteristics of this obstacle.

Associative interpretation emerges from the patient's free associations when it is carrying the latent preconscious and consequently comes close to "mestizos" and through them to derivatives of the unconscious. This type of interpretation carries, implicitly or explicitly, the history that in any case needs to be explicated, since associations are usually disguised deformations of this history: a past that has become present. Interpretation must send them back to the past.

Symbolic interpretation utilizes universal symbols* in order to open new associative paths. They sometimes orient the patient in relation to the meaning of a symptom or a dream, but they tend to be incomplete. We could say that they are just another weapon in the psychoanalytical therapeutic arsenal.

It is sometimes also possible to interpret a dream literally when the analyst has thorough knowledge of its previous circumstances and perceives that the meaning of the words of manifest content* refers to it (*The Interpretation of Dreams*, 1900).

Anagogic interpretation was described by H. Silberer, but Freud considers that it is not psychoanalytical. This interpretation seeks the meaning of a dream in a more elevated abstraction within the psychical. Freud considers it an intellectualization, something the patient already does, and resistance to knowledge of the unconscious. The psychoanalyst seeks depth in the unconscious, in repressed infantile sexuality, rather than in beautifying preconscious abstractions or metaphors.

Interpretation collaborates with construction*, the other psychoanalytical therapeutic weapon *par excellence*. Interpretation may move on to a construction, and one construction may generate another. This enriching, dynamic interplay takes place constantly in an analytical process. It is only interrupted by moments of resistance, due to transference or not, and negative therapeutic reactions, all of which may be modified, some more than others, by interpretive work.

INTROVERSION OF LIBIDO

Ger.: Libido Introversion. – Sp.: introversión libidinal. – Fr.: introversion libidinale. – It.: introversione libidinale. – Port.: introversão libidinal.

This withdrawal of libidinal cathexis* from preconscious presentations* generates distance from real objects*, which are replaced by phantasy* objects, all mechanisms corresponding to secondary repression of the neuroses referred to as historical or transference* neuroses. Libido* withdrawn from objects (from their preconscious presentations) then cathects preconscious daydreams; since cathexis is not withdrawn from unconscious thing-presentations, unconscious sexual object desire persists, is repressed, and seeks ways to reach the preconscious.

Preconscious daydreams (mestizos between primary process* and secondary process*) express repressed wishes as fulfilled wishes by camouflaging secondary process: their formal aspects are retained, but phantasies are ruled by the pleasure principle* (hallucinatory wish satisfaction*), rather than the reality principle*.

In introversion, retreat from reality* is not total, as it is in narcissistic libidinal withdrawal. Unconscious cathexis of the desired object persists and returns from the repressed* through the phantasy that fulfils the disguised object wish.

Then, what was unconscious cathexis of the desired object remains as a phantasy, part of thought* activity. Phantasy has no hallucination; partial regression* to perception is managed by the ego* and never reaches the sensory intensity of a hallucination*. Return to reality* occurs simply through reality testing (blinking, for example).

As we said, the fact that unconscious cathexis of the object persists distinguishes introversion of libido from narcissistic withdrawal. In the latter, libidinal cathexis stanches the ego and takes refuge in it.

Introversion of object libido forms a rich culture medium for neurotic symptom* formation, dreams*, and so on, whereas preconscious phantasies are repressed to the unconscious.

INVOCATION

Ger.: Berufen. – Sp.: invocación. – Fr.: invocation. – It.: invocazione. – Port.: invocação.

This form of negation* (a preconscious process attempting to reinforce unconscious repression*, also the key to access to the repressed presentation*), preceded by some type of "no", announces the reappearance of the repressed, substitute formation*, symptom* or something similar, in a manner that seems to unconsciously "invoke" its presence.

Negation opens the way in this case to the reappearance of a presentation, until this time successfully repressed and therefore forgotten, which returns first as a negation and then as return of the repressed*.

Freud's example in a footnote to his article, *Negation* (1925), is that of the patient who says, "How nice not to have had one of my headaches for so long" (p. 236) when an attack is felt to be imminent and appears to be called up, "invoked", but in which he is unwilling to believe.

ISOLATION

Ger.: Isolieren o Issolierung. – Sp.: aislamiento – Fr.: isolation. – It.: isolamento. – Port.: isolamento.

Isolation is the defence mechanism* or form of secondary repression produced by the unconscious ego* in response to the anxiety signal* it feels in response to Trieb* which has been prohibited by the superego*. The Trieb's thing-presentation*, however, may access the word-presentation* (and thereby the preconscious and conscious ego) as long as it remains free of affect; for this reason it is isolated from all its possible connections (associations* and bindings* with others). In this way the ego exerts a repressive effect on Trieb whereby access to the specific action* is blocked; however, the presentation is not rejected and relegated to the unconscious since its isolation severs its connection with the remaining presentations. In this sense, the mechanism is effective.

The patient's actions represent the disconnection of links between presentations*.

Freud explains:

> It, too, takes place in the motor sphere. When something unpleasant has happened to the subject or when he himself has done something which has a significance for his neurosis, he interpolates an interval during which nothing further must happen – during which he must perceive nothing and do nothing.
>
> (1926*d*, p. 120)

It is as if bridges connecting what is isolated had been broken, leaving the individual exactly like an island. The subject's acts represent this fact (such as the secret "hopscotch" the obsessional neurotic plays with sidewalk squares or the obsessional patient's difficulty in finding relations between one theme and another in session or between one session and another, for example).

When isolation is successful, the presentation is deprived of its affect (quantum of affect is given by the presentational cathexis and its potential for association with other presentations; when these circuits are broken by isolation, the presentation loses its affect) and it is unable to participate in associative commerce or thought* activity. Therefore, it is out of reach of the preconscious ego, which is consequently unable to use it.

Isolation is a defence mechanism typical of obsessional neurosis*.

It is one of the mechanisms of secondary repression: the removal of preconscious cathexis, except that, instead of de-cathecting the word or displacing its cathexis* on to another word-presentation or a bodily innervation, the word remains in the preconscious, but without its corresponding affect and cut off from its associative bridges with other words. It may even admix with or join other mechanisms such as displacement on to the trivial or others. Moderate isolation utilized with plasticity is a part of normal thought; it is part of the tendency to put things in order, a sublimational anal trait.

In its pathological counterpart, when taken to an extreme, it forms the *délire de toucher* (delusion of touching) which in part configures its essence since presentations must not touch; this injunction has been extended to dictate that nothing must be "touched".

J

JEALOUSY

Ger.: Eifersucht. – Sp.: celos. –Fr.: jalousie. – It.: gelosia. – Port.: ciúmes.

This normal affective state is directly related to Trieb for mastery*, an aspect of sexual Trieb*. It is connected with intimacy sought by the amorous couple, since sexual Trieb is asocial in this respect. Sexual love* can only be shared with the subject's partner.

Freud described three degrees of jealousy: (1) competitive or normal; (2) projected; (3) delusional.

The first is composed of mourning* for the object* of love thought to have been lost and for the narcissistic wound suffered. There may be feelings of hostility towards rivals and a greater or lesser amount of self-criticism. Although it is normal, it is irrational.

> [I]t is rooted deep in the unconscious, it is a continuation of the earliest stirrings of the child's affective life, and it originates in the Oedipus or brother-and-sister complex of the first sexual period.
>
> (1922, *Some Neurotic Mechanisms in Jealousy, Paranoia and Homosexuality*, p. 223)

It is often experienced even bisexually, for example jealousy among friends.

In the second type, projected jealousy originates in the subject's own infidelity whether practised, fancied, or repressed, and then projected for relief of the ego* before its moral conscience* and the pounding of the repressed.

"The jealousy that arises from such a projection has, it is true, an almost delusional character; it is, however, amenable to the analytic work of exposing the unconscious phantasies of the subject's own infidelity" (Ibid., p. 225).

The third type or layer of jealousy (Freud considers them different types or strata although they may coexist or sum up) also springs from repressed yearning for unfaithfulness, but in this case objects of fantasy* are of the same sex; sexual differences are previously disavowed* and then repressed in a very special way involving some decathexis of the thing-presentation* and then projection of the unconscious* wish* on to the object*. This form of paranoia* disavows the homosexual impulse not accepted by the ego; that is to say, the "masculine protest", the bedrock*, so deep in paranoia, which makes its therapeutic access so difficult. Jealous paranoia disavows the homosexual impulse which returns from the projected with the phrase: "It is not I who love the man – she loves him" (*Psycho-Analytic Notes on an Autobiographical Account of a Case of Paranoia (Dementia Paranoides)*, 1911, p. 64) (in men) or "It is not I who love the women – he loves them" (Ibid.) (in women).

"In a delusional case one will be prepared to find jealousy belonging to all three layers, never to the third alone" (1922, *Some Neurotic Mechanisms in Jealousy, Paranoia and Homosexuality*, p. 225).

JOKES

Ger.: Witz. – Sp.: chiste. – Fr.: mot d'esprit. – It.: scherzo. – Port.: chiste.

In this intellectual procedure, rapid use of primary process* saves part of the expenditure of incestuous sexual Triebe*, destructive Triebe*, and derivatives of both demanded by repression*. The energy thereby saved is discharged, producing the pleasure* of laughter which, depending on the type of joke (for example, off-colour jokes) may be hearty or even a guffaw.

The method utilized for an instant is the use of primary process whose form is similar to a dream* but without formal regression* (from word to perceived image) but treats the word as if it were a thing-presentation* or plays on a word's different meanings as well as the variety of things to which it alludes.

Sometimes a letter or a syllable is changed or words are broken down into syllables through condensations* and displacements* that make use of contiguities*, analogies*, homophones (analogies in sound), or oppositions*. These superficial word associations* (formal analogies) conceal deeper associations (of meaning).

Actually, the individual plays with words just as the infant played while acquiring language*, a manner in which words, more than representing things, are themselves things.

There are several types of jokes: we progress from infantile word play to innocent or abstract jokes whose effect is never excessive laughter; they generally produce no more than a smile. Jokes that produce more pleasure tend to be off-colour jokes born from the gross banter and merry sexual insults of groups with little culture or inhibitions. In off-colour jokes, hidden by condensations and displacements, the aim is to sexually attack (undress) or simply to attack someone (to discredit or degrade an authority figure, for example). A third party is needed to listen to the joke: the person who will experience the most pleasure with the discharge of laughter.

Therefore, off-colour jokes require three components: (a) the creator who tells it; (b) the person about whom the joke is told (generally absent or imaginary, except in rude obscenities); and (c) the third party who enjoys it. For the author or teller of the joke, pleasure is at first very small but grows intense by contagion (identification* with the person enjoying it). This complex mechanism gives the joke its intended social effect; it needs a spectator since it cannot be enjoyed alone.

The best jokes balance disguise with what the third party can understand; if they are too complex, they demand too much effort since they lose their pleasurable effect when they require effort. If a joke is too easy, the third party must be in a jovial mood with inhibitions already low and disposed to gross obscenity, cultural level reduced. The third person enjoys it most because the creative intellectual operation, abrupt and momentary use of primary process inserted into secondary process* discourse, is given freely by the author and therefore demands no effort of creative wit. By means of the other's intellectual operation, the third person obtains a certain level of satisfaction for Trieb* prohibited within the psychical apparatus.

However, the author also needs the third person in order to enjoy his joke, since as we said, a joke in solitude produces no pleasure; only when laughter is provoked in the third party may the author feel pleasure through contagion of identification with the other's laughter. This turns the joke into a social phenomenon *par excellence*, which differentiates it from humour*, a similar type of pleasure but with narcissistic libido*. In humour, the subject may smile at him- or herself or at problems in reality*, joking about them and thereby diminishing their importance, whereby the ego* becomes momentarily omnipotent: humour needs no third parties; although they may also enjoy it, the subject does not need them to enjoy humour.

Jokes are a safety valve that permits disinhibition of Trieb without involving action. It may be supported by a comical appearance (cf. comic*) which prepares the atmosphere for the pleasure of the joke.

JUDGEMENT OF ATTRIBUTION

Ger.: Urteilsspruch or Urteil fallen. – Sp.: juicio de atribución. – Fr.: jugement d'attribution. – It.: giudizio di atribuzione. – Port.: juízo de atribução.

This function or type of thought* activity attributes or does not attribute a property to a thing*.

Originally, the ego* (the purified pleasure ego*) accepts everything pleasurable as its own and identifies the unpleasurable as the external world. It recognizes as ego everything to which it attributes the production of pleasure. This ego makes a judgement of attribution previous to judgement of existence.

With development of secondary process*, study of the thing's attributes becomes more complex. Opposition between good and bad had depended on satisfaction or non-satisfaction by the object*. Later, better understanding* of the object is achieved by copying it and putting oneself in its place.

The object's attributes are centred on its actions, movements, and way of performing them. These movements are imitated and put through a cathexis of the subject's own body, thereby becoming attributes of the subject's own ego. Only then are they understood. At the beginning, actions themselves are utilized – primary judging* – and subsequently, presentations* of these actions. Comparison of the latter with the memory* of what was once an action produces an attribution of useful or harmful (good or bad). If this comparison allows a saving of cathexis* of presentation – that is to say, if the cost of the object's action in relation to our memory is exaggerated – it may have a comical* effect.

JUDGEMENT OF CONDEMNATION

Ger.: Verurteilung o Urteilsverwerfung. – Sp.: juicio de condenación. – Fr.: jugement de condamnation. – It.: rifiuto de parte del giudizio; condamna. – Port.: juízo de condenação ou desestimação.

Through this type of judgement of attribution*, an action corresponding to fulfilment of a certain wish* is consciously prohibited or left aside.

This is one of the loftiest ways to tame Trieb* when it is a product of intense associative commerce with full knowledge of Trieb, binding* between the thing-presentation* and the word-presentation*, and links with many other word-presentations by which Trieb is consciously known (its presentational content and their great strength). The preconscious ego accepts it as its own, but decides not to put it into action, since it may be unadvisable for many reasons.

However, in negation*, a judgement of existence* does not accept Trieb as a part of the preconscious ego, although repression* has partly been overcome once this Trieb has acquired a word-presentation with which to express itself. Then, if negation is lifted, the ego may still condemn it consciously and impede its passage into action.

Judgement of condemnation involves acceptance of the existence of Trieb. Although it is considered the ego's own, it is not allowed to advance towards action.

It obviously differs from repression. The latter involves presentational ignorance, a removal of cathexis* from the word-presentation (secondary repression) belonging to the Trieb derivative; for this reason, the word representing the thing-presentation associated with it unconsciously does not reach consciousness* (forgetting*). Repression is primary process* utilized by the unconscious ego which produces Trieb ignorance. In contrast, judgement of condemnation is secondary process* that involves knowledge, an ego selecting and taming the satisfaction of its Triebe.

JUDGEMENT OF EXISTENCE

Ger.: Urteilende Denken. – Sp.: juicio de existencia. – Fr.: jugement d'existence. – It.: giudizio d'esistenza. – Port.: juízo de existência.

This type of judgement is also a function of the conscious ego's thought* activity; the ego must accept or reject the existence of a presentation* in reality*, the real existence of a thing* in the world, or belief* in it. It does so when the ego clearly distinguishes a given perception* from a wish-presentation, a presentation that in the last analysis originates in memories*.

Judgement of existence is a function of the preconscious ego, inhibitor of hallucination* of the wish* presentation, of the definitive reality ego* originating in the initial reality ego*.

The desired object* with which the desired sensation was produced is sought to be "refound". Identity with what is desired is therefore sought, but in a realistic manner, accepting the limitations of reality and its difficulties.

Then, different levels of identity appear between what is desired and what is perceived; this identity depends on more or less difference between them.

What is most important is recognition of the difference between wish-presentations and the perception (which implies acceptance of existence or non-existence of the perception), and recognition of an inside and an outside, a psychical space and a real external space, of an ego and a not-ego, all of these differences ruled by secondary process* and the reality principle*.

This judgement may become fissured. During the period of phallic erotogenic predominance in boys initial recognition of sexual difference is of possession versus non-possession of a phallus. For a boy, the reality of castration (at this moment) implies a possibility that it may occur, and castration anxiety* ensues, felt as possible punishment if he persists in his desire for phallic sexual activity.

He may then resort to disavowal* of the existence of castration: a contradictory judgement of existence, a definite "it does not exist" which, if it persists as a predominant form of ego functioning, generates deep alterations (cf. alteration of the ego*) in the ego, even its splitting*.

JUDGING

Ger.: Urteil. – Sp.: juicio. – Fr.: jugement. – It.: giudizio. – Port.: juízo.

This developed thought* process mainly utilizes word-presentations* to enables the subject to analyse a perception*, compare it, and differentiate it from the desired presentation*. The reality of its existence is thereby determined, and the characteristics of its attributes are studied.

In response to presence of the perceived, thought activity inherent to the preconscious ego* breaks it down into an unchanging part of it, its features, for example, which may be compared to the subject's own unchanging parts. These are also understood by performing them, imitating them, putting them through the subject's own body, as Freud explains in his *Project for a Scientific Psychology* (1895–1950). "Cognitive or judging thought seeks an identity with a bodily cathexis" (p. 332).

The unchanging part of what is perceived is called the thing*. It is not understandable and cannot be referred to an action of one's own. The changing part is constituted by the thing's attributes, understandable since they may be performed by the subject so long as they possess cathexes related to the erotogenic zones* involved.

Problems arise in relation to sexual Triebe*. We recall that they have thing-presentations* at first, then word-presentations as erotogenic zones in the link with the object* are gradually awakened. For this reason, an experience of excitation involving an erotogenic zone before its period of predominance is traumatic: it therefore remains anticathected and fixated. Since this experience cannot be referred to any other experience, it cannot be bound or understood.

Quantity of excitation* corresponding to the traumatic situation*, which occurred when there were no presentations to bind it, may return in a deferred* manner. Now they exist, but they are insufficient, since these experiences also bring along quantity of cathexis corresponding to the previous event; consequently, they are traumatic and must be fought off continually.

The classical example is the primal scene*, seen or heard during the first phases of sexuality (the oral or anal phase, for example), as is the case of the "Wolf Man" (*From the History of an Infantile Neurosis*, 1918); at this point, Freud also proposes phylogenetic origins as a hereditary schema of this primal phantasy*.

If this activity of judging is to develop, there must be an ego inhibiting hallucination and primary process*. The greater the wealth of preconscious presentations in order to compare what is perceived, the better this secondary process* activity functions.

More presentational wealth brings greater ability to understand and to put the object's attributes through the subject's body.

The activity of repression* or any other process of presentational decathectization* impoverishes the activity of judging by withdrawing cathexes from many word-presentations (in transference neuroses*). The thought activity of the preconscious ego is therefore unable to utilize them in order to compare them to what is perceived.

K

KEY NEURONES

Ger.: Schlüsselneuronen. – Sp.: neuronas llave. – Fr.: neurones clef. – It.: neurone chiave. – Port.: chave neuronio.

Freud resorts to this theoretical concept in his *Project for a Scientific Psychology* (1895–1950) when, in the context of its positivist logic, he needs a material quantitative explanation for what creates the sensation in the memory of pain (fear, anxiety). He then refers to this source as the key neurones.

At the moment of pain, the painful sensation is produced by the quantity inherent to the object breaking into the psychical apparatus. However, in the moment of its memory*, where does this quantity come from? The object is no longer present, but the sensation of pain is quite similar. What is the source of this sensation? He then resorts to this contrivance, as if there were neurones which segregate substances producing the sensation of the painful or anxiety-generating memory. These are key neurones.

This reasoning approaches some neurosciences, and is a product of the wish to find a quantitative-material explanation for everything. Freud never published this text (its publications was posthumous), nor did he ever mention this concept in the rest of his works.

L

LANGUAGE

Ger.: Sprache. – Sp.: lenguaje. - Fr.: langage. – It.: linguaggio. – Port.: linguagem.

The subject of language, studied by the pre-Socratics (Heraclites and Parmenides) and later by thinkers such as Plato and Aristotle, was considered capital in classical philosophy, as well as in Leibnitz among others, to such an extent that the history of the philosophy of language may be superimposed upon the history of philosophy, and language considered either a moment of "logos" or logos itself. In contemporary philosophy, the study of language reappeared with Hegel and acquired commanding importance with the studies of Wittgenstein and even Bertrand Russell. Linguistics finally took shape as the science of language with the works of Ferdinand de Saussure, then R. Jakobson, C. Morris, N. Chomsky, and many others. Contemporary Centro-European philosophy considers language the central figure in its debates (Heidegger, Gadamer). The works of Freud were already in full development when Saussure appeared on the scene, and linguistics had not yet been born. Lacan's "reading" of Freud's works is strongly supported by Saussurian linguistics (among other groundings).

Freud made important contributions to knowledge of the subject of language considering that his general conception of the psyche was based on its alterations, concluding in the conception of its function in relation to the normal psyche. When Freud refers to language, he usually refers to spoken language, to speech in words, especially to word-presentations* belonging to the preconscious* ego*. This does not mean that he thought there was no pre-verbal language; his conception sometimes extends to mimicked expression, for example (as in his explanation of ego regression* in symptoms* of conversion hysteria*) *Panorama of the Transference Neuroses*, 1915 – or when he explains the phenomenon of the comical* – *Jokes and Their Relation to the Unconscious*, 1905 – and we could even consider the same in relation to certain thing-presentations* (usually images) with a certain level of binding* superior to that of primary process* and therefore having some secondary process*, at the dawn of thought* activity of the ego in the early psyche*. This type of thought, which he refers to as reproductive thought, enables the baby to distinguish its beloved mother from other people, to recognize differences between what is desired and what is perceived, before learning language in words, and even before recognizing her as an object* of desire*. That is to say, this level of thought participates in the constitution of the first levels of the definitive reality ego*, based on an initial reality ego* and despite the superimposition of a purified pleasure ego* ruled by the pleasure principle*.

Freud closely connected language, which he valued as one of the major creations of human culture*, with what he considered different levels of thought activity: (a) thought produced with presentations* of images (as in babies and in adult dreams*, and of course as in his greatest discovery, the unconscious*, the latter ruled only by primary process); (b) thought effected by movements (movements of babies at the breast which lead infants to form a Gestalt with figure and background, and enable them to recognize the identity of the breast, both front and profile). We may include mimicking expressions as a form of language of this type; (c) language itself, a human creation, language spoken with word-presentations, the origin of what is referred to as the symbolic universe.

In *On Aphasia* (1891) and in his *Project for a Scientific Psychology* (1895), Freud discusses thing-presentations*, word-presentations*, and formal differences between them. Concerning the former, he explains that they are constituted from traces left by the perceptual sign (especially visual signs, produced through all the erotogenic zones* and sensory organs), but also have very broadly interconnected: they are "open": one is the other quite easily because of the many attributes through which they may connect. In contrast, the intertwining of word-presentations is comparatively closed, each word having only a small number of feasible connections with other words, which makes the establishment of secondary process and binding of (libidinal) energy which cathects these presentations more possible.

In his *Project for a Scientific Psychology* (1895), he describes how biological bodily discharge (internal alteration*) produced in response to the invasion of quantities of excitation* into the psychical apparatus, originating the expression of emotions, when understood (cf. understanding) by extraneous help*, becomes a call; added to words emitted by the mother to her infant and to the experience of the infant's own screams emerging in experiences of pain*, sounds are gradually connected with experiences, thereby forming the base for access to language, called "maternal" for this reason. Words thus acquired in this imitative-identification link first acquire a concrete sense of things and then a sense of their meaning; they advance further and further with growing complexity of tongues, acquiring symbolic distance. This process of moving away from the concrete aspect of things culminates in adolescence when the possibility of abstract thought* is attained. This Freudian explanation includes a biological base (expression of emotional discharge) which in a dynamic manner, with fundamental participation of the maternal object, is gradually transformed into the social, generating spoken language, the remarkable way in which human beings understand each other.

However, there is another perspective in Freudian theory. Language also arises so that consciousness* may learn of desires which would otherwise retain their original, unconscious status. This knowledge is acquired by moving cathexis* from thing-presentations to the emission of sounds that signify them. Consciousness is thereby able to "hear" its desires as it does any perception*, and also to "hear" the many relations between presentations (logical relations, for example, which at the same time limit them since, as mentioned, they are "closed"), in this way permitting change in the repetition compulsion* inherent to Trieb*, and also change in the conception of the subject's own body and its history as a lovable or hateable object (narcissism*). All this creates surprising levels of specific action* since instinctual repetition may vary symbolically. Although specific action* is predetermined by previous histories, it arises as a "creation" because it always differs from the original history.

However, this is not all: what is lacking is perhaps the most important part of the Freudian discovery. Just as words constitute the highest level of Trieb binding, of knowledge of it, withdrawal of cathexis from the word-presentation is a very effective mechanism for ignoring it. It is therefore one of the central mechanisms of secondary repression, an ignorer of Trieb and desire, which sends them into the repressed unconscious.

How is this cathexis extracted from the preconscious word-presentation? By displacing it onto another presentation (a word, mimicry, or conversion) and utilizing the latter to reinforce the previous anticathexis* belonging to primary repression*. How is this displacement* produced? By utilizing the laws of association* (contiguity*, analogy*, opposition*). When the latter correspond to thing-presentations, they utilize attributes of the object represented.

However, when primary process is able to filter through gaps in secondary process, words no longer connect through their meaning but instead associate by the similarity of their sounds (homophony) or their writing (the order of their vowels, structure or similarity of their syllables, even contiguity between one syllable and another), as if they were concrete things connected by their forms rather than signifiers related by what they signify. This and other similar phenomena described by Freud in *The Interpretation of Dreams* (1900), *The Psychopathology of Everyday Life* (1901) and *Jokes and Their Relation to the Unconscious* (1905) show the case of repression by virtue of withdrawal of the repressed* due to the multiple meanings of words and utilization of their form (sound and writing) for their unconscious meaning.

The work of psychoanalysis is to set out, paraphrasing M. Proust, "in search of the lost word" by reconstructing the road by which it was lost, in order to find the meaning of dreams*, parapraxes*, forgetting*, transference repetitions (cf. transference* and repetition compulsion*), symptoms, and so on. The original word (historical truth*) represented the unconscious wish (of repressed infantile sexuality*), the one that due to the vicissitudes of human history (and also individual history) became anti-culture. This created the paradox that human beings were obliged to lose (repress) this word, which was a qualitative cultural leap, in order to access culture*.

LATENCY PERIOD

Ger.: Latenzperiode / Latenzzeit / Aufschubsperiode. – Sp.: período de latencia. – Fr.: période de latence. – It.: periodo di latenza. – Port.: período de latência.

This period of human life divides sexual development into two stages. It is established at the end of the Oedipus complex (around six years of age) when the latter and infantile sexuality* are nearly completely dissolved* and the superego* is established; it continues up to puberty. The term "latency" refers to a decrease in quantity of Trieb excitation* during this period and the suspension of problems arising with the Oedipus complex: they are as if frozen, reappearing in puberty and adolescence with all their previous strength and problems. Freud presents the hypothesis that human beings descend from a species of animal that culminated its sexual development at five years of age (*Moses and Monotheism: Three Essays*, 1939) and that, as a product of events narrated in *Totem and Taboo* (1913) in relation to parricide and generation of the fraternal alliance or band of brothers*, the superego was established in the psychical apparatus of those who then became human beings; this resulted from successful repression of sexual Trieb* and its postponement in their development, even undoing what was already attained. Human beings are the only animals having this latency period, sexual retardation, and development of sexuality* in two stages.

In general, the latency period is not very conflictive, therefore tending towards some degree of sublimation* (useful for "being loved" by the object), with successful defence and apparent health (1896).

With respect to the freezing of sexual Trieb, this period of life is more marked in boys than girls, probably because of differences in the formation of their superego. In *The Ego and the Id* (1923) and the manuscript discovered recently among Sandor Ferenczi's papers, the *Overview of the Transference Neuroses* (1915), he shows the analogy and phylogenetic connection between the latency period and the period of glaciation, a concept also discussed by Ferenczi in his *Thalassa*.

In *Moses and Monotheism: Three Essays* (1939), Freud presents its analogy with the development of the religious conception of monotheism, which began in the Egyptian period of Pharaoh Akhenaton, then fell, reappearing later in the Jews through Moses. He refers to this intermediate period as a latency period, comparing it to the concept we are discussing.

He also mentions a latency period in the neuroses* in a different sense and context, since it occurs between the moment of a precipitating frustration* and the appearance of symptoms*.

LATENT CONTENT (OF DREAMS)

Ger.: latenter Inhalt. – Sp.: contenido latente (del sueño). – Fr.: contenu latent (du rêve). – It.: contenuto latente (del sogno). – Port.: conteúdo latente (do sonho).

The many associations*, ideas, memories*, and thoughts* the dreamer expresses through the manifest content* of a dream*; it is composed of day residues*; that is to say, elements taken from events that occurred the day before the dream, although it may contain much older memories.

The latent content or "dream thought" is much larger than the manifest content. The latter has been condensed (cf. condensation*) in the process of "dream work"* until the manifest content is finished.

By analysis and working through* of latent content, the meaning of the dream is reached: knowledge of the unconscious* wish* fulfilled through it.

By extension, the unconscious meaning may also be considered latent content (Freud himself seems to have done it sometimes), but in the strict sense the latent corresponds to preconscious* thoughts on the basis of which the analyst may reach repressed unconscious wishes. Latent content is reached by complying with the fundamental rule*. To call for it, the analyst asks the patient to remove attention* cathexis* from conscious censorship* and to let him or herself be led by whatever comes to mind in relation to the manifest content. The fundamental rule is not a strict law for patients to obey, at least not solely; they obey even when they apparently do not want to do, because everything that occurs to them after describing the manifest content must be taken in this sense by the analyst, since these ideas are preconscious and constitute the latent content of the dream. They facilitate the way to find its unconscious meaning.

LETTER 52 (TO FLIESS)

Ger.: Brief 52. – Sp.: carta 52. – Fr.: lettre 52. – It.: lettera 52. – Port.: carta 52.

One of the most famous letters from Freud to Fliess (cf. Fliess papers*), dated Vienna, December 6, 1896. In it, he outlines an arrangement of presentations*, more or less processed traces left in the psychical apparatus by experiences; they lead him closer to defining his first topic while at the same time he formulates other important ideas that endure throughout the rest of his works.

Here, he mentions that the wish-presentation* is generated by a process of stratification which also undergoes repeated rearrangement and retranscription.

Memory* is not simple but rather multiple. It is registered in diverse varieties of signs.

First, the neurones* register perceptions*. The first registration is the perceptive sign, which associates by simultaneity. Then it passes into the unconscious* where perhaps causal connections intervene; here, traces are memories* of concepts. In this last globalizing sense, we could infer its correspondence with what he later refers to as thing-presentations*. These may return to consciousness* by translation into a third type of transcription linked to word-presentations* corresponding to the official ego*, which is also referred to as the preconscious*.

This letter describes the path leading from perception, its form of registration in the psychical apparatus, and its initial connections with other inscriptions, to its potential memory and evocation through words.

It also explains the mechanism of repression*, relating each of the forms of transcription to different periods of life. For Freud, in the translation from one transcription to another, a defence is normal if the transcriptions correspond to the same psychical phase. However, there is a pathological defence against a memory trace* not translated from a previous phase.

This defence* is called repression and occurs in relation to sexuality* because of sexuality's special place in development. Genital* stimulation is understood or "felt" in the corresponding period but not in previous periods; the deferred* phenomenon occurs by which it is not understood before the genital period, with a quantity of excitation that originated in the previous excitatory episode, by which it becomes traumatic; this unpleasure* generates defence or repression.

We return now to the previous paragraph to clarify some points.

Freud considers that one transcription is translated into another. He considers that thing-presentations are translated into word-presentations in order to reach consciousness. If the events that occurred, leaving thing-presentations, were previous to the possibility of possessing word-presentations that "understand" (cf. understanding*) these thing-presentations, they correspond to an erotogenic zone* not yet psychically developed and therefore to traumatic situations* that these thing-presentations commemorate. In this case, then, repression is only anticathexis* (cf. anticathexis*) given that there is no word to be decathected (cf. decathexis*). If the thing-presentation finds sexuality corresponding to the level of the erotogenic zone adequately developed and understood, "having received a bodily cathexis", and word-presentations with a certain level of elaboration and connection between them, normal defence may be established; if not, repression, the pathological but most common defence, is utilized.

In the same letter, Freud tries to relate memories of experiences to the cause of neurosis*, hysteria*, obsessional neurosis*, and paranoia*, "the repressed memories relate to what was current in the case of hysteria between the ages of 1.5 and 4, of obsessional neurosis between 4 and 8, and of paranoia between 8 and 14" (1896, p. 236).

Another consequence of premature experiences is perversion* whose condition seems to be, at this point in theory, that the defence has not taken place before completion of the psychical apparatus, or that there is no defence at all. Later, in *A Child Is Being Beaten: A Contribution to the Study of the Origin of Sexual Perversions* (1919) and in the case history of the "Wolf Man" (*From the History of an Infantile Neurosis*, 1918 [1914]), he understands that this affection is produced by a different type of repression or defence in response to recognition of sexual difference which appears in the phallic phase during the Oedipus complex (phallic–castrated), a phase and period to which the subject is fixated; this fixation* based on disavowal* of this difference must from that time forward be sustained, producing splitting of the subject's ego*.

LIBIDINAL WITHDRAWAL

Ger.: Libidoentzüg. – Sp.: retracción libidinal. – Fr.: rétraction libidinale. – It.: ritrazione libidinale. – Port.: retração libidinal.

This is the basic metapsychological mechanism by which different types of narcissistic pathology are configured.

It is the process by which libido is decathected from thing-presentations* or presentations of unconscious object* wishes*; this libido then cathects the ego*. Object libido thereby becomes narcissistic libido.

In *schizophrenia** it shapes the least noisy but specifically pathological manifestations of illness: "detachment of libido from its objects and, further, megalomania, hypochondria, affective disturbance and every kind of regression" (*On Narcissism: An Introduction*, 1914, p. 86).

It must be differentiated from libidinal introversion. In the latter, libidinal cathexis* is withdrawn from some preconscious object presentations whereas the unconscious presentations remain cathected. Therefore, one preconscious presentation is displaced* to another. Phantasies* or daydreams* are configured in this way; they are disguises more or less concealing unconscious thing-presentations of repressed wishes. The unconscious object wish is intact in them, at most hidden to the preconscious ego's own repressive defence mechanisms. Therefore, in introversion we observe no regression to narcissism*.

This regression does exist in libidinal withdrawal. In this case it is a question of stanching a wounded ego with all of the libido available to do so.

In *melancholia**, unconscious cathexis is also withdrawn, but through a mechanism of regression*, the object presentation goes back to behaviour characteristic of the oral-cannibalistic phase, becoming, as then, identification*. For this reason, "the shadow of the object falls upon the ego", and the hate* of the superego* also falls upon it, although the preconscious ego does not know that this hate is aimed at the object. In any case, by virtue of identification, some cathexis of the presentation of the object wish (regressed to hate) remains in the unconscious. This object cathexis (although it is identification, we recall that it is the "first form of love") becomes a security for the psychical apparatus which saves it from having to resort to restitution* in order to reconnect with the object (once the acute episode of illness has passed). Thus, the subject is free of the psychical deterioration left by a preconscious ego having words cathected but not supported by cathected thing-presentations, which would incurably distance it from reality* (the restitution delusion* is a caricature of the object link produced in schizophrenia and paranoia*).

The danger of melancholia is different: destructive Trieb* lodged in the superego may succeed in destroying the ego.

In the other forms of *narcissistic pathology* this withdrawal of cathexis is more partial. In *sexual perversions** cathexis is withdrawn from the thing-presentation that might signify castration, and therefore objects which may belong to the other sex are no longer desired (by unconscious desire), despite recognition of their existence in the preconscious* with word-presentations* but with unconscious desires.

Borderline patients have an especially labile unconscious libidinal object cathexis which makes it easy to break off through libidinal withdrawal: they also easily make narcissistic identifications* with the object's attributes and also rapidly recompose the link. Object cathexis cannot be clearly differentiated from identification in any of these processes.

LIBIDO

Ger.: Libido. – Sp.: libido. – Fr.: libido. – It.: libido. – Port.: libido.

This psychical* sexual energy is the transformation of quantity of excitation* of somatic sexual energy. This energy accumulates, and when it goes beyond a certain threshold, it enters the psychical apparatus* and cathects presentations*. At this point it becomes psychical, and libidinal wishes* result.

When it cathects unconscious* thing-presentations*, libido moves from one presentation to another quite freely, ruled only by laws of association* (contiguity*, analogy*, and opposition*), forming condensations* and displacements* with and between presentations. When it enters the preconscious*, libido cathects word-presentations*, thereby reaching a new level of binding* with which it acquires the characteristic of bound energy* proper: strongly cathected energy whose displacement is weak.

Libido therefore constitutes psychical or presentational sexual energy. There are two types of these presentations: of the ego* (originally the body itself and gradually its variably complex and variably abstract attributes) and of the object*.

Libido which cathects the ego (including the ego ideal*) constitutes ego libido or narcissistic libido, satisfied in adults mainly by pleasing the ego ideal and consequently enhancing self-esteem* (a derivative partly of infantile narcissism* and partly of "the omnipotence which is corroborated by experience" [1914, p. 100]; that is to say, fulfilment of the ideal and success; and lastly, proceeding from objects, from being loved by them).

Before its establishment in a psychical apparatus possessing a superego-ego ideal and a developing ego, narcissistic libido is satisfied mainly by autoerotic play with the child's own erotogenic zones and, after the first levels of recognition of the object as a source of pleasure* (but not recognition of sexual difference), by the object relation (parental love); at this juncture it partly becomes object libido.

However, a tiny part of narcissistic libido was object libido from the start (erotogenic zones are first stimulated by the object and by the initial reality ego; this stimulus is partly recognized as being external) due to its anaclisis* in satisfaction of the ego's self-preservative Triebe* (therefore not sexual, having not libido but rather interest*). The self-preservative Triebe form a base from which the libidinal plus arises which later becomes cathexis of object presentations, gradually recognized as major sources of pleasure.

Homosexual libido, recognizing no sexual difference, is halfway between object libido and narcissistic libido. This type of homosexual libido not only guides narcissistic object choices* in what are referred to as "narcissistic affections" such as homosexuality*; it also rules links in which sexual difference is left aside or disavowed: social bonds, paternal-filial relations, and so on. Establishment of the superego-ego ideal even basically requires this homosexual libido proceeding from the link with the parents. When this link is transformed by identification* into an ego trait, homosexual libido becomes narcissistic.

Object libido *par excellence* recognizes the object as a source of pleasure and accepts its sexual differences. Pleasure offered by the object link with the different sex overcomes narcissistic castration anxiety* caused in childhood by acceptance of sexual difference.

The subject's sexual apparatus possesses these three libidinal types or levels (narcissistic, homosexual, and object), each differentiated by its proportions and different forms of situating libido.

In the second Trieb theory, libido practically becomes life Trieb* when it acquires the name of Eros*. Hence, it comes to include self-preservative Triebe of the ego which do, however, retain their specificity. As life Trieb, libido is opposed to death Trieb*, in a complex way, since it is also fused* with it.

LIBIDO, PHASES OF THE

Ger.: Libidophasen. – Sp.: fases de la libido. – Fr.: stades de la libido. – It.: fasi della libido. – Port.: fases da libido.

Libido* is psychical sexual energy* gratified by stimulation, friction, and even the sight of erotogenic zones*, whose pleasure* extends throughout the entire body. However, it goes through diverse stages in which one erotogenic zone predominates over the others.

The first predominant zone is the mouth. It is stimulated mainly by the sucking of oral mucous membranes and by the act of biting when teeth emerge; for this reason, this phase is called the "oral-cannibalistic" stage.

As muscle control increases (and with it, the possibility to control sphincters), the predominant phase is the sadistic. In it, the object* is gradually recognized as a separate source of pleasure, to which the child may offer its first "gift" (faeces) in exchange for being loved, sought in order to soothe fear of object loss and to receive the object's love*, but mainly to avoid invasion by tension of need. Fear of object loss precipitates the first anxiety signal*, cultivated by the ego* in order to deal with Triebe*.

These vicissitudes are associated with anticathexes*, generators of libidinal fixation points*. Since this fixation is in relation to the mode of satisfaction of the erotogenic zone, the anticathexis* generates its opposite: the subject is fixated, but the anticathexis produces disgust for what was fixated; it does the same at the level of object recognition, with each related erotogenic zone and type of history experienced with the object, including the object presentation*.

One of these phases is related to Triebe of observing and being observed, sadism and masochism*, which arrive in the period of the anal phase between one and three years of age. In all these stages, the skin is eminently important.

In pre-oedipal phases, the tendency is perverse polymorphous, since no Trieb* aim predominates greatly over the others or at least enough to gain supremacy to unify them. Stimulation of a zone motivates pleasure in this zone, isolated from the others, extending neither to the body nor to the ego* as a whole.

When the phallic phase is reached (given the magnitude of its sensations in boys), the previous phases submit to its supremacy and become part of phallic-urethral erotism*. This moment coincides with global recognition of the object as such (now incestuous) and its choice, apart from the first recognition of sexual difference (phallic–castrated). The period of the Oedipus complex* is entered, the ego's castration anxiety predominating. The father is recognized in his full dimension and acquires the characteristics of a rival in the boy's positive Oedipus complex. In girls, the phallic phase involves clitoral erotism, which perishes due to penis envy*. Then they recognize castration, and their mother complex* begins. They blame their mother for their disability, and try to restore their wounded narcissism* with the unconscious phantasy of having a child with their father. Only then do they enter the positive Oedipus complex.

The concept of libidinal phases or stages was described by Freud, but did not acquire special importance in his theoretical development as it did in some post-Freudians who, like K. Abraham, may have schematized this concept too much, perhaps giving libidinal development too rigid a formality. Freud viewed infantile sexuality as being perverse polymorphous throughout this period. This means that part Triebe* in each erotogenic zone are constantly boiling, even when one is predominating over the others. Although erotogenic zones are labelled oral, anal, or phallic, this does not imply that there are no others such as vision, skin, or the whole body. For this reason, in order to describe these themes more amply, we prefer to place them, as Freud does in *Three Essays* ... (1905), in the chapter on erotism: oral, anal, and phallic-urethral.

LIFE TRIEB

Ger.: Lebenstrieb. – Sp.: pulsión de vida. – Fr.: pulsion de vie. – It.: istinto o pulsione di vita. – Port.: pulsão de vida.

This is the tendency to return to a previous state in mental life governed by the pleasure principle, and therefore to an experience of satisfaction* or pleasure*, from the moment a stimulus enters the psychical apparatus* (coming from Trieb* itself, although it may also proceed from the external world or, from the external world, activate Trieb by stimulation of an erotogenic zone*).

Like all Trieb, it is preservative, but what it aims to preserve is a previous state in life. Return to the inorganic (death) is the aim of death Triebe*.

Life Triebe or Eros* includes sexual Triebe* with object, homosexual, and narcissistic libido*, and self-preservative Triebe*.

Life Trieb in general and sexual Trieb in particular tend to produce progressively larger integrations. We may understand this trend as a tendency to generate more and more binding of libidinal energy with presentations* (especially thing-presentations), as opposed to death Trieb which tends to break the levels of binding that create wishes*, and consequently, leads to their decathexis*.

Decathexis of unconscious thing-presentations* is one way to shorten the path towards the inorganic. When the presentation is decathected, the level of presentational quality* is lost, including psychical quality of Trieb and of wishes which are motors of the psychical apparatus, and it consequently becomes pure quantity (approaches the inorganic).

Also, when cathexis* is withdrawn from the presentation, the wish to perceive the perceptual quality inherent to it is lost. Loss of the desire to have new experiences paralyzes action; the stillness achieved in this way is also conducive to the inorganic.

The object presentation* becomes essential in the constitution of life Trieb. This presentation ultimately results from traces left by experiences with the object.

This description shows that life Trieb is growing complexity which has arisen from the inorganic. All phenomena of life, especially those connected with objects, prolong the path towards death. The opposition between these two types of Trieb is played out between different levels of fusion which seek to neutralize the tendency to death; in this way, complex phenomena of life arise among which object desire has a notable role.

Life Trieb is noisy. Death Trieb, mute; it is only heard through diverse noises produced by life Trieb.

LIFTING (OR UNDOING) OF REPRESSION

Ger.: Aufhebung der Verdrängung. – Sp.: levantamiento de la represión. – Fr.: levée du refoulement. – It.: Sollevamento della repressione. – Port.: cancelação da repressão.

The lifting of repression is the principal objective of Freudian psychoanalytical treatment. With it unconscious wish* tendencies acquire word-presentation and thereby access to consciousness*. This is produced when the analyst is able to reconstruct traumatic events which originated this repression in the analysand, and the latter discovers which defence mechanisms* or repression* the ego utilized for this purpose and the reason for which they were being repeated.

The lifting of secondary repression generally produces relief of neurotic symptoms, although they are also associated with general improvement and changes of behaviour after the transference neuroses and negative therapeutic reactions that tend to appear have been overcome.

In contrast, in order to produce more radical changes, changes in the character* and in the general tendency to suffering stemming from early periods of life and events corresponding to the Oedipus complex* proper, primary repressions* must be lifted. That is to say, it is necessary to fluidify fixations* originating in the period of infantile sexuality, to which events experienced in this period contributed heavily; they have a certain universal characteristic but also an individual peculiarity in each individual. To "lift" primary repression is perhaps simply an expression: primary repression proper cannot be lifted, at least not totally; however, it is important for the subject to know of its existence, its reasons, the traumatic events that caused it and which generated libidinal fixation points and thereby not only tendencies but also character. However, this is not all. These different histories must be linked together, given a logical sequence, with their counterparts, conflicts, current repetitions (transference being one of these).

As Freud explains:

> Actually, there is no lifting of the repression until the conscious idea, after the resistances have been overcome, has entered in connection with the unconscious memory trace. It is only through the making conscious of the latter itself that success is achieved.
>
> (*The Unconscious*, 1915, pp. 175–6)

Finally, the lifting of repression is an arduous task, it is psychoanalytical work *par excellence*; with it, repression* is moderated, becomes less rigid and more manageable by thought, since the subject possesses words, their corresponding bindings and possible bindings in order to bring understanding of reality*, for example, into secondary process. The lifting of repression is not just one, nor are repressions alone; they are tied to historical facts of the subject's life and may be numerous (multidetermination). Therefore, lifting repression is not just one action but the result of many such liftings, some more important than others, whose meanings must be tied to secondary process, in other words, given binding*. In any form and gradually, it is something quite concrete, which produces effects, is effective, when it is successful. It is what produces real changes. In the subject's behaviour, providing greater freedom in the relation with the individual's Triebe and desires, and consequently less anxiety and fewer symptoms as well as better possibilities for ethical behaviour, having deeper knowledge of unconscious wishes and Triebe and also the tendency to superego self-punishment. The effect of lifting repression is enrichment of the ego, increase of signified presentations of current signifiers, and expansion of capacity for thought. This process has nothing to do with the sexual liberation postulated at one time, but with a more mature, better bound sexuality, an ego better able to reason. Achievements of the ego are gradual, advancing as construction* advances. This is the true Freudian road to the "cure".

LONGING, CATHEXIS OF

Ger.: Sehnsucht/besetzung der Sehnsucht. – Sp.: añoranza, investidura de. – Fr.: nostalgie, investissement de la. – It.: nostalgia, investimento di. – Port.: saudade, investidura de.

Here we have an intense cathexis of object libido* produced in response to the irreparable reality* of object* loss. Longing is due to hyper-cathexis of the wish for the object; since it is no longer present, hence no satisfaction is possible, an accumulation of psychical pain* is produced during the mourning process.

In the case of physical pain*, Freud describes a quantity of excitation* originating in the "moving masses" in the external world (*Project for a Scientific Psychology*, 1950) which entered the body through a break in its surface. It may also occur due to illness in one of its organs, and is associated with a quantity of libido that crowds into the painful organ (1925).

Something analogous occurs in the case of psychical pain. There is a very intense pile-up, not of object libido, but the cathexis of longing. Reality shows that the wish* for the lost object will never again be satisfied as before, which intensifies it and clashes with this real impossibility, a situation every time the lost object is evoked. The mourning process consists mainly of gradually detaching the cathexis of longing from reality. This process can take place when the predominant cathexis has been of object libido, since if previous object* choice was predominantly narcissistic*, libidinal withdrawal is produced upon which libido returns to the ego* as in the case of melancholia*. In this latter affection, the ego's sense of guilt* occupies the place of longing for the object.

LOVE

Ger.: Liebe. – Sp.: amor. – Fr.: amour. – It.: amore. – Port.: amor.

In *Instincts and Their Vicissitudes* (1915*c*) Freud defines love as "the relation of the ego to its sources of pleasure" (p. 135).

The sources of pleasure* of the ego* may be in its body, in itself, or in the object*. When the sources are in its body, this is called autoerotism*. Once the body is constituted into an ego and libido* is located in it, we speak of narcissism*. The libido that finds pleasure in the ego is called narcissistic pleasure. Narcissism is a form of love: love for the ego.

When the object begins to be recognized as the ego's principal source of pleasure, libido that seeks pleasure in the relation with it is called object libido*. In this way the highest love is constituted, love *par excellence*: object love. It may possess different nuances, classes or forms. Capacity for object love develops gradually, together with the ego, in a complex manner.

> When the purely narcissistic stage has given place to the object-stage, pleasure and unpleasure signify relation of the ego to the object. If the object becomes a source of pleasurable feelings, a motor urge is set up which seeks to bring the object closer to the ego and to incorporate it into the ego. We then speak of the "attraction" exercised by the pleasure-giving object, and say that we "love" that object.
>
> (1915, pp. 136–7)

In the first infantile stages love is ambivalent; it is not totally distinguished from hate. Being* is also not distinguished from having*. Therefore, the first form of affective tie is identification*. The analogous model is that of cannibalism, in which the loving tendency towards the object implies incorporating it; therefore, its disappearance and transformation into part of the individual's being. It is a type of love that implies the destruction of the object as such. In the mastery of the anal stage (cf. anal* erotism and Trieb of mastery*) there is less but more evident ambivalence, and the differentiation between the categories of *being* and *having* is greater. When synthesis of the sexual instincts* is complete and the genital stage is established (cf. genital*), love becomes the opposite of hate and coincides with the total sexual aspiration.

We observe a broad spectrum of possibilities in the phenomenon of love. During the period of the Oedipus complex*, the child finds a first object of love in one of the progenitors; all the sexual instincts that demand satisfaction come together on this object. Repression*, which occurs later, obliges the child to renounce most of these infantile sexual aims and leaves a sequel: a deep modification of the relation with the parents. After this effect, the child remains tied to them but with instincts that are necessarily called "aim inhibited". The child's feelings towards these loved persons receive the term "tender".

This "aim-inhibited" love or tenderness is the affect able to create more enduring ties between human beings, which is explained by the fact that they cannot be fully satisfied.

Sensual love is destined to be extinguished by satisfaction; in order to persist it must be admixed from the outset with purely tender components – that is to say, aim inhibited – or undergo a change in this direction.

Aim-inhibited love is what binds members of the group* and is an essential factor in the generation of Culture*. Sensual love is antisocial in this sense; the sexual couple requires intimacy and does not share its love; if it does so, we speak of sexual perversion*.

Freud also observed that children (and adolescents)

> derived their sexual objects from their experiences of satisfaction. The first autoerotic sexual satisfactions are experienced in connection with vital functions which serve the purpose of self-preservation. The sexual instincts are at the outset attached to the satisfaction of the ego-instincts; only later do they become independent of these, and even then we have an indication of that original attachment in the fact that the persons who are concerned with a child's feeding, care, and protection become his earliest sexual objects; that is to say, in the first instance his mother or a substitute for her.
>
> (1914*c*, p. 87)

In other cases, he notes, the object is not chosen on the model of the mother but of the subject: "We say that a human being has originally two sexual objects – himself and the woman who nurses him" (1914*c*, p. 88). From these two derive the models of object choice*: the anaclitic* type (most commonly masculine*) and the narcissistic type (more typically feminine*).

Therefore, we could say that love derives from growing complexity of the ego accomplished by the vicissitudes of the sexual instinct. This produces in turn complex mixtures with a tendency to return to the inorganic inherent to the death instinct*.

The main obstacle – we could almost say the only one – that the death instinct encounters in its path towards the inorganic is this complication that arises for it with the phenomena of life, of which the principal exponent is love.

As complexity grows, different phenomena appear, the sexual instinct admixes with the death instinct, and by doing so is able to master it, though only partially. The genital sexual act taken to its genital aim, sensual love, is the principal form of mastery of pure quantity (cf. quantity of excitation*), of non-quality, and the death instinct.

Culture is edified basically on suffocation* of the sexual instinct, specifically of incest. Repression* makes a beachhead in the repression of incest and then extends over all possible sexuality, using for this expansion the laws of association* between representations*. The destructive instinct* which results from a first level of mixture with the sexual instinct in which hate is not distinguished from love, is also suffocated; they are also not well distinguished in some types of aggression or in mastery (in the former the domination of the destructive tendency over the loving tendency is perhaps more clearly seen at times, but we must remember that in order to conquer the object of love a certain level of aggression is needed; in the latter, the object of love is retained without consideration of the harm to the object involved in this retention).

The libidinal ties on which cultural groups are based are aim inhibited. All cultural creations are products of this libido that we could call sublimated. There is less mastery of the death instinct in these creations since some death instinct remains unmixed. Thus, a paradox arises: this complication encountered by the inorganic generated by the phenomena of life, from which in turn culture was born, carries within itself fairly free and unmastered death instincts in the very essence of the creation of the cultural fact. Therefore, in this culture it seems that sometimes the destructive tendencies of human beings predominate over those of love.

M

MAGIC

Ger.: Magie. – Sp.: magia. – Fr.: magie. – It.: magia. – Port.: magia.

This technique and strategy of animism* (*Totem and Taboo*, 1913) predominates in primitive humans and in children; it is produced in part by the need to master the world, is ruled by the pleasure principle* and wish fulfilment* put into action (taking a step past mere fantasy). It also expresses omnipotence of thought*.

Magical incantations seek to eliminate the enemy by destroying a similar doll or something belonging to the person; hunting is also propitiated by drawing a picture of the action.

This mechanism is also utilized in children's play. Their games are phantasies* fulfilling wishes acted out or represented by toys or real fetishes representing idealized figures of adults. The most common fantasies are of being grown-up like the parents, doing the things they do or what children suppose they do. When boys play at being a hero*, they unconsciously fulfil parricidal wishes. In girls, playing with dolls, besides fulfilling the wish to be grown-up, are active-aim Trieb satisfactions. Figures, dolls, toys, or fetishes utilized for acts of magic are chosen according to laws of association*: by contiguity* in some cases: something belonging to the enemy, treated the same way the person wishes to treat the enemy; or by analogy* (drawings or toys), related to something more symbolic.

Magic and children's play utilize mechanisms halfway between primary process* and secondary process*: reality* is both accepted and disavowed*. Therefore, neither magic nor children's play is limited to mere presentation. There is overvaluation of the psychical presentation* above things in reality; and yet it is put into action. This action is not a specific action* which would satisfy Trieb*, although in some cases it may be a form of preparation leading to it. Even children's play gradually acquires these characteristics by virtue of sublimation*. For example: from the wish for mastery of objects fulfilled by a drawing, a person may fulfil this wish as a graphic artist, thereby transforming a magical mechanism into a specific action proper.

MANIA

Ger.: Manie. – Sp.: mania. – Fr.: manie. – It.: mania. – Port.: mania.

This clinical picture corresponding to narcissistic pathology is explained by Freud as a characteristic of melancholia* or a defence in response to it, which transforms it into the opposite. Mania and melancholia struggle with the same "complex" to which the ego* succumbs in melancholia, whereas mania has dominated it or pushed it aside (*Mourning and Melancholia*, 1917).

Although manic excitement implies triumph, what has been defeated remains hidden from the ego.

Mania is characterized by euphoria, a jubilant affect, and more readiness to undertake any type of action.

> In mania, the ego must have got over the loss of the object (or its mourning over the loss, or perhaps the object itself), and thereupon the whole quota of anticathexis which the painful suffering of melancholia had drawn to itself from the ego and "bound" will have become available. Moreover, the manic subject plainly demonstrates his liberation from the object which was the cause of his suffering, by seeking like a ravenously hungry man for new object cathexes.
>
> (1917, p. 255)

The object* has been overcome, and is now identified* with the ego. Now, the subject *is* the ego ideal*, or is again the ideal ego*. The individual now possesses everything, as occurred with the infantile or primitive ideal. This was the infantile hypothesis regarding paternal omnipotence or the idea of primitive humans with respect to the primal father of the primal horde*, who possessed the objects by which he was loved, and had no need to love.

The objects or the cathexes of object presentations* have lost their transcendence, the subject has become emancipated from them, there is no more mourning and no more self-reproach*; self-esteem* has risen to the level of megalomania*. The subject *is* the ideal, *is* "His Majesty the Baby" (1914, p. 91), voraciously choosing toys.

Cathexis* of object presentations is constantly sought; however, this seeking involves lack of desire*, weakness of unconscious* object cathexes, depreciation, devaluation, and emancipation from the object; also, passage of libidinal cathexis to the ego, cathexis of its presentations and of the part of it corresponding to the ideal and the ego's identification with it.

MANIFEST CONTENT (OF DREAMS)

Ger.: manifester Inhalt. – Sp.: contenido manifiesto (del sueño). – Fr.: contenu manifeste (du rêve). – It.: contenuto manifesto (del sogno). – Port.: conteúdo manifesto (do sonho).

This is the dream* as perceived by the patient and, by extension, as the patient tells it to the analyst.

As something perceived, the first case is a mental process that has undergone work by which it returns to images, received as perception* by the subject's consciousness* during sleep. The dream expresses a repressed wish* that is fulfilled in a disguised form.

As a narration, the dream is the return to words of what was perceived as an image. Secondary elaboration* intervenes in both cases. When patients tell their dreams, they cover them with a blanket of intelligibility at the service of censorship* which may make the meaning more obscure to consciousness.

Freud writes in *The Claims of Psycho-Analysis to Scientific Interest* (1913): "The dream as we remember it after waking is described by us as its 'manifest content'" (p. 170).

MASCULINE

Ger.: männlich / maskulin. – Sp.: masculine. – Fr.: masculin. – It.: maschile / mascolino. – Port.: masculino.

This term is applied to characteristics of men, although they may also be found in some women.

Pre-oedipal* children are only slightly differentiated in terms of activity-passivity, sadism-masochism, although we could say that in boys the active predominates over the passive. However, all Trieb is active in the sense that it actively seeks discharge; notwithstanding, its specifically active or passive (cf. active–passive*) aspects are observed in the form of this discharge, in its Trieb aim. The masculine arises from the transformation of the active element of the Trieb aim before recognition of sexual difference, at the moment when this difference begins to exist.

In any case, masculine refers to secondary, social, sexual characteristics: characteristics of the behaviour of men, not of women, throughout the history of culture, which is neither organic nor biological.

Almost all Freudian theory is developed from the masculine perspective (Freud's perspective), and concerns the masculine. In this sense, there is little to add beyond a reference to this fact. The importance of the difference of the development of the feminine appears late in Freud, as befits the philo-masculine society in which this theory was organized (despite Freud's disagreement with these social characteristics). Only in articles such as *Femininity* (1932) or before, in theoretical discussions such as *The Economic Problem of Masochism* (1924) or *A Child Is Being Beaten* (1919), does theory require the creator of psychoanalysis to explain the feminine and with it, the problems specific to women.

Among other points, he states that the superego* is established earlier in boys, is more unconscious* than in women, and that the ego ideal* demands that the ego* sublimate; for example, it demands that men be "heroic", "be a man", to be Oedipus, and that their conscience* will punish them if they are not all this, and even more if they are. He emphasizes the prolonged pre-oedipal* period in girls and describes the castration complex* which leaves traces in their personality and contributes to the occupation by women of "second" place.

The masculine in women may be a caricature of men in some cases, with levels of relation with some types of homosexuality; in others, necessary elements acquired by identification with masculine characteristics of the men in their lives (father or brothers), characteristics traditionally exclusive of men and therefore considered masculine. A woman must struggle to acquire them or to persuade society to allow her to utilize them, since they are rooted in social history, such as intelligence and clarity of thought. Therefore, the apparently clear specificity of the masculine is in reality problematic.

The masculine develops in puberty, when the question of sexual difference is essential; in previous stages, development presents preparatory antitheses: active–passive, sadistic-masochistic, not castrated-castrated, which generally lead to the masculine–feminine theme in puberty and adolescence.

MASOCHISM

Ger.: Masochismus. – Sp.: masoquismo. – Fr.: masochisme. – It.: masochismo. – Port.: masoquismo.

In the strict sense, this is a type of sexual perversion* consisting in obtaining sexual pleasure* from physical or moral pain*, either by debasement, abuse, submission, or unconditional obedience, gagging, physical blows, bonds, and so on.

In a broader sense, which includes the former, it takes three forms: "as a condition imposed on sexual excitation, as an expression of the feminine nature, and as a norm of behaviour. We may, accordingly, distinguish an erotogenic, a feminine and a moral masochism" (*The Economic Problem of Masochism*, 1924, p. 161).

Erotogenic masochism is primary. A fragment of death Trieb* expelled by a muscular path was converted into destructive Trieb*. Another portion remained in the psychical apparatus, partly free and partly fused with libido*. This Trieb fusion then results in Trieb for mastery and sadism*, later directed towards Trieb aims such as reversal into the opposite* and turning round upon the subject's own self*; by these means, sadism may return to masochism secondarily, in which case another individual is needed to occupy the sadistic position whereas the subject becomes the object of that person's sadism.

Pleasure experienced in the sadomasochistic couple is always masochistic, since pain can only be felt in the subject's own body and then be extended to sexual pleasure. The sadist knows that the masochist feels this pain because he remembers his own pain and the sexual excitation generated by it. He then identifies with the masochistic suffering and is able to feel pleasure while saving himself any real suffering.

There is an intermediate step in these Trieb vicissitudes in which sadism is turned round upon the subject's own self without need of an object. This is self-punishment* or self-torture rather than masochism (*Instincts and their Vicissitudes*, 1915).

In feminine masochism, the primary erotogenic stimulus is joined by secondary masochism proceeding from what had become sadism. A certain level of sexual difference (phallic–castrated) needs to have been recognized. Thus, the deepest phantasies of the feminine masochist are to be castrated, possessed sexually, or to deliver a child, phantasies attributed to femininity but not limited to women.

Moral masochism as behaviour is detached from sexuality* and therefore also from the masochistic experience of sexual pleasure. It is associated with an unconscious sense of guilt*, and is involved in the negative therapeutic reaction. Suffering is what matters, not its source, whether this may be the lover, another person, or impersonal circumstances. This moral masochism depends on the constitution in the psychical apparatus of a superego which is sadistic towards the masochistic ego*.

MASTERY (CF. TRIEB FOR MASTERY)

MASTURBATION

Ger.: Masturbation. – Sp.: masturbación. – Fr.: masturbation. – It.: masturbazione. – Port.: masturbação.

In this form of autoerotic satisfaction of sexual Trieb*, pleasure is obtained by rhythmic self-stimulation of erotogenic zones* of the subject's own body.

Freud describes three periods which derive in three levels of masturbation. The first corresponds to the autoerotism* of babies and organ pleasure. The next period originates when the phallic zone takes supremacy over the other erotogenic zones, with which they acquire unity and deferred* meaning. In the meantime, formation of the ego's* bodily source completed: the definitive reality ego* is constituted when all the erotogenic zones are united, an achievement which also involves definitive recognition of the object* as the seat of pleasure. Object choice*, also culminating at this time by virtue of anaclisis* in part on satisfaction of self-preservative Triebe*, falls to the mother. The baby now possesses speech, establishment of repression* begins, play* is utilized as a magical formula for Trieb satisfaction, and phantasy life therefore exists. Phantasy* is a mestizo production between primary process* and secondary process*; it is almost hallucinatory wish fulfilment* constructed on the basis of thought* with words and their inherent characteristics.

During this second period of masturbation, the pleasure of stimulation of an erotogenic zone is joined to a wish-fulfilling phantasy, wishes for the object, and therefore proceeding from object libido*; this libido is satisfied autoerotically, but now in the psychical sphere, fulfilling a phantasy of object desire. The problem is that this object wish became incestuous when the phallic level was reached (cf. phallic-urethral erotism*), which is dangerous. Castration anxiety* appears then, and the oedipal drama unfolds entirely, concluding in the formation of the superego* and passage into the latency* period. All of the previous infantile period is forgotten, especially incestuous phantasies developed at that time, which remain dissolved* forever.

With puberty, quantity of sexual excitation* frozen during latency reappears, and with it, what is usually considered masturbation proper. Then, phantasy returns, disguised. In allusions to these masturbatory phantasies, however, we may infer the involvement of derivatives of incestuous wishes and of all infantile sexuality*.

Construction of these masturbatory phantasies also includes previous vicissitudes of Trieb, fixation* points generated by shifts from predominance of one erotogenic zone to another, traumatic* situations experienced with objects inducing hyper-excitations in certain erotogenic zones, the origin of fixations to the erotogenic zone and characteristics of the object, which for this reason also influence subsequent object choice*.

Masturbatory phantasy also has other, later vicissitudes such as sublimation*, by which it may be transformed, when not repressed, for example, into works of art, creating new realities. Then, it moves away from the autoerotic* and comes closer to the social.

Obsessional thought itself has masturbatory characteristics. For example, in compulsive doubting, the act of thinking itself is eroticized; for this reason, instead of preparing for action, it replaces it.

Neurotic masturbation precipitates a sense of guilt*. In adolescents, this guilt is conscious and generates a vicious circle: masturbation – guilt – firm resolve not to repeat the masturbation – falling back into it – guilt again. Freud considers it the "primary addiction", comparing it to alcoholism, to which we could now add drug addiction.

This sense of guilt is apparently connected with pleasure derived from phantasies which fulfil object wishes in construction up to adolescence. In psychoanalytical treatment, like symptoms*, they must be unwoven, disassembled, and reconstructed, until the real phantasies, the roots of this sense of guilt, are reached: those related with incest, the discovery of sexual difference, castration anxiety, formation of the superego, and those of infancy and the period of oedipal conflict.

MATERIAL TRUTH

Ger.: materielle Wirklichkeit oder Wahrheit. – Sp.: verdad material. – Fr.: vérité matérielle. – It.: verità materiale. – Port.: verdade material.
Material truth refers to the external world, to things* of the world, which Freud in the *Project for a Scientific Psychology* (1895–1950) calls "masses in motion and nothing else" (p. 308).

These are things in themselves, those that the subject cannot ultimately know. However, the thing is knowable as it is known by the subject, not as it is in itself. We understand the thing's attributes, but not the thing. Our knowledge of things is experiential historical truth*: what we experience with them or the way in which we experience them (involving affect*); thus, they become psychical reality* or truth.

Notwithstanding, in our investigation during psychoanalytic treatment, we try to come close to what we assume has been material truth, in the knowledge that in reality we obtain levels of historical truth* in which the perceptual apparatus, quality* and therefore also subjectivity, participated, thereby changing the type of truth from an external truth, inaccessible in and of itself, into the psychical representational world. "What we call *things* are residues which evade being judged" (Ibid., p. 334).

This Freudian statement implies that we cannot know the thing of the world; it is something we do not understand because we are unable to put it through a bodily cathexis or to put ourselves in its place, to imitate it, or to identify with it; the preconscious ego* has no presentations with which to compare these things in order to test reality*. For this reason, the thing of the world to which material truth belongs is by definition unknowable, and may therefore belong to the order of the traumatic, since it has no psychical presentation.

MATRIARCHY

Ger.: Matriarchat. – Sp.: matriarcado. – Fr.: matriarcat. – It.: matriarcato. – Port.: matriarcado.
In Freud's hypothesis in *Totem and Taboo* (1913) and confirmed in *Moses and Monotheism: Three Essays* (1939), this stage of humanity falls between parricide and final establishment of the fraternal alliance* or band of brothers, with its social contract renouncing Trieb, recognizing mutual obligations, and establishing sacred institutions, in sum, the inauguration of law and rights; in this period, most of the complete power left vacant after the elimination of the father passed on to the women.

Matriarchy left traces in the form of maternal deities, probably previous to male gods (all later than totemism*); both (maternal and paternal gods) are preserved afterwards. With the establishment of the fraternal alliance, maternal law was replaced by a restored patriarchal regime in which power was shared by many members; until the advent of monotheism when one masculine god recovers the omnipotence of the primal father.

MEGALOMANIA

Ger.: Grosenwahn. – Sp.: megalomania. – Fr.: mégalomanie. – It.: megalomania. – Port.: megalomania.
This anomaly occurs when the ego* is overly cathected* by libido* proceeding from the id*.

The narcissistic wound having decreased self-esteem*, narcissistic libido compensates by hastening to restore the ego, doing so excessively.

Passing megalomania may be normal. When it is more constant, it constitutes certain typical character traits* or even character pathologies. When it is mitigated, it is joined to arrogance as a character trait. Then, the ego's wound, or rather the diminished self-esteem from which arrogance defends it, is constant.

Megalomania is common in narcissistic affections and some perversions* (feelings of superiority in some homosexuals*), and in narcissistic affections themselves: nearly all the psychoses, especially paranoia* and paranoid schizophrenia*.

In melancholia*, megalomania is negative: the ego's grandeur is its feelings of guilt for all the world's evils.

In schizophrenia it is part of delusions* of grandeur, even the persecutory delusion that perceives the ego as being so important that it is persecuted by organizations, for example.

In contrast, in transference neuroses*, feelings of inferiority tend to predominate (quite probably the narcissistic wound, which always exists, is not in these cases large enough to need to offset it with the opposite, and may instead be felt; here, the object's attraction continues to predominate even though it may have wounded the ego).

In some character traits or in real character pathologies, pride, arrogance, and haughtiness appear as reaction formations* against feelings of the ego's inability, or as satisfaction for symptoms acquired as character traits (in obsessional character pathology, pride in cleanliness or ethics, values fought for). In any case, these traits indicate more or less severe narcissistic wounds.

The narcissistic affection in which megalomania appears in its prototypical form is mania*, which Freud considers a reaction to melancholia. In mania, cathexis is withdrawn from the object* presentation* concealed behind a mad, incessant search involving debasement, lack of desire*, weakness of object cathexis, and passage to ego cathexis, basically of the ego ideal* and identification* with it.

MELANCHOLIA

Ger.: Melancholie. – Sp.: melancholia. – Fr.: mélancolie. – It.: malinconia. – Port.: melancholia.

In this narcissistic affection *par excellence*, symptomatology is similar to mourning*: severe unwellness, loss of interest in the external world, inability to love, and generalized inhibition* of action. To this is added an important inhibition of self-esteem*, the emergence of self-reproaches* and self-debasement, even a delusional expectation of punishment which may lead to suicide, none of which is part of a normal mourning process.

In melancholia, unlike in mourning, loss of a loved one or any other object of a more ideal nature is unnecessary, although it is sometimes precipitated by this type of situations, in which case it configures pathological mourning with a melancholic base.

What is essential in melancholia is the lowering of self-esteem; in this sense, the loss has occurred in the ego*, a loss of value for the subject.

Other striking characteristics are a lack of shame in self-reproaches in the presence of others, unlike the case of a person in the process of mourning. In contrast, melancholics exhibit cruel frankness, finding pleasure in denuding themselves, since these individuals have lost all respect for their ego.

In the mechanism of melancholia cathexis is withdrawn from unconscious* object* presentations* (thing-presentations*) and is placed into the ego. Previously, there has been regression* to the stage of object love when this object was considered the ego (pure pleasure ego*) because it was loved: identification*. By virtue of this identification in the unconscious ego, object love* (now hate* through regression) obtains a disguise; the object's "shadow has fallen upon the ego". This unconscious ego is now the object, unknown to the melancholic's preconscious ego. By identification, the patient has a regressive relation with the object in which hate is not distinguished from love; the superego utilizes this situation to discharge all the death Trieb* it has "cultivated" onto the ego. This is observed clinically as self-reproaching. In negative megalomania, the sense of guilt* is megalomaniacal. The object is no longer desired. The tie with the object has become the tie between the superego and the ego in which the object is included, unknown to the subject. The ego *is* (cf. being*) the object, has identified with it, *is* it, as it did at the "dawn" of psychical constitution. In its sadism* towards the ego identified with the object, the superego may become a "pure culture of death Trieb" and raze the self-preservative Triebe*. Melancholic identification is secondary* and narcissistic*, since it is generated after objects have been recognized as such and becomes part of the ego, though only for a limited period: as long as the melancholic episode lasts.

MEMORY

Ger.: Gedächtnis. – Sp.: memoria. – Fr.: mémoire. It.: memoria. – Port.: memória.

Freud did not specifically study the subject of memory. However, we could say that he did make substantial contributions to it, especially in regard to its way of functioning, some of its mechanisms, and also some of its defects, at least those with psychical causes. However, in the *Project for a Scientific Psychology* (1950), he does provide some definitions of memory. When he refers in this text to facilitations* of the connection between neurones*, he calls it the power of an experience to continue to produce effects. Then, when he refers to memory as a property of the nervous system: "a capacity for being permanently altered by single occurrences" (p. 299).

He also explains that neurones whose contact-barriers* allow quantity of excitation to pass with difficulty – that is to say, neurones that retain information reaching them from perception* – result in a possibility to represent memory. Below, he adds: "Memory is represented by the facilitations existing between the ψ neurones" (Ibid., p. 300). He immediately adds complexity: "memory is represented by the differences in the facilitations between the ψ neurones" (Ibid.). This definition is dynamic since it conceives of a memory in which connections between neurones must be related in order to function correctly and for their comparison; from this point to presentations and connections between them …

Freud considers memory essential to development of the psyche. Presentations (together with quantity of excitation* or affect* cathecting them) are the essence of the psyche (cf. soul*), conceptual processing of memory traces*; therefore, they are memories of perception (historical truth* rather than material truth*). Therefore, we could say that Freud does not explain what memory is. Who has been able to do it? However, he considers its way of functioning, which he explains to some extent, as a base from which to explain other concepts such as forgetting*. However, he does provide a highly important contribution, perhaps undervalued, to the understanding of memory in general.

In regard to the functioning of memory, Freud describes one of its essential mechanisms: association. In this sense, he is an associationist. Memories arise from analogies or contiguities between new perceptions and old perceptions remembered. We recall that the apparatus constantly searches reality to find what it desires. For this purpose, it needs to remember what it desires (the experience of satisfaction*, not necessarily the first one, but may be any of them) in order to compare the memory to the perception and, in order to find thought identity*, to compare what is now perceived to what was perceived before and is now memory*. It must differentiate between the perception now and the desire that emerged previously, when it was also a perception.

However, all this is even more complex: some experiences of satisfaction in the past changed sign after going through the Oedipus complex period (this is the essence of what Freud called primary repression*): what was satisfactory became traumatic and consequently, all the memories of infantile sexuality (also the birthplace of adult desires) were sent to the unconscious*, became unrememberable, and therefore, all current perceptions that might remind us of them are repressed (avoided, disavowed), as well as thoughts (phantasies*) which also might produce memories that must remain unconscious in order to avoid activating the infantile trauma, thereby generating anxiety (castration anxiety, fear of object loss, and so on, depending on previous fixation points formed in experiences with predominant castration anxiety which tries to include the other, but sometimes fails to do).

When Freud explains the mechanisms of repression*, he also explains the functioning of memory. Repression acts principally on word-presentations* which the conscious psyche utilizes for thinking. If a word is repressed, it goes to the unconscious*, and conscious efforts to evoke it are in vain. Consciousness* functions basically with words, although they, being present, refer to images of things. In forgetting, only the image may be in consciousness (Signorelli, the example of forgetting proper names analysed by Freud) but, lacking the word to name it, he cannot mention it or even think it, except in vain attempts by consciousness to remember.

Once repression is established, conflict is installed: what is desired is also what is feared, which leads to many attempts to overcome this highly unsurpassable obstacle; among these attempts we find culture* no less, through sublimation*, but also the discontent it involves. It is from this theory of implicit memory that Freud derived the bases of the key to psychoanalytical treatment; lifting repression; that is to say, going with the analysand back down the road to repression established in the psyche by infantile oedipal conflict; recovering its memory: remembering in order to stop repeating. When presentations from the infantile past are remembered, the unconscious wish and the conflict that repressed them may be thought, similarities and differences may be found in relation to the actual conflict, but mainly, the force and unmanageability of the unknown may be removed; when it is known, it may be handled better with reason and ethics*. On the road back, the endeavoured lifting of repressions is produced.

MEMORY (MNEMIC) TRACE

Ger.: Erinnerungsspur o Erinnerungsrest. – Sp.: huella mnémica. – Fr.: trace mnésique. – It.: traccia mnemonica. – Port.: traço mnémico.

This trace is what remains in the psychical apparatus* following each experience or each perception* of it. Some perceptions are very important, at first the experience of satisfaction* and the experience of pain*. The experience of satisfaction leaves three types of traces: the image of an object; the image of a movement and a sensation of pleasurable discharge* registered in the nucleus. When these three traces are mutually facilitated (cf. facilitation*), they form a wish* presentation*. This wish is for repetition of this experience whenever cathexis* of Trieb excitation returns. As for the experience of pain, what is facilitated is a tendency to discharge and also an image of the hostile object* and of movements made.

At the beginning memory (mnemic) traces form presentations of things with which the psychical apparatus* is going to operate. These traces undergo several transcriptions and linkages by laws of association*, and are finally registered as concepts (cf. Letter 52*).

Other traces are superimposed onto these thing-presentations*; these traces also enter through the perceptual apparatus, but with a higher level of complexity, since they represent or symbolize the former to consciousness*. These memory traces of words generate word-presentations* necessary for thought* activity, secondary process*, the ego*; in sum, the highest functions of the human psychical apparatus.

METAPSYCHOLOGY

Ger.: Metapsychologie. – Sp.: metapsicología. – Fr.: métapsychologie. – It.: metapsicología. – Port.: psicología.

Although this term was created by Freud in 1915 for a book to be entitled *Preliminary Works for a Metapsychology*, this book was not published in this form, but with only five of the works (six others disappeared, and one was found among Ferenczi's papers) he attempted to coherently organize theoretical ideas that were organized separately in each of his previous works, together with new ideas. Then, as his investigations made his thought more complex, this complexity grew geometrically, and his theories were disseminated throughout his works. Therefore, we consider metapsychology the theoretical aspect of Freudian psychoanalysis dispersed throughout his works from beginning to end without omitting any of his development, which in spite of their complexity continue to preserve their coherence. Freud wrote his works not only to be understood but also to show his trajectory as he discovered phenomena in human beings that he tried to explain with his theory; this accounts for part of the complexity of his reading despite his brilliant, clear prose.

Metapsychology is a psychology "that leads us behind consciousness". It is a psychology that takes us towards the unconscious and then centres its study on this unconscious; from there it sets out to examine the way it influences human behaviour and conscience. Speech is closely related with it. In other words, it is reason, human logos, trying to explain its own "irrational" origin (seen in this way by a consciousness unaware of its base which in reality simply belongs to a different logic unknown to consciousness). Metapsychology arises from observation and its interpretation, from interrelations between multiple observations and even from some speculation which assembles a coherent whole to explain the functioning of the human soul.

Metapsychology postulates a dynamic psychology in constant movement, generated by energy proceeding from the external world or the subject's own body, directed towards a motor discharge (specific action) that is also secretory (affects) through presentations (which Freud considers former perceptions and with which this energy acquires the name of libido, life Trieb) or without them, in which case the aim is total discharge (death, death Trieb). Energy and presentations unbind only rarely, and therefore remain fused in diverse ways, one predominating over another depending on the case. Energy is its quantity (only measurable as "more" or "less") which takes or seeks a perceptive quality directed by presentations (thing- and word-); therefore, metapsychology possesses an economy. It also occurs in a space, neither visible nor measurable, we would also say immaterial; its laws, conflicts, splitting, and other aspects are different; it has a topic (or rather two topics; the second is structural, adding complexity to the first and including it). Libido may aim towards the ego which in turn must comply with the ideal: this is narcissism. Finally, human life transpires in a society constructed by humanity in its relations between human beings, persons more or less important to each individual, whose subjective presentations of their experiences in it, of others' image of them, and of the social in general construct the individual psyche; peculiarly human modes of constructing the social are edified on this base.

First, we would say that this construction begins with recognition that non-rational, affective, Trieb, infantile sexual desire exists and participates in diverse ways in each person's present time, although it originated in the individual's infantile past. Second, an attempt is made to bring it back from this unconscious to reason, to return to it words lost by the mechanism of repression, thereby multiplying the ranks of the rational ego, the person's self-knowledge, and the potential to incorporate into thinking presentations previously held in the unconscious.

This describes the prehistory of the subject's constitution according to Freud's unique notion regarding history (history experienced with objects, experiences that remain not only in forgotten memory but also seek to be repeated; that is to say, history that seeks to make itself present and a present which seeks its history) in which what becomes present (in disguise) does so unknown to this subject's consciousness.

But this is not all; here, he describes the nature of Trieb, the manner in which wishes are generated because wishes are motors of psychical functioning, and also narcissism, love of the ego, both the high point of health and also of the severest pathologies.

Second, therefore, Freud attempts to recover this history or historical truth, in order to utilize it to find the historical and hence individual meaning of actual reason; in this way to restore the subject as the master of its own discourse and action.

Metapsychology's detailed description of the manner in which these processes occur concomitantly generates theoretical concepts for their understanding in order to enable us to exchange ideas clearly on ways of functioning of the human soul. These mechanisms become more complex as their description deepens, but they never cancel what went before, which remains standing. Freud starts with a historical evolutionism of the subject (*Three Essays* ...) which partially conflicts, since 1920, with the discovery that all Triebe are preservative Triebe (which we may infer when reading the *Project* ...), that they tend to return to a state previous to the appearance of the stimulus, that creation belongs not to Trieb but to the fact that its real repetition is impossible. He then goes on to describe a structured psychical apparatus centred specifically on the history of the Oedipus complex and its commemorative monuments in the apparatus. Identification is added or subsumed with the presentation as bricks in this "construction", which adds further complexity to the nth degree and a new twist to the theory of anxiety and others. The social has entered the apparatus through the superego, although it had already done so since the first moment of life, the ego itself being a precipitate of the social, and all this in different ways and forms. Conflict between its parts is at the core of the human soul. Freud overcomes without overcoming, in the Hegelian manner (aufhebung). The object relation is dialectic, constant, and fluid in spite of the protective apparatus against stimuli embodied by its very psychical structure.

Freud's works culminate in the study of the social sphere; we could say that he hypothesizes, in the form of a myth on human origins. Human groups gather together around a leader and the members of this group identify with each other. He delves into the ills of culture and rethinks history through the figure of Moses.

All this analysis takes place in metapsychology, Freud's masterpiece, which provides a new perspective on the study of human beings. Through metapsychology, psychoanalysis is not only a psychotherapeutic technique (the best and the most complex), but also a science which influences other sciences and generates a turning point in all knowledge about ourselves.

MEYNERT'S AMENTIA (ACUTE HALLUCINATORY CONFUSION)

Ger.: Amentia (Meynerts). – Sp.: amencia de Meynert (confusión alucinatoria aguda). – Fr.: amentia de Meynert (confusion hallucinatoire aigue). – It.: amencia di Meynert (confuzione allucinatoria acuta). – Port.: amencia de Meynert (confusão alucinatoria aguda).

This type of psychosis* is mentioned by Freud several times in his works and described by one of his teachers, the psychiatrist Meynert.

It is a type of acute psychosis produced as a reaction to the loss of a loved one (perhaps with previous incomplete discrimination between the ego* and the object*) when perception* of this painful aspect of reality* is disavowed. Freud cites the example of the mother who has lost her baby and continues to rock a piece of wood, and another: the abandoned fiancée who continues to await the arrival of her beloved with each knock at the door.

Object* loss is disavowed*, and the object continues to be perceived, or rather the memory* of its image is received as a perception. There is alteration of the ego* and therefore the ego withdraws cathexis from the conscious perceptual end (Pcpt.-Cs.) and instead functions under the sway of the pleasure principle* instead of the reality principle for which the perceptual apparatus is so necessary; the Trieb phantasy* is thus mistaken for the presence of the object and the real perception of its absence.

Meynert's amentia differs from other types of psychosis. For example: in hysterical psychosis, phantasies* perceived as hallucination* are repressed (disguised, anxiety-producing, they return from the repressed*) whereas in amentia this is not the case; quite the contrary, they are loved by the ego.

In schizophrenia*, cathexis is withdrawn from the thing-presentation, and the unconscious wish for the object, a motor for the psychical apparatus*, is lost. For such an event to take place or as a consequence of it, the ego is practically demolished and is even projected into the external world and perceived hallucinatorily, returning from it (voicing of thoughts), also through orders sent by machines (symbols* of the body, the origin of the ego) or critical observations (the superego* which is also projected and perceived hallucinatorily as a perception) of its acts.

In amentia there is less, shallower, and more limited withdrawal of cathexis from the unconscious object presentation than in schizophrenia, or it may not occur at all; consequently, the clinical picture of alteration of the ego and ego regression is also milder. The main affection is nonacceptance of the perception of the absence of the object in reality; for this reason, the clinical picture is more reversible, although intermediate pictures mixing the two or one clinical picture that becomes the other are also observed; this depends basically on the degree of alteration of the ego* and regression*.

MNEMIC SYMBOL

Ger.: Erinnerungssymbol. – Sp.: símbolo mnémico. – Fr.: symbole mnésique. – It.: simbolo mnestico. – Port.: símbolo mnémico.

Freud proposed this term for certain neurotic symptoms*, usually of conversion hysteria, whose form of production is something like a symbolic commemoration; that is to say, they have an analogous relation with certain repressed unconscious meanings which are therefore not recognized by the ego* as its own wishes*. The meanings of symptoms, in these cases, are accessible through symbolism expressed by the symptom itself, and therefore it is unnecessary to ask the patient for associations or to utilize them to reconstruct events that conceal or contain thing-presentations* of unconscious wishes as we commonly do.

For example, a facial neuralgia symbolizes a slap to punish a forbidden wish (Cäcelie M.*); a limp, "the impossibility to take a step" towards the repressed wish (Elisabeth von R.*); and others.

Another example of this type of substitute formation* as an origin of symptoms: the "Rat Man" when he suffers an obsession to lose weight. His fiancée was staying at that time with a cousin named Dick, a word which also means obese, and the patient obviously wanted to get rid of him. The interpretation was derived from the patient's associations* or from the analyst's previous knowledge of his circumstances.

This type of expression of the meaning of a symptom is more common in some patients than in others. It also occurs in an isolated form or may be mixed with other meanings.

The latter may be repetitions of scenes from the patient's history (historical truth*) which may not have a symbolic explanation: at most, a change of interpretation from the logic regarding the meaning of events of the past.

When the symptom is produced by a mnemic symbol, it may be interpreted rapidly when the analogy* between one presentation* and the other is understood with no need of associations from the patient.

Associations are needed for understanding* through constructions* of historical truths in the other type of symptom formation referred to by Freud at the beginning of his works as "associative functional" (*Studies on Hysteria*, 1895).

These two types of substitutive formation may combine and present in a mixed form; the analyst is advised not to consider the analysis of the meaning of a symptom complete until after having utilized all the possible associations arising from any of the symptom's elements, since it is over-determined and therefore new meanings may appear leading to new levels of the problem which in turn account for other phenomena belonging to this complex network of meaning that is the psychical apparatus*.

In Freud's works we find several examples of this approach: (1) the astasia-abasia* of Elisabeth von R., studied on the basis of her associations in connection with different parts of the symptom. When all her associations are interrelated, the presentational store of the preconscious ego is enriched with the return of word-presentations* for memories* of past events which acquire a new meaning that is expressed symbolically through the symptom, "not take a step towards her brother-in-law, despite her wish to do so"; (2) the "Wolf Man's" actual constipation merits a construction-interpretation. Through it, Freud reconstructs a large part of the episodes of infantile sexuality connected with anal erotism* and the way it fits into recognition of sexual difference, which the patient began to recognize with the advent of the phallic phase; consequently, predominantly masochistic Trieb becomes feminine. This produces the phantasy of giving his father a child as a feminine phantasy, one of the symptom's meanings; also, by analogy*, as a mnemic symbol of the phantasy of giving birth, typical of feminine masochism* in general.

The interpretive level is thereby enriched with the recovery – by virtue of the construction* based on the patient's associations – of the mnemic store of infantile sexuality*, origin of the symptom and of essential characteristics of the character of this patient's ego (such as passivity and difficulties in managing money, for example).

Thus, levels of analysis of the symptom and also of the ego are deepened (*From the History of an Infantile Neurosis*, 1918).

Freud also utilizes the expression "mnemic symbol" in other ways. In *Inhibitions, Symptoms and Anxiety* (1925), the anxiety signal* is a mnemic symbol of anxiety of birth trauma: the entry of large quantities of excitation* into the psychical apparatus. This mnemic symbol of automatic anxiety*, a signal of danger of the latter, is utilized by the ego to defend itself through repression* in the broad sense of the term, or defence mechanisms*, in an automatic and unconscious* manner, before any access of id* Trieb* to the ego and therefore against the ego's acceptance of Trieb (or the unconscious wish implicit in it) as its own.

Anxiety* as a clinical phenomenon is partly a mnemic symbol of actions that were once the subject's own specific actions* (the birth trauma which made the subject breathe) or those of humanity, even hysterical attacks in prehistoric times, all phenomena that lost their specificity but retained a form of expression that commemorates them symbolically, now as a simple expression of affect.

MOTHER COMPLEX

Ger.: Mutter Komplex. – Sp.: complejo materno. – Fr.: complexe maternel. – It.: complesso materno. – Port.: complexo materno.

A particular type of relation established by the daughter with her mother, the daughter's first sexual object choice* by anaclisis of sexual Trieb* over self-preservative Triebe*. It is previous to entry into the oedipal period (preoedipal*), and in this period becomes negative oedipal when sexual difference acquires experiential value.

In the course of this intense link, more prolonged than in boys, the girl's ambivalence* grows slowly, especially when she enters the oedipal period. It is then that she must leave it behind and recognize sexual difference (on this phallic level of erotogenic zone*, recognize that she is castrated), and change object*, turning to her father from whom she could receive the wished-for penis-child.

Throughout this time, the link with her mother becomes more hostile, sometimes generating fixations* that make passage to the father difficult (thus, at first the link with the father is transference from the former link with the mother) or this passage may carry nuances belonging to the former link.

The girl only reluctantly accepts this new situation. She needs to break off with her mother (up to that time her prime object choice) and also make her responsible for her handicap, in the face of which she is barely able to leave her.

This passage is very painful, and if it is not overcome, it returns in adolescence and becomes stormy.

As always, this overcoming, which is always so humanly relative, involves the complemental series.

When a mother hinders or arrests a daughter's sexual activity, she is fulfilling a normal function whose lines are laid down by events in childhood, which has powerful, unconscious motives, and has received the sanction of society. It is the daughter's business to emancipate herself from this influence and to decide for herself on broad and rational grounds what her share of enjoyment or denial of sexual pleasure shall be. If in the attempt to emancipate herself she falls a victim to a neurosis it implies the presence of a mother-complex which is as a rule overpowerful, and is certainly unmastered. The conflict between this complex and the new direction taken by the libido is dealt with in the form of one neurosis or another, according to the subject's disposition. The manifestation of the neurotic reaction will always be determined, however, not by her present-day relation to her actual mother but by her infantile relations to her earliest image of her mother.

(*A Case of Paranoia Running Counter to the Psycho-Analytic Theory of the Disease*, 1915, pp. 267–8)

MOTOR END

Ger.: Motilität / motorisches Ende. – Sp.: polo motor. – Fr.: pole moteur. – It.: polo motore. – Port.: polo motor.

In the schematic picture in Chapter VII of *The Interpretation of Dreams* (1900), this is the place Trieb stimulus must reach in order to attain discharge through action carried out by utilizing the muscular apparatus.

Action is regulated by the preconscious ego*. In theory, the ego must guide it, lead it, and decide on it; however, action receives pressure from several flanks: the id* fights for satisfaction of its Triebe, whereas the superego* counters them with a powerful "reaction formation"*. The unconscious part of the ego (the defence mechanisms*) also sometimes force certain automatic actions which the preconscious ego must make an effort to explain through rationalizations and, finally, the difficulties of reality* place a limit on its possibility of action.

Cornered in this way, the preconscious ego, by utilizing thought*, the reality principle* and its power of synthesis, must devise actions to generate pleasure* and gratify narcissism* without involving the sense of guilt*. It is only sometimes successful, and then only relatively so.

At the moment of action, discharge is effective. Energy is unbound, leaves freely, and the level of quantity of energy in the ego decreases. This is the final moment, the sought for moment that produces pleasure.

MOURNING

Ger.: Trauer. – Sp.: duelo. – Fr.: deuil. – It.: lutto. – Port.: luto.

This is a normal, painful process produced by the loss in reality* of a desired, loved object* or of "an abstraction which has taken the place of one, such as one's country, liberty, an ideal, and so on" (*Mourning and Melancholia*, 1917, p. 243). It is characterized by a painful mood, loss of interest in the external world – unless it recalls what has been lost – the loss of capacity to love, work, and so on. This manifests the effort the ego* must make to carry through the painful process of detaching itself from the wish* for the presence of the loved object, the same object that reality shows is no longer there.

It is a process of object libido* that finds no solution, since the object no longer belongs to reality, which in turn produces an increase of longing* (belonging to object libido) for it. Therefore, mourning is a more or less prolonged process the ego needs in order to accept definitive object loss in reality. It must detach its wish for it from each of the moments that recall it: those in which it has left its trace.

Sometimes this affective process is long, almost interminable. However, in general, with time and psychical work accomplished in its course, this pain is gradually mitigated until it nearly disappears, leaving in the ego a commemoration, a trait that belonged to the object, an identification*, a regression* to a wish to be* the object, since the ego can no longer have* it. At the same time, libidinal introversion withdraws libido from anything not corresponding to the lost object or memories relating to it. In each situation when the object was hyper-cathected*, the situation of psychical pain* is reproduced when reality confirms the impossibility of satisfying the wishes thereby reactivated.

As the cathexis gradually detaches from the presentation* of the lost object, it passes onto another object that replaces it, together with a process of ego identification with attributes of the lost object which facilitates or enables giving up the object.

"It may be that this identification is the sole condition under which the id can give up its objects" (*The Ego and the Id*, 1923, p. 29).

The loss of a loved one may unleash a neurosis or any other type of pathology, configuring different types of pathological mourning. A severe form is psychotic disavowal* of the loss of the loved one, with hallucination of its presence, as in the case of Meynert's amentia*. Another may be due to different forms of neurosis*; these were doubtless latent and asymptomatic, now emerging in symptoms* as hysteria*, obsessional neuroses*, and so on.

Mourning must be differentiated from physical pain, although if the latter is caused by a bodily loss, it may secondarily generate a situation of mourning for loss of part of the ego, which is then narcissistic mourning.

The psychical pain of mourning is caused by hyper-cathexis* of longing for the object added to impossibility to satisfy it, which generates the helplessness* that characterizes the subject going through this process. It is as if, because it has become aware that it will no longer have the object, the ego aimed to recover all the pleasurable moments experienced with the object, even those that were fancied, all in an ideal way governed by the pleasure principle*; for this reason, among other things, the virtues of the deceased person tend to be remembered. When cathexis of longing is mitigated and the object wish successfully replaces the lost object, psychical pain decreases.

Melancholia* is not necessarily unleashed by a mourning process. It is instead a problem of narcissistic libido between the superego-ego ideal* and the ego, which causes the ego to suffer. In this agency, the unconscious form of a link of hate* with the object appears, since the latter is inside the ego and is usually an object belonging to the history of infantile sexuality* that was smuggled in by virtue of identification. The general mood of melancholia is phenomenologically similar to that of mourning, except that self-reproaches* predominate over longing for the object. Self-reproaches are unconscious reproaches addressed to the object which, without the ego's knowledge, is within it.

MYTH

Ger.: Mythus. – Sp.: mito. – Fr.: mythe. – It.: mito. – Port.: mito.

Although this concept pertains to social psychology, Freud perceived continuity between social and individual psychology, utilizing myth. Myths are expressed through the phantasies*, poetic embellishment, and archaic memories of peoples, in the manner of individual screen memories*, which erase memories painful to national or popular sentiment.

Myths belong to the first type of world conception, the animistic* conception, which projects psychology onto the external world, nature, and the inanimate.

Although a myth is a distortion of historical truth*, its core may always be reconstructed* by psychoanalytic technique and theory, as it does for dreams*, parapraxes*, screen memories, phantasies, or symptoms*. Examples of this type of constructions in Freud's works are found, for example, in *Totem and Taboo* (1913), in *The Acquisition and Control of Fire* (1932), and even in *Moses and Monotheism: Three Essays* (1939).

The type of distortion in a myth is the same as dream distortion. The myth, however, resorts to universal symbols*, those formed gradually over the course of human history in times before or during the period of creation of speech, and later forgotten. Myths are also formed from primal phantasies* such as the primal scene*, seduction*, castration*, return to the womb, and the family romance*. They are also shaped by processes of condensation* and displacement* typical of primary process* and of intermediate products of the primitive period with predominance of omnipotence of thought*, as in animism and magic*.

Freud sees myths as disfigured relics of wishful phantasies of entire nations, secuñar dreams of young humanity.

The myth of the hero* often explains the origin or is the "myth of the origins". In these presentations embellished by the poet, the hero occupies the place of the fraternal alliance (the poet identifies* with the hero); in this alliance, the brothers banded together to defy and kill their despotic father; they devoured him and with this act created a new social order; they incarnated the father's prohibition, forbidding incest and parricide (out of guilt* and longing* for having killed the father) forever (primarily repressed). With this, a specialized part of the ego* formed in the psychical apparatus* of each member of human culture; Freud calls it the superego*, in charge of compliance with these laws, from that time forward felt to be natural as a result of repression which induces forgetting of the original circumstances.

Psychoanalytic interpretation* of myths utilizes scientific thought* in the manner of dream interpretation. It attempts to surpass animistic thought and enter metapsychology*. Thus, in *Moses and Monotheism: Three Essays* (1939), from the Biblical myth he extracts a hypothetical reconstruction of the origins of the Jewish people. In *Totem and Taboo* (1913), the study of diverse primitive customs and myths enables Freud to theorize on human origins and to create his own "scientific myth". In *The Acquisition and Control of Fire* (1932), he utilizes the Greek myth of Prometheus, punished for having stolen fire from the gods of Olympus, in order to discuss the control of Trieb in the period of predominant phallic-urethral eroticism*, taking the line of thought that culture is edified on the suppression* of Trieb.

N

NAMES

Ger.: Name. – Sp.: nombre. – Fr.: prénom. – It.: nome. – Port.: nome.

Children and primitives, who give words their full thing-meaning, consider a person's first name an essential piece and important treasure of their personality. Children believe consciously that when two things have names that sound the same, this indicates a deep concordance between these two things. The same is true in adult patients, but refers to their unconscious* meaning.

In a different context, some primitive societies forbid pronouncing the name of dead persons, as if this mention alone might resuscitate them (*Totem and Taboo*, 1913).

We notice that temporary forgetting* of names is the most frequent of our parapraxes (*The Psychopathology of Everyday Life*, 1901). We now examine this more closely. The attempt to reproduce it is disturbed, and in the disturbing complex there is either a pre-existing connection or else one has been established by a law of association* (analogy*, contiguity*, and opposition*).

The most effective disturbing complexes show that they are referring to the subject (personal, family, professional) (1901).

Among the motives for disturbances generated by memory* and those against which the ego* defends itself by forgetting, Freud highlights the purpose of avoiding unpleasure* produced by the memory, which is not unconnected from aversion towards the person possessing this name.

Another phenomenon of group psychology*, studied very little, is the fact that the forgetting of names is highly contagious. In a conversation it is usually enough for one person to mention having forgotten a certain name for others to withdraw it from memory as well. It is as if one person's unconscious had given a clear signal and the unconscious of the others had understood it quite well.

NARCISSISM

Ger.: Narzissmus. – Sp.: narcisismo. – Fr.: narcissisme. – It.: narcisismo. – Port.: narcisismo.

In strictly metapsychological terms, narcissism is libido* cathecting* the ego*; that is to say, "love* of the ego".

The subject of narcissism is definitively presented in his theory in his work, *On Narcissism: An Introduction* (1914), written after his work on Schreber and in the context of polemics with Jung. Freud considers that Jung is wrong when he thinks that libido is not sexual but instead a unique, vital energy and motor of life. Jung also disputes the concept of libidinal introversion, misunderstanding it and mistaking it for libidinal withdrawal* (Freud considers the latter but not the former to be the possible generator of schizophrenia*).

In 1914, Freud upholds his libidinal theory as a sexual theory, but adds complexity by subdividing it into object libido which is pleased with its link with objects, and narcissistic libido which is satisfied in the ego. Object libido arises by anaclisis* on the object of satisfaction of the other Trieb*: self-preservative or ego Trieb*, from which it gradually separates until it finally opposes it.

With this presentation in society of narcissistic libido, the ego is also considered a libidinal object and, despite self-preservative Trieb, problems begin to centre upon narcissistic libido and object libido.

Concerning libidinal introversion – misunderstood by Jung – Freud considers it the commonest mechanism in the neuroses*. It is object libido that takes refuge (becomes introverted) in objects of phantasy*; that is to say, in object wishes* fulfilled imaginarily. These phantasies form preconscious daydreams* which, if repressed, become unconscious* and generate symptoms*, dreams*, and other phenomena.

What Jung fails to understand is the difference between libidinal introversion and narcissistic libidinal withdrawal. Freud refers to the latter in the Schreber case (*Psycho-Analytic Notes on an Autobiographical Account of a Case of Paranoia (Dementia Paranoides)* (1911); in this text, he explains that in withdrawal the unconscious object presentation* is decathected*, the wish for it is unconsciously and categorically broken off, it is no longer desired in phantasy, and this libido now cathects the ego.

A wounded ego needs libido if it is to stop bleeding. The ego may be wounded by an offence from the object on which it depended to uphold its self-esteem*, probably because libido did not reach it either primarily (infantile narcissism) or from the ego ideal*.

The effect of libido withdrawn from object wishes and placed in the ego appears in clinical work as hypochondria* (the bodily origin of the ego), as megalomania* (ego libido proper), or as an experience of the end of the world (a consequence of breaking off from the object wish).

Organic illness may also increase narcissism. The diseased organ attracts all the (narcissistic) libido to itself, leaving little libido for objects.

In love life, narcissism is involved in the unconscious motives for which the subject chooses its objects, based on anaclisis on those that satisfy self-preservative Trieb (nourishing mother-protective father) or on characteristics of the ego itself. Some of the object's traits are chosen by anaclisis whereas others may have a narcissistic base with anaclisis on the subject's own ego. In different and varying proportions, this choice is generally both object and narcissistic (except in quite firmly structured character pathologies in which everything is more rigid).

In object choices* with a narcissistic base, the subject depends more on the object for self-esteem; these choices may predominate in subjects with self-esteem damaged previously, in early moments such as in the castration complex* (one of the causes of its predominance in women) or in the pre-oedipal* phase (usually with oral fixation* points).

Therefore, in object choices with a narcissistic base (such as the homosexual*, for example), the ego is more humiliated when the object fails and frustration* ensues.

In these cases, if unconscious desire for the object is broken off and the ego is cathected libidinally, narcissistic pathology is generated.

Infantile narcissism is expressed as a delusion* of grandeur, an expression of children's omnipotence of thought* which makes primary objects part of their ego and enables them to carry out all the desired specific actions*.

A previous state of *primary narcissism* is inferred hypothetically: the ego *is* everything pleasurable (purified pleasure ego*), in this sense, an ideal ego*; the ego was the object of pleasure, or equally, the object of pleasure (the mother) was considered ego. Unpleasure* was non-ego, although an initial reality ego* functioned which distinguished between ego and non-ego, depending on whether a muscular movement repulsed or failed to repulse a stimulus. How do we understand the child's primary narcissism, not objectless but in reality secondary to the object link (*The Ego and the Id*, 1923)? It happens that recognition of the object as well as of the ego is a complex act which takes place partially at the outset (initial reality ego, pleasure ego) and also gradually builds up with experience (definitive reality ego*).

Love* for this definitive reality ego, finally constituted in the period of predominant phallic-urethral* eroticism (with all its oedipal problems, anatomical sexual difference, and castration complex), is what is called narcissism. At this point, all this autoeroticism* and the pre-oedipal is discovered to be in reality narcissistic (the latter actually homosexual), since at this time the ego is discovered as such and therefore the object (or vice versa) as well. From this moment forward, object libido, whose action has been increasing, pushes more vigorously towards the object; as a consequence of oedipal conflict, the superego* is constituted in the psychical apparatus, which binds a good deal of previous homosexual and narcissistic libido (love for both parents, especially the father).

What is left of infantile narcissism remains as the ego ideal (longing for the past delusion of grandeur) which demands the same perfection as the father of infancy, capable of anything ("You ought to be like this (like your father)" (*The Ego and the Id*, 1923, p. 34). Secondary identification* with the parents reinforces primary identification*, in turn generating conscience* ("You may not be like this (like your father)" (Ibid.). The conscience is in charge of watching and punishing the ego to make sure it complies with the ego ideal; if the ego does so, it again becomes the ideal ego (pleasure ego and omnipotence of infantile thought) that it once was.

Narcissistic gratifications accompany satisfaction of the ego ideal, "omnipotence corroborated by experience" (*On Narcissism: An Introduction*, 1914), gratifications tending to belong to the sphere of sublimation* (desexualized*).

Finally, narcissistic gratifications are also obtained from the object link, as we mentioned concerning narcissistic object choice.

Freud's discussion on parental love is interesting. He places it in the narcissistic type of object choice. It is in reality a homosexual link (aim-inhibited with non-recognition of sexual difference and therefore homosexual), an object link in which the object is the ego. This is true for the mother, for her love towards her child (perhaps because the child relieves her own castration complex, and since it fulfils the wish that takes her into the positive Oedipus complex*: to receive a penis-child from her father), but also for the father who would like to relieve all his frustrations and fulfil his unsatisfied wishes through his child: all that Freud summarizes in the figure of "His Majesty the Baby" (*On Narcissism: An Introduction*, 1914, p. 91).

NARCISSISTIC IDENTIFICATION

Ger.: Narzisstische identifizierung. – Sp. identificación narcisista. – Fr.: identification narcissiste. – It.: identificazione narcisistica. – Port.: identificação narcisista.

Narcissistic identification refers to everything in the ego* which therefore constitutes it; everything in which certain attributes of the object* become part of a subject's ego. We may say that all identification is narcissistic, so long as we understand narcissism* in the strict sense as libido* in the ego; we see that some identifications do not belong to it or that the ego considers them ego-dystonic. By definition, some hysterical* identifications constitute symptoms* but do not constitute the ego: they are simply vehicles of expression of return of the repressed*.

Of course, primary identifications* are narcissistic, as are also secondary identifications* constituting the superego*, since this agency is a special part of the ego. However, all identifications added to the paternal or maternal line are also secondary, such as teachers, leaders, and heroes, which constitute the ego and superego and form some of the subject's character traits.

Some narcissistic identifications (which become part of the ego) are fleeting, such as those produced in group* links in which egos are diluted in favour of an "expanded ego" having the same ideal, constituted by a leader or an abstraction. Within these fleeting narcissistic identifications we include the pathological, such as melancholia in which "the shadow of the object fell upon the ego" (*Mourning and Melancholia*, 1917, p. 249). These last as long as the melancholic attack (cf. melancholia*). In obsessional neurosis*, the ego and superego are partly compromised (in self-reproaches*, in doubts), but identifications are also considered foreign to the ego as uncontrollable compulsions*. We could say that this type is only partly narcissistic.

The prototype of narcissistic identification is that of melancholia, even the manner in which it makes the link with the object unconscious. Here, the ego is apparently hated*, but in reality it is the object with which the ego has identified that is hated.

NEED

Ger.: Bedürfnis / Not. – Sp.: necesidad. – Fr.: nécessité. – It.: bisogno. – Port.: necessidade.

Freud assigns this term to endogenous stimuli; that is to say, those proceeding from the subject's own body and generating somatic needs: hunger, breathing, and sexuality. When these needs are bound to presentations*, they become desires*. However, the term "desire" was limited in practice to sexual desires. The latter are formed by libido* cathecting (cf. cathexis*) presentations. Energy cathecting self-preservative Triebe is referred to as "interest"*.

Individuals are exposed to "exigencies of life"; that is to say, stimuli proceeding from the person's own body, which must be satisfied by specific actions*.

In his *Project for a Scientific Psychology* (1950), Freud proposes that needs originating in endogenous stimuli are constantly being formed in intercellular substance and only periodically become psychical stimuli. By accumulation and summation and having passed a certain threshold, they enter the psychical apparatus* where they bind to presentations (Freud utilizes the concept of neurones*, but subsequently, in the same text, he refers to them as presentations, a term he chooses definitively in Chapter 7 of *The Interpretation of Dreams*, 1900), thereby completely entering psychology; these presentations exhibit what were once perceptions*, principally experiences of satisfaction* or pain*.

Traces of satisfaction are transformed into psychical wishes (object* wishes in the case of sexual Triebe*), and constitute object libido. These object wishes depend heavily on experiences with objects in which the object must be differentiated from the ego, among other things.

Need corresponds to biological quantity which Freud considers could be chemical, and which constitutes the motor for Trieb*: *Drang*: the peremptoriness or urgency for transformation into action and successful discharge.

Need becomes desire and Trieb when it enters the psychical apparatus and binds to presentations. Stratification of these presentations (first thing-presentations*, then word-presentations*) is so complex that it generates the complexity of the subsequent course of Trieb and desire.

The road they take is in principle that of sexual Triebe. They send stimuli to psychical life from both organs deep inside the body and on the body's surface: the erotogenic zones*. In this way, the body's interior and exterior interrelate.

Stimulus proceeding from inside the body before binding* with presentations is referred to as "somatic sexual tension" or "tension of need".

NEGATION

Ger.: Verneinung. – Sp.: negación. – Fr.: (dé) négation. – It.: negazione. – Port.: negação.

Adverse judgement of the preconscious* ego* which does not accept that word-presentations* evoking repressed* thing-presentations* belonging to the unconscious* are its own. These thing-presentations obtain word-presentations which enable them to access consciousness*, but the preconscious ego adds the "no"; this "no" does not exist in the unconscious but does in the preconscious. In this negated form, the wish* may be thought but not accepted by the ego; in this way, the wish is separated from the affect*, one of the objectives of repression*.

Negation acts on a higher level than repression*, since it belongs to the preconscious ego and therefore to thought* activity for which it is the entryway from the repressed. It involves the lifting of repression, yielding to the preconscious ego, and judging activity which rejects its truthfulness.

All lifting of repression probably involves a passage through negation: the word-presentation corresponding to the Trieb tendency first enters the preconscious on condition that it is negated; however, this condition enables it at least to be thought and perhaps, at some point, to be accepted by the ego.

An undesirable intermediate effect sometimes intervenes in which negation is overcome by mere intellectual acceptance, unassociated with its corresponding affect which would emerge with true recognition of the repressed unconscious tendency.

Some classical examples presented by Freud in his article, *Negation* (1925), refer to patients' verbalizations: "'Now you'll think I mean to say something insulting, but really I've no such intention'" (p. 235). Or in reference to a dream*, "'You ask who this person in the dream can be. It's not my mother'" (Ibid.). Or even in relation to an interpretation*: "'I didn't think that', or 'I didn't (ever) think of that'" (Ibid., p. 239).

NEGATIVE THERAPEUTIC REACTION

Ger.: negativ therapeutische Reaktion. – Sp.: reacción therapéutica negativa. – Fr.: réaction thérapeutique négative. – It.: reazione terapeutica negativa. – Port.: reação terapéutica negativa.

This type of paradoxical reaction occurs in certain patients in the course of a psychoanalytic treatment. It consists in the worsening of the patient's symptomatology when the meaning of a symptom* has been revealed or when the historical meaning of an ego characteristic has been understood; it is an unconscious ego* defence mechanism in response to an onslaught of Trieb or a certain unconscious wish*.

That is to say, when improvement or relief of illness is expectable, the opposite occurs. To some extent, a slight, transitory worsening of symptoms is common in all treatments in the period when the repressed presentation* enters consciousness, as an expression of the struggle of resistance; however, this resistance* is usually overcome, and another level of the process is gradually entered.

However, in some cases the worsening of the illness becomes strong and nearly invincible. The patient clings to it desperately as if through the suffering involved in the illness a debt were being paid or a guilt unknown to consciousness expiated; loss of illness would leave the subject without possibilities to pay it back or to expiate it. Perhaps an unconscious suspicion arises that the guilt might be worse than the illness. There is some truth in this; the 'mysterious masochistic tendencies of the ego'; meaning: death Trieb* fused with sexual Trieb* as erotogenic or primary masochism*, added to the need for punishment* produced by the unconscious part of the superego* (as binding of reintrojection of the destructive Trieb now aimed against the ego) now supports need for punishment* or suffering through illness.

Need for punishment, also incorrectly called unconscious sense of guilt*, together with primary masochism, join forces to sate themselves with suffering produced by illness; for this reason, its cure is unwelcome and is instead rejected, especially when its possibility seems to be nearing.

This is a question of proportions or of quantitative struggles, and also depends on the degree of structural change the analysis aims to achieve, as well as each patient's 'bedrock'* (*Analysis Terminable and Interminable*, 1937).

Both primary masochism and need for punishment are present, also in different proportions, in the human psychical apparatus*. They are inherent to the form of its structuring, especially in the establishment of the superego.

Freud states that it is quite likely the strongest resistance to the cure and the most difficult to overcome. In *Inhibitions, Symptoms and Anxiety*, 1925, he calls it "resistance of the superego".

It is possible to overcome the need for punishment when it is the product of identification with someone who was at some time the object of an erotic cathexis*: that is to say, when it is "borrowed" (*The Ego and the Id*, 1923, *n.* p. 50).

"There are certain people who behave in a quite peculiar fashion during the work of analysis... Every partial solution that ought to result, and in other people does result, in an improvement or a temporary suspension of symptoms produces in them for the time being an exacerbation of their illness; they get worse during the treatment instead of getting better. They exhibit what is known as a 'negative therapeutic reaction' (Ibid, p. 49)."

NEURASTHENIA

Ger.: Neurasthenie. – Sp.: neurastenia. – Fr.: neurasthénie. – It.: nevrastenia. – Port.: neurastenia.

An affection described by G. Beard, its characteristic symptoms* are psychical fatigue, dyspepsia, cephalea, constipation, spinal paraesthesia, and impoverished sexual activity.

Freud categorizes it as an affection whose cause is not related to repressed historical presentations* or memories* (psychical causes), but rather to actual motivations of a mechanical character. That is to say, it is one of the actual neuroses*. In neurasthenia, the problem lies in excessive and inadequate discharge of somatic sexual tension (basically, an effect of sexual discharge of excessive masturbation*, beyond what would correspond to a transference neurosis* due to masturbatory phantasy*).

Freud attempts to distinguish between neurasthenia and other clinical pictures. In anxiety neurosis*, for example, the major symptom is anxiety* in the form of anxious expectation* as an attack of anxiety or in the form of generally somatic equivalents of it. It is still an actual neurosis: somatic sexual tension is not connected, for diverse reasons, with presentations. It has accumulated.

It did not become libido*. The mechanical effect of this accumulation of a state of anxiety (resulting, therefore, from automatic anxiety*, which lacks presentation).

Melancholia* is not an actual neurosis although it may seem to be clinically; in the Fliess papers*, Freud differentiates it from anxiety neurosis: in melancholia, it is not somatic sexual tension that is stagnated but rather psychic tension (a need to be loved, but with sexual anaesthesia).

Although neurasthenia and actual neuroses were Freudian themes mainly in his early thinking, his conceptualization was preserved up to the end of his work. In this sense, he understood them as the actual-neurotic nucleus of all transference neurosis and also as mixed neuroses.

NEURONES

Ger.: Neuronen. – Sp.: neuronas. – Fr.: neurones. – It.: neurone. – Port.: neuronios.

Freud presents this neuropsychical unit in his manuscript, not published in his lifetime, *Project for a Scientific Psychology* (1895–1950). This presentation is based on two major ideas: (1) quantity of energy circulates in the psychical apparatus* through material particles; (2) these material particles are the neurones.

Some neurones (which he refers to as ϕ) receive stimuli from the external world. They are subjected to very intense excitations which render them permeable ("pervious") to excitation, so much so that no vestige is left of it. In contrast, ψ neurones retain quantity and thereby keep a trace of the way excitation passed through them. These neurones therefore possess memory. They also have no direct contact with the external world, are protected from quantities of excitation* proceeding from it by a protective shield against stimuli*, formed partly by ϕ neurones themselves.

Ψ neurones, however, have free contact with endogenous stimuli proceeding from the body. They have a direct relation with nuclear ψ neurones which in turn connect through contact-barriers* with the ψ neurones of the pallium, receiving information about quantitative aspects of the external world through the ϕ neurones.

A third type of neurones, the ω or W (*Warhnemung* [perception*]), registers perceptual* quality when stimuli are within a quantitative range limited by a minimum and a maximum quantity, below which they are not perceived and above which they are perceived as pain*. These neurones register the periodicity of neuronal movement, the rhythm of its movement per unit of time; a period translated as quality or non-quantity.

There are also motor neurones in charge of transferring action to the muscles, and key neurones, producers of "affect"* following the experience of pain.

As mentioned, the neurone schema was gradually left aside in the *Project* …, and neurones were re-conceptualized as presentations*; presentations arising from processed derivatives of perceptions. They are described in this manner in Chapter VII of *The Interpretation of Dreams* (1900), although Freud had already discussed them in *The Conception of the Aphasias* (1891). In *The Interpretation of Dreams* he finally breaks away from the anatomical schema, but also develops and deepens many of the ideas in the *Project* …, moving them to the presentations, the "psychical cells".

NEURO-PSYCHOSES OR PSYCHO-NEUROSES OF DEFENCE

Ger.: Abwehr Neuro-Psychosen. – Sp.: neuropsicosis de defensa. – Fr.: psychonévroses de défense. – It.: neuropsicosi da difesa. – Port.: neuropsicose de defesa.

Freud uses this term to refer to neuroses whose cause is psychical or presentational. They arise as a result of the ego's* defence against incompatible or unbearable presentations*, whether because the ego considers them so, or because incompatibility is caused by traces left by events of the subject's own history. They generally refer to traumatic* situations of a sexual origin which the ego wishes to fend off in diverse ways; this type of neurosis* originates when its endeavour partly fails.

They are curable by psychical treatment if the meanings of their characteristic symptoms*, produced by "incompatible presentations", are found.

Freud described them in two articles, one in 1894 (*The Neuro-Psychoses of Defence*) and another in 1896 (*Further Remarks on the Neuro-Psychoses of Defence*).

They are characterized by a defence* (which he sometimes refers to as repression*, although thirty years later, in *Inhibitions, Symptoms and Anxiety*, 1925, he again calls it "defence") against a presentation the ego considers unreconcilable. Consequently, in a hysteria* this presentation becomes a somatic innervation expressing a mnemic* symbol of this incompatible presentation. The latter arose from a trauma* of sexual origin: a passive seduction* had produced genital irritation in childhood, and had only become traumatic in puberty, in a deferred* manner.

Obsessional neurosis* comprises several steps. First, an active episode of seduction is originally experienced with pleasure*, perhaps following a previous passive episode. The active episode was repressed but returned as self-reproaches*, the origin of obsessional ideas* which is a different category of secondary symptoms aimed at stopping self-reproaching.

In Meynert's amentia*, the presentation the ego finds incompatible was part of reality*: usually a painful loss for the subject, a loss from which the ego defends itself in a hallucinatory way.

Freud describes a case of paranoia* in which the unreconcilable presentation is also a repressed childhood sexual experience which returns from the repressed* with a certain distortion that makes it unrecognizable, such as hallucinations* and self-referential delusions*, all of these disguised forms of self-reproach.

These neuro-psychoses of defence are characterized not by the fact of being neuroses or psychoses* but by a common feature: they are the ego's defence against an unreconcilable presentation, which returns from the repressed in diverse ways and originates in childhood sexual experiences.

The category "neuro-psychoses of defence" is therefore the opposite of "actual neuroses". In the latter, the cause is actual and sexual: problems originating in actual discharge of somatic sexual tension (rather than psychical, in the sense of presentations of past experiences). In the neuro-psychoses of defence, presentations incompatible with the ego have been repressed, and conceal the meaning of actual symptoms.

NEUROTIC ANXIETY

Ger.: neurotische Angst. – Sp.: angustia neurótica. – Fr.: angoisse néurotique. – It.: angoscia nevrotica. – Port.: angústia neurótica.

Unlike realistic anxiety*, this anxiety* is not felt in response to perception of external danger, or rather is not produced by it but is provoked by danger that is internal but unconscious*; that is to say, it is unknown to the conscious ego.

This is the ego's anxiety in response to its Trieb* following the installation of primary repressions that convert the possibility of their satisfaction into something that produces anxiety since they are welded to external danger implied by Trieb (loss of object, castration, loss of the object's love) as the ego is increasingly distinguished from the object* of pleasure* when presentations of Trieb press to obtain satisfaction.

In children, during the period of the Oedipus complex*, castration anxiety* is realistic; in adults, it is a reminder signal of that anxiety; thus it becomes anxiety that generates ego defence mechanisms* which, when they fail, may produce symptoms*.

Therefore, neurotic anxiety is both a product and an origin of neurosis.

Actual neuroses* are quite another matter; in them, anxiety is not bound to presentations* but is an automatic expression of quantity of excitation*.

Anxiety in schizophrenia* occurs in a manner similar to actual neuroses, although its causes are different. In this narcissistic psychotic affection, the destruction of the psychical apparatus* by quantity of excitation produced in response to decathectization* of its unconscious thing-presentations* leaves this quantity of excitation unbound or with very weak binding, because the word-presentation is not supported by the thing-presentation which is now decathected and projected (as for example in paranoid delusions).

NEUTRAL ENERGY

Ger.: Verschiebare Energie / indiferente Energie. – Sp.: energía indiferente. – Fr.: énergie neutre. – It.: energia indifferente. – Port.: energia indiferente.

This neutral type of energy (neither erotic nor destructive) is displaceable; when added to a qualitatively differentiated erotic or destructive impulse, it raises its quantity of total cathexis*.

This energy may be in the id* or in the ego*. In the ego it is desexualized, aim-inhibited Eros*, which is generally the type of energy cathecting the ego.

> [T]his displaceable libido is employed in the service of the pleasure principle to obviate blockages and to facilitate discharge. In this connection it is easy to observe a certain indifference as to the path along which the discharge takes place, so long as it takes place somehow.
>
> (*The Ego and the Id*, 1923, p. 45)

It is much more difficult to explain indifferent energy in the id, since to have a psychical character with psychical quality, an energy must bind to a presentation. The presentation is what gives it quality that was perceptual and is now a memory of it, which makes it belong to the pleasure principle. An energy that is not bound to a presentation is no longer indifferent but seeks to return to the quantitative, to the inorganic, beyond principles. Without the presentation, it is mere quantity. In any case it may be qualified at the perceptual-conscious Pcpt.-Cs. end as unpleasure*, or even as automatic anxiety*. The indifference of this energy could be postulated in relation to the increase of impulses of love* or hate* which at the beginning of psychical life are almost indistinguishable, and are only differentiated in the phallic stage. The hate that is initially undifferentiated is part of libidinal Trieb* at that time.

In his first Trieb theory, Freud questions the existence of psychical energy without differentiation between sexual libido* and self-preservative Trieb*. Here, the problem centres on whether the character of energy is defined by its binding to a certain thing-presentation*; if it did, then the sexual or self-preservative character of the latter would determine the attributes of this energy.

NIRVANA PRINCIPLE

Ger.: Nirwanaprinzip. – Sp.: principio de nirvana. – Fr.: principe de nirvana. – It.: principio del Nirvana. – Port.: princípio de nirvana.

This tendency of death Trieb* in the psychical apparatus lies beyond the pleasure principle* with which it sometimes tries to fuse but at other times it openly opposes.

It seeks to return to the absolute zero that characterizes the inorganic, not life. In its effort to discharge stimuli, it sometimes resembles the pleasure principle, although the latter seeks to discharge the last stimulus that entered the psychical apparatus in its endeavour to experience satisfaction* or pleasure*, depending on what experience has taught it to be the more adequate aim. This wished-for repetition remains within life; it is not a return to absolute zero but instead to the relative zero of the moment previous to entry of the quantity of stimulus into the psychical apparatus.

Barbara Low borrowed the expression "Nirvana principle" from Buddhism and Schopenhauer's philosophy in which a return to nothingness implies the loss of individuality and union with the universe. That is to say, return to the all.

After 1920, in Freud's works it becomes the third principle governing mental functioning. It cannot be seen directly; it is instead inferred from complex repetitive behaviour of patients that leads them "daemonically" to suffer, to withdraw from quality*, to separate from the presentation*, to return to pure quantity, and ultimately to death, to the inorganic.

NODAL POINT

Ger.: Knottenpunkt. – Sp.: punto nodal. – Fr.: point nodal. – It.: punto nodale. – Port.: ponto nodal.

In this type of condensation* many other presentations* come together at the end of complete chains of thoughts*, and possess great psychical significance. It may be part of a dream*, a symptom*, or a parapraxis*, for example. In dreams, this condensation is not manifested in any sensory type of character, but rather in the intensity of presentational content. Thus, what is most important, most meaningful, what condenses most meanings, is expressed in the dream, for example, as being larger but not clearer to the senses.

Each nodal point is therefore a presentation linking many others, the departure point of many roads and the point of arrival of many others which are key elements in the analytic process and also in the analysis of a particular dream.

It is part of the unconscious* mode of functioning, with free displacement* of psychical energy* among presentations, following laws of association* and forming this type of condensations, which are more significant than the rest.

O

OBJECT

Ger.: Objekt. – Sp.: objeto. – Fr.: objet. – It.: oggetto. – Port.: objeto.

Psychoanalysis considers that the fellow human being is the object, as in classical psychology: the opposite of the subject and the opposite of the ego*.

The object is situated, we could say, as a central point in Freudian theory, since all the vicissitudes of unconscious Trieb's link with it through the ego are extremely complex, even though the object itself is not the Trieb aim but only the means to reach this aim.

The Trieb aim* is actually to return to the state previous to the appearance of the stimulus, the link with the object being the best means to achieve this.

Freud considers that the purpose of the psychical apparatus* is to administrate or mitigate the exigencies of life* in response to pressure from Triebe proceeding from the body. Among these, at first self-preservative* Triebe predominate, their satisfaction requiring a nourishing object.

Sexual Triebe* depend anaclitically (cf. anaclisis*) on self-preservative Triebe; the former Triebe take pleasure in the link with the object as well as others (autoerotic), also sexual, which take pleasure in the subject's own body.

Freud's hypothesis is that the psychical apparatus tends to hallucinate* conditions of satisfaction and pleasure*, and also to consider everything pleasurable as being ego (purified pleasure ego*) given its extreme defencelessness and total dependence on the object, from which it will never again separate (*Inhibitions, Symptoms and Anxiety*, 1925), and as a way to defend itself from the object, since the experience of satisfaction* has taught it that the tension of need* is relieved by the presence of the pleasure-generating object which for this reason is thenceforward desired. Desire*, the motor of the psychical apparatus, is constituted in this way.

Autoerotism* is satisfied quickly with simple movements. But object desire is more complex: the object is independent of the ego, generating fear of object loss and longing* for it when it is absent. When the object is present and loves us, the pleasure felt is much greater then autoerotic pleasure.

This desire continuously requires knowledge of reality* since the object is there (is part of it), and therefore pleasure is there, although pain* may also be encountered there.

In this constant interplay, the vicissitudes of libidinal development are produced with object desire predominating as well as narcissistic libido* or an intermediate stage which is homosexual libido: starting with the phallic stage, infantile libido not recognizing the sexual difference of the object. In the phallic stage the Oedipus complex* is generated, the ego is finally constituted and therefore also narcissism*, as well as the ego ideal*-superego*, which becomes a major source, from that moment forward, of libido for the ego, so long as the ego complies with its conditions.

The object remains the place where object libido takes pleasure. Narcissistic libido proceeds in part from the object, nourishing the subject's self-esteem* and feeding libido to the ego (other sources of narcissistic self-esteem are the id* with its presentations* of the past of infantile sexuality; that is to say, the pre-oedipal period, the castration complex* and its consequent traces; also, of course, the ego's actual "successes".

Libido is utilized predominantly in search of the object or to stanch the wounded ego, depending on the ego's vicissitudes and narcissistic wounds (the most important of these relate to the castration complex). In narcissistic pathology, the wounded ego "is bleeding", and this outflow must be stopped in a most immediate measure to put an end to its loss. This is what narcissistic libido does when it withdraws from object presentations and cathects the ego.

An intermediate point runs through narcissistic object choice* in which the link with the object does not please object libido predominantly but needs more to support narcissism or self-esteem. Any affront caused by the object may lead to refuge in narcissism, libido then being withdrawn from unconscious object presentations and placed in the ego, in its presentations.

The link with the object is, Freud considers, highly complex and subject to numerous and changing alternatives, certain aspects predominating at some moments and others at other times. In all these circumstances, history intervenes, associated with attempts of the psychical apparatus to repeat this history (history of the erotogenic zones* and of the ego with the object), either its libidinal aspects or not (those beyond the pleasure principle*).

The ego, which is the opposite of the object, arises partly from sensations and presentations of the subject's body but also from identifications*, at first primary identifications* with the object (the pre-oedipal, the direct), then secondary identifications*, produced from transformations of object cathexes*, sometimes their loss or the loss of others taken as models (whose prototype is the father of childhood) which generally come to constitute a part of the ego called the superego*-ego ideal*, which may clash with the ego, especially when the latter is associated with Triebe prohibited by culture*.

In these cases, the object or its characteristics become ego characteristics. They partly originate the subject's character*, a way of being; that is to say, the object may be not only what the ego desires but also what constitutes the ego itself.

The object presentation is the main part of the thing-presentation inherent to the unconscious*: it is what constitutes unconscious desire, which is therefore unconscious object desire. This desire may be accepted by the ego and put into action with the superego's permission. (If the action is "disobedient", the superego punishes it with sense of guilt*; if what is "disobedient" is a preconscious phantasy or a phantasy repressed to the unconscious instead of action, punishment consists in a need for punishment*.) The wish goes into a state of repression* when its preconscious cathexis is withdrawn and it is left without a word-presentation*, which is the main condition for being known to the preconscious ego, at least at a certain point in the individual's development.

Therefore, the unconscious object wish may have several vicissitudes: (a) to reach its aim; (b) to generate punishment or need for punishment* in the ego; (c) to be repressed and thereby deprived of the word providing access to the preconscious (neurosis*); (d) to be decathected* in the unconscious (experience of the end of the world, schizophrenia*); (e) to be cancelled and projected to the exterior (paranoia*); (f) to be decathected in the unconscious and transformed into narcissistic* identification (melancholia*). If there is object loss*, it may be foreclosed, but foreclosure* takes all this reality away (acute hallucinatory confusion or Meynert's amentia*); if the loss is accepted in reality, suffering is produced by cathexis of longing*, the origin of the psychic pain of mourning*.

The object's absence at first produces fear of object loss, then anxiety for loss of its love* (the counterpart in women of male castration anxiety*); because of castration anxiety, boys accept mastering their Triebe in exchange for object love*, since they discover that it is indispensable to relieve automatic anxiety* produced by invasion of the tension of need in the psychical apparatus. It is on this principle that sphincter control first and then all education in general is based.

OBJECT CHOICE

Ger.: Objektwahl. – Sp.: elección de objeto. – Fr.: choix d'objet (ou choix objectal). – It.: scelta d'oggetto. – Port.: escolha de objeto.

The child's recognition of the object's* importance for obtaining pleasure* is neither a simple nor a lineal process. Children partially recognize it as such from the outset (initial reality ego*, self-preservative Triebe*) although it is predominantly confused with their ego* (sexual Triebe*) insomuch as it produces pleasure* (pleasure ego*) and is not distinguished from zones of their own body which also produce pleasure (autoerotism*).

This first libidinal stage is narcissism*: when the subject's own body unifies all its erotogenic zones* and forms a definitive ego. Recognition of an ego is recognition of not-ego; that is to say, an object, a major source of pleasure that soothes the tension of necessity.

Later, this object is chosen by anaclisis* to the object recognized by self-preservative Triebe, or rather in the erotogenic zone through which the link with this object was established.

This is the first level or primary object choice, a choice that falls on the nourishing mother. When the link with her is defective, the incipient ego may take refuge in autoerotism, the cradle of narcissism. Even autoerotism needs a minimal previous object link to "inaugurate" it, which it preserves from then on; narcissistic object choices may predominate, seeking to reinforce the very weak ego's link with the object, this motivation prevailing in the type of choice.

Since the Oedipus complex* soon arrives – with its concomitant recognition of sexual difference (phallic–castrated), castration anxiety*, and the castration complex* – this initial object choice becomes incestuous. It partly succumbs to repression* and partly persists as tenderness, its aim inhibited, and desexualized.

In adolescence, when the thrust of Trieb (*Drang*) is reinforced, they return

will again choose an object, now a secondary choice bearing the marks of that repressed primary unconscious* choice.

The other type of object choice already mentioned proceeds from narcissism. Attributes of the ego or the ego ideal* are chosen in the object; such is narcissistic object choice. Anaclitic object choice is intimately related to it and is often found mixed with narcissistic object choice, one of them predominating.

Anaclitic object choice is closely related to the vicissitudes of object libido*; narcissistic choice is related to narcissistic libido but also to object libido, since it provides a refuge when difficulties arise with the other type of choice, and may even originate in identifications* with objects.

OBSESSIONAL CEREMONIAL

Ger.: Zwang Zeremoniell. – Sp.: ceremonial obsesivo. – Fr.: cérémonial obsessif. – It.: cerimoniale ossessivo. – Port.: cerimonial obsessivo.

A complex compulsion* to which the person with obsessional neurosis* is sometimes subjected. It serves, without the person's knowledge, to control anxiety*. This anxiety appears if for any reason the completion of the ceremonial is prevented. Although it tends to be bothersome, the patient is unable to prevent it.

Freud presents the example of an eleven-year-old boy:

> He did not go to sleep until he had told his mother in the minutest detail all the experiences he had had during the day; there must be no bits of paper or other rubbish on the carpet in his bedroom in the evening; his bed had to be pushed right up against the wall, three chairs had to be placed in front of it, and the pillows had to lie in a particular way. In order to go to sleep he was obliged first to kick both his legs out a certain number of times and then lie on his side.
>
> (*Further Remarks on the Neuro-Psychoses of Defence*, 1896, p. 172, Footnote)

The ceremonial has an apparently rational basis although it is absolutely irrational. Its unconscious motivations may in most cases be reconstructed (cf. reconstruction*) and its meaning thereby be found, which makes it possible to return the ego's* thought* activity to rationality.

The case of this boy

> was explained in the following manner. Years before, a servant-girl who put the nice-looking boy to bed had taken the opportunity of lying down on him and abusing him sexually. When, later on, this memory was aroused in him by a recent experience, it manifested itself in his consciousness in a compulsion to perform the ceremonial I have described above. The meaning of the ceremonial was easy to guess and was established point by point by psycho-analysis. The chairs were placed in front of the bed and the bed pushed against the wall in order that nobody else should be able to get at the bed; the pillows were arranged in a particular way so that they should be differently arranged from how they were on that evening; the movements with his legs were to kick away the person who was lying on him; sleeping on his side was because in the scene he had been lying on his back; his circumstancial confession to his mother was because, in obedience to a prohibition by his seductress, he had been silent to his mother about this and other sexual experiences; and, finally, the reason for his keeping his bedroom floor clean was that neglect to do so had been the chief reproach that he had so far had to hear from his mother.
>
> (Ibid., pp. 172–3, Footnote)

The obsessional ceremonial is an expression of ego defence mechanisms* such as undoing what has been done* and isolation* whose progressive failure increasingly enables the return of the repressed*; that is to say, it is an expression of obsessional neurosis, although in some normal anal characters* the tendency to order sometimes acquires certain ceremonial characteristics.

> Neurotic ceremonials consist in making small adjustments to everyday actions, small additions or restrictions or arrangements, which have always to be carried out in the same, or in a methodically varied, manner. These activities give the impression of being mere formalities, and they seem quite meaningless to us. Nor do they appear otherwise to the patient himself; yet he is incapable of giving them up, for any deviation from the ceremonial is visited by intolerable anxiety, which obliges him at once to make his omission good. Just as trivial as the ceremonial actions themselves are the occasions and activities which are embellished, encumbered and in any case prolonged by the ceremonial – for instance, dressing and undressing, going to bed or satisfying bodily needs. The performance of a ceremonial can be described by replacing it, as it were, by a series of unwritten laws.
>
> (1907, *Obsessive Actions and Religious Practices*, pp. 117–18)
>
> Thus in slight cases the ceremonial seems to be no more than an exaggeration of an orderly procedure that is customary and justifiable; but the special conscientiousness with which it is carried out and the anxiety which follows upon its neglect stamp the ceremonial as a "sacred act". Any interruption of it is for the most part badly tolerated, and the presence of other people during its performance is almost always ruled out.
>
> (Ibid.)

We have given Freud the floor since his description is so clear. We only highlight the character of the obsessional ceremonial as sacred action, which makes it more akin to a religious ceremonial. However, when it is slight it may go unnoticed or be kept secret, a crisis of anxiety arising when some external cause blocks it. Finally, the involvement it usually acquires with normal everyday acts related to touching the body, the erotogenic zones* and the sight of them or their embellishment makes these chores interminable and tortuous (bathing, dressing, going to bed, eating, and many more).

OBSESSIONAL COMMANDS

Ger.: Zwangsgebote. – Sp.: mandamientos obsesivos. – Fr.: commandements obsessifs. – It.: comandamenti ossessivi. – Port.: mandamentos obsessivos.

Compulsive orders felt by the preconscious ego* of the obsessional neurotic to be its own (not as coming from the external world, as in the case of auditory hallucinations*), which generate anxiety* if they are not obeyed. They may be a positive expression of Trieb satisfaction or a negative expression of superego punishment.

Examples of these commands are those of the "Rat Man" (1909): to sit for an examination on the first day possible, which later becomes the command to cut his throat with his razor (superego punishment), and then the idea of killing his lover's grandmother who was guilty of having caused him to separate from her momentarily (murderous wish*).

In all these examples, obsessional* ideas cause anxiety due to aggressive content which the patient's ego is unable to accept as its own, much less in reference to amorous Trieb. In order to control them he resorts to "protective measures" such as undoing ceremonials* and others. Anxiety, first and foremost, is an unconscious* signal of the unconscious ego in response to danger of superego* punishment. When it overflows, quantity of excitation* (automatic anxiety*) momentarily invades and rapidly obtains presentations (wish-presentations it attempts to repress or superego presentations, all regressed to the anal-sadistic phase).

OBSESSIONAL IDEA

Ger.: Zwangsidee. – Sp.: idea obsesiva. – Fr.: idée obsédante. – It.: idea ossessiva. – Port.: idéia obsessiva.

Although this idea imposes itself on the subject's consciousness, the ego does not accept it is its own, which generates deep unpleasure* and anxiety* for the ego.

The obsessional idea expresses return of the repressed* in obsessional neurosis*. In early childhood, reaction formation* (anticathexis*) in response to anal Trieb* had been the way to establish primary repression*, generating the consequent fixation* point and its "successful defence and apparent health". It now returns due to frustration* or reactivation of Trieb (for example, puberty or adolescence), and it does so by the expression of ideas; that is to say, with word-presentations* whose peculiarity is to keep their thought connections isolated from the rest. For this reason, they are felt to be foreign to the ego which does not recognize itself in them, finds them foreign to it and to its "way of being" (its character, marked by reaction formation), and reacting to them with anxiety*. In any case, they generally denote a repressed wish* which for some reason is returning.

Classical examples: the "Wolf Man's" compulsion* to say or think dirty words such as "poop" whenever sacred things related to religion came up in the period of his "saintliness" (1917); or the "Rat Man's" idea that the rat torture would be suffered by his fiancée or his father (1909).

The obsessional idea, an expression of return of the repressed, also evidences the particular feature of obsessional repression* which does not withdraw cathexis* from the preconscious presentation* but instead isolates it (cf. isolation*). That is to say, it severs its associative and affective connections, which enables the word to become conscious but not to be felt as the subject's own wish. This generates ego anxiety (carrying the mark of anticathexis of repression).

This struggle between the repressed and the repressor expresses affective ambivalence* in the symptom. The repressed gradually takes preponderance in action (but not in consciousness) and the symptom* no longer produces anxiety. It is progressively assimilated into the ego by virtue of its secondary benefits*. It is then able, by another route, to take over certain dimensions of character traits and therefore of ego* resistance to psychoanalytical cure. It may even restore narcissism (by obeying certain ideals of cleanliness, for example) and even Trieb satisfaction may predominate (hand-washing at some point is close to compulsive masturbation).

In situations of frustration the obsessional idea may return from the repressed. It then stimulates in the ego the same anxiety that generated this idea.

OBSESSIONAL NEUROSIS

Ger.: Zwangsneurose. – Sp.: neurosis obsesiva. – Fr.: névrose obsessionnelle. – It.: nevrosi ossessiva. – Port.: neurose obsessiva.

This psychical affection is perhaps the one Freud studied most. We could even say that it is his nosographical creation; although Krafft-Ebbing had mentioned an obsessional presentation in 1867, the term "obsessional neurosis", its clinical, psychopathological, and metapsychological descriptions and explanations are Freud's.

At first (1894–6), Freud places it within the *neuro-psychoses of defence** since psychical ego* mechanisms act in response to incompatible presentations* from which it defends itself; a highly complex process.

The development of all individuals includes a stage of "infantile immorality". In the future obsessional neurotic, traumatic sexual experiences occur, first passive and then active; the former make repression* possible and the latter return subsequently as self-reproaches* (those passive experiences lead to the formation of hysteria* that lies behind all obsessional neurosis).

This period is ended by repression and substitution by a primary defence symptom* (a character trait* such as scrupulousness or a certain distrust). The subject achieves an apparent state of health which is really successful defence.

In the period of illness, repressed memories* return due to failure of the defence. At the price, however, of an alteration: compromise formations, expressions of return of the repressed*, the ego defends itself in turn through actions and symptoms referred to as "secondary defence" which are "protective measures" but may also become compulsive and lead to obsessional actions.

Secondary defence generates the compulsion* to brood, to think about supernatural things, a compulsion to count, or the mania of doubting. Other defence may be expiatory (ceremonials*), or preventive manoeuvres (phobias, superstition, pedantic meticulousness) and others. In 1905, in *Three Essays on the Theory of Sexuality*, Freud describes infantile sexuality* and the erotogenic zones*. Of these, the stage of predominant anal erotism* is also the phase of muscular development and mastery. The anal zone possesses the pleasure* corresponding to mucous membrane but also to sphincter (muscular) control, a pleasure that may increase, as mastery of the muscles advances, through the retention of faeces, the compression they exert on anal mucous membrane, and concomitant pain. This pain, within certain limits, produces sexual excitation and pleasure.

Sphincter control is muscular, and is achieved by domination of the striate muscle apparatus. Through it, babies are able to perform a certain level of action that enables them to recognize growing levels of object*. They begin to recognize that they *are* (cf. being*) not the object, and that the latter is highly valuable, nearly indispensable, since pleasure is derived from it. Therefore, the baby attempts to *have** the object. At this time, sadism* and Trieb for mastery develop, together with early attempts at verbal language*.

In the link with the mother, the equation faeces-penis-child-gift appears, with renouncement of Trieb satisfaction in exchange for the mother's love*. This renunciation in exchange for the mother's love keeps fear of object loss* at bay.

In *Character and Anal Erotism* (1908), Freud demonstrates that characteristics developing in the history of this erotogenic zone and their connection with the mother through this zone or anything related to it become, by way of sublimation*, character traits in the adult, traits that in other cases may be products of reaction formations*.

The more anticathexis* the reaction formation possesses, the more fixation* points it generates in the anal erotogenic zone, or the stronger the fixation originating in it will be, which gives these traits (tendencies to saving, order and tenacity) the rigidity and intensity of pathology (stinginess, scrupulousness and stubbornness).

In *Obsessive Action and Religious Practices* (1907), Freud establishes similarities and differences between obsessive ceremonials and religious ceremonies.

In 1909, he publishes *Notes Upon a Case of Obsessional Neurosis* in which he theorizes while narrating the case history of the "Rat Man" and the vicissitudes of his treatment. This work is probably the most important one that has been written on this affection through a clinical case. This patient is fearful that something may happen to loved ones, has obsessive impulses and prohibitions, and struggles incessantly against these ideas. In this text, Freud shows the importance of events during the periods of infantile sexuality and the latency* period, charged with pleasurable sexual hyperexcitation (with the female servants) on the one hand and unpleasurable on the other (he complains to his mother about painful erections, for example), with intense wishes* and voyeuristic actions and subsequent ideas of punishment; also, "delusions"* that his parents might recognize his ideas although he did not express them.

Together with his actual obsessive fears, sanctions and obsessional oaths appear: oaths he must obey although he does not know why.

He also constantly expresses thoughts of uncertainty. An observer might think that his fears regarding what might happen to his loved ones and most of the rest of his symptoms reveal unconscious wishes. But he feels they are merely "thought connections", as if verbal presentations were isolated from affects*.

The patient shows ambivalence*, mainly in reference to the paternal complex*, since ideas that something might happen to his father arise whenever he has sensual desires, but this ambivalence also exists in his link with women. Around the time he consults with Freud, he has the obsession that his fiancée might suffer torture. What type? With rats. The rats get into the anus of the tortured person. This phantasy produced intolerable anxiety, but it conceals an anal-sadistic wish in relation to his fiancée, taking pleasure in her suffering. This phantasy also occurred to him in relation to his father.

Commands arise as suicidal or criminal obsessions or compulsive demands, such as a protective compulsion or compulsion to count or to understand, which Freud reconstructs one by one and finds several meanings for each.

Adolescent onanism is quite singular in this patient. It begins following his father's death and dissipates quickly; his onanistic phantasies usually referred to a rebellion (stubbornness placed in the paternal complex).

Freud describes the characteristics of obsessional* thinking with its wishes, temptations, impulses, reflections, doubts, commands, oaths, and prohibitions. Then he describes the characteristics of the obsessional preconscious presentation, generally lacking in affect, and of "obsessive delusions". Obsessional substitute formation* deforms them by omitting steps (ellipsis).

The obsessional neurotic's superstition differs from that of primitive peoples in that it is partly believed by the ego and partly not, as if there were two diverse and opposite conceptions; he believes and disbelieves at the same time. For example, he believes in premonitory signs, in the possession of prophetic thoughts, and at the same time possesses an apparently hyper-rational thought* structure.

His tendency to uncertainty generates his aversion for clocks or anything that might provide certainty, the choice of ambiguous or unsolvable themes such as paternal filiation, the length of life, life after death, and memory. All these mechanisms correspond to omnipotence of thought*.

In the obsessional personality, hate* is usually repressed in favour of love (reaction formation) together with a strong constitutional development of the sadistic component of love.

In the obsessional neurotic there is regression* from acting to thinking (ego regression); thinking substitutes action instead of preparing for it. In this sense, obsessional thinking is similar to infantile (autoerotic) onanism.

In the "Rat Man", there is premature repression of Trieb of seeing and knowing*. For this reason, the thinking process is sexualized, and pleasure, instead of referring to thought contents, resides in the act of thinking itself. With the help of Trieb for knowing, action may progressively be replaced by preparatory acts of thought. Therefore, thoughts undertaken with an expense of energy that should be destined to action become compulsive. Action is replaced by thought.

Finally, the case is replete with interpretations* linked to the patient's history, and even includes fragments of sessions that give us a glimpse of a certain style of Freud's work (cf. psychoanalytical technique*).

In 1912, in *Totem and Taboo*, he compares the taboo*, a primitive social phenomenon, to obsessional neurosis, which he calls the "illness of taboos" in view of the quantity of prohibitions, commands, and oaths that govern obsessional thought.

Prohibitions are unmotivated and their origin is enigmatic, but they have emerged and must now be upheld due to uncontrollable anxiety* not produced by threat of external punishment but because their violation would bring on unbearable ill fate to a certain person in his circle.

Prohibition of contact is the guiding and core prohibition of obsessional neurosis; it begins with direct contact and expands to "coming into contact". Anything leading thought towards the forbidden, provoking any contact with thought, is just as prohibited as direct body contact.

Some obsessive prohibitions are understandable, others are unimaginable or senseless, such as certain ceremonials. Obsessional prohibitions are characterized by being quite displaceable, and consequently, impossibility may invade everything.

"Obsessional patients behave as though the 'impossible' persons and things were carriers of a dangerous infection liable to be spread by contact on to everything in their neighbourhood" (1913, p. 27). Association* is generally by contiguity.

Freud draws attention to the ambivalence in the taboo against contact: the person desires and also abhors effecting this action. The prohibition is precise and conscious whereas the pleasure of contact is unconscious because of repression; therefore the reasons for the conscious prohibition are unknown and all rational attempts to destroy it fail.

This prohibition is intense, precisely, because of its unconscious counterpart, "the unsatisfied pleasure that persists in what is hidden". Its transferability and capacity for spreading are reflections of a process that shows that the unconscious wish is seeking pleasure, facilitated by the psychological conditions of the unconscious* (primary process*, condensation*, and displacement*).

Trieb pleasure is displaced in order to avoid being thwarted, and generates substitutes for what is prohibited.

> In consequence of this, the prohibition itself shifts about as well, and extends to any new aims which the forbidden impulse may adopt. Any fresh advance made by the repressed libido is answered by a fresh sharpening of the prohibition.
>
> (1913, p. 30)

However, this tension seeks discharge in the same obsessive acts which increasingly enter the service of Trieb and gradually approximate the action originally prohibited.

The prohibition of contact is at first related to contact with the genitals (onanism) and then to the object link, prohibiting the initiation of any type of mastery, any attempt to use a person or a thing. Freud also mentions ambivalence of sentiments (love–hate), especially when he explains the taboo of the dead. He relates obsessive self-reproaching after the death of a loved one with unconscious hostile wishes which were repressed by a strong, contrary, loving reaction formation which is what is conscious* as an ego character trait. Therefore, the subject finds this hostility inexplicable.

Freud states that the predisposition to obsessional neurosis includes an elevated quantity of this primitive ambivalence of sentiments.

Finally, he describes another characteristic of primitive thought and of neurotics in general, but especially the obsessional neurotic: overvaluation of psychical acts. Because of repression of the sexual, a new sexualization has occurred, that of thought, which renders it omnipotent, a fulfiller of wishes (disguised), and far removed from reality* (from specific action*).

Animism*, the first conception of the world, and its technique, magic*, are part of this omnipotence of thought that governs the obsessional neurotic, neurotics in general, children and primitive peoples.

In the seventeenth of his *Introductory Lectures on Psycho-Analysis* (1917), Freud discusses symptoms and immediately chooses obsessional neurosis to exemplify them, first describing the general phenomenological picture:

> Obsessional neurosis is shown in the patient's being occupied with thoughts in which he is in fact not interested, in his being aware of impulses in himself which appear very strange to him and in his being led to actions the performance of which give him no enjoyment, but which it is quite impossible for him to omit.
>
> (p. 258)

These patients feel obliged to think, to the point of exhaustion, the most extravagant things, which they feel are foreign to them and sometimes fill them with anxiety, but which they never carry out in reality.

It also complicates the simplest everyday actions such as going to bed, bathing, or going for a walk until they become bothersome and nearly insoluble tasks. "Certainly this is a crazy illness" (Ibid., p. 259).

He also cites examples of obsessive rituals and shows their unconscious sense, discovered by psychoanalysis. The task of the psychoanalyst is this: "simply to discover, in respect to a senseless idea and a pointless action, the past situation in which the idea was justified and the action served a purpose" (Ibid., p. 270). This is a historical, singular interpretation of the meaning of the symptom. However, typical symptoms perhaps originate in a typical experience, common to all human beings, as well as in a universal reaction imposed on the patient by the nature of the pathological alteration, such as repeating or doubting, in this case.

In *From the History of an Infantile Neurosis* (1918) he presents another famous patient: The "Wolf Man". As an adult, he seemed to be predominantly obsessional. Freud traces the history of the appearance of the obsessional neurotic in him, whose origin he places in the period of latency. At that time he manifested a certain religious beatitude, an identification with Christ and compulsive ideas that generated anxiety, such as having to say "poop" whenever he mentioned God, or thinking about the Holy Trinity whenever he saw three piles of manure, symptoms that in themselves express his ambivalence.

It is extremely interesting to follow Freud in his analysis of the symptom of obstinate constipation. He interconnects anal erotism with oedipal-castration* problems, and offers the best example of why hysteria always underlies obsessional neurosis. It is a conversion* whose meanings are gradually revealed in the manner of layers of onion in connection with many moments of the history of his infantile sexuality* (the cloacal theory*) and his repressed negative Oedipus complex*

In *On Transformations of Instinct as Exemplified in Anal Erotism* (1917), he shows the identity in the unconscious between the concept of poop (money, presents), child, and penis, which may be permuted among themselves. He also shows the paths by which this takes place, and thereby again interconnects what is anal with castration and the birth of children; from this arises the cloacal theory in children and masochistic* phantasies in adults.

Finally, in *Inhibitions, Symptoms and Anxiety* (1925) he again deeply analyses defence in obsessional neurosis in view of his conceptualizations of ego, id* and superego*, anxiety signal*, and ego defence mechanisms*. He attributes the obsessional character to reaction formation, with love as the anticathexis of hate, and "being clean" as anticathexis of the anal. Reaction formation usually originates quite early, and therefore we could take it as an example of primary repression*, the origin of a repressed fixation point. Isolation* seeks to block relations between word-presentations*, exaggerating a task of normal thought to the point that it succeeds in forming unconnected islands. The paradigm is the *délire de toucher*. It is also part of the "taboo against contact" of primitive peoples.

Undoing what has been done* utilizes magical means in order to "not make room" for something that has already happened, as if it could be erased by magic. The fact is related to a Trieb phantasy or wish, and undoing is opposition to it. In this way, symptoms in two steps originate, as well as some ceremonials and oaths.

Another mechanism typical of this neurosis is displacement on to the trivial, by which small details may be placed on the same level as important ones, making obsessional thought extremely muddled, costly and ineffective.

Freud also discusses regression from phallic problems to anal erotism*, thereby producing a certain defusion of Triebe when erotic components are segregated from the genital aim.

We have the following sequence: an individual who because of reaction formations has a certain character (for example, extremely kindly) has compulsive ideas which he feels are foreign to his being and cause him anxiety: sadistic ideas the unconscious ego tries to control or undo through magical mechanisms (although the subject may in appearance be quite rational) or at least to isolate the affect. Trieb regression produces in turn a hyper-severe (regressive) superego. What was erotic Trieb has become an aggressive* compulsion, and "the struggle against sexuality will henceforward be carried on under the banner of ethical principles" (1925, p. 116). Libidinal regression has reinforced the conflict* in two directions: the defender has become more intolerant, and what is attacked has become more unbearable.

OBSESSIONAL THOUGHT

Ger.: Zwangsdenken / Zwangsgedanke. – Sp.: pensamiento obsesivo. – Fr.: pensée obsessive. – It.: pensiero ossesivo. – Port.: pensamento obsessivo.

This type of thought* utilizes an overload of cathexis* generated by cathexis withdrawn from the current corresponding to action. Non-obsessional thought develops by planning action (and subsequently executing, postponing or condemning it), whereas obsessional thought is tied up because it is eroticized thought (regressively, to anal erotism*) because of its content and also because its hyper-cathexis* prevents desexualization*; it is thought that replaces action since it consumes all libido* itself. It is not planning to subsequently carry out action or not, but is instead hyper-cathected wish fulfilment* which condenses punishment and reproach.

Phantasy* or daydreaming is a mixture of primary process* and secondary process* whereas obsessional thought possesses all the structure and logic of secondary process, obtained through word-presentations*. Its strong binding* and weak displacement* only serve a defensive anticathexis against Trieb*.

This type of thought either alters the ego* or is a product of the ego's alteration.

It possesses other characteristics: omnipotence of thought*, magical thought, and expressions of the anal character: scrupulousness, a tendency to avarice, and total paralysis of action, an expression of the ambivalence* (a product of anal-sadistic fixation*) typical of the type of preconscious thought of obsessional neurotics.

The characteristic result is therefore intense, exhausting, scrupulous thought constantly deviated towards the trivial, getting stuck on details, and becoming muddled and extenuating for the subject who complains about it and sometimes even uses it as resistance to treatment: "I don't want to think anymore!"

Another difference compared to phantasy or daydreaming is precisely that the latter state requires less cathexis, is freer, and even more pleasurable (although it may also be anguishing). However, the extreme binding of obsessional thought also reveals primary process utilized by the ego in its attempt to defend itself from Trieb.

OBSESSIONAL VOWS

Ger.: Zwangsfluch. – Sp.: juramentos obsesivos. – Fr.: serments obsessifs. – It.: giuramenti ossessivi. – Port.: juramentos obsessivos.

An important element of obsessional preconscious thought, it may be a type of undoing*. A premise occurs to the obsessional neurotic that he must fulfil an obligation no matter what, in spite of the also quite strong tendency to disobey it. This is partly an expression of ambivalence* characteristic of anal erotism* inherent to the predominant fixation* point of the obsessional neurotic, and partly an expression of the struggle of the superego* which is obeyed in this case by the ego* in response to the presence of Trieb originating in the id*.

The "Rat Man" (1909), in his famous episode during war manoeuvres, when the pince-nez he had bought through the mail had been paid for, he felt on the one hand a "sanction": to not return the money; if not, the rat fantasy would fall upon his father and the lady; immediately, a command in the form of a vow followed: "You must pay back the 3.80 kronen to Lieutenant A." (p. 168). The patient debates his thought and action like a soldier who must obey two contradictory orders.

This example shows clearly how, due to libidinal regression*, the fight against sexual Trieb is transformed into an ethical struggle (paying back the debt as a banner of honesty).

In response to the intensity of sexual Trieb, debased and disfigured into aggressive Trieb, we see the superego's cruelty (and regression), the ego serving its two masters with contradictory acts and with them expressing in part obsessional doubt (getting on and off the train, an act repeated in all the stations during his journey back to Vienna).

The vow is a compulsive preconscious* element which places a powerful block against Trieb. It is impossible for the individual not to keep it. Failure to do so is paid with anxiety*. It therefore involves an automatic ego defence mechanism whose failure generates ego anxiety in response to the Trieb impulse from the id; not only failure but also any compliance less than meticulous, not "word for word". This description shows erotization of obsessional* thought. Words are overburdened with energy that should correspond to action; they have acquired the value of facts.

OCEANIC FEELING

Ger.: Ozeanischesgefühl. – Sp.: sentimiento oceánico. – Fr.: sentiment océanique. – It.: sentimento oceanico. – Port.: sentimento oceãnico.

This type of feeling is described by Romain Rolland in a letter to Freud which the latter transcribes at the beginning of *Civilization and Its Discontents* (1930). This feeling, according to R. Rolland, is the true origin of religious sentiments in human beings.

> It is a feeling which he would like to call a sensation of "eternity", a feeling as of something limitless, unbounded – as it were, "oceanic". This feeling, he adds, is a purely subjective fact, not an article of faith.
>
> (p. 64)

Freud answers that he is not quite sure what Rolland means, but he utilizes this concept in terms of his own conceptions to refer to "an indissoluble bond, of being one with the external world as a whole" (Ibid., p. 65).

Then, he describes the development of the ego*. He begins with the initial reality ego* and continues by centring on the pure pleasure ego*. The latter does not distinguish itself from the external world because it *is** pleasure*; the category of *having* does not yet exist for it: ego is everything that produces pleasure; therefore, the ego is the object*, even though the perceptual apparatus indicates bodily limits. Its "egoness" is not defined by bodily limits but rather by pleasure.

In this regard, we may speak of a certain oceanic feeling, a lack of limits, or oneness with everything.

This type of ego or ego functioning belongs to the ego's developmental history and may therefore be chosen as a mechanism of ego regression* in some pathologies and also in group psychology*. The mechanism behind this Freudian conception is identification*.

OEDIPUS COMPLEX

Ger.: Ödipus Komplex. – Sp.: complejo de Edipo. – Fr.: complexe d'Oedipe. – It.: complesso di Edipo. – Port.: complexo de Edipo.

The culminating period of infantile sexuality* when sexual object Trieb* reaches full development, acquiring incestuous characteristics since it is supported by self-preservative Trieb* and therefore chooses as its object* the same object that satisfied this Trieb*. From this beginning, different types of problems ensue, since the prohibition of incest is one of the basic pillars on which human culture* was built.

It takes place during a period of the child's development between approximately four and six years of age. After that time, the child enters a period of latency* of sexuality* similar to glaciations in the evolution of the planet. That is to say, human sexual evolution takes place in two waves: from birth to the culminating period of the Oedipus complex, its later repression* or dissolution* together with all previous infantile sexuality* (which generates infantile amnesia*) and a second, definitive wave in puberty and adolescence. In the interval between them, the period of latency.

Repression or dissolution of the Oedipus complex, centred on incest and parricide, is a condition for access to culture. In its place, as a "commemorative monument", a structure called the superego*is established in the psychical apparatus*.

It is the "nuclear complex of the neuroses" since all presentational psychical pathology arises from different forms of defence utilized by the psychical apparatus against conflicts that appear directly or indirectly in this period of life.

During infantile sexual evolution, entry into the period of predominance of the phallic erotogenic zone*, now the principal locus of pleasurable sensations, brings several changes. First, all the previously predominant zones (oral, anal), with partial satisfaction and isolated from each other, fall under phallic supremacy, thereby unifying different bodily sensations and consolidating the formation of an ego* whose origin is basically bodily.

At the same time the ego completes its formation; when it is a reality ego*, the object* does the same; it has been recognized as such on different levels: with the progress of the muscular apparatus, in childhood playing* and language* acquisition, which "began" in the stage of predominance of anal erotism*.

As we said, the object is fully recognized (or its recognition has come to a first level of conclusion) as the principal source of pleasure*, is also accepted (with advances and setbacks) as not being the subject (unlike the pleasure ego*), and is therefore desired.

The advent of the category of having* over that of being* implies recognition of ego-object opposition; it begins with the initial reality ego*, becomes firmer in the anal stage and is confirmed in the phallic phase with the addition, at this time, of sexual difference, as well as the presence of the rival.

There is a first level of object choice*, after which this object is recognized as the principal source of pleasure, supported in part by self-preservative Triebe* and in part by narcissism* coming from the object (an object not yet recognized as such but rather as ego, to the extent that it produced pleasure). Therefore, the first object chosen by both girls and boys, whether this choice is narcissistic or anaclitic, is the mother.

In girls, the pre-oedipal* maternal link is firmer and more lasting than in boys; different routes derive from this fact which may already have been glimpsed in active and passive aims of Trieb (cf. active–passive* and Trieb, aim of*), which later diverge even further.

The definitive arrival of the reality ego forces autoerotism*, previously predominant, to yield to narcissism; this may be desexualized and thus become love* of an abstraction arising from the subject's own body (its principal seat) but which is not the body but rather the ego. From what body is the ego born? From a body possessing history and language, able to speak about itself, think of itself, remember itself and even love itself. It is a human creation, a product of human history, and also of traces left by that history in this body.

The phallic phase brings the fall of previous infantile sexual theories* such as the theory of the cloaca* and of the phallic mother*. Boys and girls face a first level of sexual difference in which the masculine is valued narcissistically as the only genital. This is traumatic: girls feel they do not have it and boys feel they are in danger of being deprived of it. Sexual difference in this period is presented in terms of phallic–castrated.

Recognition of sexual difference, necessary for the evolution of object libido*, is a crossroads for narcissism; that is to say, libido satisfied in the ego. This ego, consolidated with phallic predominance, finds it difficult to overcome the possibility of losing something that focused narcissism: self-love; the latter is also the weapon that utilizes object libido to love the object and be loved by it. Consequently, the castration complex* arises, accompanied in boys by castration anxiety* and in girls by penis envy*. In girls, castration seems to be consummated, whereas in boys it is presented as being possible; in boys the positive Oedipus complex is configured gradually: the wished-for object is the mother and the feared castrator is the father (the latter borne out by phylogeny).

Therefore, the boy begins to recognize that his mother is castrated, and is attracted to her by object libido; identification*, taken mainly from his father, becomes hostile, and he begins to fear castration; this castration would be carried out at the hands of this progenitor or a substitute, generally an animal (a totemic relic) which is the origin of infantile animal phobias*.

The case presented above in its abbreviated and typical form describes the positive Oedipus complex in boys, object libido predominating over narcissistic libido. However, all human beings possess constitutional bisexuality, and the difficult vicissitudes of the link with the object sometimes cause narcissistic libido to predominate. In this case, for example, support of narcissism requires secure possession of the penis itself in view of the danger of its loss, not only as a means of loving the object. In these circumstances, extreme defences are called upon when sexual difference is recognized.

The difference between the sexes (phallic–castrated) is disavowed*. If this occurs, where is the subject to return if not to the infantile theory of the cloaca?

Disavowal is usually partial, which generates splitting of the ego*; in this way sexual difference is simultaneously accepted and not accepted. In these cases, the object sought is the parent of the same sex; this may later derive in homosexual fixation* which may in turn be the origin of a subsequent sexual perversion* or may generate rejection by the ego in the form of "masculine protest" and produce the castration anxiety signal*, which may be repressed by the same ego in diverse ways (through different defence mechanisms* or repressions in the broad sense).

This anxiety is castration anxiety since, on this level of the infantile psyche, assuming a feminine position in the link with the father involves the boy's acceptance of his own castration.

In view of this danger, all the above may be repressed (homosexual fixation including disavowal), after which a fixation is constructed on the Oedipus complex developed in this manner; this fixation drives subsequent hysterical neuroses*, phobias*, or obsessional neuroses* (for example, "Dora" and the "Wolf Man"); and of course, paranoia* and psychosis* in which other mechanisms intervene (Schreber).

The positive Oedipus complex is superimposed on the negative in diverse proportions, together configuring the "complete" Oedipus complex. Both positive and negative aspects include fear of castration at the father's hands and, in neurotic fixation, castration anxiety is perceived as realistic anxiety* when the Oedipus complex appears.

The ego utilizes this anxiety later as a signal to set into motion defence mechanisms against Trieb with more or less narcissistic libido and more or less object libido (the ego partly recognizing and partly knowing nothing about sexual differentiation).

These defence mechanisms sometimes generate pathological character* traits that derive in character pathologies or in neurosis* when their objectives are not reached.

More or less solidly structured homosexuality* or fetishism* may result when disavowal of sexual difference predominates and the objective of not producing castration anxiety in the ego is reached; or when the need for reassurance that castration is impossible exceeds the limits of tolerance of castration anxiety.

The girl's vicissitudes are different. Her preoedipal* link with her mother lasts longer and runs deeper (up to the age of four or five), to the point that we could say that the woman's link with the mother object begins by being pre-oedipal and gradually becomes negative oedipal. Throughout this initial infantile period there is repudiation or foreclosure* which then progressively becomes disavowal of sexual difference. When the girl begins to accept this difference (that is to say, her castration in the terms of her infantile psyche), the port of arrival of the positive Oedipus complex begins to take shape. When she discovers the difference between her clitoris – the reigning zone of erotism in the girl's phallic phase – and the penis, she feels she has been the object of injustice; she feels handicapped; this in turn is perceived as punishment, and later includes other girls, then her mother, and finally women in general.

Comparison of the clitoris to the penis leads her to feel mutilated; she envies the boy his organ, feels dispossessed of it, and wants to recover it: this envy impels her to rapidly suffocate clitoral masturbation.

Her feeling of impairment leaves deep traces in the female character and, together with previous predominance of passivity as a Trieb* aim, helps her psychical apparatus to form more as an object than as a subject, which adds to difficulties in the constitution of the ego of many women.

If her feeling of impairment is repressed and the feminine is mistaken for the castrated, she is unable to overcome this mistake, precisely because it is repressed and out of reach of her thought* activity.

Then, the feminine is synonymous with what she depreciates (agreeing with boys): she possesses a masculine ideal she will never access. She then falls prey to phallic envy and tries, for example, to be a boy or to do everything boys are supposed to do, as a means to obtain the wished-for penis (playing with dolls also involves a certain active form of possessing a penis).

Her narcissism suffers a fundamental wound at this time of definitive formation of her ego, a wound that, as we said, leaves indelible marks on feminine character: her great need to be loved, greater than in boys, her clinging to the "natural", her weaker sublimational imperative, more limited autonomy, and consequent dependence.

Just when she recognizes castration as a universal feminine characteristic and therefore the non-existence of the phallic mother, the girl blames precisely her mother for her impairment, and aggressively breaks off the pre-oedipal and negative oedipal link with her, which goes into a state of repression. At the same time, she seeks out her father in the endeavour to get a penis. By the symbolic equation faeces-penis-child, she slowly diverts this wish towards the wish* to get a child from her father. Thus, she enters the period of the positive Oedipus complex, which also lasts longer than the boy's, since there is no castration anxiety to force urgent repression (fear of loss of love is felt in relation to her father and draws her nearer to him rather than repelling her).

Gradually, a more lenient and more preconscious* (Prec.) superego than the boy's is established which is also more dependent on real external circumstances and more delayed in forming.

All along this path, the girl discovers sensations connected to the rest of the female genital apparatus and thus develops her adult femininity, an opportunity to recover her narcissism diminished by the castration complex. The latter is repressed to the unconscious* where it may later cause depressive, paranoid, or generally neurotic periods at moments when for some reason the quantity of excitation* increases (as for example in adolescence or menopause).

After the period of the Oedipus complex (returning to our discussion mainly of boys), as a result of castration anxiety, all infantile sexuality is repressed as well as all the primary repressions* and anticathexes* to which the incipient ego had appealed to defend itself against traumatic facts previous to the Oedipus complex but later understood in a deferred way.

Thus, a psychical apparatus is finally structured with an id*, an ego and a superego. The id is unconscious; the other two have unconscious, preconscious and conscious sectors. Incestuous sexual Trieb, in the "normal" or ideal case, is dissolved and partly disappears;

one part is integrated into the ego as desexualized libidinal energy, forming part of character traits. This same desexualized energy may also derive into sublimations* through ego actions.

However, if it is repressed, it generates pathological character traits or, when the repressed returns*, neurosis*.

As a "commemorative monument" to the Oedipus complex – the most traumatic period of infantile sexuality – the superego is installed in the psychical apparatus; this differentiation of the ego demands that the latter be like the ego ideal* that emerges from the parents' narcissistic aspirations for the baby and from previous infantile narcissism.

This superego is formed as an immense anticathexis against infantile sexual Trieb through secondary identifications* with the parents and with the parental superego-ego ideal.

Establishment of the secondary identification "superego" is added to the previous primary identification* (located first in the ego), reinforcing the character and, in boys, their masculinity as well, which we could also say "truly" originates here.

OMNIPOTENCE OF THOUGHTS

Ger.: Allmacht der Gedanken. – Sp.: omnipotencia de los pensamientos. – Fr.: toute-puissance de la pensée. – It.: omnipotenza del pensiero. – Port.: omnipotência do pensamento.

Freud observed this originary hyper-cathexis* of thoughts in children, primitive human beings, and neurotics. Thought activity (eroticized, not very desexualized or sublimated) prevails over or conditions facts of reality*. In neurosis*, libidinal hyper-cathexis is produced through regression (cf. regression*). Although it is common to all the neuroses (historical or transference neuroses) and of course to the psychoses*, in its strict sense, it characterizes obsessional neurosis*.

The famous "Rat Man" – an obsessional patient – coined this expression "as an explanation of all the strange and uncanny events by which he, like others afflicted with the same illness, seemed to be pursued" (*Totem and Taboo*, p. 86). He was just thinking about a person when he appeared before him, as if he had conjured him up; if he suddenly asked about the health of someone he hadn't seen for a long time, he was informed that he had died in the last few days, which led him to believe in telepathic announcements; if he proffered a curse on a stranger who didn't even take it seriously, he was sure that he would die soon, burdening himself with responsibility for his death. Omnipotence of thoughts is intimately linked with obsessional superstition and, therefore, with its animism*, magic*, and other symptoms.

> But we must not be led into supposing that it is a distinguishing feature of this particular neurosis, for analytic investigation reveals the same thing in the other neuroses as well. In all of them what determines the formation of symptoms is the reality not of experience but of thought. Neurotics live in a world apart, where, as I have said elsewhere, only "neurotic currency" is legal tender; that is to say, they are only affected by what is thought with intensity and pictured with emotion, whereas agreement with external reality is a matter of no importance.
>
> (Ibid.)

In the different world-visions through which humanity has passed, we may trace the vicissitudes of omnipotence of thoughts:

> At the animistic stage men ascribe omnipotence to themselves. At the religious stage they transfer it to the gods but do not seriously abandon it themselves, for they reserve the power of influencing the gods in a variety of ways according to their wishes. The scientific view of the universe no longer affords any room for human omnipotence; men have acknowledged their smallness and submitted resignedly to death and to the other necessities of nature.
>
> (Ibid., p. 88)

It is characteristics of omnipotence of thoughts that thinking replaces action instead of constituting a means for it. Thinking retains the cathexis* corresponding to action and, thereby hyper-cathected, becomes a rumination of thoughts that never materialize in action and may become bothersome and even produce anxiety in patients, especially if their compulsive characteristics predominate.

OPPOSITION

Ger.: Widerspruch. – Sp.: oposición. – Fr.: opposition. – It.: opposizione, contrasto. – Port.: oposição.

In this law of association* a presentation* is linked to another because it means the opposite or because its formal difference is opposite.

In *The Interpretation of Dreams* (1900), Freud states that if the meaning of a dream* is not understood, it is sometimes better to turn it around and give it a meaning opposite to the apparent meaning. He does this in the famous dream of the "Wolf Man" concerning the tranquillity of the dream scene, interpreting that this stillness represents a great deal of movement. He does the same with the same patient's screen memories*; the latter vaguely remembered sexual scenes from childhood in which he believed he had attempted to seduce his sister. Based on different indicators, Freud presents the hypothesis that what happened was just the opposite: his sister seduced him, later corroborated by the patient (once he got over the narcissistic wound involved in acceptance of this affront); this advance enables Freud to continue reconstruction of the developmental twists of his infantile sexual Trieb*, which changed after this traumatic seduction from active to passive and from passive to masochistic* and from masochistic to homosexual*. In the same case history, he says that the patient's frequent use of opposition as a path of unconscious association indicated the sexual inversion (homosexual) of unconscious Trieb predominant in him.

ORAL EROTISM

Ger.: Oralerotik. – Sp.: erotismo oral. – Fr.: érotisme oral. – It.: erotismo orale. – Port.: erotismo oral.

This type of erotism consists in obtaining pleasure* by stimulation of mucous membranes of the mouth and lips. It is the human child's first erotism. In the oral stage of libidinal development, the natural object* is the nipple of the mother's breast. At first, oral erotism is unified and even mistaken for self-preservative Trieb that satisfies hunger and provides it with anaclisis (cf. anaclisis*). It gradually separates from it by virtue of a "surplus" of pleasure remaining after satisfaction of hunger. The baby obtains pleasure from sucking, first the mother's breast (which "initiates" it), then any part of the infant's body that may satisfy it (fingers, toes, and so on). In the latter case, pleasure is autoerotic.

In this first type of infantile sexuality*, the aim is to devour the object, subsequently taken as a model for the psychical process of identification* (*Group Psychology and the Analysis of the Ego*, 1921).

The first erotogenic zone* is opened whose excitation produces a particular feeling of unpleasurable tension and a centrally conditioned sensation of itching (*Three Essays on the Theory of Sexuality*, 1905) which diminishes with the action of sucking.

The oral link with the mother is fundamental for the vicissitudes of object libido* which is born during this period. For this reason we could say that when the object is chosen, apparently for the first time in the phallic stage, this is already a second choice, an object that is "refound" (cf. refinding the object*).

Traumatic events at this time (due to excessive stimulation or its lack) originate fixation points: reasons for a tendency to satisfy sexuality by oral suction of the genitals. When this tendency becomes predominant, it may configure perversions*.

Fixations due to anticathexis* (primary repression*) cause disgust* which is a dam for oral and anal erotism. It is typical to pathological degrees ("Dora", 1905) in hysterical characters. The background of these individuals always involves an especially problematic maternal link, and oral fixation always lies just beneath the surface.

The first experiences of satisfaction* and pleasure as well as of pain* occur in the oral stage; both types of experiences are departure points for a series of subsequent experiences. All these traces of experiences with the object gradually acquire the form of thing-presentations.

In this period the foundations of language* are formed by affective discharges of internal alteration* understood by the mother as calls from her child; in this way the mother–infant link is constituted.

At this time recognition of the object as a source of pleasure is not accepted by sexual Triebe* which function under the aegis of the pleasure principle*, and everything that produces pleasure* is recognized as ego; therefore, this type of ego includes what in reality is the object. The psychical apparatus functions with the category of being*. The category of having* is not inaugurated until the anal stage. Freud calls this type of mental functioning the pleasure ego*.

In any case, this lack of recognition of the object as not-ego is defensive, since before the pleasure ego, an initial reality ego* which distinguishes I from not-I based on bodily boundaries, perhaps because at that time self-preservative Triebe and their governing reality principle* predominate.

Part of oral erotism corresponds to Trieb of mastery*, expressed essentially by its aim of devouring the object; for this reason it is also described as "cannibalistic".

It may begin with teething and emerge simultaneously with a higher level of recognition of I and not-I in regard to sexual pleasure. Another expression of Trieb of mastery* in this period can be seen in the pleasurable, rhythmic pulling on the earlobe of some babies as autoerotic activity.

Oral erotism doubtless generates character traits* in adults, though not in such an obvious way as anal erotism. Some of these traits are built on those relating to passivity and others (riding on anticathexis*) seem to be the opposite (distrust or arrogance, for example). Cannibalistic characteristics may be added to anal sadism* and may even elaborate sexual perversions. Sublimations* (kissing is one of the main expressions of tenderness) sometimes generate character traits (in the period of predominance of the oral zone, direct primary identifications* are produced). Partial pleasures of oral erotism are also steps in normal sexuality when subjected to genital primacy.

ORDINARY THOUGHT

Ger.: Gewohnliches Denken. – Sp.: pensar común. – Fr.: penser du commun. – It.: pensare commune. – Port.: pensar comum.

In this type of observing thought* signs of quality* (perceptual quality, the spoken word) are not evoked or are evoked only sporadically; the cathected* ego* automatically continues its associative course from which conscious thought results; although the latter has intermediate links outside consciousness, they may return to it. Our most common form of thought* is preconscious*. It possesses words and binding* and is not as strongly cathected by the qualitative perception* of words but may acquire it as soon as the ego cathects it with attention*, so long as it does not come too close to presentations* deriving from the repressed unconscious*, since in this case it may enter the state of repression and be forgotten as occurs so often in the course of the day.

Extraneous thoughts and sudden occurrences actually proceed from the above process in which the associative chain, left outside consciousness because its cathexis of attention was withdrawn, suddenly provokes an idea that evokes qualitative signs (word-presentations* cathected with attention) and becomes conscious, abruptly appearing in consciousness as if it had come out of thin air. All the steps in the associative course remained outside consciousness, which registered only the end of the process and perceived it as a sudden occurrence.

ORGAN PLEASURE

Ger.: Organlust. – Sp.: placer de órgano. – Fr.: plaisir d'organe. – It.: piacere dell'organo. – Port.: prazer de órgão.

Freud utilizes this term to refer to pleasure*ascribed to a specific organ of the body*. It is pleasure accessed by stimulation of this organ (any of them, but especially an erotogenic zone*) without any concomitant psychical stimulus. It is autoerotic at first, but also may not be. Pleasure at first is also pregenital* if the organ stimulated is not the individual's genitals. Rubbing of the genitals also produces organ pleasure which may culminate in genital orgasm.

This concept underscores the organ's inherent erotogenic character, produced by its stimulation, generally tactile, corresponding to the rubbing of mucous membrane, depending on the organ. Pleasure corresponding to psychical phantasy in the presentational object link is built on this organ pleasure, organ pleasure being previous to this phantasy in children.

ORGAN-SPEECH

Ger.: Organsprache. – Sp.: lenguaje de órgano. – Fr.: langage d'organe. – It.: linguaggio del'organo. – Port.: linguagem de órgão.

This alteration of speech* is described by Freud in the early phases of schizophrenia* or in some of its clinical forms (simple and hebephrenic). In it, phrases undergo a certain syntactic disorganization that renders them incomprehensible, and mention organs or bodily innervations.

The relation with the organ is constituted in substitution for all thought* content.

"Here the schizophrenic utterance exhibits a hypochondriac trait: it has become 'organ-speech'" (*The Unconscious*, 1915, p. 198).

The whole thread of schizophrenic thinking is dominated by this expression whose content is a bodily innervation; reference to the word-presentation* also predominates over allusion to the thing-presentation*. The word-presentation is no longer a mention in consciousness* of the thing-presentation, but instead *is* the thing-presentation and is treated as such, with the same proximity between thing-presentations and concrete things* in the world.

> In schizophrenia words are subjected to the same process as that which makes the dream images out of latent dream-thoughts – to what we have called the primary psychical process. They undergo condensations, and by means of displacement transfer their cathexes to one another in their entirety.
>
> (Ibid., p. 199)

Substitute formations* are formed by similarity between word-presentations themselves, not by what they refer to.

All these processes may occur because, on account of the subject's frustrations* with actual and historical objects*, fixated to the latter, the subject withdraws cathexis* from unconscious object wish presentations* (we recall that cathexes of thing-presentations of the unconscious object constitute unconscious wishes, motors of the psychical apparatus*).

Since the ego is originally and basically bodily, any word-presentations kept cathected acquire this bodily content, the character of concrete thing-presentations, and their primary process* processing, since they now occupy the place of what they mean.

Organ-speech is consequently an effect of narcissistic libidinal withdrawal* of cathexis from the thing-presentation. It may also be an unsuccessful attempt to recover, through word-presentations, some kind of link with objects, to reconstruct the world, ruled of course by primary process, with words treated as things: as body organs from which the ego originated.

In response to this type of speech tied into the organic, limited to words which utilize primary process to relate to each other, automatic anxiety* arises, since this speech has not even the slight solidity of Trieb binding sometimes provided by a delusion* as a form of conciliation with Trieb* or even having dominated it somewhat, by virtue of which anxiety* may be lower. The clinical example presented by Freud is a female patient treated by V. Tausk; she says, complaining about her lover who tries to change her point of view: "My eyes are twisted".

ORIGINAL GUILT

Ger.: Urschuld. – Sp.: culpa primordial. – Fr.: culpabilité primordiale. – It.: colpa primordiale. – Port.: culpa primordial.

In the Freudian hypothesis, this is the original guilt of human culture* felt by the sons, the band of brothers* who murdered the primal father of the primal horde*.

Since the ambivalent relation with the father included admiration and therefore love*, after hate* was discharged, longing* and guilt emerged, and consequently incestuous and parricidal Trieb were definitively suffocated and the superego* was established.

These events, deduced by Freudian logic and supported by anthropological studies of the period – Darwin, Atkinson, Robertson Smith – but advancing beyond them following the discovery of unconscious meanings of his patients' symptoms, must have occurred in prehistory. Freud considers that they are inherited by all subjects and "made their own" during their Oedipus complex*. Then, death wishes towards their father tend to be displaced on to an animal (a totemic relic) and originate infantile phobias.

Original guilt was generated by these acts which made culture possible by virtue of this same guilt. Humanity is obliged to pay eternally for this conquest by going through this unpleasurable sensation incarnated in each individual when re-experiencing a similar history during the oedipal period.

Religions speak of "original sin". In Christianity, a religion of the son, this son offers his life as redemption to pay for an offence committed by humanity against God the Father. What could this offence paid by death, be if not death itself? (the talion principle). The death of the father of the primal horde derives first into a totem, a sacred animal, and then recovers its human form in God the father.

This guilt generates morals, religions, ethics, and the maximum prohibitions of all cultures: incest and murder, first the father and then all the human race.

OVER-DETERMINATION

Ger.: Überdeterminierung. – Sp.: sobredeterminación. – Fr.: surdétermination. – It.: sovradeterminazione. – Port.: superdeterminação.

Freud emphasizes this concept at the origins of his works (*On Aphasia*, 1891; *Studies on Hysteria*, 1895) and maintains it throughout (cf. determinism*). Various factors intervene in the aetiology of every psychical fact. Every psychical fact has numerous origins and causes, some more important than others, which converge in it. It may even be somatically over-determined (for example, in hysteria).

This theoretical concept is also practical: for example, Freud does not stop at the initial clarification of a symptom, but goes on searching for other determinants that combine to produce the same result. The panorama thereby gains in precision and the construction* in depth, the consequent lifting of repression* producing a broader effect and leading to more lasting improvement in the patient. For reconstruction, Freud goes back along the path the symptom took during its formation, step by step, station by station, leaving nothing aside on the grounds of just one explanation. Each station, each point, belongs to and refers to it; in any case, the way it takes this path must also be revealed for a global and gradual construction, now understandable for the analysand, who was utilizing this symptom or character trait to defend him or herself. This review invariably leads back to infantile sexuality*, to its repressed traumatic events, and to all the other factors added to it from that moment forward, arriving at this outcome. Construction of this path is not limited to symptoms but includes all psychical products that may be analysed in the same way, since they are always over-determined, the complemental series* flowing together. This of course does not mean that constructing or interpreting is a matter of summing causes, but rather that one single saviour must not be sought. The whole path of the patient's associations must be travelled (in this sense Freud is an associationist), associations that tend to run through certain periods of life when the events that repression avoids remembering consciously happened. Once they are analysed, others follow, and thus the patient gradually improves as the therapist goes along untying them and thereby brings into secondary process each of the once-forgotten memories of these situations that were traumatic at the time and are now feared. That is to say, rather than one explanation or meaning of a symptom, several are found which combine and are repeated, in some way, in the subject's history.

P

PAIN

Ger.: Schmerz. – Sp.: dolor. – Fr.: douleur. – It.: dolore. – Port.: dor.

Physical pain consists in an invasion of the psychical apparatus* by large quantities of excitation*. Any sensory excitation, even of the superior sensory organs, produces pain when the stimulus passes a certain threshold. Pain is also felt if continuity of the perceptual-conscious system (Pcpt.-Cs.) is broken when the protective shield* is overwhelmed. Finally, when a painful stimulus originates in an internal organ, the external periphery is replaced by the internal, and the quantity of excitation generating pain comes from the subject's own body.

The cause of pain in the psychical apparatus is a large increment of quantity of excitation which is, within certain limits, felt initially as unpleasure*. Beyond this limit, it is perceived as pain.

Freud explains pain on two levels: pain itself and the experience of pain. Pain leaves only an inclination to discharge*. The experience of pain leaves, in addition to this tendency, which is certainly less important, a facilitation* between this experience and the memory trace* of the pain-causing object*.

The trace of the experience of pain triggers affect* (in this respect, the same is probably true of pain alone, except that in absence of any no memory trace, it cannot be connected to an experience or presentation): fear, anxiety, origins in turn of primary defence, and the tendency to escape from any situation referring to or similar to the painful experience.

Up to this point, we are describing physical pain, which may participate in sexual excitation. For example, in the stage of anal-sadistic* erotogenic predominance, by virtue of the Trieb of mastery*, physical pain has an important part in this excitation.

With anal-sadistic fixations*, for example in the case of sadistic* or masochistic* perversions*, pain becomes a prime element for excitation, not because it is sought as an aim in itself but because through it the individual is sexually aroused and able to feel pleasure*.

Pain itself is sought in moral masochism, although in this case what is sought is preferably psychical pain: abuse, ill-treatment. This moral masochism is one of the more or less visible forms of fusion of life Trieb* with some degree of fusion with death Trieb* and destructive Trieb*; it always involves guilt* which serves as an expiatory mechanism.

We now discuss the psychical pain felt in the mourning* process. As in physical pain, cathexis* is concentrated, although the libido* of physical pain is narcissistic whereas in mourning it is object libido. It is cathexis of longing* for the presentation* of the wished-for object whose impossible satisfaction is indicated by reality testing*. This cathexis is repeated in each situation analogous to one in which the object was intensely cathected. In each of these situations, the ego* must work to withdraw libido from the object's presentation, a moment when psychical pain returns, since the level of object libido longing rises together with recognition of the real impossibility of its satisfaction.

Finally, pain is also caused by hysterical conversion*, a substitute formation* for repressed fantasies* that return as a mnemic symbol* or by historical association, as in the case of Cäcilie M.'s* facial neuralgia, which expressed her phantasy of a slap on the cheek, or Elisabeth von R.'s astasia-abasia, a product of associations by contiguity* which, taken all together, symbolically expressed an incestuous phantasy with her brother-in-law. All these fantasies contain satisfaction of Trieb and also its punishment by virtue of condensation*.

PANIC

Ger.: Panik. – Sp.: pánico. – Fr.: panique. – It.: pánico. – Port.: pánico.

A type of group anxiety* of great magnitude, it is produced mainly in artificial masses* when for some reason libidinal ties between its members are diluted. These members are interrelated in the same way as presentations* in the psychical apparatus*. Libidinal ties through identification* among their egos and through identification* of the group's leader with the ego ideal* of all its members predominate among them. This explains the immensity of anxiety liberated when these libidinal ties are broken; it is similar to what occurs in the individual when thing-presentations* are decathected and automatic anxiety* appears.

The group (especially the artificial group) acts by binding the libido* of each of its members, and these bonds are a type of social, not intrapyschic, taming of Trieb. In this sense a group member may be "cured" of his neurosis* by the simple fact of belonging

to an artificial group (at least so long as the person is a member of it), since it acts by binding libidinal energy which would otherwise produce effects of return of the repressed* in the subject's apparatus, generating neurosis. The more the group is constituted with libido proceeding from the repressed and in a predominantly free state, the more it is transformed into panic if the group is dissolved.

The causes by which a group may disintegrate may be external, producing realistic anxiety* precipitated by a traumatic situation* entering from external reality*, or may be internal to the group (for example, loss of the leader). The latter case proves the importance of the binding of previous libidinal ties of the group's members with their leader, since when these are broken, the disproportionate phenomenon of panic results. Freud compares the latter situation or group phenomenon to individual neurotic anxiety*.

PARANOIA

Ger.: Paranoia. – Sp.: paranoia. – Fr.: paranoia. – It.: paranoia. – Port.: paranóia.

In this type of psychosis* a delusional system has been established in the ego or, in other words, delusional ideas dominate the ego.

From the beginning, Freud considered it a neuropsychosis of defence*, and therefore a type of defence* established by the ego in response to the appearance of presentations* it considered incompatible. In the neuropsychosis of defence, the ego defended itself from traumatic events of the infantile past by projecting* them in order to feel that what was in reality internal proceeded from the exterior. In this sense, paranoia was a neurosis of defence (as opposed to an actual neurosis* whose cause resided in an actual fact of sexuality*, specifically, its mode of discharge).

Freud's experience revealed the grave compromise and alteration of the ego* in this defence which made treatment very complex and difficult. Later, this finding leads him to place it in what we could consider a sub-division of the neuro-psychoses of defence: what are now called narcissistic neuroses (or psychoses). The others are transference neuroses*.

In the case history of Schreber, Freud develops his theory on paranoia quite clearly. He describes an intermediate phase between autoerotism* and object love*, which he refers to as narcissism*, in which libido* cathects a psychical structure that forms gradually and is called the ego.

As the existence of this ego is progressively being recognized, the object is also recognized: both are sources of pleasure*. At first, objects are recognized as being similar to the ego, having intrinsic thing-parts (which the subject's ego cannot understand in the sense that it cannot make them its own or imitate them by a physical action; for example, traits or features) and its understandable attributes (attributes that may be imitated by actions); lacking sexual differences (infantile sexual theories*) and therefore cathected with homosexual libido.

When sexual differences are recognized, the heterosexual object is chosen. The remaining homosexual libido is sublimated, desexualized, and either becomes part of social bonds or facilitates further sublimations*.

In paranoia an unconscious homosexual fixation* to the object is produced. Subsequently, if for some precipitating reason this homosexual libido increases, a regression* to that fixation point may take place, re-sexualizing sublimations and social ties already acquired, in response to which the ego resorts to extreme mechanisms for its defence.

Freud then describes different ways in which the ego counters the sentence: "I love him" (in the case of men). In the persecutory delusion* love is transformed into hate*, and the latter is projected on to the object's unconscious*. Then, several steps follow: unconscious object presentations are decathected*, love is regressively transformed into hate and projected on to the object's unconscious. In this way, the paranoiac, who has regressed to sexualization of his narcissistic homosexual fixations and lost his sublimations, now defends himself from his Triebe*, feeling that they are alien and instead proceed from the object (transformed into hate), all of which he believes to discover in small indicators, parapraxes* and other actions of the object which express his natural ambivalence.

In erotomania, love is not transformed into hate but displaced* from the object and projected. In this case the paranoiac perceives that a certain woman is in love with him, that he is loved, which he believes he can confirm in view of certain indications he feels are "messages". He thereby contradicts the sentence "I love him" with this one: "I do not love him – I love her – because she loves me".

In regard to delusions of jealousy*, love for men is contradicted by projecting this love on to a woman: "It is she who loves him". He is then suspicious of the woman's relations with all the men he is unknowingly tempted to love.

In delusions of grandeur, libido is placed only in the ego. Here, the contradiction is; "I love no one, I only love myself". The delusion of grandeur is also part of the other delusions and they are mutually interchangeable. Jealous and persecutory delusions produce the most anxiety in the subject. Erotomania must be differentiated from acute hallucinatory or Meynert's amentia* and hysterical psychosis*, since their clinical forms are sometimes similar. Hallucinations in different types of paranoia are predominantly auditory; in the other two, they are visual; those in amentia are pleasurable and in hysteria are anguishing.

Paranoiac delusion, however, is an attempt to cure the illness just when the object presentation is unconsciously decathected, which produces a break with the unconscious wish, experienced by the ego as "the end of the world", the end of wishes* relating to the world of objects.

Preconscious word-presentations* are utilized in an attempt to restore this link with objects that has been broken in the unconscious.

This is the content of the delusion, formed with difficulty by utilizing the laws of primary process* which allows word-presentations* to be utilized as if they were thing-presentations*; Schreber provides an example of this mechanism. In this way, a certain reconciliation is reached with homosexual Trieb (Schreber feels that the homosexual link is a "request from God" who has chosen him to redeem humanity and give birth to children) (*Psycho-Analytic Notes on an Autobiographical Account of a Case of Paranoia (Dementia Paranoides)*, 1911).

In *A Case of Paranoia running Counter to the Psycho-Analytic Theory of the Disease* (1915),

Freud discusses a female paranoia, which he had already described in *The Neuro-Psychoses of Defence* (1894). In this new case, it is interesting to see how the strong fixation to the mother figure (displaced onto the employer), by preventing definitive displacement on to the male figure to access the "positive Oedipus", produces ego breakdown and delusion, as well as the loss of achievements of sublimation and social ties. In *Some Neurotic Mechanisms in Jealousy, Paranoia and Homosexuality* (1922), he again discusses jealous paranoia added to normal and neurotic jealousy, also describing certain characteristics of the paranoiac patient who seems at times (perhaps depending on the quantity of excitation* in the subject's psychical apparatus) able to consciously "condemn by judgement" these delusions and even to depreciate and devalue them. He mentions in this text that there is no dreaming in paranoia: at most, dreams* with repressed homosexual phantasies*. The paranoiac is a preconscious* category, a type of rejection of the homosexual phantasy in paranoiac or neurotic patients.

Freud attempts to define paranoia proper as a chronic affection dominated by restitution and an attempt to reconstruct the world instead of breaking relations with it. Delusion prevails over narcissistic withdrawal expressed as an experience of the end of the world*. This situation is preponderant in schizophrenia* in its simple and hebephrenic clinical forms. In any case it is difficult to distinguish clearly between paranoia and paranoid schizophrenia; in the latter, the delusion is perhaps less rigid and compact and therefore less successful.

In acute hallucinatory confusion or Meynert's amentia*, the problem is withdrawal of cathexis from the perception* in order to disavow* the existence of an intolerable presentation in it (mourning*). It is similar to the case of hysterical psychoses in which the intolerable presentation is sexual, imposing itself in a hallucination, disguised by the repressed, but still producing anxiety*.

In these cases the ego is less compromised than in paranoia and, in these acute affections, the delusion is transitory.

In chronic paranoia, the hallucinatory mechanism does not prevail, although it does appear in acute attacks, associated with high anxiety. Then, it is predominantly auditory: the patient hears voices describing, for example, what the subject is doing ("now he's moving his hands") as if someone were watching, pointing out all the subject's actions and also insulting and threatening the subject indirectly or even directly. Regression to perception of the superego function which originated in maternal vigilance has taken place.

Also of interest is Freud's observation concerning hallucinations* of paranoia in Draft K (1896): when they are visual, they correspond to the memory*, which returns from the external world, of events the patient experienced in the past, which were traumatic considering the moment of sexuality when they occurred. As for the "voices", auditory hallucinations, the affect for having partly enjoyed the traumatic experience returns in them in the form of accusatory reproaches, of course from the superego, now perceived by the perceptual apparatus*.

The sonification of thought* is another way for the subject's own thoughts to regress to perception, their origin, but now felt to be hallucinations.

PARAPRAXIS

Ger.: Fehlleistung. – Sp.: acto fallido. – Fr.: acte manqué. – It.: atto mancato. – Port.: ato falho.

An apparently erroneous act on the part of the official ego* (Prec. and Cc.) whose meaning is the fulfilment of repressed wishes*.

It is not in reality an error but an act whose performance may be extremely complex but is considered or judged by the conscious* or rather by the conscious ego as foreign to its intentions.

The intentions are those of the unconscious id* which, by virtue of symbols, analogies, or contiguities between presentations*, are able momentarily to command action and in some way produce perceptual identity*.

In this way, primary process* filters into secondary process* through an act (speaking is also an act); the conscious ego considers it an error.

Freud describes different types of parapraxes such as forgetting*, in speech or in action, of proper names, foreign words, names and phrases, impressions and intentions: stammering, slips in reading or writing, misplacing things, chance and symptomatic actions, errors in general, and combined parapraxes.

Like dreams and symptoms, they are fulfilments of repressed unconscious wishes unrecognized by the official ego as belonging to it.

Freud's explanation of this phenomenon is based only (as in the case of dreams and symptoms, with rare exceptions) on the first topic and the first Trieb theory, but it may be enriched by the theory of death Trieb* and the structural theory (cf. psychical apparatus*) by using his explanations of similar phenomena: this is the case of punishment dreams* explained as " fulfillments of wishes, though not of wishes of the Trieb impulses but of those of the critical, censuring and punishing agency in the mind" (*New Introductory Lectures on Psycho-Analysis*, 1933a, p. 27) or in humour*. In the same line of thinking, Freud describes persons with this need for punishment*, inferred from their propensity to accidents, self-destructive illnesses, and the like. These punishments are usually attributed to fate. They come from the unconscious superego* or are sought out unconsciously by the ego in order to expiate the sense of guilt* produced by the superego.

Unlike the classical parapraxis, they satisfy self-punishment* produced by the sadism of the unconscious superego or by masochism of the ego. They are involuntary acts, also experienced as errors, which produce failure, punishment, or self-destruction, and should be categorized as Trieb defusions*; they are therefore actions beyond the pleasure principle*, ruled by the Nirvana principle*, pure repetition compulsion*.

Parapraxes may also express resistance* produced by defensive anticathexis* of the unconscious ego; therefore they do not satisfy Trieb but instead the defence* against it without belonging, at least completely, to the need for punishment, but rather to the unconscious defensive part: ego resistance. This mechanism may produce, for example, forgetting to come to a session, arriving to it late, or mistaking the time and many more, all acts experienced as errors by the patient's conscious ego but in reality produced by unconscious causes opposed to satisfactions of unconscious wishes mixed with other types of satisfaction, those of Trieb and the need for punishment.

PART TRIEB

Ger.: Partialtrieb. – Sp.: pulsión parcial. – Fr.: pulsion partielle. – It.: pulsione parziale. – Port.: pulsão parcial.

This form in the evolution of sexual Trieb* corresponds to the period of infantile sexuality* previous to predominance of the phallic* erotogenic zone* and the consequent establishment of the Oedipus complex.

Its type of satisfaction is predominantly autoerotic; although Trieb pleasure* in the object* link exists from the outset, its anaclisis* is in self-preservative Triebe*; through caregiving the object gradually awakens pleasurable sensations of the erotogenic zones which become Triebe* and sexual object wishes* in childhood.

The ego* gradually acquires more recognition of the object as the main source of pleasure, with the consequent appearance of anxiety signals* of danger of losing it, beginning with fear of object loss*.

Once phallic supremacy is reached, part Triebe are subordinated to it (castration anxiety* also appears as a danger signal for the ego in response to the possibility of losing the "central" concern of narcissism* and the weapon with which object love* is obtained).

This situation is accentuated later when the genital level* is reached, in puberty and adolescence, when part Triebe become part of forepleasure* and foreplay in the genital sexual act.

Other vicissitudes may also be dissolution* (becoming an object cathexis through identification* and consequently, an ego characteristic), as well as return from the repressed*, which generates neuroses* or psychoses*, or their transformation into sublimation*.

When fixation* of the object presentation* corresponding to a part Trieb is not associated with repression* but instead with disavowal* of sexual difference, part pleasure prevails or even replaces the pleasure of genital discharge (tendency to perversion*).

All sexual Triebe corresponding to the different erotogenic zones of infantile sexuality are part Triebe not corresponding to a totality, which is attained gradually insomuch as they begin to belong to an ego that unifies them: this ego (the definitive reality ego*) is in reality a process whose first level of culmination occurs in the phallic phase, a moment when autoerotism* becomes narcissism.

However, some Triebe are part Triebe in themselves and are complemented through the object link although they may later belong to totally genital Trieb and be part of it; for example, sadism* and masochism* and the pleasure of looking and being looked at. One Trieb vicissitude complements the other. Sadistic pleasure results from identification with the object's masochistic pleasure, and the pleasure of looking with that of being looked at. These are primitive vicissitudes of Trieb and also a first line of defence* against it in connection with its aim, which was active but becomes passive or vice versa (sadistic pleasure becomes masochistic or "voyeurism" becomes exhibitionism). This in turn is related to previous traumatic situations, the origin of fixation* points, which occurred during this prehistoric period of life.

Both Trieb of looking and that of being looked at, the sadistic and the masochistic, are gradually subordinated to genital primacy and become part of fore-pleasure and fore-play in the genital* link or are repressed, and may be a potential source of neurosis (hysterical* blindness or obsessional neurosis*, for example). They may also lead to sexual perversions. Another possible vicissitude is their sublimation.

PATHOGENIC NUCLEUS

Ger.: Patogenen Kern. – Sp.: núcleo patógeno. – Fr.: noyau pathogène. – It.: nucleo patogeno. – Port.: núcleo patógeno.

In *The Psychotherapy of Hysteria (Studies on Hysteria IV)* (1895), Freud describes the technique to follow in order to obtain the deepest meaning of the symptom; he mentions a "triple psychical stratification" (foreseeing perhaps the later psychical "topics", which are also triple), specifying the place where analyst and analysand, respectively, should work and the dynamic process produced during this analysis, a process in which the deep psychical structure hidden within the symptom is discovered. He represents it figuratively as a circle with which the analyst is confronted. The symptom and its associations* are on the periphery of this presentational circle which represents the patient; the latter are on the second level of the strata. Then, a *theme* develops, associations of the same type corresponding to memories* of different periods of the patient's life, some more closely related than others, but never part of a structure with logical meaning. In this figure, Freud places these associations lineally. The psychoanalytic function is to enter this circle radially and to interrelate the different memories logically, thereby gradually finding a structure of meaning that now forms zigzagging, broken lines in this geometric figure which it is increasingly difficult to enter due to layers of resistance, also situated lineally but with a different degree of depth. The more the radial direction advances towards the nucleus of this imaginary circle, the greater the resistance. The end point is the pathogenic nucleus, defended by strong layers of resistance. By finding the logic of the relation between memories, the analysis draws nearer to this pathogenic nucleus, though not without overcoming resistances on the way; as the meaning, or rather, multiple meanings of the multi-determined symptom gradually come into view, this symptom becomes diluted.

Freud continues to value this explanation of the analysis of a symptom throughout the development of his theory, and we could say that it reaches its maximum expression in *From the History of an Infantile Neurosis* (1918) in which the "radial interpretation" achieves surprising depth, explaining not only the patient's symptoms but also the entire development of his infantile sexuality*, including the explanation of his character* as an adult.

PENIS ENVY

Ger.: Penisneid. – Sp.: envidia del pene. – Fr.: envie du pénis. – It.: invidia di pene. – Port.: inveja do pênis.

Painful affect felt by girls when they discover the first level of sexual differentiation (phallic–castrated), thereby entering the stage of predominance of phallic erotism* and discovering the difference between the central organ (the clitoris) and its sensations and the boy's (the penis, which has phallic but not yet genital characteristics).

The boy's possession of the phallus is felt by girls as their own castration; that is to say, humiliation and helplessness*, an invasion of anxiety that has no other discharge except as automatic anxiety*. Then, she hates* the boy she feels is privileged because he has not been castrated, mastery Trieb* of the penis, a wish to take it away from him arises, and destructive* or aggressive* Trieb* is turned against her "little brother" who possesses the organ she feels deprived of. Girls also resort to defence mechanisms such as disavowal* of sexual difference, which, so long as it lasts, softens her feelings and lowers her anxiety*; however, it does not usually last (if it did, it would lead to a psychosis* of the type of Meynert's amentia*), generating splitting of the ego* on which fixations* are established which may later generate sexual perversions* such as homosexuality* or fetishism*.

Penis envy may therefore originate subsequent psychopathological disorders, depending on the way the psyche deals with it; if a sense of guilt* and unconscious feelings of having been castrated as a personal punishment for some historical-individual cause predominate, they may generate repressive fixations and the formation of an asexual character*, with difficulties in links with men and a predominance of libidinal introversion which in some cases may lead to narcissistic withdrawal of libido*. In this case, differentiation may be accepted as a personal punishment not suffered by other women, of course not by her mother, who continues to be phallic (cf. phallic mother*).

Gradually, within the limits of normality, the girl accepts castration, first in herself, then in other girls, and finally in her mother. When she accepts it in her mother, she does so by fighting with her and blaming her for making her this way, thereby leaving behind the negative Oedipus* with her and beginning to console herself with the penis-child equation by which she wishes to have a baby, now by her father, thus entering the positive Oedipus complex on the way towards femininity; she arrives there in puberty and adolescence when she accesses the masculine–feminine sexual differentiation of the genital stage*.

Of course, envy is an affect not limited to girls, although it is reinforced by anatomical sexual differentiation and infantile narcissistic appreciation of the only genital recognized as such in the period of predominance of phallic erotism, and may leave more or less severe traces in the formation of her ego* and therefore her narcissism*. It is also a cause of eventual neuroses* when the repressed returns*. The major problem in girls is historical: vicissitudes in the link with the object* that generated this envy during infantile sexuality* and formed her repressed unconscious*; for this reason, that past may become actual at any present moment if it is frustrating.

PERCEPTION

Ger.: Wahrnehmung. – Sp.: percepción. – Fr.: perception. – It.: percezione. – Port.: percepção.

It is with this function that the psychical apparatus* (especially the conscious ego*) utilizes the body surface, the five senses, and therefore the erotogenic zones* to register stimuli entering from the external world and changes in quantities of excitation within the organism. They are registered, respectively, as perceptual quality and pleasure or unpleasure* quality*.

In the *Project for a Scientific Psychology* (1895), when Freud explains this register of quality, he introduces the time factor into movement of the stimulus, which he refers to as "period"* or periodicity.

This register of period, a quality of movement inherent to quantity of energy, transforms quantity into quality at the very instant it is perceived by the perceptual system.

If perception is to function correctly, the perceptual apparatus* must be cathected previously. Experience has shown the importance of registering the maximum quantity of perceptions since what is wished for may be among them. Consequently, two levels of attention* cathexis* are utilized: reflex and copious. The former is free, avid for perceptions, at least in connection with what is wished for, since the appearance of a perception which arouses the memory* of a wished for or feared presentation* provokes immediate dispatch of more cathexis* of attention* (copious attention) to the perceptual apparatus, whereupon this perception becomes sharper and more conscious*.

Perception is influenced by wishes* and also by their vicissitudes, one of which is repression*. In this case, when a perception reminiscent of something wished for or forbidden appears, anticathexis* is placed on the perception. Consequently, what is wished for or forbidden is not perceived or alternatively, its perception is depreciated or understood in a different and non-conflictive sense (for example, sexuality with incestuous overtones in hysteria).

Although the perceptual apparatus is always free to receive perceptions, it also possesses an apparatus for previous selection (positive or negative), which is to say that it tends to favour or reject certain perceptions depending on the way they are structured.

Each perceptual register leaves traces: "perceptual signs". It is gradually transformed into thing-presentations* and word-presentations* which must subsequently be differentiated from each new perception.

When presentations are perceived as perceptions, they are called "hallucinations", normal in dreaming but pathological in psychoses*. In perversions* the existence of sexual difference is disavowed* but not by perception: sexual attraction is between subjects of the same sex or through a fetish which may be considered a split-off part of the ego (cf. splitting of the ego*). It is a problem of the preconscious ego rather than of the perceptual apparatus; the preconscious ego simultaneously accepts and does not accept the reality it perceives, unknowingly producing constant contradictions in its thought* activity. In any case, it avoids perception of the female genital, considered repulsive, and of anything symbolizing it (or castration) which might generate anxiety*.

PERCEPTUAL END

Ger.: Wahrnemung-system. – Sp.: polo perceptual. – Fr.: pole perceptuel. – It.: polo percettuale. – Port.: polo perceptivo.

In the schematic picture in Chapter VII of *The Interpretation of Dreams* (1900), the part corresponding to mental dynamics is represented by a path that begins at the perceptual end. This is simply the body surface, the sensory organs (sight, hearing, taste, touch, and smell), which also constitute erotogenic zones* where pleasure* and unpleasure* are perceived.

Entry of a stimulus into the psychical apparatus* is perceived as unpleasure by the perceptual end; once inside, it is converted into Trieb* since it has psychical presentation*.

At the origin of the psychical apparatus, an action was created to eventually produce something: to eliminate unpleasure generated by the stimulus, producing pleasure in the same erotogenic zone where it had arisen, for which the intervention of an object of the external world was important.

When the apparatus grew more complex with the development of human culture*, the presentation to which the stimulus was bound underwent other vicissitudes (repression*, sublimation*, and so on), and its transformation into pleasure became growingly complex. In any case, the original cycle remains and all stimuli enter the psychical apparatus through the perceptual end or perceptual-conscious system and attempt to reach the motor end*.

PERCEPTUAL IDENTITY

Ger.: Wahrnehmungsidentität. – Sp.: identidad de percepción. – Fr.: identité de perception. – It.: identità di percezione. – Port.: identidade de percepção.

The objective sought by primary process* is a perception identical to the one desired. To reach it, it resorts to hallucination* or to mistaking an actual perception for the one desired, simply because the former possesses an attribute that makes it analogous, contiguous, or opposite to the latter; these categories need secondary process* in order to differentiate themselves from identity.

The desired perception* is one of those that were once experiences of satisfaction*. When a new influx of quantity of excitation* penetrates the psychical apparatus* and cathects (cf. cathexis*) memory traces* of one of these experiences, then the desire or rather the desired presentation* is configured. The wish-presentation has three parts: an object* (which is reactivated first), movements of discharge, and the pleasurable sensation upon discharge in the nucleus.

In the first type of psychical functioning, the Freudian hypothesis (primary process) explains that, when the wish is reactivated, it is perceived directly as being fulfilled. Therefore, the object is perceived as a hallucination, and movements of discharge* occur. However, what is missing of course is the sensation of discharge: all to the contrary, quantity of excitation grows.

Primary process seeks identity with the experience of satisfaction or pleasure* at any cost; since it is impossible, the ego* is obliged to inhibit* this tendency to perceptual identity.

Therefore, perceptual identity is a failed hypothetical, primitive mechanism forcing the psychical apparatus to operate on a more complex level of functioning: secondary process. It too seeks perceptual identity, but through thought* (thought identity*), and must consequently resign itself to partial identity: to parts or symbols of it.

Self-preservative Triebe* and the reality ego* (in which self-preservative Triebe predominate) quickly adopt secondary process with its thought identity. Sexual Triebe* are more reluctant, given the possibility of autoerotic satisfaction (cf. autoerotism*) and the existence of narcissism*. Identity may be found in the content of dreams*, in neurotic symptoms*, in some parapraxes*, and of course in psychosis*, all of these being different degrees of failure to establish secondary process and its effort towards thought identity.

PERIOD

Ger.: Periode. – Sp.: período. – Fr.: période. – It.: periodo. – Port.: período.

This temporal characteristic of movement of the stimulus registered by the perceptual apparatus* gives the stimulus the character of quality* when it is perceived. Freud presents this hypothesis in his *Project for a Scientific Psychology* (1895) and in a similar work, *The Economic Problem of Masochism* (1894), when he attempts to define the experience of pleasure*. This experience consists not only in discharge but in the way it is produced in relation to a unit of time. Therefore, period is a property of quantity, of the time it takes energy to move, and as such is propagated in a different way. The sensory organs filter stimuli, since they admit stimuli only of certain processes with definite periods. In the *Project* ..., perception* of the period of Q quantity corresponds to the W neuronal system (ω) in charge of perceptions of conscious quality.

PHALLIC MOTHER

Ger.: phallische Mutter. – Sp.: madre fálica. – Fr.: mère phallique. – It.: madre falica. – Port.: mãe fálica.

The phallic mother is a (pre-oedipal*) infantile sexual theory previous to the recognition of sexual difference (phallic–castrated) corresponding to the phallic period. For this reason, the lack of a penis in females is not recognized; differences between persons are recognized, but these peculiarities are individual; neither universal differences nor two types of human beings with different bodies and sensations exist. It corresponds to the cloacal theory* according to which children are born through defecation, like faeces (equation faeces = child); therefore, all human beings are the same and may bring children into the world. This theory is hardly conflictive and occurs in the Eden of pre-oedipal infancy (seen as such through adult eyes); in it, the only anxiety* possible (except the terrible automatic anxiety*) Is fear of object loss in the maternal-filial link, the father not yet perceived by the child as a rival, but only as a figure with which the infant endeavours to identify primarily (cf. primary identification*). During the conflictive oedipal period, castration anxiety* appears, since the sexual difference starting to be accepted refers to possession or non-possession of a phallus. In this phase, this difference may be disavowed*, accompanied by regression to previous theories: the cloacal theory and the theory of the phallic mother.

With access to the Oedipus complex*, infantile sexual theories are repressed, including that of the phallic mother. However, this theory, like everything repressed, seeks to return from the unconscious* and appears diversely disguised through myths*, fairy tales, dreams*, symptoms*, even social links formed with desexualized homosexual libido (not recognizing sexual difference). Of course, the figure of the phallic mother is central in pathologies whose core problem is disavowal, as in sexual perversions*; also in narcissistic pathology which defends against fixations* of homosexual libido, and in paranoia*.

PHALLIC PRIMACY

Ger.: phallisches Primat. – Sp. primacía fálica. – Fr.: primatie phallique. – It.: primazia fallica. – Port.: primazia fálica.

This characteristic potential of the phallic erotogenic zone* to be the height of infantile sexuality* enables this zone to marshal the Trieb aim* of all the previous erotogenic zones. The intensity and quality of sensations produced during phallic primacy are such that the phallic zone, which after puberty becomes the male reproductive organ, subsumes the other erotogenic zones. In the phallic period, the object* is finally recognized as a source of pleasure* for what is now displaced object libido*; all the previous erotogenic zones bearing their histories experienced with objects are also recognized, and configure stations of the phallic corresponding to parts of a new entity called the ego*, the residence of narcissism*. As soon as there is object libido, an initial level of sexual object choice* follows, a choice whose anaclisis (cf. anaclisis*) is self-preservative Triebe*; for this reason, it falls to the maternal nurturing object.

The sensations produced in the penis urge the boy "to do something violent, to press in, to knock to pieces, to tear open a hole somewhere" (*On the Sexual Theories of Children*, 1908, p. 218).

Trieb* leads towards the object and to discovery of the vagina in women, but collides with narcissism, dominant (though never exclusive) until then. Precisely at this time, the centre of narcissistic values, given the quantity of sensations it produces, is centred on the presence of the phallus, and the child cannot easily accept the existence of persons that do not have it, since in that case threats of castration* received at one time could be realities. This is joined by infantile sexual theories attributing possession of the penis to all beings, including women and mainly the mother: here, we are well into the oedipal period. First, sexual difference is disavowed*, a difference that may gradually be accepted.

The level of acceptance of sexual difference produced in this period of infantile sexuality reveals phallic primacy, since what is accepted is the existence of only one sexual organ, the phallus. Some people possess it and others were deprived of it by castration. The resulting sexual difference is therefore phallic–castrated. The phallic is appreciated and the castrated depreciated.

This sexual differentiation is dissolved* in the unconscious together with all infantile sexuality. It re-emerges in puberty, when it must be replaced by the more real "masculine–feminine" corresponding to genital primacy. In any case, part of the former type may remain repressed* and fixated* in the unconscious* where it may generate conflicts in subsequent sexual development in both girls and boys.

On the other hand, it may also be partly disavowed and lead to eventual splitting of the ego*, which implies contradictions in secondary process*, the seed of possible sexual perversions such as homosexuality* or fetishism*, pathologies based on disavowal of sexual difference.

PHALLIC-URETHRAL EROTISM

Ger.: Urethral-phallische erotik. – Sp.: erotismo fálico-uretral. – Fr.: érotisme phallique-urétral. – It.: erotismo fallico-uretrale. – Port.: erotismo fálico-uretral.

Phallic-urethral erotism is related to pleasure* derived from rubbing the genital apparatus. It predominates in the phallic stage of infantile sexuality* corresponding to the Oedipus complex*. It is intimately related to all the phallic problems and subsequently to the genital problems in this complex.

The autoerotic satisfaction of urethral erotism is what is commonly called masturbation*.

This masturbation in reality develops in three stages: one produced occasionally in the previous oral and anal stages when the pleasure obtained was organ pleasure and was almost only autoerotic.

In a second period corresponding to the phallic stage, the main focus of our discussion, phallic-urethral erotism predominates; however, a psychical apparatus* is now also configured, possessing thing-presentations* and word-presentations* and a weak but growing shield of repression*; the subject is in the midst of the problem of recognition of sexual difference and therefore of the Oedipus complex; in the positive case of boys, they have a well-defined object choice*: their mother. Destructive Trieb* is freed, aimed at the father whose real function in the family has now been discovered.

Therefore, satisfaction of phallic-urethral erotism is associated with extremely traumatic facts. Girls face it with the castration complex*: depreciation and envy they feel when comparing their clitoris to the male penis which they feel they have been deprived of.

Autoerotic urethral pleasure is related to manual rubbing partly involving Trieb of mastery.

In this stage, manual rubbing of the penis is already associated with preconscious presentations* (daydreams) including incestuous and parricidal phantasies*. All this dissolves or is brutally repressed when the Oedipus complex is resolved and the superego* is established. Masturbation is interrupted at that juncture, and a period of latency* is entered until puberty. At this time, it reappears with renewed vigour and in general is the only masturbation adults remember, which they consider the cause of their sense of guilt* and feelings of inferiority. They have forgotten (because of repression) the onanism of the Oedipal period (phallic-urethral erotism) whose phantasies are the unconscious* base of daydreams in puberty.

Sublimation* of urethral erotism generates ambition as a character trait. This fact may be related in part to the oedipal problem centred on possession of the mother and mainly rivalry for her, even intra-subjectively, with the father.

In the phallic stage, individuals may defend themselves from the threat of castration by disavowing it, in order to avoid renouncing masturbation, since through that mechanism the threat of castration is no longer dangerous. This disavowal* is partial. The ego* splits. On the one hand, it satisfies the id* and on the other hand, it submits to the superego. It accepts and does not accept the existence of castration. This may form a base for ulterior sexual perversions such as fetishism*.

When phallic-urethral pleasure predominates, the other erotogenic zones bow to its supremacy. The road to genitality begins while the perverse polymorphous character of the previously dominant erotogenic zones is unified; the formation of the ego ensues, an ego that emerges from the individual's own bodily sensations.

Some impulses not entirely understood by the child are connected with excitation of the penis and its urethral erotism: "obscure urges to do something violent, to press in, to knock to pieces, to tear open a hole somewhere" (*On the Sexual Theories of Children*, 1908, p. 218), led certainly by object libido in search of the vagina. These impulses collide with narcissistic libido that postulates the existence of the penis in women. The unsolvable character of this problem contributes to its repression and dissolution and consequent forgetting*.

In girls, phallic erotism is located in the clitoris, the bodily site of infantile masturbation, which may decline more commonly than in boys for various reasons; perhaps the most important is the narcissistic wound produced by penis envy in the comparison with the boy, but also because of the passive trend with which the girl ends her fight with her mother: by recriminating her for having made her castrated, which produces the desire to have a penis and then a child, which produces the passage to the father, thereby inaugurating the specifically female Oedipus complex. Girls must therefore repress phallic erotism and replace it, in adolescence, with vaginal erotism or the specifically feminine desire to be penetrated by a penis, no longer the father's but as transference of it.

PHANTASY

Ger.: Phantasie. – Sp.: fantasía. – Fr.: fantasme. – It.: fantasia. – Port.: fantasia.

This psychical product is a half-breed formed (like dreams*) by elements of the unconscious* and (like thought*) by the preconscious*.

Phantasy is logical thought, assembled with perfect syntaxis of words and expression of all the links between words representing things. However, it is also an image of fulfilled wishes. By virtue of this regression to images, its perceptive registers are facilitated, precisely as transitory wish fulfilment; although this satisfaction is instantaneous and comes in only a few doses, it sometimes gains momentary belief*, but never real belief, since it does not achieve hallucination*. The degree of perception of images is similar to that of a memory*: clear but less vivid than a dream*. This is why they are half-breeds: they are at the boundary between secondary process* and primary process*. They are secondary process "wish fulfilment" of predominantly sexual or ambitious wishes in men and sexual wishes in women, which are represented as being fulfilled.

Because of their sometimes repressed sexual content, phantasies are at the root of neurotic symptoms when they are repressed, and of many dreams of which they form the main part. When they become unconscious, they lose their secondary process structure and also their word-presentations* which gave them access to the preconscious. The thing-presentations* remain in a state of repression with unconscious cathexis.

Phantasies or daydreams also support artistic creation. Artists are fanciers that allow themselves this luxury since their talent enables them to transform their phantasies into new levels of reality*: works of art*.

Masturbatory phantasies deserve a chapter of their own. The subject, by introversion of object libido* and also autoerotic manoeuvres, obtains sexual pleasure* from phantasies related to object or homosexual libido*. Since these are not accepted by the moral conscience*, they subsequently cause guilt* feelings although the phantasies may not be acted upon, and into a sense of guilt*, added to the former if they are put into action.

Onanistic acts provoke guilty feelings and even guilty conscience in a deferred* way; in reality, this guilt originated in the second stage of masturbation* during the Oedipus complex*, a period when masturbatory phantasies were incestuous. The subject acquired diverse degrees of fixation* to them, and now they return, transformed or disguised to some extent, in adult phantasies.

Some masturbatory phantasies are of beatings*, an expression of feminine masochism in both men and women. They are formed in several stages and tend to cause sexual impotence in men.

Since these incestuous phantasies or their masturbatory derivatives are systematically rejected by the censorship* of consciousness*, free association* is difficult in psychoanalytic treatment, mainly in patients with structured character disorders or with certain obsessional characteristics. An ego* is impoverished when its energy is spent on anticathexes* to prevent access of phantasies into consciousness* and on the criticism of free phantasy by the ego's censorship.

Phantasy is the most common type of thinking, governed by the pleasure principle*.

It does not lead to a specific action* as does practical thought* or cognitive thought*: when it succeeds in doing so (in a work of art, for example), it is no longer phantasy. In the meantime, it has no pre-defined aim; even reaching an aim is not pre-defined. It is separate from action and replaces action, by which it reaches, at moments, certain levels of pleasure.

PHOBIA

Ger.: Phobie. – Sp.: fobia. – Fr.: phobie. – It.: fobia. – Port.: fobia.

This system of avoidance in anxiety hysteria* functions as a third-line defensive parapet against emergence of the substitute formation* of repressed Trieb* (the phobogenic object). To the harder repressed Trieb pressures to return, the more the substitute formation* expands (according to the laws of association*), as well as the phobia's system of avoidance.

Phobia is an ego* regression* to infantile mechanisms. The child suffering from fear of object loss requires the presence of its mother to defend the child from feeling helplessness*. In phobia the subject regresses to the need to be accompanied caused by the danger of the phobogenic object; that is to say, the object that is a presentation of the repressed presentation. The accompanying person takes the place of the mother who protected the child from the dangers of external reality*.

The phobic rampart is a "third-line" defence* reassuring that the anxiety-generating scene will not be produced; its mechanism is formed by anticathexes of attention* of secondary repression in the perceptual conscience system (Pcpt.-Cs.) which separate the ego from emergence of castration anxiety* which is what is feared in the phobogenic object, just as it was once feared in the father of childhood.

The repressive mechanism in anxiety hysteria, of which phobia is a part, both succeeds and fails. It is successful with respect to the original presentation*, but does not eliminate the affect* the latter originates; instead, it persists but is displaced (cf. displacement*) onto another presentation. Through phobic avoidance and the presence of the accompanying person, anxiety* is partially overcome.

Anxiety hysteria involves displacement: from the presentation of Trieb not accepted by the ego onto another presentation that becomes a substitute formation* and anticathexis against emergence of the original presentation. Then, the phobogenic avoidance mechanism is established: another level of anticathexis that functions as a sentinel guarding the frontier.

PHOBIC RAMPART

Ger.: schutzende Wall. – Sp.: parapeto fóbico. – Fr.: parapet phobique. – It.: parapetto fobico. – Port.: parapeito fóbico.

A complex secondary expansion of the substitute formation* or symptom* of anxiety hysteria*; it begins with the appearance (by displacement*) of an anticathexis* of secondary repression (a repressor and also generator of rationalization*) in the external world.

This anticathexis replaces Trieb* feared by the ego*. This Trieb proceeds from the phallic* erotogenic zone* and its oedipal problems (positive or negative), which generate castration anxiety* in the ego; the ego is unwilling to accept it and defends itself from this Trieb by displacing it on to the external world or a presentation* of it linked to it associatively (by virtue of which it may be reconstructed) which is anticathected and becomes an anticathexis. From this point on, it is enough for it to be close, or even just to be mentioned, to provoke anxiety*.

This anticathexis gradually expands (by association*) secondarily and produces an inhibition* in the ego which then avoids future encounters with presentations in any way reminiscent of the initial anticathexis; thus, it is progressively more distant and anxiety is less likely to emerge. For example, in the case of Little Hans, the conflicting "father" presentation is displaced on to a fear of horses, from horses to carriages, from these to the fact of going out, even accompanied, and so on. In this way the rampart of avoidance expands.

Other elements of this gradually formed presentational rampart may be the need these patients start to have of being accompanied as when they were children in view of the dangers of the world (ego regression*).

The phobic rampart is never completely successful, however widely it may expand, since on the one hand it imposes extensive hindrances on the ego's freedom and on the other hand, the ego may succumb to anxiety in response to any unexpected appearance, since the presence of anxiety-provoking objects may escape its knowledge.

PLAY

Ger.: Spiel. – Sp.: juego. – Fr.: jeu. – It.: gioco. – Port.: jogo.

It is difficult to define the essence of the activity of playing. Freud would doubtless locate it in the domain of phantasy and fancied (unreal) wish fulfilment. In any case, it differs from simple fantasy because it is not limited to the terrain of the psychical, as occurs in solitude; because it is an action in reality that produces wish fulfilment in a symbolic manner, only the type of fulfilment is psychical. However, we could include many activities in this type which are not playing, unless we take such a broad concept of play that it may include for example art* (as Huizinga does), and if we do, we could include nearly all human activity. Something of this kind occurs with the advance of capitalism and the professionalization of different games, since they have basically become specific actions* or sublimations* in fact, rather than part of the road leading to them. However, we shall not refer to this aspect now beyond a mention of it.

We focus now on child's play, which Freud discusses in Chapter II of *Beyond the Pleasure Principle* (1920). In this text he mentions the first game, created by a one-and-a-half-year-old child who is also beginning to babble meaningfully. The child plays by throwing a spool on a thread and then pulling it back; he accompanies the first action with an "oooh" and the second with a "Da", which is the part that most pleases him. Freud understands that the child is referring to "fort" (it went away) and "Da" (here it is); the theme of the game is therefore leaving and returning. The person who leaves and returns is his mother. With his game, the child is renouncing Trieb satisfaction from his mother.

By virtue of the game he is able to accept her departure without protest. He compensates by producing the scene of her disappearance and return by himself and with objects available to him. We could say that it is a symbolic way to decide when his mother is leaving and when she returns, by virtue of the power of doing the same with an object belonging to her (the spool of thread) or symbolizing her, a way that does not exist in reality; his mother goes out, and this is what he is learning to accept with the help of his game.

Up to this point, the game follows the pleasure principle. However, Freud also observes that the child insistently repeats the first part of the game ("fort") much more than the second part ("Da"). The first part of this circuit is the one that does not give him pleasure. Why repeat this one more than the second one? What about the pleasure? Was it not pleasure seeking that guided everything? This acute observation, together with those of other observers of human behaviour, lead him to the conclusion that it involves something beyond the pleasure principle that also guides it and against which it struggles constantly. The game may well also belong to repetition compulsions of traumatic situations. When and to what extent it is one or the other, or whether one predominates over the other, depends on each subjectivity ("the magnitudes in conflict").

Games of chance, which may lapse into addictions, lie in a different direction: Freud compares them to the masturbatory cycle (cf. masturbation*), the struggle between the preconscious and its "healthy" intentions against Triebe, a struggle inevitably won by Trieb*.

Why do children play, then? They need to do it, since through play they are able to "appropriate" their world, the object world (their mother in particular); they do it with symbols (taken by analogy or contiguity) of the object and their stories, in order to change them or to repeat them. Children play at doing what grown-ups do, and adult play has infantile connotations. This apparent paradox motivates a concept useful in child analysis as a means of communication and understanding and also a royal road to access infantile problems, as fantasy, dreams, and symptoms provide in adult analysis.

PLEASURE

Ger.: Lust. – Sp.: placer. – Fr.: plaisir. – It.: piacere. – Port.: prazer.

This feeling is produced at the moment of Trieb discharge, the end of the cycle initiated when sexual Trieb* entered the psychical apparatus*.

Discharge was made possible by a specific action* carried out with Trieb*, more or less involving changes in relation to the original discharge, as in sublimation* (in which the pleasurable feeling belongs to narcissism* – although it also results from the object relation* – is lower, more diluted and lasting).

With greater erotization, pleasure is generally greater, although with some exceptions. It is not only the action of discharge that counts but also how long discharge lasts.

In sublimation, as we said, intensity of pleasure changes due to the desexualization* that defines it.

Narcissistic libido* also produces the same effect in adults when for example the ego* cathects the ego ideal*.

In these latter cases it is more complicated to bind pleasure to Trieb discharge so clearly.

Many of these more lasting, pleasurable feelings of gratification enable a feeling of well-being, of "feeling well", which is different from the acuteness of pleasure.

In all cases, these types of pleasure are linked to specific actions, some erotic, others sublimated or desexualized, but all situated at the motor end, in action.

PLEASURE PRINCIPLE

Ger.: Lustprinzip. – Sp.: principio de placer. – Fr.: principe de plaisir. – It.: principio di piacere. – Port.: princípio de prazer.

This tendency of psychical functioning attracts towards pleasure* and repels unpleasure*. If the psychical apparatus* is conceived of as an intertwined complex of presentations* interconnected by an amount of energetic cathexis* (sexual libido* in the unconscious, desexualized or sublimated in the preconscious ego*), the type of displacement of energy seeking immediate discharge is ruled by the pleasure principle. This displacement is produced from presentation to presentation, generating in turn the vertiginous condensations* and displacements inherent to primary process*.

The pleasure principle may also be taken in a broader sense if it refers to a hallucinatory perception* of the wished-for object that the subject believes*, producing actions as if wish fulfilment* and the assumed presence of the object were real, which generates consequent frustration*.

Both cases involve perceptual identity*. In the first case, small, similar attributes are taken to mean that different things are the same thing (condensation), or else wished-for identity is found among different presentations by way of simple analogous or contiguous attributes (displacement). In the second case, identity is found between wish and perception.

It was perhaps because of the frustration generated by a system that functions under the rule of this principle that Freud first called it the unpleasure principle and then unpleasure-pleasure (Chapter VII of *The Interpretation of Dreams*, 1900); in 1911, in his paper on *Formulations on the Two Principles of Mental Functioning*, he gave it the definitive name.

In any event, although no psychical apparatus* could function only under this hypothetical principle, it remains a fact. The pleasure principle needs the reality principle in order to carry out its function. The ego's self-preservative Triebe* (not the rebellious sexual Triebe*) lead towards the reality principle* which is never definitively established but is obliged to develop throughout life, emerging to tame the pleasure principle and adapt it to reality*.

In the last analysis, it continues to rule the tendency of the psychical apparatus as a whole and the interconnection between presentations, not only id* Triebe but also those of the unconscious ego; the unconscious ego calls upon it for help in forging its unconscious defence mechanisms* (repression*), utilizing the anxiety signal* to force libidinal cathexis to withdraw when by virtue of some law of association* a presentation is associated with another that may lead to the danger of castration (a real danger in childhood, not in adults).

In this case the ego or its unconscious part is again ruled by the pleasure principle, avoiding unpleasure.

The functioning of the superego* or of its unconscious part may also participate in this principle. The need for punishment* satisfies the superego's pleasure principle, to which destructive Trieb* (which takes things "beyond") is added, reintrojected, and bound by the superego and "obscure masochistic tendencies of the ego".

The pleasure principle is the transformation of the principle of inertia when Freud introduces it into psychology. It is ultimately the tendency of the psychical apparatus to return to the state previous to the appearance of a stimulus or to get rid of it in order to repeat past models of success (wishes born from experiences of satisfaction*) to which it tends to return.

For this purpose, it needs to resort to a certain contradiction: to inhibit it in order to adapt it to reality.

The inhibiting ego, secondary process*, thought* activity, and language* intervene, forming a cycle that must culminate in specific action* when it is successful. However, at this point reality has already been indicating the possibility or impossibility of reaching pleasure, and this has led to the reality principle.

The pleasure principle rules free energy* (a term coined by Breuer). The reality principle (a complex form of the pleasure principle) rules bound energy*.

PRACTICAL THOUGHT

Ger.: praktisches Denken. – Sp.: pensamiento práctico. – Fr.: pensée pratique. – It.: pensiero pratico. – Port.: pensamento prático.

This type of thought* lies, so to speak, behind all other types of thought.

In it, the word-presentation* is more or less directly bound to the thing-presentation*, and reaching action requires a minimum of mediation.

We could say that it is not a high level of thought, is more tightly associated with things and material reality*, but its objective is common to all types of thought and must form the base of all of them to prevent them from wandering so far from the facts as to become delusion*.

All thought must involve the study of reality in order to find thought identity* with what is desired and to refind the object* in it, thereby reaching action, the aim of all thinking.

In this sense all thought is practical. The difference resides in its mediations, more or less temporal postponement, the degree of metaphor in identity achieved, and the scope of this identity.

PRECONSCIOUS

Ger.: Vorbewusst. – Sp.: preconciente. – Fr.: préconscient. – It.: preconscio. – Port.: preconsciente.

One of the provinces or "psychical places" of the first topic, it is also a state of presentations*, especially of word-presentations. Although the latter are outside consciousness* they may access it easily by means of attention* cathexis*.

This psychical place possesses laws of functioning and characteristics of its own described by Freud in the first topic and sustained in the second. They consist essentially in government by secondary process*, thought* activity, and the search for thought identity: however, some mestizos from the unconscious infiltrate the frontier: daydreams* or phantasies*. This place is composed mainly of word-presentations* (images, odours, sounds, melodies, or tactile sensations may inhabit it and be put into words by the subject's ego). These words represent, symbolize, or signify thing-presentations* which, in a fully formed psychical apparatus*, become part of the unconscious*.

Therefore, the preconscious is born together with language* acquisition. In this sense its function is to help inhibition (cf. inhibition*) of discharge (discharge previously dominated by the need of immediacy when the psychical apparatus was based on thing-presentations, basically images). At first, word-presentations signify thing-presentations. Then one word signifies another word; thus, growingly complex signifying chains progressively form, although a thing-presentation is always behind them as their ultimate guarantor. Word-presentations involve a high degree of libidinal binding; all the characteristics of secondary process appear definitively with them: contradiction, censorship*, thought activity, the ego*'s synthetic function, reality testing*, for example.

Therefore, the preconscious is an ego characteristic, presentations belonging to the ego (including the superego*) or at least part of it (i.e., the unconscious ego corresponding to its defence mechanisms*).

The preconscious ego also includes word-presentations that remain in it but are ignored or condemned by judgement* or conscious censorship, or because they are considered unimportant, in which case they may remain as day residues* which, if they receive transfers of unconscious cathexes, may form a dream by virtue of dream work*.

Certain weak paranoiac delusions may be ignored for some periods of time (*Some Neurotic Mechanisms in Jealousy, Paranoia and Homosexuality*, 1922) through condensations by judgement, thereby remaining preconscious; that is to say, possessing word-presentations and accessible to consciousness. In reality, any other type of word-presentation may also enter this state.

Preconscious presentations generally enrich the ego when they are not products of defence* but genuine presentations of unconscious wishes* Even defence may enrich it if it involves knowledge of the word-presentation of Trieb*, even though judgement may decide not to carry it into action; in this case, defence implies preconscious taming of Trieb rather than ignorance and remittance to the unconscious into a state of repression* which would empty the ego. Psychoanalytic treatment searches for repressed unconscious presentations in order to bring them into the preconscious and recover words decathected* by repression. When a previously repressed word is recovered, it enters thought and acquires the best binding for expansion of the preconscious ego.

The preconscious possesses all the characteristics of secondary process. If it is to become conscious, it needs attention cathexis. In this sense it is latent.

Once the psychical apparatus is constituted with repression* and dissolution* of the Oedipus complex* and all previous infantile sexuality*, the latter's presentations lose their connection with words; although they tend to return from the repressed* through psychical derivatives thereby able to access the preconscious as part of phantasies or by generating symptoms*. Derivatives of the repressed unconscious may also be perceived by conscious censorship and be repressed again, which may for example cause forgetting*.

Repression separates the unconscious from the preconscious whereas judgement of condemnation* separates the preconscious from consciousness. In the second topic's schematic picture, the characteristics of the preconscious schema become those of the preconscious ego in general, except censorship which belongs to the superego.

Both ego and superego have unconscious parts corresponding to defence mechanisms and need for punishment. The id* is entirely unconscious.

The preconscious forms gradually, like the ego, on the body surface, through contact, especially through language, with the external world. Although it separates from this surface, its origin is in the perceptual apparatus* and in its need to adapt Triebe to the reality principle*. Language is essential in this panorama, since it generates the possibility of social links.

Phantasies or daydreams lie on the frontier between the preconscious and the unconscious, mestizos between primary* and secondary* process, since they possess the complete form of secondary process but are governed by the pleasure principle* and have little contact with reality*. They may sometimes appear in symptoms if they are employed by repressed presentations in order to return in other sublimations* (for example, artistic creations), or they may become conscious and become masturbatory phantasies, sexual or not. They may also remain on the frontier as simple "day-dreaming" or may even be production partners of subsequent nocturnal dreams*.

PRE-OEDIPAL

Ger.: präödipisch / präödipal. – Sp.: pre-edípico. – Fr.: préoedipien. – It.: preedipico. – Port.: pré-edipiano.

This concept was described by Freud in his papers on female sexuality*. It was subsequently developed by his follower, Ruth Mack Brunswick, and taken to its ultimate consequences by Melanie Klein and her school; even by Jacques Lacan whose "desire of the mother" places it in a different perspective.

> [F]or you must know that the number of women who remain till a late age tenderly dependent on a paternal object, or indeed on their real father, is very great. We have established some surprising facts about these women with an intense attachment of long duration to their father. We knew, of course, that there had been a preliminary stage of attachment to the mother, but we did not know that it could be so rich in content and so long-lasting, and could leave behind so many opportunities for fixations and disposition. During this time the girl's father is only a troublesome rival; in some cases the attachment to her mother lasts beyond the fourth year of life. Almost everything that we find later in her relation to her father was already present in this earlier attachment and has been transferred subsequently on to her father. In short, we get an impression that we cannot understand women unless we appreciate this phase of their pre-Oedipus attachment to their mother.
>
> (*New Introductory Lectures on Psycho-Analysis*, XXXIII Femininity, 1933, p. 119)

The pre-oedipal therefore refers at first to Freud's discovery, when he studies female psychology more deeply, of the persistence and importance of the girl's love link with her mother previous to development of her castration complex*. This link is first and foremost narcissistic and therefore a narcissistic object choice with homosexual libido* unrecognizing sexual difference to the extent that phantasies* emerge of conceiving a child with the mother or having her child from her (without yet recognizing sexual difference but instead applying the cloacal theory* and the theory of the phallic mother*). On this level, the father's role is that of "protective father".

At first, primary identification* with the mother governs as the first type of affective link; then she is recognized as an object of narcissistic pleasure*; later, the girl recognizes sexual difference and breaks off from her mother, identifying with her secondarily and reinforcing primary identification.

The narcissistic love link with the mother (pre-oedipal) becomes the negative Oedipus when phallic* primacy is reached (girls arrive later than boys) and sexual difference is recognized. At first, phantasies of having a child by and giving a child to the mother remain, acquiring phallic aspects and therefore becoming negative oedipal. Later, object choice* varies, interrupting the strong maternal link. Then the girl wishes to have a child from her father (which indicates that this love link with him is in reality transference* of the previous maternal link). However, the circumstances of recognition of two types of sex (phallic–castrated) arrive only with the Oedipus complex*, negative at first and later positive (precisely, resistance to this recognition emerges early in the pre-oedipal phase; however, in any case, the pre-oedipal had already become negative oedipal).

In girls, the pre-oedipal maternal link is therefore more important than in boys. It predominates in oral* erotism but also in the anal*, especially in connection with sphincter control because of care received by nearby private parts that are stimulated and thereby awakened erotically by the mother (for which reason in some constructions* she appears as the producer of the original seduction*), generating pleasurable sensations.

During the period of sphincter training, greater recognition of the object* involves anxiety* for the possibility of its loss but not recognition of sexual difference. Trieb for knowledge in this period motivates the child to elaborate infantile sexual theories* in which sexual difference is not recognized.

The pre-oedipal maternal link extends to the boy but is less important. In any case, since it is the most primary, it opens the way to future forms of love links corresponding to subsequent periods in which other erotogenic zones* predominate until the phallic phase arrives and all the problems change.

The oral, anal, visual, and tactile link with the early, predominantly narcissistic mother (not recognized as an object but only as ego* to the extent of the pleasure she gives), later a narcissistic object choice with anxiety for losing her and attempts to appropriate her, is accompanied by a paternal link. It is on the one hand protective but also acquires characteristics of identification*, now differentiated from object cathexis* but still primary. The child wishes to be like him, to contain his omnipotent attributes (as seen through the child's eyes).

Thus, gradually and not exempt from accidents, the Oedipus complex is entered and the pre-oedipal left behind as the libido aims towards one of the sexes, at which time the progenitor of the other sex becomes a rival.

The superego* is established as a product of secondary identifications* (following recognition of the object of sexual desire and of the rival) which reinforce primary identification.

The importance of the notion of the pre-oedipal is that it deepens the study of infantile sexuality*. Developmental differences between boys and girls before recognition of sexual difference and its implications, all of which is prepared in the pre-oedipal period, may be seen more clearly.

PRESENTATION

Ger.: Vorstellung. – Sp.: representación. – Fr.: représentation. – It.: rappresentazione. – Port.: representação.

This term proceeds from philosophy and psychology previous to psychoanalysis. Freud gives it his own, original meanings. Presentation and the *quantum* of affect* cathecting it (cf. cathexis*) are the two famous components of the psyche.

Presentations are "psychical cells", cemented to each other by the mortar of quantity of excitation* which, in the case of sexual Triebe*, becomes *quantum* of affect or libido* through the sole fact of their cathectization.

These presentations are produced in a complex manner. Their origin, in principle is directly related with perception* and the perceptual trace it leaves in the psychical apparatus*. This relation is so intimate that it sometimes seems to be synonymous with the memory trace* and therefore also to be the register of memory. Ultimately, this is true, although not as it appears to be.

The presentation gives quantity of excitation – which when joined to it may become *quantum* of libidinal affect – a presentational or psychical quality* which enters the psychical apparatus in search of perceptual quality; when united with the object presentation, it also becomes a wish* to "refind" the object.

It had perceptual quality when it was a perception, of which a trace or perceptual sign is left; after some secondary elaboration*, this trace became presentations of the wish to repeat the same perception of that experience (so long as it was satisfactory).

Each experience also has its own complexity, as the process of its reproduction or remembering* also does, in order to become a presentation.

At the moment of the experience (the model utilized is the experience of satisfaction* described in the *Project for a Scientific Psychology* (1895 [1950]), an object's image is registered, as well as an image of movements of object and subject and the concomitant sensation of pleasurable discharge.

In essence, traces left in the psychical apparatus by this presentational complex constitute presentations* of things or of sensations felt with things, or rather objects*, together with sensations of acts performed with and by them.

Traces are dynamic, involve an object image, an action and a sensation, and enable the act of remembering (actively, as in reproductive thought, and otherwise in phantasy*); they are also dynamic in that their cathexis* presents a motion directed towards action, impelling quantity of excitation towards action, thereby producing the peremptoriness or pressure of Trieb*.

Also, the wish for a particular object is based on the memory trace of this object, by virtue of which the presentation of that thing once perceived and wished to be perceived again acquires psychical characteristics.

Thing-presentations are not therefore the thing in itself. They are a presentation of what happened to the subject with the thing during the experience and also the filters it had to overcome at the perceptual end* set up by the protective shield* (whose last barrier is strong cathexis of attention* or anxious expectation*), this perception influenced by the unconscious* and the ego*, thereby giving it subjectivity (*Beyond the Pleasure Principle*, 1920; *A Note Upon the "Mystic Writing-Pad"*, 1925; *Negation*, 1825).

At the moment of experiential perception, the latter is broken down into several parts: one part is unchanging whereas others are changing; the latter category configures its attributes.

The wish-presentation is in reality concentrated on the central thing: the sensation, sought to be felt again when an object with the same attributes that produced it is refound.

The same object is never refound; that is to say, perceptual identity* with it is never found, although some identity may be achieved through the sensation which, as we said, is the core of the thing.

With respect to the object's image and attributes, the only road is the search for thought identity*; that is to say, through study of the *perceptum* to find similarities and differences between it and what is wished for by utilizing thought*.

When we describe the complexity of the perceptive process, we demonstrate how far Freudian thought is from any intention of objectivity, since subjectivity is its essence.

Reality* is always historical reality for the psychical apparatus, and when for some reason it cannot be historical, it becomes traumatic. Material reality is unreachable by definition, since the very act of perception translates the external world's "masses in motion" into qualities (*Project for a Scientific Psychology*, 1895–1950).

Therefore, when we speak of "truth", it is in this sense: we endeavour to refind historical truth* subsequently blacked out from perception by intrapsychic defensive processes aimed against perceptions containing things or objects from previous times which became actual wishes that now (following the psychical establishment of primal repression*) originate anxiety in the unconscious ego against which it defends itself.

There are further complications: first, thing-presentations are stored by the psychical apparatus following the laws of primary process*, which freely condenses and displaces cathectic energy among them, especially the portion corresponding to the object and its attributes.

Fixation* points are also generated by the types of link between certain erotogenic zones* and objects when the former were over-stimulated by the latter, for example.

These fixation points may be attributed to anticathexes* against quantity of excitation produced during these episodes which become traumatic situations*. The first primary repressions are constituted in this way they are forerunners of definitive primary repression, which is finally established in the phallic phase following the Oedipus complex*, the culmination of infantile sexuality*, at which time a definitive reality ego* is formed; at the same time, infantile amnesia* is generated: presentations of the first experiences previous to this repression are forgotten. It is thereafter difficult – if not impossible – for them to access consciousness*.

Before the appearance of repression* following the period of the Oedipus complex, another type of presentation, the word-presentation, had emerged, also through the object link; they were not strictly presentations of experiences (although they themselves configure a kind of experience), but instead referred to experiences or signified them, thereby enabling the conscious ego to know about thing-presentations*. In this way, thought* activity was perfected by this possibility to interrelate presentations, which are now word-presentations (also proceeding from the perceptual apparatus, but only as signifiers of thing-presentations, not directly as the latter). Word-presentations* (we are now speaking of language*) reinforce the possibility of strong cathexis* and weak displacement*: the highest level of binding of libidinal energy to which human beings may aspire.

In time, thing-presentations required more and more word-presentations in order to access consciousness and, as the latter emerged, they founded the preconscious whose headquarters is in the ego.

Through the action of repression, presentations of infantile sexuality were left without cathexes of word-presentations to enable their access to the preconscious, and consequently the psychical apparatus was split into a repressed unconscious and a preconscious, belonging to the id* and to the ego, respectively. Thing-presentations (produced by registers of all the senses, but predominantly visual) belong to the unconscious, and word-presentations (most of which are signifiers of thing-presentations, although with increased complexity they may signify other words which in turn represent things, thus moving farther away from them, sometimes too far) to the preconscious.

Psychoanalysis endeavours to find the relation, lost through repression, between thing-presentations of infantile sexuality and word-presentations belonging to the preconscious.

Since repression is dynamic and demands constant pressure, it produces defects that originate returns of the repressed*, the origin of neuroses*, parapraxes*, dreams*, and other phenomena.

PRIMAL HORDE

Ger.: Urfamilie. – Sp.: horda primitiva. – Fr.: horde primitive. – It.: orda primitiva. – Port.: horda primitiva.

This hypothesis of Charles Darwin on the primal social state of human beings, together with others of Atkinson and Robertson Smith, was useful to Freud to postulate the phylogenetic origins of horror of incest, totemism*, the Oedipus complex*, and the appearance of the superego (*Totem and Taboo*, 1913; *The Ego and the Id*, 1923).

"Darwin deduced from the habits of the higher apes that men, too, originally lived in comparatively small groups or hordes within which the jealousy of the oldest and strongest male prevented sexual promiscuity" (1913, p. 125).

The primal chief or primal father was the absolute master of the women of the horde: he castrated, killed, or drove away his male offspring, forced to wander around and carry out exogamy* because of their father's jealousy*. How did the horde survive, since the primal father died at some point? The females managed to save the smallest young, and one of these would take the primal father's place when he grew old.

From this conjectural historical construction* Freud later drew his hypothesis that the exiled brothers banded together, killed the father, and devoured him, thereby forming the fraternal alliance* with which the father's law obliging them to exogamy became internal to their psychical apparatus; they felt it was natural (product of a social event) and had a strong tendency to violate it. Totemism followed, with the creation of the superego and horror of incest, all essential elements of human culture*.

PRIMAL PHANTASIES

Ger.: Urphantasien. – Sp.: fantasías primordiales. – Fr.: fantasmes originaires. – It.: fantasie primarie. – Port.: fantasias primordiais.

Inherited universal phantasies:

> [P]hylogenetically inherited schemata, which, like the categories of philosophy, are concerned with the business of "placing" the impressions derived from actual experience … precipitates from the history of human civilization. The Oedipus complex, which comprises the child's relation to his parents, is … the best known member of the class. Wherever experiences fail to fit in with the hereditary schema, they become remodeled in the imagination – a process which might very profitably be followed out in detail. It is precisely such cases that are calculated to convince us of the independent existence of the schema. We are often able to

see the schema triumphing over the experience of the individual.

(*From the History of an Infantile Neurosis*, 1918, p. 119)

There are five primal phantasies: return to the mother's womb; the primal scene*; seduction* by an adult; the threat of castration; and the family romance*.

"[S]ome sort of hardly definable knowledge, something, as it were, preparatory to an understanding, was at work in the child at the time" (Ibid., p. 120). That is to say, an *a priori* of the individual's experience was experience of the species, a preparation for understanding new phenomena by relating them to these schemas or by means of them.

"We can form no conception of what this may have consisted in; we have nothing at our disposal but the single analogy – and it is an excellent one – of the far-reaching instinctive knowledge of animals" (Ibid.).

When Freud, in *Moses and Monotheism: Three Essays* (1939), discusses the manner of responding to actual stimuli, which often seem to be hereditary behaviour rather than adequate to this experience, he advances the hypothesis that the archaic inheritance of human beings includes not only predispositions but also contents, memory traces of experiences of former generations.

The example of universal symbolism*, which is without doubt congenital, is in the same phylogenetic category; it originates in the period of development of language*, which is familiar to all children without having received instruction, and is the same in all peoples in spite of the diversity of their languages.

PRIMAL REPRESSION

Ger.: Urverdrängung. – Sp.: represión originaria. – Fr.: refoulement originaire. – It.: rimozione originaria o primaria. – Port.: repressão primaria.

This type of psychical mechanism is constituted during the period of infantile sexuality* by different types of links established with objects* through different erotogenic zones* whose predominance alternates among them and whose satisfactions are gradually held back by dams. These dams are fully established in the psychical apparatus at the end of the Oedipus complex*, when the superego* is set in place; in this way, primal repression of infantile sexuality is definitively configured, leading to its dissolution* and amnesia.

Each time predominance passes from one erotogenic zone to another, the zone left behind is subjected to some repression*. "Those that were gods in one age become devils in another" (thoughts from Goethe's *Faust*, quoted by Freud as a metaphor of this process).

This repression is itself a certain level of primal repression; it could be considered "normal" or inherent to development (not referring to the biological or at least not only the biological).

In the passage from the oral to the anal period, children tend to reject milk or cream. The faeces once so highly valued, so closely linked to the baby's pleasure and love, later become the prototype of all that is disgusting and repulsive. Infantile exhibitionism and voyeurism are also dammed up by shame; sadism and masochism are even denied recognition by the ego* as something belonging to it.

To all this we must add traumatic events also producing repression; that is to say, "quantitative factors such as an excessive degree of excitation and the breaking through of the protective shield against stimuli" (*Inhibitions, Symptoms and Anxiety*, 1926, p. 94). When quantity of erotogenic excitation is such that the psychical apparatus is unable to bind excitation with other presentations* (by interrelating them, for example), an extreme defence must anticathect these quantities of excitation*. From that point forward, this anticathexis* requires an expenditure of energy to keep it "fixated" (one of the forms of constitution of fixation* is primal repression whose only mechanism is anticathexis), whose achievement consists in transforming what is pleasurable into something unpleasurable.

The most characteristic example of anticathexis is reaction formation* which may even produce ego character traits*.

Therefore, the prehistory of infantile sexuality is the period in which these primal repressions arise, and this history is "*highly individual*" (*Repression*, 1915, p. 150). We repeat: different in each individual. Traces of events in this individual prehistory sometimes remain as primal repressions when anticathexes were needed to defend the ego from invasion by quantities of excitation. Fixation points were thereby created since anticathexis is not applied once and for all but must be maintained.

Infantile sexuality culminates, as we know, at the end of the period of the Oedipus complex, together with all the drama experienced in it ("the most traumatic fact of infantile sexuality") and the permanent effects it leaves in the formation of the psychical apparatus. Among other things, it occurs during the period of phallic primacy* over the other erotogenic zones when it subsumes the former phases and makes them part of a unit that will be the ego. This ego desires the object, an object that acquires incestuous characteristics in this period. For this reason and for other equally important ones, repression of all infantile sexuality, with all its previous fixations already established but now re-signified by the Oedipus complex, becomes indispensable in order to access culture*.

The resulting structure is a product of identification*; it is the superego* which in turn constitutes something like an immense anticathexis ("reaction formation" as Freud called it) against the appearance of Trieb* in the ego; this Trieb* has now been repressed, but pressures to return from this state.

From this point on, what has been done introduces a definitive difference: what we refer to as primal repression ("dislodging pressure"); the repression we observe in clinical work, especially in adults, comes later; it actually endeavours only to reinforce the former, and is called secondary repression ("pressure to hunt").

This repression, which seconds the first, utilizes other mechanisms to ensure its effectiveness by decathecting the preconscious presentation (in transference neuroses*), whereby the unconscious thing-presentation is unable to find expression in the preconscious, and consequently in the ego or in consciousness. The second mechanism is the anticathexis already utilized by primal repression but now preferentially placed in the perceptual apparatus, where it mainly constitutes the mechanism of resistance* of ego repression. Finally, from the unconscious, what is primally repressed attracts the preconscious presentation, aiding the repressive effect by making it unconscious.

PRIMAL SCENE

Ger.: Urszene. – Sp.: escena primaria. – Fr.: scène originaire. – It.: scena originaria o primaria. – Port.: cena primária.

A sexual scene between the parents, seen or heard by the child (whose predominant zone is pregenital*, usually the anal) who has no other way to understand it than as a sadistic, aggressive relation given the predominance of sadistic Trieb* at this time of childhood.

When this child reaches the phallic stage, the memory* of the primal scene is understood in a deferred* manner, and at that moment the scene becomes traumatic since this understanding* involves the appearance of sensations in the child's body leading to the perception of sexual difference; these sensations may be recognized at this level (phallic–castrated), a situation that brings with it the danger of castration.

Freud explains in detail the importance of the understanding of the primal scene in the case history of the "Wolf Man" (1918) which is elaborated by an anxiety* dream* whose analysis proves the child's understanding of castration on an unconscious level, especially because of the anxiety he felt when he awoke from the dream.

The primal scene is not consciously remembered by the adult, but is reconstructed from elements of the dream and its associations. Freud wonders whether the child really witnessed these scenes and, although he provides undeniable evidence that he believes he did (because of his impressive reconstruction which he would otherwise nearly have to throw into the trash by omitting the essence of psychoanalysis), he leaves the benefit of the doubt to whoever disagrees.

The primal scene phantasy* is one of the phylogenetic primal phantasies which function in the same way as Kantian categories by leading the child's associative lines of thought* in the general line of interpretation indicated by these same inherited phantasies.

PRIMARY GAIN FROM ILLNESS

Ger.: primärer Krankheitsgewinn. – Sp.: beneficio primario (de la enfermedad). – Fr.: bénéfice primaire de la maladie. – It.: utile primario della malattia. – Port.: beneficio o lucro primário (da doença).

A type of solution to which the ego* may arrive in a psychical conflict*, probably the one that is economically most convenient.

The ego is subjected to often contradictory and conflictive demands. The id* Triebe* tend to clash with aspirations coming from the superego-ego ideal.

The ego needs to find a synthesis for them which involves an arduous task of working through, and in the meantime it must defend itself from the anxiety signal* with which the superego threatens it (fear of the superego*), reality* (realistic anxiety* and social anxiety*). The ego can usually only appeal to the pleasure principle* (which in this case defends the ego from the unpleasure of the primarily repressed and therefore changes its affect) and automatically deploy unconscious defence mechanisms* or secondary repressions which generate compromises, creating neurotic symptoms*, pathological character* traits and even splitting of the ego*. The ego thereby avoids knowledge of the conflict, making it unconscious*. The primary gain is strong ego resistance* to the cure.

Therefore, psychoanalytic treatment has to bring it to light and to consciousness*, to knowledge of the prec. ego. This generates a transitory economic discomfort which derives in a liberation of the economic effort it was costing the ego to maintain the symptom.

PRIMARY IDENTIFICATION

Ger.: primäre identifizierung. – Sp.: identificación primaria. – Fr.: identification primaire. – It.: identificazione primaria. – Port.: identificacao primária.

Freud assigns this term to identification* originating mainly in the first periods of life before libidinal object* cathexis* or its recognition as a source of pleasure*: identification without previous object choice*. It is also referred to as "direct identification" because it is not mediated by recognition of the object with which it identifies as: (a) the main source of pleasure; and (b) the main obstacle (rival) to wish fulfilment*.

These identifications take certain attributes (ways of effecting actions) of primary objects – even though the predominant purified pleasure ego* does not at first recognize them as such – which eventually configure deep structural ego* characteristics.

The next type of link (at the end of the oral and early anal phase) of boys (and perhaps girls as well) with the father, previous to the Oedipus complex* is identification*. Unlike the mother, who is the pleasure object for both girls and boys (for this reason, the person who exercises this function receives object cathexis as the child gradually recognizes her as such: a source of pleasure foreign to the ego), an object the child would therefore wish to have*; the father figure, the person who fulfils this function, is what the child wishes to be* (strong, omnipotent, omniscient, as small children feel their father is, characteristics not yet related to recognition of sexual difference). For this reason, the father is an object of identification (related to learning action); this identification is primary, still in the category of being; it later becomes part of the ego and is consequently narcissistic* and of course pre-oedipal*.

In *Findings, Ideas, Problems* (1941) and *Instincts and Their Vicissitudes* (1915), Freud discusses the idea of an ego mistaken for the object so long as the latter is pleasurable: a purified pleasure ego functioning at the dawn of life with the category of being, previous to the category of having, in relation to sexual satisfaction. "I am the pleasure object or I am the breast" is the leitmotif of this type of ego. This is the major characteristic defining direct identification previous to recognition of a pleasure object, at least in the perspective of sexual Trieb*. In this sense, the latter is also primary identification in spite of its loving link with the unrecognized object; precisely for this reason, because it is not recognized, the relation "is the original form of emotional tie with an object" (S.E: V.XVIII, p. 107).

However, the initial reality ego* also functions from the dawn of life, and this ego distinguishes between ego and not-ego, mainly by determining bodily boundaries. In general, it corresponds to self-preservative Trieb*.

We therefore have two types of direct primary identifications: "I am the breast" (the category of having not yet existing) and identification with the father before recognition of sexual difference, the father not configuring a fully configured pleasure object (in this second form of primary identification, being is differentiated from having, and the ego does not want to have the father), but wanting to "be like him".

However, primary identification acquires a hostile tone in the period when phallic-urethral* erotism predominates, when sexual difference is known. Wanting to be like the father becomes wanting to occupy his place, part of the positive Oedipus complex, with definitive object recognition (the mother) as the place of pleasure and the father as the obstacle (rival) to it, so that the type of identification gradually becomes secondary*: secondary to object recognition as the main source of pleasure and as the rival, and also to constitution of the superego* to reinforce the ego in its work of suppressing* Trieb*.

This early "being the object" is a type of primary identification that constitutes the ego, previous to any libidinal object cathexis (in one case the pleasure object – the mother – and in an intermediate place, those that are not pleasure objects – identification with the father), therefore belonging to primary narcissism. When "one has been the object", its characteristics have left traces. These traces eventually constitute modalities inherent to the incipient ego (ruled by the category of being). Others become object presentations* or presentations of a wish for the object (ruled by the category of having), when they are cathected with libido*.

We observe that primary identification is a complex and dynamic concept belonging to a certain developmental moment as the characteristics of links gradually change with growing recognition of reality*, that of the subject's own body and ego as well as that of the desired object, and the appearance of the rival. All this results in the production of a different type of identification (now secondary because the pleasure object has already been recognized as foreign to the ego, and the rival as opposed to obtaining pleasure from the former), which reinforces primary identification and partly constitutes the ego itself as well as a special part of it called the superego*.

PRIMARY JUDGING

Ger.: primäre Urteilen. – Sp.: judicación primaria. – Fr.: judication primaire. – It.: giudicazione primaria. – Port.: judicação primária.

This primitive thought* activity does not utilize word-presentations* but rather, basically, actions. It is not primary process* – that is to say, a tendency to hallucinatory wish fulfilment*, perceptual identity*, and free energy* – but neither is it secondary process* which recognizes reality* and seeks thought identity* with bound energy* and word-presentations. Freud describes primary judging in his *Project for a Scientific Psychology* (1895–1950). It is a concept with similarities and differences in relation to the concept of identification*.

The first types of understanding* of the object* consist in repeating its movements and attributes. Babies imitate their mother, this imitation being their way to understand her. They move their hands as she does, laugh as she laughs, cry or scream when she does, or when they hear screaming. This imitative value of all perception* gradually constitutes primary identifications* through "introjections" (S. Ferenczi's term) of attributes or characteristics of the subject's movements. At the same time, the first type of judging forms: thought previous to words, accomplished by actions.

Primary judging is also related to reproductive thought (in which thing-presentations* predominate) involved in it (since to think or compare it is necessary to remember); however, primary judging*, unlike reproductive thought, seeks understanding of the external object and the subject's own body through actions rather than presentations*. It is precisely the latter that are left afterwards as traces of these actions, thereby moving to a higher level to become part of the complexity of the psyche's presentational fabric.

Through this process, subjects growingly need less and less action – except expressions of mimicry and the comic* – in order to think, emit judgements, put themselves in the other's place and understand the other, and to express themselves. They already possess a symbolic level acquired through language* acquisition, by which this initial concrete level is progressively transformed.

PRIMARY PROCESS

Ger.: Primärvorgang. – Sp.: proceso primario. – Fr.: processus primaire. – It.: processo primario. – Port.: processo primário.

This type of mental functioning, as its name indicates, predominates originally in babies. It is gradually overcome and partly tamed by secondary process* which develops throughout life.

Later, in adults, primary process is limited to the functioning of the unconscious* and therefore reigns in the id*, in unconscious parts of the ego* (defence mechanisms*), and perhaps in the unconscious superego*.

It is basically a type of relation between unconscious thing-presentations* which produces or results from free displacement* of energy among them.

It therefore operates with free energy*. Ruled by the pleasure–unpleasure principle, it seeks perceptual identity*. Presentations are condensed, producing very rapid identities between them through laws of association*. A presentation contiguous to another is identified with it. The same occurs when it is analogous, and even an opposite presentation becomes the other to the extent that it is associated with what is wished for. The unconscious wish utilizes laws of association to find vertiginous identities with the wished-for presentation, perceptual identities configuring identifications* with it. The analogous, the contiguous, and the opposite are identical to what is wished for: they "are" what is wished for.

These identities exist neither in space nor in time. In this sense, it is mental activity discovered by Freud which does not comply with Kantian concepts such as *a priori* categories of thought*. They do not fit into this type of thought; it is psychical activity but not strictly thinking.

Contradiction does not exist. "No" does not exist. This is a condition required of presentations proceeding from the repressed unconscious if they are to access the preconscious ego, consciousness*, and therefore secondary process.

Primary process, in sum, is a form of relation between unconscious thing-presentations, predominantly visual residues of perceptions* (although registers originating in all the other senses and erotogenic zones* may participate in their formation through the object link), which utilize laws of association (contiguity or simultaneity, analogy* or opposition*) to generate condensations* of them and free displacements of cathectic energy among presentations, following these laws of association to this end.

It seeks identity to extremes. It mistakes what is desired for what is perceived because the thing is something contiguous, analogous or opposite. It does not distinguish associations from identities. It spares itself reality testing*.

For all these reasons it is ineffective. It does not lead to specific action*. It may at most produce autoplastic* internal alterations*. It cannot change the world. Although its aim is pleasure*, it generates unpleasure*.

However, it is somewhat effective when it is repressed and manages to return from this state, acting on secondary process and influencing it to produce neurotic symptoms*, dreams, parapraxes*, and other phenomena, all of these being disguised forms of satisfaction of sexual Trieb*.

Primary process is ruled by the pleasure principle*, by means of which pleasure is never really accessed. Reality* must be accepted and the pleasure principle transformed into the reality principle*, in order to reach pleasure in reality. Since this result is not always produced, reality is often opposed to it. Therefore, for access to pleasure and specific action, primary process must be inhibited* and another, higher process with strong cathexis* and weak displacement utilized; this process takes reality into account and consequently produces changes in the real world necessary to satisfy or gratify internal Triebe.

Primary process is perhaps one of the major psychoanalytic discoveries, a form of relation between presentations, a manner of thinking but not genuine thought: acceptance of a type of psychical functioning different from what is accepted as such by the official ego's consciousness. This psychical functioning possesses its own laws or rather utilizes laws of association for its own benefit, and has every right to be considered as such, as the psychical functioning of the unconscious.

In psychoanalytical treatment, by backtracking along the path it has taken, the meaning of symptoms may be recovered, making conscious the unconscious, moving primary process containing the repressed into secondary process, inherent to the preconscious.

PRINCIPLE OF CONSTANCY

Ger.: Konstanz prinzip. – Sp.: principio de constancia. – Fr.: principe de constance. – It.: principio di costanza. – Port.: princípio de constãncia.

This law of universal movement in classical Newtonian physics was utilized by Freud to explain the movement of energy within neurones* in his *Project for a Scientific Psychology* (1895).

It complements the principle of inertia* according to which each neurone tends to discharge the quantity of excitation* entering it.

Complex organisms need a certain amount of constant energy available in order to respond to the "exigencies of life"*. They need to store energy. The main quantity of excitation* proceeds from their own body. To satisfy needs it generates, specific actions* must be carried out which usually require a larger amount of energy than what is provided by need. For this reason, the principle of inertia* must be overcome and the principle of constancy utilized. The latter includes the former (a certain constant quantity is needed to access the principle of inertia and to discharge energy proceeding from need), but is on a different level.

A given energy, therefore, remains constant. This is the Freudian theoretical grounding for the concepts of bound energy* and the secondary process*, important because they lead to the origin of the ego*. In other words, the ego functions according to this principle which, in psychological terminology, Freud subsequently calls the reality principle*, while the principle of inertia* becomes the pleasure principle*.

Since the untamed sexual Triebe* want only to follow the pleasure principle, their passage to the reality principle is much more difficult and problematic.

In contrast, the ego's self-preservative Triebe* are governed from the outset by the reality principle.

PRINCIPLE OF INERTIA

Ger.: Trägheitsprinzip. – Sp.: principio de inercia. – Fr.: principe d'inertie. – It.: principio d'inerzia. Port.: princípio da inercia.

According to this first law of universal movement, any object that is stimulated tends to return to the state previous to the stimulus. In general, it tends to return to zero (not necessarily to absolute zero but rather to the moment previous to the stimulus).

Freud introduced this law of Newtonian physics into psychology, having studied in the School of Helmholtz as a disciple of one of its famous members, Ernst Brücke, when Freud considered neurones* as material particles pierced through by stimuli in his early works.

The text of this law, in Newton's words [translated from Latin], is: "Everybody continues in its state of rest, or of uniform motion in a right line, unless it is compelled to change that state by forces impressed upon it". Freud gradually introduced this principle into metapsychology, although he did not yet utilize this term (despite having begun to use it in earlier letters to Fliess), first in his *Project for a Scientific Psychology* (1895), a manuscript not published in his lifetime. In his subsequent works, the principle of inertia became the pleasure principle* – now purely psychological – which preserves many points of connection with the former version, and its maximum expression, the Nirvana principle*.

PROJECTION

Ger.: Projektion. – Sp.: proyección. – Fr.: projection. – It.: proiezione. – Port.: projeção.

This psychical mechanism is characterized by perception* (more precisely, the subject's initial interpretation of what is perceived) of internal psychical processing in the external world. They may be affective states (for example, sadness; a cloudy or rainy day gives the subject a feeling that the atmosphere in a certain place is somehow sad).

Projection utilizes the laws of association* such as analogy* – rain=tears – and also preconscious* thoughts* (phantasies* of infidelity in normal jealousy*, known to the ego*, repressed by it, and returning from the repressed in neurotic jealousy), even unconscious* wishes* (the typical case is paranoia*; in this case the wish is decathected in the subject's unconscious and perceived in the unconscious of other people); but not only in paranoia. Each preconscious wish is supported by an unconscious wish, cathected of course. Sometimes the ego knows it and sometimes it does not. In this sense, when preconscious wishes are projected, so too are unconscious wishes, implicitly or implicitly.

Projection is a largely normal mechanism in the early moments when thought activity appears by virtue of language acquisition*. It is part of omnipotence of thought*, by which reality* is felt to form part of thought. It is at the base of animism*, the first worldview of humanity and of individuals, which persists in neurotics.

> Spirits and demons, as I have shown in the last essay, are only projections of man's own emotional impulses. He turns his emotional cathexes into persons, he peoples the world with them and meets his internal mental processes again outside himself.
>
> (*Totem and Taboo*, 1913, p. 92)

This normal and universal mechanism is utilized by the ego as a defence against id Triebe* in response to the anxiety signal* (of castration, for example), felt to be similar to automatic anxiety*, when Triebe fight to become part of the ego in order to reach action.

In this case, the unconscious ego projects the affect* it is trying to expel, or the presentation* of the object wish that causes it. Then, projection is already a defence mechanism* of the unconscious ego, or a form of repression*.

We define metapsychological differences between the diverse levels of projection: (1) one level participates in the first human worldview and therefore in normality; (2) another level generates neurosis*; and (3) a different level forms a significant part of an equally important type of psychosis* such as paranoia* or paranoid schizophrenia*, a category to which we may add borderline states between psychosis and neurosis. The first level (normal) is not necessarily defensive, at least not from Trieb; at most, it may defend from reality when it aims to qualify it (associate it with something analogous from the past, for example, in which it was a perceptual quality*). It is intimately linked with and participates in subjectivity, the way of understanding reality, of feeling and experiencing it. We may think that no mechanism of repression intervenes. There is no attempt to ignore Trieb or object wishes: reality is simply understood or seen in terms of the individual's own psychical mechanisms, translating reality into them; for this reason reality or the notion of it possesses a large subjective component. No matter how much science tries to be objective, the "thing in itself" of external reality is unknowable.

This is not to say that neurotic mechanisms have no participation in this type of projection at certain moments; phenomena do not occur in isolation as we describe them theoretically in order to understand them, but rather as mixtures.

Neither do we surrender to subjectivity nor cease the struggle to find the objective; we seek to define our limits while recognizing the loss of omnipotence of thought; ultimately, what characterizes scientific thought is that it reaches levels of truth, not the only truth.

With respect to neurotic projection, neurotic jealousy is the product of a phantasy of infidelity repressed by the subject's ego and therefore not accepted as its own but instead felt in the object. Another example is anxiety hysteria* and its phobic rampart*. However, strictly speaking, although Freud describes displacement* from one preconscious presentation to another, the fact, also mentioned and accepted by Freud, is that this substitutive preconscious presentation produces anxiety* when it is perceived in the external world, and after this moment the subject acts with this external world in such a way as to avoid coming into contact with the feared presentation.

When the incestuous sexual wish proceeding from the id aims to access the ego, a preconscious presentation cathected with a danger signal (that of castration) is then projected. The ego defends itself in this way, and danger is felt to proceed from perception of an image in the external world that was displaced from the repressed presentation; it also acts as anticathexis*, since the more contact with the phobia-generating object, a substitute formation* produced by displacement of the original presentation, is feared, there is less danger of feeling that danger may proceed from the latter.

In anxiety hysteria, the unconscious wish is intact, returning from the repressed from the exterior through the phobia* (what returns is the danger of castration* generated by the wish, in childhood realistic anxiety* and now neurotic anxiety*).

In paranoia, however, the subject's unconscious wish is projected onto the object's unconscious. In this narcissistic psychosis, unconscious presentations are decathected and the subject is thereby deprived of its own unconscious wishes, which it perceives in the unconscious of others in a distorted form (in persecutory paranoia*, transformed into the opposite*: love* into hate*). The subject "guesses", by means of "signs", repressed wishes of objects towards himself.

These object wishes are pre-oedipal*, narcissistic, and homosexual, not recognizing sexual difference which appears with the phallic phase, a type of recognition involving the existence of castration*.

Therefore, in paranoia, homosexual wishes are projected in disguise in order to conceal this homosexual characteristic from the eyes of the paranoiac's ego, which does not accept it as part of itself, just as before when it was unable to accept sexual difference. The cause was ultimately the same: if phallic sexual difference were accepted, the possibility of the existence of castration would also have to be accepted, including the danger of suffering it.

If the homosexual wish is accepted as the ego's own, its implicit premise is castration, unacceptable for the ego's "bedrock". Therefore, the only way out of this labyrinth is to break off from the object wish, so conflictive, and to pour libido* into the ego (generating hypochondria* and megalomania*), whereas the original unconscious object wish is projected.

Breaking off cathexis of the unconscious object wish produces the experience of the end of the world*: the end of the world of object wishes. It is a last defence, repression in the broad sense, as Freud understands it in the case of "Schreber".

By virtue of projection, the homosexual wish returns from the object's unconscious, distorted in several ways (producing diverse clinical forms), through which connection with the world is reconstructed by means of the delusion*, developed with word-presentations* that have taken the place of unconscious presentations or thing-presentations*. At this point, projection is different; the essence of the psychical apparatus, the "nucleus of being", the unconscious wish, the id or its most important part, is projected. Unlike projection of the preconscious wish in neurosis, it is the unconscious wish that is projected. The latter in reality remains in the ego constituted by words now emptied of their unconscious content, of their meaning: the ego is consequently left deeply altered. However, the degree of this alteration of the ego* determines therapeutic possibilities.

PROTECTIVE SHIELD

Ger.: Reizschutz. – Sp.: protección anti-estímulo. – Fr.: pare-excitations. – It.: apparato protettivo contro lo stimolo. – Port.: proteção anti-estímulo.

These shields are utilized by the psychical apparatus* to defend itself from stimuli external to the subject's body: Freud refers to them in the *Project for a Scientific Psychology* as "masses in movement". They are located on the body's surface, exactly the area of contact with this overwhelming quantity of stimuli from the external world.

The quantities of stimulus from this external world are far greater than those the psychical apparatus is usually able to endure; for this reason the protective shield is generated on the surface. It is physically composed of filters against quantities located at the perceptual end*, the sense organs, filters that seek to level off the quantity of excitation* entering from the outside to make it more bearable and susceptible to binding for the interior, the psychical apparatus.

When these quantities overflow the filters, the result is bodily pain* or an actual traumatic situation* (origin of traumatic neuroses*).

However, aside from the bodily shield, the "last resort" is the extent of anxious expectation* (the degree of tension binding attention) with which the perception* of the external stimulus is received. Perception is not simply a passive process; it is possible to perceive with a stronger or weaker previous cathexis* of attention* and even of anxiety or anxious expectation*.

The larger the quantity of attention cathexis, the greater the possibility of binding the stimulus. If the latter is not bound, if it is not transformed into quiescent cathexis* by virtue of thought* processing, its link with other presentations* (the more presentations are available for binding, the better possibility it will have to exist), becomes traumatic, and it is left at the mercy of repetition compulsion*.

Here, we are referring to actual external trauma* rather than to sexual trauma of infantile prehistory, with which it obviously has points of contact but also differences. In this actual case, a stimulus is traumatic when it surpasses a certain quantity or a certain unit of time in which this quantity may be perceived, it succeeds in overcoming the protective shield*, and is not perceived as qualitative but as quantitative, remaining in the psychical apparatus as a quantity of stimulus unable to bind to any presentation.

The dreams* of traumatic neuroses are nocturnal repetitions of the traumatic event the subject endeavours to forget during the day; it is produced in part by repetition compulsion* and also by the attempt, through the dream, for the ego* to feel anxious expectation*, the last resort of the protective shield. This allows the ego to feel it as unpleasure* and therefore as quality*, having thereby passed to the pleasure–unpleasure principle by which it may be associated with other presentations of similar past experiences, entering the presentational world once again. At this point it may also have an opportunity to enter the thought process and become quiescent cathexis.

The protective shield, composed in part by cells that "die" so that deeper strata may live, has some (sense organs) that receive news of the external world from deep connections, thereby preserving the psychical apparatus from external quantities. However, it does not do the same for internal quantities, bodily needs and Triebe*. This also provides support for the peremptory character of Trieb, pressuring for Trieb action.

One of the most primitive defence mechanisms utilized against them is projection*, with which they may be felt to proceed from the external world; the psychical apparatus may then defend itself from them in a second instance, utilizing the protective shield*. This may lead to diverse types of pathology or may remain in the sphere of normality (animism*, paranoia*, anxiety hysteria*, normal and delusional jealousy*, for example).

PSYCHE (CF. SOUL)

PSYCHICAL CONFLICT

Ger.: psychischer Konflikt. – Sp.: conflict psíquico. – Fr.: conflit psychique. – It.: conflitto psichico. – Port.: conflito psíquico.

A conflict results when two opposite tendencies clash. The notion of psychical conflict involves mental dynamics and is part of the very essence of psychoanalysis.

Of course, conflicts are not always generators of pathology. However, we may recall that any conscious conflict may reactivate subjacent unconscious conflicts and, in this case, contribute to the appearance of neurosis*. Also, an ego* whose character* frequently has a tendency to conflict is a potential source of pathology.

We consider different periods of libidinal development. In each of these a certain erotogenic zone* predominates over the others. Diverse types of conflict run through the erotogenic zones: between love* and hate* or between active and passive* (ambivalence* with respect to the object* in both cases), between object libido and narcissistic libido* or between libidinal Triebe* and the ego, which experiences anxiety and defends itself from them.

The ego must also deal with continuous conflicts with the id*, the superego, and reality*. It must mediate between all these factors and reach a synthesis. When it is unable to do so, it must split (cf. splitting of the ego*).

The conflict *par excellence* – a kind of core to which all other conflicts refer – is the oedipal, a highly "complex" complex. In boys, it originates the conflict between love and hate for his father whom he feels is his rival for a wish* that has become incestuous (positive Oedipus complex*); or a conflict between his homosexual desire for his father and the castration anxiety* it involves (negative Oedipus complex); also the conflict between accepting and not accepting the existence of castration, and others.

The ego must overcome all these conflicts through some satisfactory synthesis; if not, they are reactivated when similar situations come up in life, or when intensification of Trieb potentiates conflicts that in other circumstances had reached a certain level of solution.

Ultimately, all neurotic conflicts occur between libidinal tendencies and the exigencies of social reality, the latter located within the psychical apparatus* (the superego* and the ego itself are marks of the social in it); death Trieb* is forever stalking, seeking to create conflict.

Although libidinal tendencies belong to life Triebe*, they are always admixed in diverse proportions with death Trieb, from which degrees of ambivalence and a greater tendency to conflict probably derive. We also know that the superego is a libidinal anticathexis* that calls upon death Trieb to kill libido. This "help" may become excessive, as in melancholia.

Then, the superego becomes "a pure culture of the death instinct" (*The Ego and the Id*, 1923, p. 53).

In this complex and intricate way, in which the mute death Trieb is represented by the degree of Trieb fusion with life Trieb and its presentations*, we may then speak of conflict between life and death Triebe.

PSYCHICAL DYNAMICS

Ger.: Psychische Dinamik. – Sp.: dinámica psíquica. – Fr.: dynamique psychique. – It.: dinamica psichica. – Port.: dinãmica psíquica.

The dynamic perspective, together with the topical and the economical, grounds psychoanalytic metapsychology. The dynamic perspective explains the psychical apparatus* as something in action, with constant changes, forces seeking discharge, and other forces opposing it; with progression and regressions*; with moments of stability and discompensations; with forces and presentations* in conflict.

Triebe* generate the energy* of the psychical apparatus*. When they are bound to presentations* – first thing-* and then word-* – Triebe are gradually mastered. Free energy* has become quiescent or bound. It is utilized in general by the preconscious ego* which in turn is partly composed of it. The ego utilizes secondary process*, thought*, a minimal form of action with a low expenditure of energy and preparation for specific action* which demands large quantities of energy.

Individuals are also equipped with a protective shield* that protects them from external quantities. If the latter enter the psychical apparatus in such high quantities that it is unable to bind them to presentations, physical pain and/or traumatic situations* result.

The psychical apparatus in the Freudian structural schema is composed of an id*, an ego*, and a superego*. The ego is charged with reconciling id demands with those of the superego, generally opposite, and creating a synthesis from them; not just any synthesis, however, but one that is adequate to reality*. These are the dynamic vicissitudes accompanying each Trieb* motion and each perception* of reality that reactivates Trieb motion. The ego must find solutions with low expenditure of energy and sufficient discharge of all the opposing tendencies it faces.

PSYCHICAL ECONOMY

Ger.: Psychische Okonomie. – Sp.: economía psíquica. – Fr.: économie psychique. –It.: economia psichica. – Port.: economia psíquica.

The economic perspective is one of the three perspectives of Freudian metapsychology, together with the dynamic* and the topical or structural (cf. psychical apparatus). The economic viewpoint originates in the earliest Freudian conceptions of the psyche as being subject to the general laws of movement; for example, the principle of inertia*. In the *Project for a Scientific Psychology* (1950) he applies this conception to neurones seeking to relieve quantities of excitation*. The economic perspective, however, persists throughout Freudian theory with increasing complexity and even apparent and foreseeable contradictions.

Psychical economy refers to everything related to quantity of excitation.

In the Freudian schema, the psyche is composed of two essential elements: presentations* and energy*. There are two types of presentations (thing- and word-). Energy circulates among the presentations and in general originates from the biological body, from Triebe*: when they are sexual, they are called libido. It is stored by the ego* as energy bound to presentations; in the ego it is desexualized and bound (to word-presentations related to each other by secondary process*), cathecting* and decathecting* presentations

> in mental functions something is to be distinguished – a quota of affect or sum of excitation – which possesses all the characteristics of a quantity (though we have no means of measuring it), which is capable of increase, diminution, displacement and discharge, and which is spread over the memory traces of ideas somewhat as an electric charge is spread over the surface of a body).
>
> (*The Neuro-Psychoses of Defence*, 1894, p. 60)

The psychical apparatus receives quantities of energy bound to presentations that come from processings of direct perceptual traces (cf. Letter 52 to Fliess) of the memory traces* of experiences of satisfaction* and pain*; that is to say, of the memory of perceived facts that at some moment had perceptual quality*.

When quantity is bound to presentation, desire is generated, the motor of the psychical apparatus, which now has a certain level of quality (although it is not the perceptual quality that is desired; the presentation is the memory of this quality), a presentational quality which is the trace left by the perceptual quality and is what the apparatus wishes to recover. It is a desire to re-experience what was felt in the experience of satisfaction, which is what the apparatus attempts to repeat. It endeavours to escape from the experience of pain, which it also takes up when presentational quality is transformed into presentation. All this directionality of energy circulating among presentations (seeking to repeat experiences of satisfaction and to escape from painful experiences) is governed by the pleasure principle* which functions in a presentational world in movement.

It is quantity that is gradually qualified as it is psychologized, and it is psychologized basically in order to become specific action*. This action culminates in a discharge of the charge that generated the circuit. It is ultimately a tremendously complex reflex arc. This reflex arc is the axis of the economic perspective. The organism generates quantities seeking discharge. These quantities bind to presentations and take on the names of wish/desire, Trieb and libido. Some presentations to which they bind may be accepted by the ego and others rejected, repressed in different ways. In his 1915 papers on metapsychology, the quantity circulating among presentations is "quantum of affect"*; this term is truly the most representative presentation of Trieb (*Drang*). All the affects* are also explained as different types of discharge.

In *Inhibitions, Symptoms and Anxiety* (1925), Freud discusses a type of anxiety* that has no need of an economic explanation: the anxiety signal*, anxiety cultivated in small quantities by the ego in order to marshal its unconscious defence mechanisms. It does not need this explanation; it is a memory* or a presentation of a different type of anxiety (automatic anxiety) which does require an economic explanation and which, by means of this signal, the ego defence mechanisms attempt to avoid.

PSYCHICAL ENERGY

Ger.: Psychische Energie. – Sp.: energía psíquica. – Fr.: énergie psychique. – It.: energia psichica. – Port.: energia psíquica.

A general dictionary may define "energy" diversely as efficacy, power, ability to take action, or a cause capable of transformation into mechanical work. In Freudian thought, the addition of the term "psychical" means we are referring to energy bound to a presentation*. Hence, this energy seeks to be transformed into action, into facts, not just any facts but rather facts that relate to presentations which are in turn memories of other facts: experiences. In other terms, this energy seeks discharge by re-experiencing them.

The idea of psychical energy in Freudian metapsychology begins with the economic viewpoint, and also the dynamic and, by definition, the presentational. It is quantity with psychical quality (this in turn a memory of perceptual quality), seeking a new perceptual quality and constantly fighting against energetic and presentational defences* which are transformations of energy, originating in the body, stored in the ego*.

In Freudian terms, energy is usually utilized for the libidinal. Energy corresponding to self-preservative Triebe is called interest*.

Does death Trieb possess psychical energy? Freud considers death Trieb a tendency of organic matter to return to the inorganic. Since there is no presentation of the subject's own death in the unconscious*, binding is not possible; therefore, it has no psychical energy (presentation of another's death may exist, but as an expression of deflection of Trieb and therefore destructive Trieb*; this Trieb is Trieb fusion). It is consequently energy (what does it utilize to "tend toward" if not energy?), though not psychical energy but presentation, pure quantity. In relation to this, it seeks to separate the energy from the presentation. Death Trieb acts on different levels of fusion with life Trieb*. In order to continue life or to lengthen the road to death, it is expelled from the organism by the muscular apparatus in the form of sadism*, Trieb of mastery*, and so on. All of these are different degrees of fusion between libidinal energy and Death Trieb.

Libidinal energy binds to the presentation in two different ways: (a) by passing freely from one presentation to another (or with freedom governed by the laws of association* and the pleasure principle*) and (b) as quiescent energy* called bound energy* (although the presentation is strongly cathected*, displacement* of cathexis energy from one presentation to another is complex, full of intermediate processes, and obliged to comply with secondary process* and the reality principle*).

Free energy functions in the unconscious id* by linking thing-presentations*.

Energy is effectively bound only if preconscious word-presentations* represent thing-presentations and act in consequence, directed by the conscious ego and its secondary process.

When the specific action* is carried through, energy having undergone all this process of binding in order to reach adequate discharge* is liberated.

At the moment of discharge (specific action) or even of the charge (when a quantity of excitation* enters the apparatus and is bound to a presentation, becoming a wish), energy has small safety valves such as internal change*, generating affects*. When discharge is unspecific and bodily (internal change), the affect is unpleasurable; for example, anxiety. Anxiety is expressed by bodily discharge such as tachycardia, hyperventilation, hyper-sudoration and others, with or without its typical feeling. When bodily anxiety predominates, especially if it becomes chronic, we enter the field of psychosomatic pathology.

As we said, internal change is a safety valve for a psychical apparatus carrying excessive quantities of energy, sometimes resulting from conflicts between presentational systems (repression*, suppression*) that prevent discharge of energy.

PSYCHICAL INERTIA

Ger.: Psychische trügheit. – Sp.: inercia psíquica. – Fr.: inertie psychique. – It.: inercia psichica. – Port.: inércia psíquica.

Also referred to as "adhesiveness of libido"*, it indicates the difficulty of libido* to change objects* and erotogenic zones*, and consequently tends to hold to them as fixation points*. It is an obstacle to psychoanalytical cure, a form of id* resistance* which by clinging to its archetypes produces a compulsion to repeat them.

It is an expression of the principle of inertia*, one of the laws of the movement of bodies. It is also an expression of psychical life in general and of Triebe* in particular. Triebe tend to return to a previous state: previous to the stimulus (life Triebe*) or previous to life (death Triebe*). What unites them is the tendency to return to a previous state; they are differentiated precisely by the previous state to which they strive to return (those of life endeavour to return to a previous experience of satisfaction* or pleasure*; those of death to return to the inorganic).

The principle of psychical inertia corresponds to description from a different perspective of phenomena such as fixation and repetition compulsion*; we place it among innate characteristics of libido: libido with its own tendency to inertia, independent of traumatic situations* (which of course may be added), libido with more difficulty than usual for leaving places it occupied (presentations* of objects, their attributes, erotogenic zones), libido that tends to fixate on them.

Libido may also have opposite characteristics (persons who constantly change object choices* or the predominance of fixation points in links with objects). Then, rather than plasticity of libido, the impression is of "having written on water" (*Analysis Terminable and Interminable*, 1937, p. 241), which is the opposite problem, resulting in another form of resistance to the cure.

PSYCHICAL OR MENTAL APPARATUS

Ger.: psychischer o seelischer Apparat. – Sp.: aparato psíquico. – Fr.: appareil psychique. – It.: apparato psichico o mentale. –Port.: aparelho psiquico.

This is a model to represent psychical functioning. Freud probably extracted it from mechanicist materialism in use at the end of the eighteenth century, mainly by the School of Helmholtz, also following the example of the anatomical and physiological model (circulatory system, respiratory system, and so on). When he took it to its ultimate consequences, he soon detached it from anatomical or neuro-physio-chemical localizations without discarding the possibility that they might exist; he viewed it instead from a different perspective. His terrain was psychology that generated a new way to understand it: psychoanalysis no less. Although the model is mechanicist, his explanation of its functioning featured predominantly psychical dynamics, functionality, and systematization.

This apparatus is constituted by an intricate mechanism with different elements that link together or oppose each other. It is "constructed" gradually, becoming more complex through new experiences. Its description corresponds to Freudian metapsychology; therefore, it has a topical, a dynamic and an economic dimension.

The theory of the psychical apparatus undergoes, in the course of Freud's works, developments, confirmations, additions, rectifications and/or changes.

His manuscript, *Project for a Scientific Psychology* (1895), published posthumously in 1950, and part of his correspondence with Fliess, is contemporary with other similar attempts at that time, such as Sigmund Exner and Breuer. In the theoretical part of the Studies on Hysteria (1893–5), Breuer discusses a psychical apparatus with a certain anatomic-histological root from which it gradually separates in the course of the text. It describes neurones* that first carry presentations, after which the former become the latter. This is explicit in Chapter 7 of *The Interpretation of Dreams* (1900). In the "Project" we observe extremely rigorous methodology of thought as if a physiologist were observing psychological issues with a microscope.

In this work, ideas appear that are developed many years later, which makes their reading indispensable for the understanding of reasoning much later.

Here, he postulates a psychical apparatus composed of neurones and quantity of excitation*, a quantity they do not tolerate and want to rid themselves of, and all the complex defence* the neurone network must then develop in order to escape being at its mercy. There are ϕ neurones, ψ neurones, and ω neurones. The ψ neurones have contact with the external world and receive large excitations coming from it which it attenuates by means of defensive filters or screens; this excitation runs through these neurons without leaving traces, which are registered by other neurones in charge of memory: the ψ neurones. Finally, perceptual quality* is registered by ω neurones, which do not register quantities but rather the timing or periodicity* of their movements.

The psychical apparatus is constituted in intimate relation with the object link, since it is set into motion following experiences of satisfaction* and pain* experienced with the object*. These experiences leave in it memory traces*, mainly traces of the object: when these traces join quantities of excitation coming from paths of bodily conduction, they configure object wishes*. The birth of the wish inaugurates the pleasure principle*.

The "Project ..." also explains thought* activity, primary defence, and normal and pathological defence, a scheme that becomes progressively more complex. Freud also speaks of an ego*, the seat of secondary process*; a form of inhibition* of hallucinations* (the latter inherent to the primary process*) in order to install the reality principle* thereby generated.

Five years later, in *The Interpretation of Dreams* (1900), Freud departs finally from the anatomical model and begins to speak in terms of topics and virtual (imaginary) psychical places. He completes the psychical apparatus described in Chapter 7 of this work in 1915 with his famous *A Metapsychological Supplement to the Theory of Dreams* (1917).

The reflex arc is the dynamic basis of the scheme, which in turn possesses an entrance and an exit for quantity of excitation (generally libidinal). The quantity of excitation enters through the perceptual end*, becomes quantity of affect* and is perceived there as displeasure; it also generates a tendency that, by binding to presentations, acquires the name of "wish".

There are two types of presentations: thing-presentations* first and word-presentations* later, when the subject acquires language*. By virtue of word-presentations, the conscious* accesses thing-presentations and may therefore think with them and finally lead the libido* to the motor end* where the circuit must end in a specific action* that discharges Trieb* at the source. This discharge is then felt at the perceptual end as pleasure*.

All this occurs on condition that Trieb is accepted by the preconscious* once the censors* have been overcome. Topically, there are two censors. The first is repression*, situated at the limit between the unconscious and the preconscious; it forms the repressed unconscious with the Trieb of infantile sexuality* whose development culminated in the period of the Oedipus complex* and whose derivatives (wishes analogous or contiguous to repressed wishes and hence identified with them) are repressed in turn, which generates (when these derivatives return from the repressed due to defects in this repression) neurotic symptoms*, anxiety*, dreams*, parapraxes*, and so on.

The second censor is conscious, reinforcing the first one. It is based on withdrawal of the cathexis* of conscious attention* and is the censor the analyst asks the patient to suppress in order to comply with the "fundamental rule"* of psychoanalytic technique*.

Summing up, this new scheme is composed of unconscious*, preconscious*, and conscious*: the unconscious*, seat of infantile wishes repressed by primary repression* (with the corresponding events experienced with objects during this period of life transformed into thing-presentations which if cathected become wishes again and are therefore repressed by primary repression; the action of repression is considered the impediment preventing passage of this thing-presentation to its corresponding word), receives analogous, contiguous, and even opposite derivatives identified with these infantile wishes and are repressed for this reason by secondary repression. Both characteristics (primary and secondary) correspond to repression, the first unconscious form of censorship that splits the psychical apparatus into an unconscious and a preconscious. The second, conscious censorship is added to it as reinforcement.

The unconscious has thing-presentations. Energy* flows among them freely (primary process) following the laws of association*, seeking perceptual identities* and utilizing condensation* and displacement*.

This is the type of psychical functioning pertaining to (but not only to) dreams.

Split off from the unconscious by virtue of repression*, the preconscious (Prec.) is composed mainly of word-presentations, one of whose functions is to represent thing-presentations in the conscious, which gives them the higher level of binding, strong cathexis and weak displacement characteristic of secondary process of thought* activity, by virtue of which what is wished for may be pursued while seeking identity of thought*.

Word-presentations pertain to language*; they are a form created by the human species in order to convey wishes to perception (the conscious in the Freudian sense) where the only addition required is cathexis of attention*.

Therefore, since the word is the most appropriate medium by which to learn of wishes, it is the place chosen by repression (especially secondary repression) for its own objective which is to ignore. It utilizes the laws of association in order to replace the original word-presentations with others, contiguous or analogous, and thereby withdraw preconscious cathexis from the former presentations which then enter the repressed unconscious and remain in a "state of repression".

This withdrawal of preconscious cathexis is a mechanism of secondary repression or actually, together with the attraction (by association with presentational content) of unconscious repetition compulsion* and anticathexis* (the latter being the only mechanism of primary repression), they are the other mechanisms of secondary repression, also known as "deferred repression".

The preconscious presentation must also overcome conscious censorship in order to be spoken, expressed, and governed more firmly yet by the secondary process, since the spoken word and even the written word have a social or communicational effect. If this conscious censorship is not overcome, it may remain in the terrain of phantasy* where it is similar to hybrid preconscious-unconscious presentations governed by the pleasure principle but with words and a certain secondary process logic. These fantasies or daydreams may rapidly become derivatives of the unconscious and generate neurotic symptoms, dreams, and so on.

In his last article on metapsychology in 1915, when Freud discusses mourning* and melancholia*, the theme of identification re-emerges (he presented it in his explanation of Dora's cough and even before, when he explained understanding* as part of the fellow being complex in the baby's relation with its mother in the "Project ..."; he gradually polishes this concept whose importance he slowly discovers); he explains it again shortly afterwards as a mechanism that generates groups* in *Group Psychology and the Analysis of the Ego* (1921).

In these two works (*Mourning and Melancholia* and *Group Psychology and the Analysis of the Ego*) he reviews, with growing conceptual precision, the theme of identification and also of the ego* which is described as being constituted basically by identification. In the second work he takes it up in his conceptualization of the group leader who occupies the place of the ego ideal* of each of its members. The ego ideal is, for diverse reasons and in different ways, a differentiated part of this ego.

In 1920 he presents what is called his second Trieb theory, in which he attempts to explain repetitive behavioural phenomena that do not seem to function under the aegis of the pleasure principle but instead beyond it.

All these factors as well as clinical observation of unconscious resistance to the cure combine to expand the therapeutic objective; it becomes important not only to make conscious the repressed but also the unconscious repressor.

Although the latter is unknown to the patient, it can only belong to the ego, which led Freud to modify or add complexity to the psychical apparatus he had described up to that point, since it was no longer sufficient to explain these and other phenomena.

It became indispensable to describe the ego as a psychical structure, an important part of which is unconscious; it was also necessary to account for the ego ideal and moral conscience*, so conspicuous in some clinical pictures such as obsessional neurosis* and melancholia*. It was also necessary to recognize identification* as a central constituent of the psyche, a place hitherto reserved only for presentation*.

In *The Ego and the Id* (1923) he therefore presents the so-called second topic or structural theory. Now the psychical apparatus possesses an unconscious id*, although not all the unconscious is in the id. All Trieb originating in the body is in the id, with its thing-presentations, as well as the phylogenetically inherited. These repressed thing-presentations are only one part of the id.

The ego gradually forms on the periphery of the id through contact with reality. It is formed essentially of identifications with attributes of objects (Freud defines attributes as ways of carrying out actions; in principle these identifications are primary). The ego is in turn the main seat of word-presentations and secondary process. Its preconscious part is governed by the reality principle and therefore examines this reality*. As a consequence of the preceding, it is also the seat of thought. It possesses in turn a synthetic function which must find a synthesis between the clashing masters it serves constantly: Trieb, the superego*, and reality. In the course of this difficult task it may break down and succumb to ego splitting*. It has limited control of action.

As we said, part of the ego is unconscious. This part provides it, with the help of the pleasure principle by which it is then governed (it represses or defends itself from Trieb, since the ego feels that it pertains to anxiety) with defensive resources against the anxiety signal* cultivated by the ego itself in its "seedbed" which it emits as a sign of danger that satisfaction of Trieb coming from the id might present.

Another part of the ego splits off from it and observes, opposes, criticizes, keeps watch over, and punishes the ego if it is not what the ideal wants it to be. This part or third agency (superego-ego ideal) has a triple origin. The first source is experience inherited from the species and repeated (symbolically) in individual experience. In this phylogenetic hypothesis, Freud includes many of his thoughts regarding the origin of the human community (parricide, prohibition of incest, band of brothers*, and totemism*).

Besides the inherited, the superego-ego ideal in the adult results from transformation of infantile narcissism* for which ego was everything pleasurable (this transformation corresponds basically to the ego ideal, the second part of the expression composed of "superego-ego ideal").

Finally, the superego is again the heir, this time not of the species but of individual prehistory, his own Oedipus complex. Secondary identifications* with the progenitors remain in it as a precipitate, occupying the main position: the omnipotent childhood father and later substitutes (teachers, spiritual guides, leaders of all kinds).

Moral conscience is thereby constituted. We could say that the superego is made of aspirations and prohibitions. Moral conscience prohibits incest, parricide, and their derivatives. The ego ideal demands perfection: the perfection enjoyed by the omnipotent childhood ego.

In both a phylogenetic and a topical manner, the superego is rooted in the id. Hence the "unconscious sense of guilt" is generated, something Freud also describes as a "need for punishment", a product of Trieb defusion* generated by the desexualization* of sexual Trieb* demanded by the ego ideal through sublimation*. In this "superego resistance" (*Inhibitions, Symptoms and Anxiety*, 1926), fate puts all the therapeutic resources of psychoanalysis to the test.

PSYCHICAL STIMULUS

Ger.: psychisch Reiz. – Sp.: estímulo psíquico. – Fr.: excitation psychique. – It.: Stimolo psichico. – Port.: estímulo psíquico.

Stimulus is the quantity of energy that penetrates the psychical apparatus* (whose corresponding model is the "comb" in Chapter 7 of *The Interpretation of Dreams*, 1900) and whose path must end, after having cathected presentations indicating which path it is and what it entails, at the motor end*; that is to say, in action.

When the stimulus is inside the subject's body, we call it Trieb*, and when it is external, it belongs to actual reality*. The latter type, belonging to reality or nature, fellow beings, and the subject's own body (in the body, but not Trieb: pain and bodily illness) is specifically what we call stimulus.

Its external character in relation to the psychical apparatus, especially the subject's Trieb body, and therefore its place in external reality and its entry into the apparatus through perception*, characterizes non-Trieb stimulus.

This concept becomes more complex. Freud also states that Triebe were once external stimuli, referring to experiences of the species, a product of memory traces they left in the apparatus which became inherited presentations, experiences of specific actions* of the species. Ontogenetic presentations corresponding to each individual's own life gradually shape the subject's own Triebe which become wishes in correspondence to the individual's own experiences, fixation points, and so on, taking a path specific to each individual but also following an inherited pattern. Therefore, what was an external stimulus at some moment in infantile sexuality*, for example, may become a presentation or an identification, thereby becoming part of a Trieb or wishful path in the adult. In any case, beyond its dynamic history and the potential transformation of one thing into another, which adds overall complexity, the actual stimulus still differs from Trieb stimulus because of its origin outside the subject. This is one more example of the dynamic and complex character of Freudian thought.

Each stimulus must overcome an individual threshold between a minimum and a maximum if it is to become a stimulus; if it is below this threshold, it is not a stimulus, and if it surpasses maximum tolerance, it is traumatic.

PSYCHOANALYTIC TECHNIQUE

Ger.: Technik der Psychoanalyse. – Sp.: técnica psicoanalítica. – Fr.: technique psychanalytique. – It.: tecnica psicoanalitica. – Port.: técnica psicanalítica.

This collection of procedures and resources was utilized by Freud to psychoanalyse his patients. (They were neurotics or had character disorders on a neurotic level; for patients with predominantly narcissistic disorders, this technique and its objectives must be modified.)

Therefore, they are utilized to bring the unconscious* or unconscious wishes* to the patients' knowledge, thereby filling in memory gaps remaining in the preconscious ego since the subject's early childhood during the development of infantile sexuality*, a period when they were repressed. The preconscious ego of these persons is thereby strengthened when they bring presentations* of object wishes coming from the id* into their personal "space"; these presentations are bound with another type of presentation belonging to the preconscious ego: word-presentations* corresponding to id presentations. By making them their own, now that they are thinkable, patients may make decisions concerning them: whether or not to lead them into action. Better knowledge of the ego itself is also gained, especially of its unconscious defence mechanisms* and resistance* proceeding from them; but also regarding the history of their formation and modalities acquired by identification*, a pathway forming part of their essence, left in the ego by the object* which is also present in the modality of the individual's being and attributes.

We may recall that libido* cathecting the ego constitutes narcissism*, with participation of the ego ideal*. When the ego's origins in identification are analysed, the narcissistic problem is also analysed.

It is true that psychoanalysis also seeks to improve knowledge of the id and its Triebe* ("the core of our being"), since they are thereby enlisted into the ego's ranks. More knowledge of the superego* draws it also into the forces of the ego, especially its unconscious part which, if it is not in the service of the ego, acts as resistance to the cure, thereby satisfying the need for punishment.

This "knowledge" of the different parts of the unconscious corresponding to the id, the ego, or the superego is provided by the meaning of symptoms*, dreams*, parapraxes*, screen memories*, and other phenomena, and by associative paths they reveal; these paths are formed according to the laws of association* (contiguity*, analogy*, and opposition); as they are gradually detached from identity (since they are welded to the unconscious by primary process*), they slowly pass into secondary process*, where words and thought* activity predominate. This task also leads to construction* of historical truths* (concerning traumatic experiences originating primal repressions* and their fixation* points) that gradually determined the form of structuring of Triebe and the psychical apparatus*. Once reconstruction is complete, the degree of Trieb fixation tends to decrease, which gives the ego more freedom in the relationship with its wishes and therefore with objects.

The fundamental rule* is practised in order to achieve this objective. What does this mean? That patients must do something they cannot do when they are with others and sometimes not even when they are alone: aim their cathexes of attention* towards whatever comes to mind without conscious censorship*. Preconscious material emerges from this free association*: phantasies* or daydreams*, generally strung together by memories* and historical or linguistic associations produced by contiguity, analogy, or opposition, and also the day's events, worries, angers, narratives concerning affective and sometimes transference links, related with objects in the present.

Dreams and subsequent thoughts about them also tend to come up. The analysis of dreams is a privileged path to access the unconscious and thing-presentations; the primary process linking them appears to be just beneath their surface. This analysis may enable access to the forgotten infantile past in a fairly simple way, progressively enriching the representational content of the analysis.

Sometimes it is very difficult for patients to allow themselves to be carried away by their passing ideas, and therefore they insist that their analyst ask questions. Each patient has a particular manner which is not even a permanent manner. It varies with each person's life, sometimes depending on the analyst's manner as well.

In each individual case, the analytic attitude is one of evenly suspended attention*; the analyst tries to listen to the patient's associations or comments when they come up, to find links between these associative chains, which may in turn form new chains, or to discover them if they were not in the patient's conscious memory*.

When resistance to associating predominates, it may be due to transference resistance, something that characterizes the process of psychoanalytic treatment: the need to analyse transference* in order to overcome this resistance.

In this phenomenon, inherent to all sufficiently deep psychoanalytic processes, this "intermediate realm between illness and life", a true transference neurosis develops.

Then, a multitude of loving and hostile affects corresponding to the repressed are displaced on to the psychoanalyst, and are re-experienced with the same intensity they had when they originated; they are repeated instead of being remembered.

If this enables the analyst to corroborate previous constructions, it is a process involving an enriching crisis from which the treatment emerges unscathed and the patient's ego enriched, with good self-knowledge, a process that must be undergone and is difficult to describe. If resistance wins, the fate of the analysis hangs in the balance, and it may fail.

If analysis goes "well", new levels of meaning are gradually found which necessarily appear in relation with events from a more or less distant past, episodes in adolescence or latency* that reveal differences and similarities with current episodes.

Older memories emerge which may be set into the frame of their meaning with those already found, the latter acquiring other meanings as well. Thus, events of the present come to be understood on account of their similarities and differences in relation with pleasurable and traumatic events of the past.

Constructions* and interpretations* come nearer to the most remote infantile past, to the prehistory of the Oedipus complex*, even through repetitions in the transference link with the analyst, a link that may sometimes present a serious obstacle to the continuation of the analysis (transference resistance) but is almost always one of the major weapons for the cure.

When all these resistance episodes are overcome, during periods of "sublimated positive transference", construction of events of infantile sexuality* is possible; it results from the re-signification of remnants of memories, of re-analysed screen memories, or from the interpretation of dreams. These constructions sometimes acquire the appearance of memories*, or of the patient's convictions, whereas others are products of logical reasoning, consistent with all the former constructions and the interpretation of repetitions in the present.

Thus, a new history is gradually put together, different from the one the patient brought to analysis, capable of accounting for many aspects of the patient's life, the meaning of symptoms in the first place, of certain repetitive behaviour, and even ways of being or ego characteristics. These emerge as the "cataphylls of the onion" are peeled away and the puzzle is put together, two metaphors sometimes utilized by Freud as graphic representations of this complex process.

However, this path is not all strewn with roses; it is filled with all kinds of difficulties, especially by the patient's unconscious resistances; if the patient has fallen into this state, it is because this subject's psychical apparatus was unable to find any better defence from Triebe. Therefore, to propose to question it for the purpose of finding another, unknown way to defend it is something at least difficult to do, particularly since the process of falling ill is unknown to the preconscious ego and therefore unconscious.

Among the most complex resistances to resolve, apart from those already mentioned, are resistances coming from the unconscious superego, the origin of the need for punishment* which needs illness and ego suffering as a form of payment. The negative therapeutic reaction is produced as a result: once a construction is concluded, the patient's symptoms worsen instead of disappearing as would be expected. Resistance resulting from repetition compulsion* proceeding from the unconscious, which aims to continue repeating a facilitated path: the history of the formation of its Trieb or the history of its satisfaction-unsatisfaction. The negative therapeutic reaction is easier to deal with when it derives from identification rather than from a traumatic event of its own; that is to say, when it is "borrowed" (*The Ego and the Id*, 1923). If it is not, it is probably what is the most difficult to resolve. However, the psychoanalytic method is undaunted by this difficulty. Analysis insists on the interpretation and construction of facts or events in the analysis of this resistance in particular as it relates with the patient's history and the way this singular psychical apparatus was structured.

"Id resistance" requires working through, simply another step in the same process although more directly aimed at Triebe. For this reason it seeks to re-historicize the singular unfolding of Trieb, as Freud did in the "Wolf Man", to work through events with objects whose vicissitudes generated different paths with diverse fixation points. It is a question of producing changes or an opportunity for changes.

As their analysis progresses, patients acquire a growing notion of themselves, full and vivid; they accept their Triebe as their own, but differentiate these from action by choosing when and how to lead them to action, binding and taming them.

At the same time, the ego becomes more preconscious and is freer of superego impositions, remnants of parental mandates of childhood.

Patients therefore feel closer to their affects and wishes, now less eroticized (they form better social links). The ego is able to sublimate them and re-eroticize them whenever it wishes to do so, thereby becoming more capable of specific action*.

This is the path of the analytic cure, an arduous and difficult road for which, unlike other cures, the patient's participation is decisive. With art and experience, the analyst leads the patient to get over hurdles in the patient's own mind, but does not spare the patient from leaping over them.

As more ambitious aims are proposed, this path becomes longer, even interminable, which may constitute another paradoxical pitfall impeding the cure.

A final hurdle all patients need to overcome is their personal bedrock*, a product of infantile defence against recognition of sexual difference: ultimately, against acceptance of the existence of castration* at the moment when the definitive reality ego* is formed in the phallic phase, from which the ego does not escape untouched but having undergone some splitting. This ego splitting* tends to be inaccessible to analysis, a practically unsurmountable barrier.

In the case of narcissistic affections in general and narcissistic psychoses in particular, this technique must be modified since the problem is different. In these affections, cathexis is withdrawn from the unconscious object presentation, and therefore the wish for it is lost, this libido then cathecting the wounded ego. Work must therefore focus not on making conscious the unconscious but on recovering the unconscious itself or the unconscious object wish by generating a possibility in the patient to recathect the thing-presentation* through the therapeutic link with the aid of "scaffolding" that functions in the place of the ego – this may be psychopharmacological support, hospitalization, family therapy, day hospital and other resources – each of these depending on the magnitude and specificities of each case. In this way, the psychical apparatus* may be repaired so that the ego no longer needs to resort to extreme defences that produce narcissistic withdrawal and prevent sublimation and the establishment of social and love links; to recover the object wish without this wish creating such a feeling of helplessness* or so much automatic anxiety* in the ego. This is possible when the damage was not excessively severe.

Strengthening the ego includes the dilution, as far as possible, of the superego as a generator of guilt, which in this type of patients is closely bound with death Trieb* and may even lead to suicide at times of Trieb defusion, a danger the analyst always takes into account.

Statistics show a growing percentage of these patients in the general population, perhaps on account of more Trieb defusion produced along with cultural "progress". Work with them is tentative and thankless, since the family seldom cooperates. Families tend to demand quick results and an impossible, resounding success, both of therapist and patient (with whom they sometimes establish resistance alliances). This is part of their family and social pathology.

The need for and almost dependence on the cooperation of the family makes the road doubly difficult, but not impossible. Persistence and patience, together with knowledge of what may be accomplished as well as the limitations involved, tend to be the best virtues in these cases, usually leading to significant satisfactions. With respect to formal aspects such as the number of sessions, the type of interpretations, whether they should be historical or transference and when to communicate them, we consider that a larger number of sessions facilitates the depth of the analysis, although this estimation is not mathematical; more sessions may even increase resistance, especially if this frequency is imposed and accepted unwillingly by the patient (obsessional modality). It ultimately depends on many variables, including the characteristics of the patient's pathology and even the different moments of the treatment. The depth of the treatment may also be calibrated in function of all the variables involved. Brief psychoanalyses may be undertaken whose objectives are limited and symptoms are cured, such as Freud did, for example in the case of Katharina*, early in his practice, but also later on, as shown in this passage from a letter to Theodor Reik when his colleague asked him about his meeting with the famous composer, G. Mahler:

> I analyzed Mahler for an afternoon in 1912 (1913?) in Leyden. If I may believe reports, I achieved much with him at that time. This visit appeared necessary to him, because his wife at the time rebelled against the fact that he withdrew his libido from her. In highly interesting expeditions through his life history, we discovered his personal conditions for love, especially his Holy Mary complex (mother fixation). I had plenty of opportunity to admire the capability for psychological understanding of this man of genius. No light fell at the time on the symptomatic façade of his obsessional neurosis. It was as if you would dig a single shaft through a mysterious building.
>
> (Reik, T., *The Haunting Melody: Experiences in Life and Music*, 1953, pp. 342–3)

According to this passage, in 1935, Freud considered this therapy with limited objectives at least one type of analysis; we may of course observe that it was not a complete psychoanalytic process (since the obsessional neurotic façade remained unexplained, as he wrote), although this psychoanalytic action produced changes, precisely in the areas that most perturbed the patient and for which he requested help.

It is also possible to try to advance further in the adventure of producing structural changes in the psychical apparatus, but this process requires steps and conditions that do not always exist. Psychoanalysis is a creative occupation and therefore, always within certain parameters, knowing what must be done, a method must be created for each case in particular, adapted to each patient's individual circumstances and also to the therapist's own individuality.

PSYCHOSIS

Ger.: Psychose. – Sp.: psicosis. – Fr.: psychose. – It.: psicosi. – Port.: psicose.

This type of mental affection is characterized by the ego's* withdrawal from reality*. Apparently, the problem is between the ego and the external world, but this is not at all simple, since we need to elucidate, among other things, aspects such as the cause for which the subject has withdrawn from reality, which aspects of it are withdrawn from and in what way, whether different types of psychosis exist, and whether in this case the problems are different (cf. schizophrenia*, paranoia*, Meynert's amentia*, melancholia*, mania*).

> There are certainly good grounds for being suspicious of such simple solutions of a problem. Moreover, the most that we may expect is that this formula will turn out to be correct in the roughest outline. But even that would be something.
>
> (*Neurosis and Psychosis*, 1924, p. 149)

What most interests the subject about reality is the object*. Triebe are satisfied in the link with it; it is the source of pleasure*, and therefore the reality wished for is everything relating to the object. The subject wishes to learn about reality because the object belongs to it. Reality must be known in order to obtain the object; at least in regard to sexual*, object, and narcissistic Triebe* (in the latter due to the portion of self-esteem* contributed by the actual object's love* and the portion that proceeds from the love of objects in the past, from infantile sexuality, and also that which proceeds from homosexual libido which is partly narcissistic, from tender links and social links, even cases of sexual* perversions in which the ego's self-esteem is supported by homosexual object libido).

However, links with objects are complex: they produce pleasure, but they also generate frustrations* and even pain*. For self-defence against these latter consequences, the subject may withdraw from them and therefore also from those aspects of reality most relevant to his or her wishes. The subject may take refuge in narcissism*, for example: since the object no longer loves the ego, the id* can certainly love it, decathecting presentations* of object wishes and cathecting* ego presentations: we are in the sphere of narcissistic psychoses in which the object wish is broken off, and since there is no unconscious object wish, what is the use of reality? Libidinal withdrawal* is produced, and this libido now cathects the ego with the aim of stanching its wounds, this situation producing clinical effects such as the experience of the end of the world (as a consequence of libidinal withdrawal from object presentations, with loss of the unconscious wish for them), megalomania* (because libidinal cathexis moves into the ego), hypochondria* and organ speech* (cathexis of the ego begins with the body; language* disturbance is caused by decathexis of the unconscious thing-presentation* and persistence of cathexis of the preconscious word-presentation* but without unconscious support as a thing-presentation). What occurs is that the ego is wounded narcissistically and needs to be stanched: to be recathected with libido. There is no longer a wish for the object to do this, since the ego has broken off from the unconscious object wish. Schizophrenia, paranoia, mania, and melancholia belong to this type of psychoses, which Freud also called narcissistic neuroses.

In order to truly reconstruct the world of object relations, narcissistic neuroses need to break down the narcissistic wall of defence behind which the ego is hiding, defenceless against each new frustration, which makes it more difficult.

At other times, the object may not love us or we may lose it, it may die, and we persist in our untamed wish to possess it. In this case reality* also tends to be disavowed*, and is filled in with hallucination* of the presence of the object, at least for a certain period of time. Here, the ego is overwhelmed by the object wish proceeding from the id, and withdrawal from reality takes place in this way: the hyper-cathected unconscious wish razes an ego not strong enough to inhibit the magnitude of cathexis of the object (homosexual object) wish, and is overcome by it. This occurs in acute hallucinatory psychoses or Meynert's amentia*. In these cases, there is neither narcissistic withdrawal nor loss of object wish, but apparently the opposite: the object wish is so strong that, in response to the reality of its loss, this loss is disavowed and the psychical apparatus regresses to "hallucinatory* wish* fulfilment". It is a different type of withdrawal from reality – essentially an intrapsychical mechanism – which produces a very important difference in prognosis of the clinical picture. In Meynert's amentia it is more acute and its future is better insomuch as object loss may be recognized with pain, which at first is impossible, then difficult, because the type of previous link with the object was regressive without total ego-non-ego differentiation: the homosexual type of object choice inherent to infantile sexuality. In time the object may eventually be substituted.

Hysterical clinical pictures are severe neuroses with important alterations of the ego* in which the problem is related to repressed incestuous sexuality* returning from the repressed*, not only as conversion* symptoms* but also as visual hallucinations (Anna O.'s* serpents and the *Gradiva* perceived by the character Norbert Hanold in Jenssen's novel), producing intense anxiety* when they satisfy repressed wishes incompatible with the ego, which does not acquiesce to them.

PUNISHMENT, NEED FOR

Ger.: Strafbedürnis. – Sp.: castigo, necesidad de. – Fr.: besoin de punition. – It.: castigo, necessità di. – Port.: castigo, necessidade de.

Also incorrectly called unconscious sense of guilt*, it is a product of destructive Trieb* (deflection of death Trieb to the external world), re-introduced secondarily into the psychical apparatus* through binding* by the unconscious superego*.

Need for punishment is not perceived by the subject as anything in particular; it is inferred from behaviour or from deeply rooted persistence of neurosis.

When it is predominant or chronic, it produces pathological characters such as "those wrecked by success"* (1916, p. 316) or "criminals from a sense of guilt"* (Ibid., p. 332).

It is also one of the strongest resistances* against the cure, the origin of the "negative therapeutic reaction" (1923, p. 49) which consists of aggravation of the illness when the meaning of a symptom*, a dream*, a repetition compulsion*, or a character trait* has been reconstructed or revealed. This resistance corresponds to the superego as a psychical structure.

It may also be expressed as a tendency to accidents and even organic illnesses. In these cases, it is usually referred to as "neurosis of destiny". We may remember that destiny, for the unconscious, corresponds to the father, and ultimately to paternal punishment.

PUNISHMENT DREAMS

Ger.: Strafträume. – Sp.: sueños punitorios. – Fr.: rêves punitifs. – It.: sogni di punizione. – Port.: sonhos punitórios.

In these dreams*, superego* wishes* are fulfilled. The situation of punishment of the ego* sought by the superego and sometimes by the ego* is represented as having taken place (the superego's sadism*and the ego's masochism*). It is determined by a repressed unconscious wish proceeding from the id*. The superego accuses the ego of having this wish, even though the preconscious ego considers this disguised wish foreign to the ego.

The affect* produced by these dreams is unpleasurable, similar to anxiety* when the dreamer awakens, since the situation of punishment is remembered as a danger-situation*. During dreaming, however, the tone may be indifferent (the punishment is counteracted by relief of guilt resulting from its expiation through it) or painful.

The need for punishment* is satisfied by punishment dreams. But what is its source? Is it the preconscious* (as Freud states in *The Interpretation of Dreams*, 1900, p. 558), or does it proceed directly from the unconscious? To answer this question we need to consider that Freud subsequently postulates an unconscious part of the superego, and that he also points out (in *The Ego and the Id*, 1923, and in *New Introductory Lectures on Psycho-Analysis*, 1933) that the root of the superego is closer to the id* than to external reality*, unlike the ego whose core centres on the perceptual-conscious system.

Therefore, in spite of being fulfilment of superego punishment, it is of course wish fulfilment, and we could even say fulfilment of unconscious wishes; but we must also remember that this punishment is for something, and this something is the unconscious repressed wish; therefore, this is a complex level of a psychical apparatus* involving struggles between different systems with opposing wishes.

PURIFIED PLEASURE EGO

Ger.: Lust-Ich. – Sp.: yo placer purificado. – Fr.: moi-plaisir purifié. – It.: io piacere purificato. – Port.: ego de prazer purificado.

Freud explains that this type of ego functioning is ruled by the pleasure principle* and may be thought of as predominant in the origins of the psyche in relation with sexual Triebe*.

It is in itself a type of logic that gives a name to a form of ego functioning which may again rule mental functioning more or less in disguise, at least in part, even behind the apparent definitive reality ego*, which is even grounded by it. We could simply think that unconscious defence mechanisms function largely according to the rules of the pleasure ego, utilized, however, against any possibility of Trieb satisfaction, since primal repression* made them unpleasurable for the preconscious ego.

This hedonistic logic considers everything causing pleasure* as ego. Therefore, if the object* produces pleasure, the object is ego. With the same logic, we draw the conclusion that everything indifferent or unpleasurable is not-ego, but rather an object or the external world.

The logic of judgements of this type of ego is obviously not ruled by the reality principle* but by the pleasure principle. Therefore, it corresponds to the ego of defence*: the unconscious ego. Utilizing the same logic, this ego (in adults) rejects id tendencies that produce its anxiety signal*, withstands them, does not make them its own; they are not-ego, since they generate unpleasure*. It deploys defence mechanisms or secondary repressions against them, which already indicate a failure of primal repression and return of the repressed*, a compromise between the ego and Trieb* endeavouring to return to it; therefore the ego, on orders from the superego*, banishes it as an "internal stranger".

However, bases are thereby laid for the definitive reality ego to function, except that in its origins and its own infrastructure this pleasure ego functions against Trieb, a type of functioning in which the superego participates and does so even unconsciously, through unconscious sense of guilt* or need for punishment: guilt that requires expiation.

The purified pleasure ego functions with the category of *being**, it is or is not the pleasure; there is no *having** within its conceptions. Everything it *is*, everything pleasurable, is loved; what it *is* not, everything unpleasurable, is hated.

Thus, based on this type of ego functioning, it is possible to reach wild conclusions: for example, if the object is pleasurable and I am the object, then when part of my body produces unpleasure, I do not accept it as ego.

This ego aims to be pure, pure pleasure. It purifies unpleasure by removing it to a distance. It is ideal in this way: unpleasure has no place in it since it defines itself by pleasure.

When the subject begins to control the muscular system, this subject is no longer forced to obey this ego, since the individual may begin to perform some specific actions* and therefore no longer needs the ego omnipotence provided by the purified pleasure ego.

Then, when individuals discover their dependency on the object and the implicit possibility of frustration, fear of object loss*, and so on, it is tempting to return to the rule of the pleasure ego: to withdraw cathexes from unconscious object wishes, cathect the ego, and thereby return to narcissism*.

However, this level differs from the one we presented when we stated that unconscious defence mechanisms were ultimately ruled by the pleasure ego. In that case, the rest of the preconscious ego was ruled by the reality principle. However, narcissistic affections break away from reality*, and therefore its functioning is ruled predominantly by the pleasure ego.

PURPOSIVE IDEA

Ger.: Zielvorstellung. – Sp.: representación-meta. – Fr.: représentation-but. – It.: rappresentazione meta. – Port.: representação meta.

This is the presentation* of the objective of the wish*, whether preconscious or unconscious (voluntary or involuntary in the conscious ego). Freud explains the voluntary wish when he needs to demonstrate coherence between thought* and the movement from the aim sought to action; however, his most important discovery is that the purposive idea also exists in apparently involuntarily erroneous attitudes or parapraxes, in dreams*, in neurotic symptoms*, and other phenomena. The purposive idea ultimately corresponds to the repressed unconscious wish, which gains expression by infiltrating primary process* into secondary process* through a fissure in secondary process.

Then, the purpose sought by the unconscious wish is not tolerated by the ego*. Since this produces anxiety*, the ego resorts to defence mechanisms*. They block knowledge of the purpose sought by this wish, now repressed and therefore prevented from entering thought and, more important, from being put into action by the ego.

The concept of the purposive idea shows the unconscious* psyche as having intention and direction. Sometimes a purposive idea comes into conflict with purposive ideas belonging to other unconscious or preconscious wishes (to the superego*, for example); in this case, the former unconscious wish returns to its state of repression* in search of fulfilment of its purpose, in disguise.

Inhibition of the Trieb* aim in order to make it socially acceptable originates aim-inhibited Triebe such as tenderness, friendship, and social sentiments, which also participate in sublimation* and the shaping of the ego.

Q

QUALITY

Ger.: Qualität. – Sp.: cualidad. – Fr.: qualité. – It.: qualità. – Port.: qualidade.

A characteristic acquired by a phenomenon when it is perceived by a subject through the subject's perceptual-consciousness (Pcpt.-Cs.) system, quality is therefore perceptual, part of the subjectivization of things of the world and even a means by which the psychical apparatus defends itself from quantities of excitation entering it from external reality (nature, fellow human beings, and the biological body).

In the real external world only "masses in motion" exist (*Project for a Scientific Psychology*, 1950). The perceptual apparatus perceives them as qualities, and continues to do so until they reach a maximum beyond which they are registered as pain* and so long as they do not go beyond a minimum below which they are not perceived. Between these two extremes lie all the nuances of qualities: colours, forms, odours, movements, in sum, everything perceptible by the senses.

The Pcpt.-Cs. perceives the masses of the external world as qualities, and also perceives its own energetic changes; thus, increases of energy are felt as unpleasure* and decreases as pleasure*.

With language* acquisition, words may be perceived as an external qualitative perception* since they have been emitted in speech and have therefore been heard. Consequently, the perceptual-consciousness system (Pcpt.-Cs.) may perceive relation between its thing-presentations* by virtue of word-presentations* which symbolize or represent them, moderating passages between them, a characteristic of the secondary process* whose highest expression is thought* activity, by means of the inhibiting action of the preconscious ego*. Then, by virtue of memory of emissions of word-presentations, this process may be omitted and thought perceived without need to emit the word again, since it has become automatic. Like everything else, this shortcut has its advantages and disadvantages; among the latter we could place the process of repression which is dedicated to cut this circuit of arrival to consciousness of whatever comes from memory (the presentation) by decathecting precisely the words that represent it in consciousness.

When any quantity of excitation entering from the body binds with presentations (Trieb*, desire*, libido*), it then acquires presentational quality, which is no longer perceptual quality but psychical quality which originated in perception. It is the memory that is now wished for; it is the perceptual quality endeavoured to be refound: the object* that produced it. The specific action* is required in order to reach this aim.

QUANTITY OF EXCITATION

Ger.: Reizmengen (Erregungsquantitäten). – Sp.: cantidad de excitación. – Fr.: quantité d'excitation. – It.: quantitá d'eccitazione. – Port.: quantidade de excitação.

A quantum of energy that enters the apparatus and is perceived by the perceptual-conscious pole (Pcpt.-Cs.); it originates in the external world (nature, fellow human beings), the subject's own body or both sources combined.

The Pcpt.-Cs. is composed essentially of sense organs, among which the different erotogenic zones* are found. Whether it originates in nature, fellow human beings or the subject's own body, this energy produces an initial type of response: an internal change*, a nonspecific type of reaction, a reflex action, a relic of what in phylogeny could have been an act adequate to an aim and now expresses only an emotion, an affect*. When this quantity is perceived in the Pcpt.-Cs., it becomes a quality*: unpleasure*; with the experience of satisfaction in relation to the object, pleasure is registered. Subsequently, when the quantity of stimulus coming from the body enters the psychical apparatus, it binds with a presentation* (first an unconscious thing-presentation*; in order to reach the ego's* consciousness and be thought, thereby acquiring a possibility to carry out action, it needs a word-presentation*). When the quantity is bound to a presentation, it becomes a wish* for something which then possesses an aim (it is no longer a nonspecific change); therefore, it takes on presentational quality. If the wish is sexual it is also called libido*; if it is related to self-preservation, it is called interest*. The term Eros* includes these two, although it is true that its use – starting with Freud himself – has made Eros a synonym of libido. In reality, the latter is broader, since it encompasses life Triebe* in general which include self-preservative Triebe*. Therefore, Eros is life Trieb in opposition to death Trieb*.

Death Trieb has no unconscious* (thing) presentation of the subject's own death. Thing-presentations are mainly traces of experiences or historical truths*; there is no experience of one's own death nor can there be; there may be of another person's death and from it, through thought, consequences may be drawn, but this is called thought and corresponds to secondary process and words rather than to unconscious thing-presentations.

There may however be presentations of another's death, and when this presentation is cathected, it becomes destructive Trieb* which presses towards this destruction, aimed now at the object.

Destructive Trieb manifests in this way, with different degrees of admixture, but always after having become destructive Trieb.

Because of its mixture with Eros (basically when it cathects its presentation or is cathected by it), destructive Trieb may or may not be led to action, may also be repressed, sublimated and so on, just as hate* or Trieb for mastery* and sadism* (ultimately, they are synonymous in spite of some small differences).

However, death Trieb is also free in the psychical apparatus, without presentation, in the form of primary masochism*, whose characteristic is a general tendency to unbind quantity from the presentation in opposition to the pleasure principle*, a tendency to re-transform quality already achieved (presentational quality achieved when quantity was bound to the presentation) Into pure quantity (perilously nearing the inorganic). Ultimately, death Trieb drives towards this return to quantity, to make the world of quality disappear, since the latter is much more closely related to life Triebe. When death Trieb is deflected towards the external world by virtue of the muscular apparatus, its name is destructive Trieb, which already involves some fusion with Eros.

The psychical apparatus is able to endure only a certain quantity of excitation in it, and is built to multiply its own complexity, which tends to moderate quantities entering it from its body (Triebe) or from the external world (stimuli). We could say that this is its main function, to transform quantity into complexity or into quality (by binding them to presentations); this gradually generates the diversity of responses that stimuli may obtain from each individual psychical apparatus.

For the psychical apparatus, quality originates in conscious perception* itself, and presentation is simply a more or less distorted memory* of it. When quantity is bound to presentations, it acquires presentational or psychical quality. It seeks to recover perceptual quality (wishes for and presses towards it), and thereby to refind the object (cf. refinding the object*) (*Negation*, 1925), now wished for in the external world, in order to be able, through a more or less specific action*, to discharge the level of quantity of excitation that provided the "initial kick-off".

Energy is bound to presentations in two ways; as freely flowing energy* and as bound or quiescent energy*. As free energy it is displaced from one presentation to another by the laws of association* as identities, typical of unconscious primary process*, with thing-presentations. As quiescent energy, it has a strong cathexis*, weak displacement, and word-presentations typical of secondary process*or thought* whose seat is the preconscious* pertaining to the ego*. The word provides quality since it is in itself a conscious perception and also because it signifies, symbolizes or represents to consciousness* the presentation of the wished-for thing.

Quantity of excitation provoked by sexual Triebe* of fellow human beings produces excitations in erotogenic zones still "unawakened" in the child's life; lacking potential understanding by the psychical apparatus, they produce sexual traumas* and therefore generate fixation points of infantile sexuality*, the origin of eventual character traits*, neurosis*, and so on. When the phase of predominance arrives to this erotogenic zone, it does so with the quantum of excitation corresponding to the traumatic event, against which the ego tends to defend itself with an extreme anticathexis*. The quantity of excitation coming from the body is not the same in all stages of life. Its affluence is greater in the period of the Oedipus complex* and its 're-editions': puberty, adolescence, and menopause, when it therefore tends to trigger moments of decompensation or neurosis.

In his metapsychological papers of 1915, Freud refers to this quantity of excitation, which circulates in diverse ways because of its various types of presentations, as "quantum of affect". The vicissitudes of quantum and presentation sometimes differ: in the case of repression, for example, it is the presentation that is repressed; this may or may not produce a decrease of affective discharge since it is independent of the presentation. In any case, the more the affect* (anxiety*) decreases or disappears, the more successful repression is (in this regard, it is more successful in hysteria than in phobia* or obsessional neurosis*).

The birth trauma* consists in a massive invasion of quantity of excitation stemming fundamentally from bodily needs; in normal conditions, it is soothed by a fellow human being, by someone (a psychical object*) in the child's environment, which Freud referred to as extraneous help*; for this reason and in different ways, the individual never becomes detached from need of the object *(Inhibitions, Symptoms and Anxiety*, 1925). The different types of anxiety against which the ego defends itself (fear of loss of the object*, castration anxiety*, fear of the superego* and social anxiety*) are mediations in response to the fundamental invasion of quantity into the psychical apparatus: automatic anxiety*.

Schizophrenics are victims, at the outset of their illness (with rupture from the unconscious wish for the object and decathexis of the thing-presentation), of a massive invasion of quantity of excitation or automatic anxiety (when the quantity of excitation reaches a certain magnitude, it automatically becomes anxiety); this coincides with an experience of the end of the world, a product of decathexis* of unconscious presentation of objects that leaves the psychical apparatus helpless and unable to bind the quantity of excitation, qualify it, and make it complex (*The Unconscious*, 1915; *A Metapsychological Supplement to the Theory of Dreams*, 1917 [1915]).

QUIESCENT (BOUND) ENERGY

Ger.: gebundene Energie. – Sp.: energía quiescente (ligada). – Fr.: énergie quiescente (liée). – It.: energia quiescente (legata). – Port.: energía quiescente (ligada).

This term describes bound energy* because the possible connection between presentations* must go through severe processing and complex handling that moderate its passage into action.

Quiescent energy belongs to the preconscious* part of the ego*. It is formed essentially of libido* with diverse degrees of desexualization* and different degrees of fusion with death Trieb* which the ego sometimes calls upon to help it subject sexual Trieb*. Its fusion with different levels of sexual Trieb also enables it to keep death Trieb in check.

The strongest and true binding is obtained when presentations corresponding to unconscious Trieb* or wishes* request access to the ego, which acquiesces, receives them, and converses with them. That is to say, they are processed by thought* activity, and accepted as the ego's own, while showing them reality* (corresponding to nature, fellow beings, and possibilities of the subject's own body); consequently, reality participates in the discussion regarding their path towards action.

In sum: the thing-presentation* is bound to the word-presentation and the latter to other words. Establishment of these complex links moderates passages between presentations.

Thus, this relative quiescence of energy forms which must eventually go into action at the adequate moment and in an appropriate way.

Sometimes, the ego needs to resort to judgement of condemnation* to avoid or postpone action, always considering this Trieb or wish as its own.

One of the objectives of psychoanalysis as a treatment is precisely the ego's taming of Trieb* after recognition of its existence, the history of its formation, and utilization of secondary process* and its quiescent energy in order to choose and calibrate the mode and manner in which to satisfy Triebe based on better knowledge of reality* and also with the consent of the superego. It must connect the unconscious* to the preconscious by refinding the corresponding words to give meaning to unconscious thing-presentations; then, the latter become part of wishes, now preconscious ego wishes the ego must include in its thought activity in order to moderate their passages while recognizing reality.

Energy also becomes quiescent when fixations* in erotogenic zones* and object presentations of Trieb are produced by establishment of anticathexes*. These anticathexes may be more or less successful (compensations by character disorders, for example), but always at the cost of impoverishment of the ego, since they ignore Trieb and blindly obey the superego which proceeds to dominate the scene. In these cases, when Trieb increases defences may fail and the repressed may return*. It does so with free and compulsive energy, which is the situation of presentations in the state of repression*, generating pathology corresponding to the neuroses.

R

REACTION FORMATION

Ger.: Reaktionsbildung. – Sp.: formación reactiva. – Fr.: formation réactionnelle. – It.: formazione reattiva. – Port.: formação reativa.

This type of defence mechanism* of the unconscious ego* consists essentially of an anticathexis* (composed of the cathexis* of presentations* exactly the opposite of those of a given wish* or libidinal Trieb*, usually anal-sadistic).

An anticathexis by which the ego relieves anxiety produced by the wished-for presentation and, repressed, acts in the opposite direction in relation to satisfaction of the Trieb.

This anticathexis arises as primary repression* of aggressive Triebe* of the anal-sadistic stage, which generates alterations of the ego* that eventually constitute its character*.

It is therefore a defence mechanism that generates character traits more than defences. This product is not felt to be foreign but rather as belonging to the ego. It is usually an early resource consolidated by formation of the superego*, itself a formation of this type:

"The superego is, however, not simply a residue of the earliest object choices of the id; it also represents an energetic reaction formation against these choices" (*The Ego and the Id*, p. 34).

However, other levels of reaction formation do not compromise the ego's character. For example, in hysteria*, in response to a certain object*, in reality hated, extremely opposite actions against this hatred are taken. This reaction formation is localized, refers to a specific object presentation, and does not become a constant ego reaction or character trait. In any case, although it is circumscribed, it refers to ego actions not felt to be foreign or contrary to the Trieb wish. Reaction formation of the anal erotogenic zone* causes fixation* to it and configures the obsessional character which constitutes "*apparent* health, but actually, of successful defence" (*Further Remarks on the Neuro-Psychoses of Defence*, p. 169); so long as the repressed does not return (cf. return of the repressed*). For their part, obsessional neurotics* (in whom the repressed returns) utilize other mechanisms to reinforce the ego defence* secondarily against anal-sadistic Triebe (now also oedipal), such as undoing (what has been done)* and isolation*. Ceremonials and other actions are configured, typical of obsessional neurosis whose characteristic pathological features are obsessions, expressions of return of the repressed, with access to word-presentations*: words not accepted by the ego as its own and which generate anxiety.

Until the return of the repressed, successful reaction formation configures an ego identity syntonic with it, which it recognizes as the ego. This is in opposition to obsessive compulsive ideas and acts (expressions of returning Trieb) contrary to the ego recognized as the official ego up to the moment when neurosis breaks out.

REALISTIC ANXIETY

Ger.: Realangst. – Sp.: angustia realista. – Fr.: angoisse devant un danger réel. – It.: angoscia (di fronte a una situazione) reale. – Port.: angústia realista.

This specific, unpleasurable, affective state in response to perception* of an external danger is akin to fear, an affect* remaining after the experience of pain*.

Freud describes:

> Realistic anxiety strikes us as something very rational and intelligible. We may say of it that it is a reaction to the perception of an external danger – that is, of an injury which is expected and foreseen. It is connected with the flight reflex and it may be regarded as a manifestation of the self-preservative instinct.
> (1917, pp. 393–4)

A few lines below, he questions the expediency of the anxiety* response to danger by observing that an adequate response would be to face it or to flee. Therefore, realistic anxiety is expedient if it is simply a signal that enables the ego* to find the adequate action; if, however, this anxiety paralyzes the ego, the latter may lose the possibility to preserve itself.

In *Inhibitions, Symptoms and Anxiety* (1925) he includes among realistic anxieties those anxieties felt by children in the process of recognition of the object* as a source of pleasure*: fear of object loss and castration anxiety*.

These anxieties are realistic since (at that period) danger comes from outside. They are no longer realistic when the ego utilizes them in a deferred manner as signals based on memories* in order to generate defence mechanisms* against Trieb* coming from inside the body.

REALITY PRINCIPLE

Ger.: Realitätprinzip. – Sp.: principio de realidad. – Fr.: principe de realité. – It.: principio di realtà. – Port.: princípio da realidade.

This form of mental functioning rules the working of the preconscious and conscious ego*; it is possible only when differences between wished-for presentations* and what is perceived are recognized.

However, the ego attempts to find some identity between the perceived and the wished for, and does so by utilizing thought*, thereby reaching certain levels of thought identity*, of refinding the object*.

The reality principle arises as a need to tame primary process* (ruled by the pleasure principle*) and to take it to alloplastic* specific action* "to change the face of the earth". In this sense it is an extension of the pleasure principle, but involves real pleasure.

For this purpose, secondary process* "reality testing"* is required with its strong cathexis* and weak displacement* of cathexis among presentations in order to compare and study the object perceived, to ascertain how close it is to what is wished for or feared, and to act in consequence.

By virtue of this principle reality is recognized, both pleasurable and unpleasurable.

Sometimes, in this endeavour, the preconscious ego may make a judgement of condemnation*, a Trieb motion it accepts as its own, and postpone action.

REALITY TESTING

Ger.: Realität prüfung. – Sp.: examen de realidad. – Fr.: examen de la réalité. – It.: esame della realtà. – Port.: exame da realidade.

This is one of the great institutions of the ego*, together with its synthetic function and moral conscience* (although the latter strictly corresponds to a part that splits off from the ego and opposes it: the superego; morals themselves may partly correspond to the ego).

Its central function is to differentiate between wishful presentations* and perceptions*.

Freud explains:

> Let us, furthermore, bear in mind the great practical importance of distinguishing perceptions from ideas, however intensely recalled. Our whole relation to the external world, to reality, depends on our ability to do so. We have put forward the fiction that we did not always possess this ability and that at the beginning of our mental life we did in fact hallucinate the satisfying object when we felt the need for it. But in such a situation satisfaction did not occur, and this failure must very soon have moved us to create some contrivance with the help of which it was possible to distinguish such

> wishful perceptions from a real fulfilment and to avoid them for the future. In other words, we gave up hallucinatory satisfaction of our wishes at a very early period and set up a kind of "reality testing".
>
> (*A Metapsychological Supplement to the Theory of Dreams*, 1917, p. 231)

The ego's perception-consciousness system (Pcpt.-Cs.) does this reality testing.

It is sometimes a simple muscular action (opening and closing the eyes, for example), by which a perception can be made to disappear. At other times, it consists of a complex action, study of the perception, which determines, attribute by attribute, the difference between perception and wishful presentation.

This meticulous examination of the *perceptum* is similar to the scientist as he utilizes cognitive thought*. The largest possible amount of preconscious presentations must be stored in the ego's memory in order to compare them to the new *perceptum*, since the wish* will filter through any gaps of error.

REFINDING THE OBJECT

Ger.: Wiederfindung des Objekts. – Sp.: reencuentro del objeto. – Fr.: retrouvaille de l'objet. – It.: rincontro del oggetto. – Port.: re-encontro do objeto.

Object* libido aims at this goal on its way towards satisfaction.

The object* wish* has originated in gain of pleasure in the experience of satisfaction of self-preservative Trieb*, which also awakened organ pleasure corresponding to autoeroticism*.

Thus, the mother was chosen as the first object of pleasure. As the ego* gradually formed, it also became partly a substitute for the object, giving birth to narcissism*, and consequently, narcissistic object choice.

We partly leave aside the problem of narcissism in order to refer specifically to object choice, independent of its base in narcissism or in anaclisis* in the case of self-preservative Trieb.

At a moment in the development of sexuality – during the period of the Oedipus complex* – maternal object choice became conflictive (due to castration anxiety in boys and castration complex* with its fear of loss of love in girls), and dissolved or "sank to the bottom". Especially in boys, it lost its sensual cathexis* in exchange for the attenuation or inhibition of the aim called "tenderness".

After the latency* period, it is reborn with all its virulence in puberty and adolescence, when it again chooses the object of pleasure, a choice marked by attributes of the first infantile choice, forgotten by the preconscious, but which the unconscious seeks to "refind".

The object is now exogamic. However, the attributes of the first infantile object choice, forgotten or remembered through repetitive action unknown to the definitive reality ego* that is already established in the psychical apparatus*, "subjected" by external reality and the superego*.

> The first and immediate aim, therefore, of reality testing is, not to find an object in real perception which corresponds to the one presented, but to refind such an object, to convince oneself that it is still there.
>
> (*Negation*, 1925, pp. 237–8)

The finding and choice of object accomplished after puberty and the definitive development of sexuality is in reality a search to refind, aided by what is stored in memory, the first object and the sensations felt with it. However, this first object became incestuous when the subject accessed culture* and it became prohibited; consequently, repression's* blanket of forgetting was thrown over it.

REFLEX ATTENTION

Ger.: Reflexaufmerksamkeit. – Sp.: atención refleja o reflectoria. – It.: attenzione riflessa. – Port.: atenção reflexa.

In his *Project for a Scientific Psychology* of 1895 (1950), paragraph 15 (Primary and secondary process), Freud describes different levels of cathexis of attention in the perceptual apparatus; one remains nearly constant and produces innervation of the muscular system, bound to attention when a certain stimulus is perceived (examples: when eye muscles are innervated, vision is directed towards this stimulus; muscles of hair follicles produce "goose bumps").

This muscular reflex response acts as a signal that must be sent to the perceptual apparatus, a second level of attention cathexis*: copious attention with which the stimulus may be localized and explored, bound to previous presentations* and finally result in carrying out (or not) specific action* (to pursue it if it is a wished-for object or to flee it if it is dangerous), if real possibility allows it.

In an actual traumatic situation*, this first level of attention is devastated, thereby interrupting the normal process of constant exploration of the real, which forces the apparatus to repeat the traumatic scene, either in action or in traumatic dreams in order to obtain enough previous and necessary reflex attention to enable binding* and passage to the pleasure principle*.

Reflex attention is therefore a level previous to the copious and "psychically utilizable" attention necessary for safekeeping psychical functioning. When it is devastated in the traumatic event, the pleasure principle is unable to establish itself properly, and the Nirvana principle consequently becomes predominant.

REGRESSION

Ger.: Regression. – Sp.: regression. – Fr.: régression. – It.: regressione. – Port.: regressão.

This psychical process of the entire psychical apparatus or parts of it usually defends against id* Trieb*, repressed wishes*, frustrations* of reality* or of the object* which involve previous recognition of a topical direction (synchronic: analogous to the sense applied by F. de Saussure in relation to language*) and progressive libidinal development (diachronic, in relation to the individual's history) in the same psychical apparatus, contrary to the direction taken by regression.

Therefore, regression understood in the broad sense results from the utilization of mechanisms previous to the level reached at the time.

Regression goes back to mechanisms utilized by the psychical apparatus previously in time, or back to the original point of a quantity of excitation* which had reached complex levels of binding; to forms of binding previous to actual binding; to previous mechanisms or forms of satisfaction of infantile sexuality* or to ego* defence mechanisms* against the latter, previous in time to those currently utilized.

Therefore, aside from the broad sense of the concept, diverse types of specific regression exist. For example, topical regression is characteristic of the mechanism of dreams*, but is related to all types of regressions including temporal and formal regressions.

During sleep, libidinal regression to narcissism* does not in itself correspond to the dream mechanism but does influence it, for example, in that the main characters in the dream represent aspects of the patient's ego.

In dreams, dream work* originates a wish-fulfilling phantasy* which unites repressed unconscious wishes with day residues* which at some moment become established in the preconscious (and therefore have word-presentations*), from which they are expelled by repression*; during sleep, access to the motor end* is prohibited and therefore regression takes place at the perceptual end*.

Thus, wishes are "seen" to be fulfilled, not through actions but through images, incomprehensible to the preconscious ego given the displacements* and condensations* undergone by what are predominantly visual thing-presentations*; precisely because of the resulting disguise, the latter are utilized by repression to ignore the repressed wish implicit in them, and sometimes the punishment for this wish as well.

Topical regression takes place by regressing from the preconscious to the unconscious and, instead of completing the arc of Trieb by action at the motor end, returning to the perceptual end: both are types of topical regression. Thus, the type of presentation* changes: from the word to the thing to the image. The same may be said for the way presentations interrelate, for which primary process* is now utilized; these are formal regressions. The psychical apparatus again resorts to "hallucinatory wish fulfilment", which is both a temporal and formal regression, and is also the mechanism which in the Freudian hypothesis is the infant's first.

This hallucination* is a perception* and therefore undergoes secondary elaboration* by the preconscious ego; this is its response to all perception in its endeavour to find logical coherence in order to understand it; however, it thereby succeeds in even further disguising the repressed wish expressed by the dream's content.

Libidinal regression, related with whatever is "diachronic" and developmental, is what moves towards fixation* points emerging during the development of sexuality* as a result of traumatic events occurring in it; it may also move towards the same changes in the predominance of one erotogenic zone* over another; when an erotogenic zone has been excessively pleasurable, it becomes difficult to leave behind and, when problems corresponding to the new zone appear, it may be more difficult for the patient's ego which perhaps returns to previous mechanisms, erotogenic zones, or types of link with objects through these zones. All this occurs in a dynamic manner, and the patient tends to suffer constant ups and downs in regard to mechanisms and forms of pleasure* sought; in any case, a certain type of defence usually corresponds to each erotogenic zone. These defences are led by repression (they obey its orders, each in its own way), especially repression of the Oedipus complex*, the "greatest trauma* of infantile sexuality", upon which the constitution of the psychical apparatus is structured from that point forward.

In this way, a disposition* is configured from which the repressed* may return, and for that purpose Trieb regresses to fixation points, and from this position, bombards the ego, generating neurotic symptoms*.

The fixation point belonging to *conversion hysteria** is phallic; therefore, what is repressed in this illness are vicissitudes in the link with the object corresponding to the phase of the Oedipus complex, with its repressed incestuous object wish and the appearance of the rival, for example. Libidinal regression is to the phallic phase. However, in relation to the type of configuration of the conversion symptom, Freud adds that regression is also to a phase previous to language acquisition (*Panorama of the Transference Neuroses*, 1915), in which the predominant form of expression is bodily, or mimicry (formal regression).

In *anxiety hysteria** the predominant fixation point is the same as in conversion hysteria, but although the theme is the same, the problem is different. In the latter, the problem resides essentially in castration anxiety* (*Inhibitions, Symptoms and Anxiety*, 1925) which corresponds to the same complex and to forms of defence against it, among which displacement is the predominant type, by which a secondary defensive rampart is formed called *phobia**, in which a certain type of regression to mechanisms or forms of relation with the object common in childhood occur. These are ego regressions to a previous mode of functioning rather than to any erotogenic zone in particular. An example is the need to be accompanied for protection against dangers as when the subject was a child. This is the case of agoraphobia* and its fears of "danger in the street", dangers controlled by the presence of someone accompanying the subject as the parents did in childhood.

In *obsessional neurosis**, regression to anal-sadistic fixation is nearly pathognomonic, together with defence mechanisms typical of the ego in response to Triebe attempting to reach it from that position. Reaction formation* is perhaps the most important and successful of these, since it forms the character*. However, return of the repressed is produced partly by failures of this reaction formation; through failures of other mechanisms such as isolation* and undoing what has been done*, the repressed breaks in by way of obsessional ideas or compulsions. The problem is also oedipal but has been degraded to the anal-sadistic by libidinal regression to that fixation point.

In *narcissistic affections*, regression is to the pre-oedipal* type of link previous to emergence of disavowal* of sexual difference, or else may result from disavowal itself when sexual differences produce castration anxiety* if they are accepted.

Regression is then to narcissism or to homosexual object choice* (narcissistic, being an object chosen in relation to its sex). The last is homosexual *perversion** (an extension of which is fetishism*). If Trieb with homosexual fixation is repressed, it forms the base for subsequent transference neuroses*.

When an unconscious object presentation is decathected* in the subject and projected onto the object's unconscious*, and also reversed into its opposite* (love* into hate*), persecutory *paranoia** results in which the fixation point regressed to is homosexual object choice. The peculiarity of the paranoiac mechanism results from the type of ego defence (projection*) utilized in response to this Trieb, intolerable for the ego, but a product of the previous fixation point to which Trieb regressed, now reactivated by some type of frustration*.

In *melancholia**, the fixation point is oral-cannibalistic, with a strikingly high degree of ambivalence* dominated by hate and superego identification* with the object; the result is that all this process concludes in hatred of the ego. In this type of regression, Trieb defusion is so extreme that a "pure culture of death instinct" is generated in the superego* which may lead to suicide. A product of regression to the oral fixation point, mechanisms common in this phase reappear such as narcissistic identification, characteristic of melancholia, but also of other pathologies described after Freud's time such as borderline patients.

In *schizophrenia** regression is to phases previous to the pre-ambivalent oral phase and to autoeroticism*, both previous to establishment of narcissism. In these cases, the ego as a psychical entity has been projected outwards: it returns from the exterior through auditory hallucinations and the delusion of influence*, or is torn to pieces into what were parts of its construction: different bodily organs or different erotogenic zones; this generates regression to autoeroticism, a regression even greater than that of narcissism: total psychical castration. Unlike dreams, there is neither topical nor formal regression; thing-presentations are decathected, and word-presentations no longer represent thing-presentations but *are** (cf. being*) them; therefore, regression is not from word to image as in dreams but rather the opposite: the word is hyper-cathected, acquiring characteristics of "organ speech" (the theme referring to the bodily organ is a product of libidinal withdrawal* onto the body, the origin of the ego).

Any higher level in libidinal development involves a greater degree of Trieb fusion with death Trieb* and greater subjection of the latter; the highest level in libidinal development is therefore the genital*.

All regression "backwards" from the latter consequently involves Trieb defusion and therefore liberation of death Trieb.

The greater the degree of regression, the higher the level of aggression* (auto- or allo-); aggression in turn is so fused with sexuality* that it is very difficult to differentiate one from the other (as in sadism, for example).

Regression is very closely related with repression in its broad definition as defence. As an effect of repression, repressed wishes or Trieb regress topically to the unconscious. They are left without a word-presentation to provide them access to the ego's preconscious, but they preserve – in transference neuroses – their cathexis* in the unconscious thing-presentation (the thing-presentation is the presentation of experiences with the object through the different erotogenic zones, which had diverse levels of fixation generating unconscious wishes). From here, they seek to return to the preconscious and sometimes succeed, for example, through substitutive formations*, with word-presentations displaced from the original ones and therefore accepted by the ego.

Thus, the repressed regresses to the fixation point where it is strengthened and from which it attempts to return, depending on the fixation point in the different neuroses, and burdened with their diverse problems.

In *Inhibitions, Symptoms and Anxiety* (1925) Freud mentions a new meaning of regression when he states that the "Wolf Man's" phantasy of being devoured by his father "gives expression, in a form that has undergone regressive degradation, to a passive, tender impulse to be loved by him in a genital-erotic sense" (p. 105). Freud differentiates this from anal-sadistic libidinal regression, previous and constitutive in the "Wolf Man". One thing is a regressive expression from the genital to the oral ("to eat" may be a metaphor of the genital sexual act), although the patient's anxiety* does not correspond in reality to fear of being eaten but to castration anxiety involved in recognition of sexual difference (phallic–castrated on this level). However, the same patient's libidinal Trieb regression to the anal fixation point, which gives form to his character* and some symptoms, is quite another thing.

It is interesting to mention the development explained by Freud regarding this patient's Trieb evolution in infancy. A product of historical constructions* based on the analysis of a dream and different screen memories*, it shows different changes of Trieb* aim in function of events, generally traumatic, that occurred. The Trieb aim regressed from phallic-active to masochistic-passive (anal), and consequently Sergei Petrov – this was his name – became a naughty boy seeking his father's punishment; from this position he progresses again, but now to homosexual (here, his wish becomes passive feminine, which implies a level of recognition of phallic castration). Now, from the "bedrock"* of his ego with its "masculine protest", he experiences castration anxiety, which prompts him to repress this Trieb, thereby reinforcing his masculinity in the latency period.

Trieb returns with all its potency from its fixation point when adolescence arrives, and often generates neurosis in this period of life.

REMEMBERING

Ger.: Erinnerung. – Sp.: recuerdo. – Fr.: rémémoration. – It.: ricordo. – Port.: recordação.

The theory of remembering and of memory* in general occupies a very important place in Freud's works. We could even suggest that they are partly a theory of memory, memories, and different forms of remembering.

Since Freud conceived of presentations* cathected with a *quantum* of affect* as formers of the psyche, and ultimately of these as results of processing of traces left by experiences and therefore memories of them, we consider that the psychical consists in diverse modes of remembering; here again, we find an original and creative aspect of the Freudian hypothesis.

We consequently discuss the diverse modes of remembering described in his works, as well as the complex problems in regard to remembering that he described throughout them.

In 1895, in the *Project for a Scientific Psychology,* he writes that memory is a product of the trace left by an experience as it travels its neuronal path. This path is facilitated (cf. facilitation*), especially if it is intense or reiterated, its use thereby made easier for each new quantity of excitation*.

> Memory is represented by the facilitations existing between the ψ neurones. Or even better: ... memory is represented by the differences in the facilitations between the ψ neurones. What, then, does the facilitation in the ψ neurones depend on? According to psych[ological] knowledge, the memory of an experience (that is, its continuing operative power) depends on a factor which is called the magnitude of the impression and on the frequency with which the same impression is repeated.
>
> (1895, p. 300)

In this work, he discusses "reproductive thought", a type of remembering with some level of binding, not so much by words but essentially by virtue of the memory of the visual image which is distinguished from the perceptual image; unlike hallucinatory satisfaction of wishes*, another type of remembering which hallucinates the conditions of the experience of satisfaction*.

These two phenomena are two types of remembering, both generated by the predominantly visual-sensory image of the experience which has some degree of binding or secondary process* possibly inhibiting the hallucination*.

Both kinds of memory are conscious. In reproductive thought, it is recognized as such, whereas in hallucinatory satisfaction of wishes it is mistaken for a perception* and believed* in reality*. The phenomenon of dreams* and hyperintense memories are common examples of this type.

The hallucinations of hysterical psychoses* and those of acute hallucinatory amentia are pathological examples.

In any case, access of memories to consciousness* does not give them the clarity or the possibility of presentational interrelations produced with the appearance of language* and its major weapon, words, which may be utilized to study reality and subsequently modify it through action.

The preconscious is born in this way, and from that point on, memories may increasingly access consciousness through words, the former types of remembering being stored away "like the bows and arrows" of today's world.

At the end of the period of the Oedipus complex*, primary repression* of infantile sexuality* is finally established, and the superego* is installed in the psychical apparatus, thereby splitting it and generating, among other things, a repressed unconscious* space whose access to the ego* is blocked by removing its access to words. In this way, infantile amnesia* of sexuality is generated, and the blanket of forgetting falls over everything that has occurred during this most important period in life. The exceptions are screen memories* and some dreams of infantile scenes not remembered in waking life which are produced through displacements* and condensations* among unconscious thing-presentations*. They access consciousness in this disguised manner without consciousness subjecting them to participate in a consistent and meaningful chain of thought.

Everything that happened in this phase, especially whatever produced high magnitude and even frequency of impressions, is anticathected (cf. anticathexis*) by the ego (utilizing the same mechanisms of condensation and displacement) when it feels anxiety* and therefore decathects* the word-presentation* that might give it access to the preconscious and thus also to the ego.

This means that presentations corresponding to infantile sexuality, mainly presentations of the Oedipus complex and any others the ego may associate with them, enter the state of repression and remain in the repressed unconscious id* as cathected thing-presentations deprived of their corresponding word-presentations which would give them access to consciousness for a return from the repressed, and from there to action. In this regard, they are not remembered.

However, as we said, they are cathected in the unconscious, and therefore struggle to access consciousness, to return from the repressed*. They sometimes manage to succeed in diverse ways: in jokes*, parapraxes*, phantasies* or daydreams, and other phenomena. In other cases, they generate transference neuroses*, whose symptoms* are produced by return of the repressed through associative paths not understood by the preconscious ego – so that the ego allows them to cross the "border" although perplexed, or simply as mnemic symbols* of those events, now repressed but commemorated or remembered through symptoms.

Therefore, symptoms are another form of remembering.

Another form is repetition compulsion*: the neurotic's (neurotic in the broad sense) repetition of some pleasurable but mostly traumatic events which hugely surpass the will* of the conscious ego.

Some events in the subject's history, the cause unknown to the ego, are repeated. They are "forms of remembering" such as transference* in psychoanalytic treatment in which events of the patient's prehistory are repeated with the analyst.

This new way of remembering an event of the past through action in the present also occurs by virtue of association of presentations which seek identity. Similarity with an old object due to similarity with this object in the present is affectively mistaken for identity with the historical object, and therefore the affect* felt with the former object is felt in the present.

The ego's reality testing is partly avoided (although the ego may examine the actual perception, the information regarding the associative or symbolic source of the repressed presentation is missing), which produces a repetition instead of a conscious memory.

> [The] patient does not *remember* anything of what he has forgotten and repressed, but *acts* it out. He reproduces it not as a memory but

as an action; he *repeats* it, without, of course, knowing that he is repeating it.

(*Remembering, Repeating and Working-Through*, 1914, p. 150)

The memory overcomes repression and manages, through diverse symptomatic compromises, to reach action; it thereby deceives the ego on another level, although the ego otherwise (in regard precisely to remembering) keeps it in line.

The objective of psychoanalytic treatment, in all cases and among other aspects, is for the patient to consciously remember what the unconscious ego wished and wishes to forget, in order to work it through*, finding new and old meanings for it and new participation in associative commerce. Then the ego is able to compare them and thereby to be enriched, testing reality closer to the truth, at least the truth of the patient's own history. The subject will have more power to distinguish between wishful transferences produced by this history and the present perception, to what extent they are different, and in what way.

Then the individual is able to genuinely remember and to choose, so far as is humanly possible, whether to repeat or not.

All thought activity* has its part in remembering. Wishes* themselves are memories of experiences of satisfaction or pleasure* experienced with the object; they are endeavours to re-experience them or at least some of their essential aspects. In this sense, the search for the object is a search to "*refind* such an object, to convince oneself that it is still there" (*Negation*, 1925, pp. 237–8).

Freud considers that we think in spirals, so to speak. The ego is enriched each time it goes round the spiral, recovering the past, expanding the future, and overcoming the repetition compulsion, a characteristic of all Trieb trends.

REPRESSION

Ger.: Verdrängung. – Sp.: represión. – Fr.: refoulement. – It.: rimozione. – Port.: repressão.
This is the ego* defence mechanism *par excellence*. Freud initially referred to it as "defence"; however, in 1915, in his famous metapsychological article, *Repression*, he defined it with conceptual precision and consolidated the term "repression" that he had been utilizing since 1900 without the precise metapsychological description; in 1925, in *Inhibitions, Symptoms and Anxiety*, he considered, though without much success in Freudian psychoanalysis, that repression was just another ego defence mechanism in response to the anxiety signal* corresponding to conversion hysteria*, and whose status was the same as others, such as isolation*, undoing what has been done*, disavowal*, splitting of the ego*, and others.

"Repression" may be defined in both a broad and a strict sense; broadly, when it acquires the characteristics of a type of ego defence*. The characteristic common to each type of repression is withdrawal of libidinal cathexis* from the presentation*.

When the preconscious word-presentation is decathected, access to consciousness* of the unconscious thing-presentation is prevented. The latter remains cathected in the unconscious and from there it struggles to return; when it succeeds through substitutive formations*, transference neuroses*, the traditional object of study of psychoanalysis, ensue. Repression is also characterized by a mechanism that complements the former: that of anticathexis*, the only mechanism of primal repression*, which reinforces preconscious decathectization* in secondary repression.

This scenario is complicated by the fact that, also in 1911, in *Psycho-Analytic Notes on an Autobiographical Account of a Case of Paranoia (Dementia Paranoides)* (the Schreber case), Freud calls decathectization of the thing-presentation repression, and not quite as if to take it in this broad sense of the term, but as a type of extreme defence of a psychical apparatus being overwhelmed by Trieb* and unable to decathect its words, since the fixation point* is narcissism* returning from sublimated homosexual libido whose unconscious object wish* has been decathected and replaced by hypercathexis of the wounded ego.

In this broad sense we may therefore speak of repression even in paranoid psychoses*. But not in the strict sense, since in this case we must restrict it to preconscious decathectization and maintenance of unconscious cathexis.

In 1925, after having developed the conceptualization of such a complex form of repression that it is difficult for psychoanalysts to limit it simply, Freud returns to the broad concept of defence, considering it one defence mechanism among many others, and not the general model of all defence mechanisms.

We consider that there are differences between the diverse manners in which the ego defends itself in response to anxiety signals whose paradigm is castration anxiety*.

It is not excessively contradictory, after reaching such depth in Freud's works, especially considering one of the aims of psychoanalytic work ("to lift repression"), to continue to call the different defence mechanisms forms of repression, so long as we specify its scope and limits.

It is more controversial to maintain the concept of repression in relation to narcissistic affections showing decathexis of thing-presentations; however, if we clarify the metapsychological difference, we may do even this legitimately. In fact, Freud never corrected what he had written before 1925, particularly his text on the Schreber case.

However, we must explain that, from *Inhibition, Symptoms and Anxiety* (1925) forward, Freud limits this concept to the defence mechanism of conversion hysteria*. He quite likely does this because the issue centres on his description in this text of the way the unconscious ego* manages to hold off the anxiety signal provoked by intrusion of Trieb*. The specific feature of repression therefore resides in the expression of anticathexis and substitute formation by somatic innervation chosen by association: by contiguity or as a mnemic symbol* (analogy*), modes of formation of the hysterical conversion symptom. However, we consider that we cannot make much progress if we restrict in this way a mechanism that has contributed so much to psychoanalytic theory; experience indicates that it may continue to do so.

There are also two types of repression in both the broad and the strict sense: primal repression (the Spanish translator adds in parenthesis: "dislodging pressure") which arises in each period of passage from the predominance of one erotogenic zone* to another in infantile sexuality*, especially if traumatic events have led by anticathexis to the creation of fixation points, unified at the moment of dissolution/repression of the Oedipus complex, resignifying them in a deferred* manner, and thereby completing their establishment in the apparatus.

The result of this base is the repression we observe in adult patients (whose psychical apparatus has a finished structure, among other reasons, on account of primal repression*): secondary repression or "pressure to hunt" presentations which, by utilizing laws of association, aim to return from the repressed*, overcoming censorship* of the ego led by the superego*, and when succeeding by virtue of substitute formations, creating neurotic symptoms and other phenomena.

REPRESSION PROPER

Ger.: Verdrängung. – Fr.: refoulement. – Sp.: represión secundaria. – It.: repressione secondaria. – Port.: repressão secundária.

This is a form of ego defence against Triebe of the id*. After the establishment of primal repression*, Triebe provoke the anxiety signal* in the ego*, a reminder of the danger of Trieb satisfaction (object loss, or loss of its love*, or castration*). For this reason, these Triebe are sent into a "state of repression"; that is to say, sent to the repressed unconscious. Since the preconscious ego does not accept them as its own, its presentations* are unable to participate in secondary process* thought* activity. Repression proper, "after repression", or an "endeavour to hunt" is manifested in clinical work with the neuroses*, precisely because it fails, thereby allowing return of the repressed* through symptoms*, parapraxes*, dreams*, and other phenomena.

In response to this danger signal, the ego reinforces primal repression with after repression. Cathexis* is withdrawn from preconscious ego presentations, and an attempt is made to avoid situations that might reactivate danger from Trieb; for this purpose, anticathexis* is placed on the perceptual end*, also as a form of ego resistance*.

The metapsychological resources of repression proper are therefore: (a) decathectization* of the preconscious ego (word-) presentation; (b) anticathexis placed essentially on the attention* of the perceptual apparatus and conscious censorship*; and (c) attraction proceeding from the unconscious exerted by the primally repressed on any preconscious presentation which might become, through some law of association*, an unconscious derivative of the repressed.

We differentiate the diverse transference neuroses* by the varied forms of decathexis of the preconscious presentation, which originate the specificity of defence mechanisms* or after repressions.

In *conversion hysteria** cathexis is withdrawn from the preconscious presentation and placed into a bodily cathexis with which it is associated by laws of contiguity* (associative symptom*) or analogy* (a symptom deriving from a mnemic symbol*), thereby creating substitute formations* through bodily dysfunctions towards which the subject experiences a *belle indifférence**.

In *anxiety hysteria**, cathexis withdrawn from the preconscious presentation is displaced (cf. displacement*) onto a presentation which substitutes it, also through laws of association* whose presence in perception* provokes an attack of anxiety*; it is as if Trieb* had become what is now a phobogenic presentation; for this reason, a secondary defensive rampart is constructed against the possibility that its presence might be perceived by the perceptual apparatus (in which case the anticathexis is functioning). In *obsessional neurosis**, the preconscious presentation remains cathected, but is isolated from its associative and affective connections with other presentations; therefore, it is considered a foreign body within the preconscious and consequently foreign to the ego. Magical resources may even be utilized against it such as undoing of what has been done* and so on, forming obsessive ceremonials*. The character trait* of meticulousness, typical of the anal character, leads to displacement onto the trivial, another type of anticathexis that blocks emergence of the important presentation which the ego is endeavouring to repress.

In *perversions** and *narcissistic pathology* in particular, the form of after repression changes radically: in perversions, disavowal* of sexual difference predominates, leading to ego splitting*. In *schizophrenia** the unconscious wish is lost when its thing-presentation* is decathected. In *paranoia**, this wish is also projected onto the unconscious of objects*, and its recovery attempted through delusion*. In *melancholia**, the ego identifies with the object as a way to make it unconscious.

Therefore, in a broad sense, all these ego defence mechanisms are also forms of after repression or repression proper.

REPRODUCTIVE THOUGHT

Ger.: reproduzierendes Denken. – Sp.: pensamiento reproductor. – Fr.: pensée reproductrice. – It.: pensiero riproduttore. – Port.: pensamento reprodutor.

This is perhaps the most original type of thought* intimately related to memory* itself, especially conscious memory which has no need of words (at least in what we could call the initial levels of the early psyche* with some level of binding) in order to have signs of quality*.

Therefore, it is both productive and a product of the first collateral cathexes, the origin of the subsequent definitive reality ego* and of the first levels of the preconscious ego* of the psychical apparatus*. In this way, the tendency to hallucination* of primary process* is gradually inhibited and secondary process* generated, now able to distinguish between a memory* and a perception*, between one perception and another, and what is more difficult, between a wish* and a perception.

In any case, we may reflect that if the ego developed no further than these conditions of functioning it would be quite imperfect. We would have no true conception of our associations*, particularly of the ties connecting representations with each other.

Although reproductive thought is able to utilize words, it is always tightly anchored to the thing-representation*, which makes its access to consciousness difficult (in the example of Signorelli, Cf.

Forgetting*, Freud recalls facial features hyper-clearly, but not the name); as we see, this characteristic may be utilized by repression* to prevent remembering.

It is closely related to phantasy but has a higher degree of binding – therefore more reality criteria – and is not mainly wish fulfillment in this sense, unlike phantasy.

RESISTANCE

Ger.: Widerstand. – Sp.: resistencia. – Fr.: résistance. – It.: resistenza. – Port.: resistência.

This clinical expression of unconscious defence* is an automatic ego response to Trieb* or to the anxiety signal* produced by the possible emergence of Trieb, about which the official (preconscious) ego seems to know nothing.

This may occur during psychoanalytic treatment and originate negative periods in this process in which the patient's knowledge of the unconscious does not progress, since the patient's ego is absorbed at this time by defending itself rather than knowing itself, on account of the danger signal that reappears unconsciously.

One of the ways this ego resistance is established is through transference* which then acquires a negative characteristic and becomes an obstacle to advance of the analysis. However, just as it is a serious obstacle, analysis of transference becomes one of its major therapeutic weapons, since repressed traumas* of childhood are re-experienced through the link with the therapist. Thus, transference neurosis* develops, the "intermediate state between illness and life" whose analysis gives psychoanalytic therapy a certain specificity.

Resistance to the cure may also be due to the superego* which strives to satisfy its need for punishment* of the ego by maintaining illness; it may even be due to the id*, the same Trieb* whose conservative tendency and repetition compulsion* make it strongly resistant to giving up historically acquired fixations*, much less its biological archetypes (cf. primal phantasies*).

Classical ego resistance is a direct expression of the mechanism of repression*, its anticathexis* exerted on possible emergence of a cathexis* belonging to an unconscious thing-presentation in the ego's preconscious.

Obsessional pathology is founded on anticathexis of the presentation* fixated in the form of satisfaction of the anal-sadistic erotogenic zone*, the origin of reaction formation* which produces most of the typical character traits of the anal character*.

In *conversion hysteria** we observe a special type of alteration of perception which consists in "not seeing anything sexual" or anything possibly referring to it. This trait, typical of this type of personality, could be understood partly as ingenuousness. It is produced by anticathexis of after repression* established in the perceptual apparatus*, by virtue of which it is possible to avoid (by "not understanding it in this sense" or "not realizing it") any perception* that might refer to the incestuous sexual fixation of this type of neurosis. This hysterical characteristic was termed a "scotoma" by Laforgue (1926).

In regard to *anxiety hysteria**, anticathexis is also placed on perception, on its attention cathexis*, in being alert to staying far from perception of the object* that generates castration anxiety*: the subject's unconscious wish impulse is displaced* from the presentation of the original object or person from which punishment is feared to come. For this purpose, a phobic rampart* is constituted, growing in complexity with each attempt of Trieb to return from the repressed, and finally becoming an integral part of the phobia* itself.

Another type of ego resistance is the gain from illness*; it may be primary (the best economic solution to conflict achieved by the ego up to this time; it only relinquishes it if it is offered a better one), or secondary (the ego accepts the illness and derives benefits from the object on account of it). With respect to superego resistance and the need to punish the ego that it needs to satisfy, knowing it is ill, this is one of the most difficult to cure. There are no special recipes for its treatment but to continue to utilize psychoanalytic therapeutic weapons, attempting to reconstruct the childhood past and the period of constitution of the superego as far as possible.

The same is true regarding id resistance for which Freud's precise instruction is to "work through" (*Durcharbeiten*), to achieve recognition of the history of Trieb, fixations and events connected with them, their relation with repetitions in the present, in real life and in transference, in search of new meanings, new relations between presentations*, and more associative commerce, which transform id into ego.

RESTITUTION

Ger.: Rückgase / Rückerstattung. – Sp.: restitución. – Fr.: restitution. – It.: restituzione. – Port.: restituição.

This process is a pseudo-reconstruction of the world of object wishes* following the experience of the end of the world* in schizophrenia*.

It follows decathexis* of unconscious thing-presentations with libidinal withdrawal* and withdrawal of libido into the ego*. The latter is hyper-cathected* due to its previous wounds in an attempt to stanch them with narcissistic cathexis*. Unconscious object wishes are abandoned.

Afterwards, the ego sometimes attempts to reconnect with the object world (for example, in paranoid schizophrenia, partially in hebephrenia, but not in simple schizophrenia in which restitution is minimal) by utilizing what remains cathected: word-presentations* belonging to the preconscious ego. They configure delusions* in paranoid schizophrenics and in paranoia, and organ speech* and disaggregation of thought* in hebephrenic schizophrenia.

In all these clinical forms, there may be hallucinations* of words corresponding to the subject's own thoughts or to memories of words once spoken by objects, which belong to the ego or the superego* and were projected (cf. projection*) to the exterior and therefore perceived by the perceptual end* as voices proceeding from the external world.

When projection comes from the ego, a delusion of influence is usually configured, and when the superego prevails, the (persecutory) delusion of being observed. Auditory perception of thought is an intermediate phenomenon between the two projections (the ego's and the superego's).

All these attempts to reconstruct the object link configure noisy symptoms* of illness, although they are the patient's attempts to achieve a cure (in the sense of reconnection with objects), utilizing what remains of the patient's psychical apparatus* after its break (which is certainly not free of a considerable quantity of hate*) from the unconscious wish for objects, a wish that structured it and gave it a reason for being.

This is therefore accomplished in the manner of hysteria (hallucinations) or of obsessional neurosis (delusions) (*On Narcissism: An Introduction*, 1914).

RETURN OF THE REPRESSED

Ger.: Wiederkehr des Verdrängten. – Sp.: retorno de lo reprimido. – Fr.: retour du refoulé. – It.: ritorno del rimosso. – Port.: retorno do reprimido.

This is the third phase of repression* of the unconscious Trieb impulse. When it is reactivated for some reason, a substitute formation* is created, and the censorship* of repression is thereby avoided, giving form to neurotic symptoms*.

Freud considers that transference neuroses* are constituted in this way. They are in reality different types of failure of repression, and for this reason the repressed re-emerges from the unconscious* in disguise, achieving a sufficiently distorted form of expression in consciousness to render it unrecognizable. It is therefore a form of expression of sexuality*, "degrading a process of satisfaction to a symptom" (*Inhibitions, Symptoms and Anxiety*, 1925, p. 95).

The repressed returns from the fixation* point; therefore, it possesses the affective tone, defence mechanisms*, traumatic histories compulsively repeated and so on, corresponding to this erotogenic zone* and to the type of object* link also belonging to it. Now, some elements of the oedipal drama also participate from the moment when all the previous erotogenic zones and their fixations yielded to phallic* supremacy; at least in the world of the transference neuroses. In other, more narcissistic affections, the nuances are different.

Return of the repressed is therefore closely related with regression* to the libidinal fixation point and the return of presentations* repressed at that point by the anticathexis*, but now in disguise, as a neurotic symptom. Neurosis is synonymous with return of the repressed and of failed repression. Successful repression does not originate symptoms, more closely resembling a dissolution* of Trieb. This process is dynamic: there are usually periods in which repression is successful and others in which on account of different exciting causes (frustrations*), return predominates.

A neurotic symptom is an expression of Trieb that is returning to the ego*, even though the ego is still defending itself from it through illness. An increase of Trieb (or its increase due to external excitation exerted on Trieb) has generated decompensation of "defence achieved or apparent health" which dominated the scene.

> The third phase, and the most important regarding pathological phenomena, is failure of repression, of *irruption, of return of the repressed.* This irruption starts from the point of fixation, and involves regression of libidinal development back to that point.
>
> (*Psycho-Analytic Notes on an Autobiographical Account of a Case of Paranoia (Dementia Paranoides)*, 1911, p. 68)

The repressed may also return in other ways: for example, in dreams*, jokes*, parapraxes*, and other phenomena. These safety valves give repression a rest by allowing some passages of the repressed into word-presentations* and thereby also into the preconscious, passages accepted by the superego* and culture*.

In narcissistic psychoses* the repressed (in the broad sense) returns in positive symptoms of illness, those that endeavour to refind the object* somehow, even if only through mere words (paranoid delusions*) by which attempts at restitution* take shape.

REVERSAL INTO THE OPPOSITE

Ger.: Verkehrung ins Gegenteil. – Sp.: transformación en lo contrario. – Fr.: renversement dans le contraire. – It.: conversione nell'opposto. – Port.: transformação no contrario ou inversão (da pulsão).

This vicissitude of sexual Trieb* is previous to the establishment of the superego* and repression* of the Oedipus complex*, in the bloom of infantile sexuality*.

It comprises two types of processes: (a) the transformation of Trieb from activity to passivity and (b) the reversal of its content; both depend on primal ambivalence* of sexual Trieb towards the object*, in terms of active–passive and love–hate.

Although this mechanism arises in a predominantly narcissistic* period (in that the object is not recognized as the source of pleasure* but rather as part of the ego*), and also belongs to autoerotism*, these vicissitudes of Trieb begin to show the importance of the object as a generator of pleasure.

The ambivalence mentioned above corresponds to the type of link established with the object through the different erotogenic zones*; Freud utilizes one of them as a paradigm: the anal zone (sadism-masochism) and the Trieb of sight (scopophilia-exhibitionism), although it extends to all the others; that is to say, to caress-to be caressed, to smell-to be smelled, to devour-to be devoured, to touch-to be touched, and so on, with different nuances and in different proportions.

The term "reversal into the opposite" describes the Trieb's change of aim (whereas "turning round upon the subject's own self" describes the change of object, since the ego becomes the object and the object becomes ego). In response to the same object, active aims (sadism-scopophilia) are exchanged for passive aims (masochism-exhibitionism). This mechanism is a means for the ego to defend itself from the pressure (*Drang*) of Trieb and its peremptory character; it expands its form of discharge but never loses it, something which does occur when a repressive anticathexis* is utilized.

In this case, a characteristic of Trieb has simply been changed, but Trieb is satisfied, although in a form opposite from the original one.

The disorder of sadism* consists of several phases. In the first, it is deflection outwards of death Trieb*, accomplished through its fusion with muscular erotism. First, there is a violent action, an affirmation of power aimed at another person as an object. Then this object is given up and replaced by the subject's own person (thereby changing the Trieb aim from active to passive). It is an intermediate step called self-punishment* or self-torture. Then, another object is sought which, as a consequence of the change of Trieb aim, acts in the subject's place; this is what we now define as masochism*.

Since masochism is characterized by pain*, it must be experienced in order to be sadistic. Only the subject that has experienced it understands (cf. understanding*) what it involves and is then able to feel the pleasure of sadism, which results from identification* with the object's masochistic pleasure.

Moral masochism provides no pleasure of any kind (perhaps narcissistic pleasure, but not produced by Trieb discharge); at most it may afford relief due to expiation of guilt provided by punishment. In other types of masochism the pleasure is not in the pain itself but in the sexual excitation it produces indirectly, especially if it includes debasement of the erotic object*, narcissistic omnipotence, and other factors.

Reversal of Trieb into its opposite consists in Trieb's return to passivity; on this road it finds the object, and the result is one of the ways to make narcissism more complex and break away from it. However, there may also be regression* to it, at least to the narcissistic type of object choice*.

Freud gives us an excellent example of change of the Trieb aim in the case history of the "Wolf Man". It was due to traumatic* situations in the infantile period, such as passive seduction by his sister after a period of libidinal regression following the threat of castration by the object when the child proposed to be active towards it. From that time on, passivity began to predominate as an aim, which generated symptoms* and even character traits* in his adulthood.

Concerning Trieb of looking, it may be previously narcissistic (autoerotic), apart from the active pleasure of looking at sexual organs and the subject's organ's being looked at by another person (exhibition). Triebe also intermingle, and therefore the pleasure of looking and of exhibiting may join those of touching, caressing, and others.

What occurs with the contents? We observe reversal into the opposite in the case of love* into hate*, as in persecutory paranoia* in which unconscious homosexual love is perceived by consciousness* as destructive persecution, an expression of hate, felt to proceed, due to the mechanism of projection*, from the object's unconscious.

S

SADISM

Ger.: Sadismus. – Sp.: sadismo. – Fr.: sadismo. – It.: sadismo. – Port.: sadismo.

This is the counterpart of masochism* in the pair: sadism-masochism. Sadism is also a type of deflection of death Trieb*, the latter considered by Freud as inherent to all living beings. This deflection is produced through development of the muscular system by which aggression* and the drive for mastery* are able to unfold in object* links. Sadism involves a certain degree of defusion* of this Trieb that is liberated to the exterior in this way.

Sadism is part of sexual Trieb*, especially in its first pregenital* levels (of these, anal eroticism*manifests it most), but some degree of sadism is involved in all sexual relations in the form of aggression and mastery.

In the strict sense, sadism may configure a sexual perversion*: pleasure in striking, hurting, dominating without conditions, denigrating, or causing suffering to the sexual partner; however, it also has a broader, desexualized sense, acquiring obscenely cultural "specializations" which may include some of the above, especially in everything connected with the struggle for power between human beings.

In *Three Essays on The Theory of Sexuality* (1905), Freud states that any stimulus beyond a certain amount may acquire characteristics of sexual excitation, including pain*. In this case, the sadist is seeking to inflict not only pain but also sexual excitation provoked by it. However, there are degrees, and sometimes the intention to produce pain in the other may be almost independent of sexual pleasure (though never absolutely, since narcissism*, which includes power relations, is always involved).

Freud explains that sadistic pleasure, the inflicting of pain or suffering, is learned first in the subject's own body*: the individual does not feel the other's pain (therefore this type of pleasure is in itself masochistic), but afterwards, by identification with the object's masochistic pleasure, feels sadistic pleasure.

Masculine sexuality usually includes sadism and feminine sexuality, masochism (in both men and women), although Freud does not refer to "masculine sadism" as the counterpart of feminine masochism (in my opinion, for the above reason: because pleasure is masochistic in both cases; the sadist does not feel the other's pain in his own body but identifies with the other's masochistic pleasure whereas the pain is in the other's body; for this reason he addresses it within a classification of masochism – feminine, moral and erotogenic masochism – and does not create a category for sadism.

The fact that pain itself (not the pain that generates sexual excitation) may produce pleasure generates an economic problem in the theory. This economic problem results from pleasure produced by an increase in quantity, but not in the case of sadism, since the sadistic individual is spared from feeling pain which the masochist does feel, and only identifies with this particular type of pleasure. Sadistic pleasure is masochistic pleasure felt by identification. In our case, then, rather than a problem, it is a theoretical confirmation of the need the psychical apparatus has to expel quantity of excitation*, which of course causes a different type of problem, but not an economic problem.

SCHIZOPHRENIA

Ger.: Schizophrenie. – Sp.: esquizofrenia. – Fr.: schizophrénie. – It.: schizofrenia. – Port.: esquizofrenia.

This name, created by Bleuler, was chosen by psychiatry for the mental disorder that Kraepelin called "dementia praecox"; Freud tried but failed to call it paraphrenia (a term adopted for a certain type of organized delusion).

Freud considered it one of the narcissistic neuro-psychoses; that is to say, affections with wounded narcissism* and a wounded ego* by which both are obstructed, which raises the level of libido* in the ego.

In his metapsychological papers of 1915, Freud explains that in schizophrenia libidinal cathexis* is withdrawn from the unconscious thing-presentation*; that is to say, from the place it must be in order to enable sexual wishes* for objects; that is to say, to enable energy to become object libido.

Quantity of excitation* acquires psychical quality* when it is bound to presentations*, and becomes more complex by acquiring relations with other presentations through laws of association*. This complexity and presentational quality thereby achieved by the psyche by virtue of the presentation, is one of the ways in which the psychical apparatus fends off quantity of excitation. Therefore, when the cathexis is withdrawn from the unconscious thing-presentations, this level of quality and of complexity achieved by binding is lost. The energy, in part, reverts to pure quantity. Another part of this energy is now aimed at cathecting the ego, object libido then becoming narcissistic.

The first part, which was simply unbound from unconscious presentations and became quantity, provokes terrible automatic anxiety* when this quantity of excitation is unbound from a presentation, generating a situation of helplessness* similar to that of the birth trauma. This situation of withdrawal of object libido*, plus the invasion of quantity suffered by the psychical apparatus, metapsychologically explains the end of the world experience, paradigmatic of schizophrenia. The other part of libido, withdrawn from presentations of objects* and therefore from objects themselves (or rather, actions aimed at them) now cathects the ego, seeking to recover narcissism, and shows how the world is to be reconstructed.

When libidinal withdrawal predominates over reconstruction, regression* may return to autoerotism*, the period previous to an ego (reality ego*) which constitutes narcissism by uniting erotogenic zones*. This clinical form of schizophrenia is called "simple".

In "hebephrenic" schizophrenia, the subject attempts to reconstruct the world of object wishes by cathecting parts of the ego with narcissistic libido, such as word-presentations*. Therefore, words no longer signify thing-presentations but only occupy their place and are consequently treated like them (with primary process*): not in a transitory sense as in jokes* but instead in a lasting way, the preconscious ego's desperate attempt to restore a presentational world decathected by the unconscious*. Consequently, the ego is fractured. The normal ego is essentially words representing wished-for things, aiming towards these things, and leading to action. These words are empty of meaning, only useful for internal alteration* or for approaching the object, but not for specific action* whatever it might be. It does not matter, for example, if the object is unable to understand, since it is not meant to express the individual's wish. Why would it matter, considering that the object no longer exists?

Therefore, there are no thing-presentations backing up these words which only represent themselves before consciousness*. Therefore, they are words without that ultimate meaning (perhaps with a dictionary meaning but even without it), plain words, simple sound images linked to each other by primary process*. The syntaxes of sentences or even words themselves are altered in this way; since they are cathected with narcissistic libido, they take up a hypochondriac theme (the origin of the ego is the body and its words now return to it), forming "organ speech"*.

In paranoid schizophrenia, paranoid reactions, and paranoia*, the libidinal fixation* point is less regressive: it is homosexual object choice.

The process is approximately the following. A narcissistic object choice was made for the sake of the individual's megalomania*, not entirely delusional (we should consider questions such as "is megalomania ever not delusional?" but we could cite arrogance as a character trait*), given that it is based on experience in the link with reality* and objects. The object involved injured the subject's narcissism by no longer supporting his megalomania. Therefore, the subject withdrew the libidinal cathexis from the unconscious object presentation and did not bind it to another thing-presentation or from there to preconscious phantasies* of objects. This homosexual object libido (without knowledge of sexual difference) became absolutely narcissistic and then proceeded to cathect presentations of the ego (including its primary and secondary identifications) as described in the aforementioned clinical forms. These words which no longer seek things (objects) are dedicated to restoring the ego by utilizing primary process to relate to each other. Delusions of grandeur or megalomanic delusions are constructed in this way.

All these instances of withdrawal of libido into ego presentations (presentations of the subject's own body and history) present clinically as hypochondria on the one hand and megalomania on the other.

In paranoid schizophrenia (more than in other clinical forms) words are utilized in an attempt to reconstruct the world of object presentations; in discourse (if it could be considered discourse), alterations in the sentence content function by associations of contiguity*, analogy*, or opposition, enabling the subject to ground the reasons for his or her delusion. This disorder must disqualify the homosexual object wish that went back to erotization, lost the ego's inhibition* of its aim, and with it capability of sublimation, and (when it was projected) even lost its place in the ego.

How was this withdrawal of cathexis from the unconscious object presentation accomplished? In a very particular way. Cathexis of the unconscious presentation (the wish) was projected (cf. projection*) into the object, and the subject was left without its own wishes and Triebe*. The object now possesses both wishes and Triebe: all of the libido. In the object, wishes and Triebe undergo diverse forms of disguise in which different forms of delusion are constituted; for example: delusions of jealousy, persecutory, erotomanic, and megalomanic delusions. In the male patient, all these constructions aim at disqualifying the declaration: "I love him". Therefore, by virtue of the mechanism of projection, the homosexual wish is not perceived as the patient's own but as belonging to the object (involving lack of subject-object discrimination due to the depth of the projected), and also undergoes different transformations depending on the clinical form. In persecutory delusions (at the root of all the rest), love* regresses to hate*.

We have not explained another type of delusion: that of being noticed or observed. This delusion originates, in adult schizophrenics, in a regression to perception* of words spoken by the parents during the patient's childhood when they observed their child critically. At that time, the child felt they were watching him to keep him from masturbating* or as a preparation for threats of castration; in sum, something coming from a sentinel looking for evidence with which to accuse him (father as a rival) rather than to protect him (protective father). Therefore, the original words that formed the preconscious superego* are hallucinated, describing the child's acts one by one ("Now he's thinking about that again", "Now he's going away"). In any case, it manifests clinically as a form of persecutory delusion but is metapsychologically attributable to part of the disorganization of the psychical apparatus as previously achieved bindings regress to their origins. What once constituted moral conscience* in the psychical apparatus is again perceived as entering from the outside as it did in childhood. Based on this perception, the subject's conclusion is that he is being observed in adult life, which derives into a persecutory delusion.

Finally, a particular form of persecutory delusion is the "delusion of influence" which includes machines that take over the subject's thoughts and actions. According to V. Tausk, these machines symbolize the body and therefore the ego. This ego is projected to the outside (in this case without regression to perception, without hallucination) which is its main origin (extraneous help*, primary identifications*, secondary identifications*, and so on).

Therefore, in paranoid schizophrenia, the unconscious thing-presentation is decathected as belonging to the subject and projected to the outside, which leaves the subject without desire for objects; in any case, it is the objects that desire him (due to the transformation of love into hate, the persecutory form of wishes is harmful). An attempt is made to reconstruct the world of object wishes consequently "destroyed" by utilizing libidinal cathexes of word-presentations (belonging to the ego) with which delusions are constructed; these delusions utilize primary process to disqualify the homosexual wish (simultaneously regressing to infantile sexual theories* such as that of the cloaca). Sublimated homosexual libido (desexualized) establishes social ties, which are thereby damaged and transformed into persecutory ties in paranoid schizophrenia.

Schizophrenia is a narcissistic affection. It is psychosis* *par excellence.*

SCREEN MEMORIES

Ger.: Deckerinnerung. – Sp.: recuerdo encubridor. – Fr.: souvenir-écran. – It.: ricordo di copertura. – Port.: recordação encobridora.

This type of disperse memory* corresponds to early childhood: derivatives retained by preconscious memory in spite of the adult's infantile amnesia*.

Their characteristics are predominantly visual-sensory. They may also be remarkably hyperintense, especially in some aspects usually having little significance in relation to their content, and therefore are "often of dubious or enigmatic importance" (*Screen Memories*, 1899, p. 303). In regard to these memories, it is difficult to find their sequential place in logical reasoning or to relate them with other events in the same period when the subject apparently remembers having experienced them.

We could almost say that they are to some extent isolated*, at least in relation to the subject's own history.

They may be more or less complex: simple images in the form of flashes, or scenes with a certain story which in any case have little meaningful value in consciousness*, and whose persistence in memory is enigmatic.

On occasion they may be composed of memories of important events, but in this case they are more or less confused, which already indicates a disguise (*From the History of an Infantile Neurosis*, 1918).

These screen memories do not always belong to early childhood. When they do not, they are mistaken for retrospective phantasies.

Childhood screen memories are constituted after the period of the Oedipus complex* and the subsequent establishment of the superego*; they are exceptions to the infantile amnesia remaining after these traumatic events. They are formed in the manner of dreams* and symptoms* by condensations* and displacements* among unconscious* thing-presentations* ruled by laws of primary process* which allow them to avoid the censorship* of repression*.

Since they are products of displacement, they have little psychical value in themselves, or at least the ego's* consciousness cannot find it. Displacement is produced by laws of contiguity* in time and space in relation to other presentations* which have intense significance, or by analogy* with some attributes of these presentations or of others.

The sensory hyper-intensity of these memories, which conceal many sensations and thereby also many histories and meanings, may be attributed to condensation; as if something neutral from this period had been chosen to represent in disguise a buried dramatic history that has left behind these screen memories and other "archaeological artefacts".

If psychoanalytic work is productive, these many meanings are reconstructed, retracing the path of their construction; that is to say, guided by associations* by historical and linguistic contiguity or analogy that the patient allows to emerge. Sometimes the analyst is aided by universal symbols*, but is always struggling against different strata of unconscious ego resistances.

In this way, based on screen memories, a logical and vivid history (present-day vividness is repeated in transference*, for example) is reconstructed, explaining a large part of levels of meaning of actual symptomatology or certain ego character traits* and their types of behaviour.

Some memories are configured in a different way: for example, their content may correspond to infancy, whereas substitutive affects* or sensations correspond to subsequent years. Freud refers to them as "retro-active" or "retrogressive" memories.

Those in which a recent, neutral impression is linked to a previous experience are more frequent; in this case they are referred to as memories that have "pushed ahead" or have been "displaced forward".

A memory may be connected "with the impression that it screens, not only through its content but also through contiguity in time: these are contemporary or contiguous screen memories" (*The Psychopathology of Everyday Life*, 1901, p. 44).

SECONDARY GAIN FROM ILLNESS

Ger.: sekundärer Krankheitsgewinn. – Sp.: beneficio secundario de la enfermedad. – Fr.: bénéfice secondaire de la maladie. – It.: utile secondario della malattia. – Port.: beneficio o lucro secundário (da doença).

A type of ego resistance* to the cure; that is to say, to making conscious the unconscious* and thereby to fill in mnemic lacunae and integrate them into the ego* following working through*.

It is based on a certain integration into the ego* of the symptom*, especially if it is lasting, by virtue of which attention* or caregiving is obtained, as well as some love* from objects* that otherwise might not have been obtained (at least this is what the patient tends to feel).

It is neither the root nor the cause of the illness, appearing secondarily, but contributes to sustain it and even acts as a motivation to cling to it or as a resistance to relinquishing it.

Freud describes it.

> When a psychical organization like an illness has lasted for some time, it behaves eventually like an independent organism; it manifests something like a self-preservative instinct; it establishes a kind of modus vivendi between itself and other parts of the mind, even with those which are at bottom hostile to it; and there can scarcely fail to be occasions when it proves once again useful and expedient and acquires, as it were, a secondary function which strengthens its stability afresh … What corresponds in the case of neuroses to a secondary exploitation like this of an illness may be described as the secondary gain from illness in contrast to the primary one.
>
> (*Introductory Lectures on Psycho-Analysis*, 1915–17, p. 384)

In *Inhibitions, Symptoms and Anxiety* (1925), Freud includes it as one of the three ego resistances, together with those of repression* and transference*; aside from those belonging to the id* and the superego*.

SECONDARY IDENTIFICATION

Ger.: Vater Identifizierung. – Sp.: identificación secundaria. – Fr.: identification secondaire. – It.: identificazione secundaria. – Port.: identificação secundária.

This type of identification* is produced after recognition of the object* as a source of pleasure* and the rival as a source of hostility, since it is opposed to obtaining pleasure from the object. It participates in the definitive constitution of the psychical apparatus because it is the mechanism of formation of the superego*, reinforcing primary identification*; the latter acquires a hostile tone that it had not yet manifested; from this hostile tone the father complex* is born.

From this point on, identification processes are secondary and quite diverse. Some join the ranks of the ego* as additions to basic primary identifications, whereas others join those of the superego. Some simply constitute symptoms* – such as hysterical symptoms – which are not part of the ego (unless they form character traits* as in obsessional neurosis and even in hysteria*). In melancholia*, however, they are not only part of the ego but even monopolize it. Identifications with traits of the lost object produced in all mourning* also become part of the ego.

Neither hysterical identifications ("Dora's" cough, 1901) nor obsessional identifications (compulsive exercising as a fantasy way to eliminate Dick – body fat – in the "Rat Man", 1909), nor even melancholic identifications constitute the ego but are fleeting visitors. They last as long as the symptom or the melancholic attack lasts, although some enter the ego and others are rejected by it.

Identifications generated among members of a group* and with its leader through common objectives, as well as those produced with artists and their works of art*, are secondary.

SECONDARY PROCESS

Ger.: Sekundärvorgang. – Sp.: proceso secundario. – Fr.: processus secondaire. – It.: processo secondario. – Port.: processo secundário.

The most highly developed form of mental process, the official preconscious ego* considers it its own. It possesses Kantian categories of time and space, non-contradiction, has a tendency to synthesis, leads to specific action*, and recognizes reality* which it takes into consideration before drawing conclusions.

It is also a type of relation among presentations*: the type that is rigorously referred to as thought*, characterized by strong cathexis* and weak displacement*, which makes energy interconnecting presentations quiescent or bound.

The demand to act upon needs and wishes* produced by Triebe* involves another need: to inhibit* primary process*. The latter considers wishes (and even needs) fulfilled on the strength of the simple fact that the consequent presentations have been cathected or that actual perceptions are associatively related to what is wished for. This leads to frustration*, which is clear and immediate in relation to self-preservative Triebe* and less clear and slower for sexual Triebe*.

Secondary process* functions like something between birth and slow metamorphosis to tame primary process and lead it to specific action producing changes in the external world which in turn produce discharges of the Trieb source, and also defend it from danger; in this case, it counters Trieb satisfaction because this would be dangerous, or postpones its satisfaction for a more adequate moment than the present; it may also make a judgement of condemnation* regarding the Trieb impulse, and block it from reaching action.

In general, it is synonymous with thought, and it resides in the ego's preconscious. It is basically constituted by complexly interconnected word-presentations* constituting the highest level of energetic binding attained by the psychical apparatus* (word-presentations supported by their signifiers: thing-presentations*, not word-presentations alone).

However, although word-presentations are the highest level, they are not absolutely indispensable for binding. Freud describes reproductive thought with a certain level of binding which he differentiates from simple wish-fulfilling phantasy; in the former, words hardly intervene, but rather the sentence or logical construction they involve. He also describes a primitive type of cognitive thought* based on action by which through imitative actions the fellow human being is understood*: subjects literally "put themselves in the other person's place". These early levels of secondary process thought, levels of presentational binding previous to language* acquisition, form a base for subsequent and more complex levels.

Secondary process is operated by preconscious and conscious parts of the ego. It therefore recognizes reality and is perturbed by contradictions; when it accepts reality, it accepts the imposed *no*, beginning with the simple fact that it is not part of the subject, and moderates the passage from one presentation to another precisely for this reason (one thing is not the other thing because it is analogous to the first: it is only analogous; the same holds for the other associative laws which are not mistaken for identities as in primary process).

Moderation of the passage of libidinal energy from one presentation to another produces weak displacement, and the intensity of this passage produces strong cathexis. These two characteristics (strong cathexis and weak displacement) define bound energy.

The reality principle* governing secondary process is opposed to the pleasure principle*; it is instead a moderation of the former, adapted to reality. It unceasingly searches for identity of the perceived with what is wished for, but utilizes thought to do it; that is to say, it studies reality and compares it with what is wished for: in what way it resembles or is different from it; searching for thought identity*, it seeks to "refind" (cf. refinding the object*) the object, to "convince oneself that it is still there" (*Negation*, 1925, p. 238), of course by thinking.

Symptoms*, parapraxes*, free associations*, repetition compulsions*, even more or less pathological character traits*, are products of substitute formations* ruled by primary process, and therefore are not recognized by the ego's secondary process as its own (except character traits and some repetition compulsions). The psychoanalytic process must reconstruct the meaning of these intrusions of primary process into secondary process, products of unconscious defence mechanisms* the ego utilizes to defend itself from anxiety signals* of danger (castration, loss of love, superego punishment, and social punishment), then to recover these presentations lost by the ego, to reincorporate them, enriching its secondary process, increasing its quiescent energy, the ego then choosing whether or not to take specific action.

SECONDARY REVISION

Ger.: Sekundäre Bearbeitung. – Sp.: elaboración secundaria. – Fr.: élaboration secondaire. – It.: elaborazione secondaria. – Port.: elaboração secundaria.

This is a reaction of the ego's* perceptual-conscious system (Pcpt.-Cs.) to all the imperfections, inconsistencies, errors, and suchlike of perceptions* and even of thought* activities. It tends to fill in, cover up, or not perceive these defects and to give them a coherent and logical form adequate to secondary process*.

In *The Interpretation of Dreams* (1900), Freud considers secondary revision the fourth factor in dream work*, alongside condensation*, submission to dream* censorship*, and consideration for figurability. However, in other articles such as *On Psycho-Analysis* (1923) and *An Evidential Dream* (1913), he states that it is not strictly part of dream work but is instead work of the ego in response to the dream hallucination* and therefore a perception it believes* and tries to understand at the very moment of perception and even at the moment when its manifest content* is being narrated.

The effect achieved is the opposite of what the conscious ego apparently seeks since secondary revision makes the dream formally more coherent but makes its logic less understandable. This serves the aims of censorship since it more effectively conceals the repressed wish*. Neurotic symptoms* also resort to secondary revision, especially those in phobias* and obsessional neurosis*, in which it is mistaken for rationalization*. It is also a very important part of the elaboration of paranoiac delusions*.

SEDUCTION

Ger.: Verführung. – Sp.: seducción – Fr.: séduction. – It.: seduzione. – Port.: sedução.

This is one of the innate primal phantasies*, the others being the primal scene*, castration, return to the womb, and the family romance*.

The phantasy of seduction of a child by an adult is more common than that of children by other children.

In the origins of psychoanalysis, phantasies of seduction emerged in all the hidden meanings of symptoms* as the content of traumatic scenes brought to light by the method of abreaction*, achieved by hypnosis.

In the final stage of his correspondence with Fliess, Freud stopped believing them, although their importance returned with the increasing complexity of theory, mainly the theory of trauma*, especially sexual trauma.

Viewed more closely, there is a first moment when the traumatic event occurs without psychical presentation (since the ego has no presentations* concerning the erotogenic zone* involved with which to form bindings, and also lacks previous cathexis of this erotogenic zone). At a second moment, when the corresponding erotogenic zone is cathected in a *deferred** manner and is linked to actual presentations, it becomes compulsive. Thus, anticathexes* generated produce fixations* which reinforce the original anticathexes that appeared when the first event occurred; these original anticathexes are practically pure quantities of stimulus in an unprepared zone, not cathected with attention, and having no presentations or any type of signification that might act to process or protect it against stimuli.

In the second moment, now having presentations and able to bind* with them, as well as copious attention, some level of "understanding"* of the event may be reached, if only unconsciously. From that moment on, repetition compulsions* are produced, ruled by the pleasure principle* in general (since if the quantity of excitation* passes a certain threshold, they go "beyond" it), at least the pleasure* of one of the systems into which the psychical apparatus is now split.

In any case, phantasies of seduction by an adult are rooted in each individual's ontogenetic historical truth*. The erotogenic zones awaken in the period of maternal caregiving of the infant when feeding, cuddling, caresses, baths, and changing of clothes provide pleasurable experiences that stimulate the baby's erotogenic zones.

In this sense, these seductions are not only inherited phantasies but also products of an interpretive construction of the individual's own history, including nuances of the histories of the father's and especially the mother's erotogenic zones.

> The anatomical situation of this region, the secretions in which it is bathed, the washing and rubbing to which it is subjected in the course of a child's toilet, as well as accidental stimulation ... make it inevitable that the pleasurable feeling which this part of the body is capable of producing should be noticed by children even during their earliest infancy, and should give rise to a need for its repetition.
>
> (*Three Essays on the Theory of Sexuality*, 1905, pp. 187–8)

These seduction phantasies may also be constructed as retrospective phantasies or may be hidden in screen memories*. In any case (whether or not the seduction occurred), phylogenetic primal phantasies and historical facts of awakening of erotogenic zones by maternal caregiving lend the primal phantasy of seduction historical and singular truth.

SELF-ESTEEM (SENSE OF SELF)

Ger.: Selbstgefühl. – Sp.: autoestima (sentimiento de sí). – Fr.: auto-estime (sentiment de soi). – It.: autostima (sentimento di se). – Port.: auto-estima (sentimento de si).

In general terms, this is a form of satisfaction of narcissistic libido in adults. It produces a feeling of indefinite well-being not directly related to discharge of Trieb; it is instead a basic state intimately related to self-confidence, to mood or state of mind, self-regard and self-respect. In these aspects, it is a basic pillar of ego health and strength.

One part of the sense of self is primary, a residue of childhood narcissism*. It stems from autoerotism* and infantile, essentially narcissistic, object relations (at the beginning of life there is no distinction between the ego* and the object* of pleasure*). These object relations, more or less pleasurable, more or less traumatic, leave different types of traces in the structuring of the ego and the psychical apparatus. Thus, children who have felt predominantly loved by their parents obtain primarily a level of self-esteem that gives their ego strength to reach further levels of self-esteem or to endure their subsequent lack of satisfaction more successfully.

All this may vary as a consequence of passage through the Oedipus complex*, which may leave severe narcissistic wounds that constitute eventual "bedrock" in the structuring of the psychical apparatus.

In women, the castration complex* often leaves a feeling of self-depreciation that sometimes becomes a basic character trait, especially if the woman has not attained a good level of sublimation*; in this case, it forces her to raise self-esteem in later ways; that is to say, by satisfying the superego-ego ideal (for this reason women are generally more docile and better adapted to social reality*) or by creating the need to receive a large amount of narcissistic satisfaction from object libido (she is more dependent on the object and its love*).

To recapitulate: part of the sense of self or self-esteem is primary, a residue of infantile narcissism. There are two other parts. One stems from actions carried out by the ego in compliance with mandates of the ego ideal*, which generally refer to sublimation. Of course, they also refer to other accomplishments such as having children, mainly in women, but also in men due to the mandate for descendants (we recall Schreber). All of the ego's success in complying with superego mandates raises self-esteem and leaves a deep, pleasurable feeling connected with the feeling of narcissistic omnipotence.

The other part springs from love received from objects or loved ones; it consists of the type of narcissistic satisfaction produced by the object relation: feeling loved by the object.

Falling in love is a flowing over of narcissistic libido into the object which empties the ego and therefore decreases self-esteem. It is recovered by being loved.

A severe disorder of self-esteem withdraws libido from objects and places it in the ego in order to stanch its wounds; it thereby transforms lowered valuation of the ego into its opposite which is expressed as diverse character traits* such as haughtiness and arrogance. The most severe cases produce delusions* of grandeur or megalomania*. This is the case of narcissistic affections in general and mania* and paranoia* in particular.

In transference neuroses* self-esteem tends to be decreased since libido cathects presentations* of object wishes* in phantasy which are impossible to satisfy since they have been repressed. This empties the ego of cathexis* which consequently lowers self-esteem.

In psychoanalytic treatment of transference neuroses, when repressions* are lifted by making conscious the unconscious*, libidinal cathexes that were anticathexes* are freed upon which they reinforce the ego (more precisely, its possibility to think what was previously repressed), which increases its self-esteem and therefore its capacity to love.

A special case of decrease of self-esteem is melancholia* in which death Trieb is defused. The object is mistaken, by identification*, for the ego. Then, hate* for the object appears in consciousness as hatred of the ego.

SELF-OBSERVATION

Ger.: Selbstwahrnemung. – Sp.: autoobservación (observación de sí). – It.: auto-osservazione. – Port.: auto-observação.

This is a function of the superego*, together with the ego ideal* (in charge of what the subject "should be") and moral conscience* (of what the subject "should not be"). This particular task is observation of the ego, its thought and actions. This observant attitude involves on the one hand a caregiving aspect and on the other hand a certain threatening attitude that relays the punitory superego aspect to moral conscience*. This observation endeavours to ensure that everything is correct and that there is no manifestation whatsoever of repressed Triebe; it is a watchman procuring to block any differences between the ego and the ego ideal, and if they do arise or appear, to punish them with a sense of guilt*.

Self-observation is evident in paranoiac hallucinations that point out what the subject is doing ("now he is looking"), which includes a veiled threat (in this case, to the one looking, for example, to "make sure" that it does not involve the primal scene*); it may also be addressed to what the subject does, for example, with his hands ("he has them on the table") in order to avoid masturbation*.

SELF-PRESERVATIVE TRIEB (EGO)

Ger.: (Ich) Sebsterhaltungstrieb. – Sp.: pulsión de autoconservación del yo. – Fr.: pulsion d'autoconservation du moi. – It.: pulsione d'autoconservazione del io. – Port.: pulsão de autoconservação do ego.

This part of life Triebe* is dedicated to protect the ego* and to help it to "die only in its fashion" (*Beyond the Pleasure Principle*, 1920) or to do so in the manner immanent to it, avoiding shortcuts to reach the inorganic for which death Trieb* is fighting.

In the Freudian scheme, breathing and hunger are models of self-preservative Triebe. They sometimes oppose sexual Triebe* and are fused with the latter at other times.

Self-preservative Triebe force the subject to rapid recognition of reality* (initial reality ego*), even the object recognized as such, since it cannot be replaced by hallucination*, presentation*, or phantasy*. In this sense, it is peremptory and immutable, and serves as anaclisis* for subsequent object choice of sexual Triebe*.

When self-preservative Trieb is sexualized, its satisfaction becomes part of sexual problems (anorexia, bulimia); an apparent loss of self-preservative Trieb may also occur in severe affections (attempted suicide in melancholia, schizophrenia, or hysteria).

In all cases, self-preservative Trieb is weak or poor in human infants, which explains part of their helplessness and dependency on the object. The ego's problems depend on the vicissitudes of narcissistic libido* belonging to sexual Trieb and cathecting the ego.

SELF-PUNISHMENT

Ger.: Selbstbestrafung. – Sp.: autocastigo. – Fr.: auto-punition. – It.: autocastigo. – Port.: autocastigo.

An intermediate phase of reversal into the opposite (transformation of activity into passivity) of sadism*, Freud discusses this concept in *Instincts and Their Vicissitudes* (1915). Here, we observe turning round upon the subject's own self but without passivity towards another. This is the first part of the transformation of sadism into masochism* when the presence of an object* to take the role of the sadistic subject is unnecessary.

In the self-punishment typical of obsessional neurosis* (but which may be found in any neurosis*), the active verb does not change into the passive verb but rather into an intermediate, reflexive verb. The object is renounced and replaced by the subject.

Self-punishment goes further than self-reproaches*, since it involves action (punishment) but is not quite masochism, which requires the presence of a sadistic object.

Self-punishment falls within the category of narcissism*; masochism needs at least a narcissistic object choice* but does involve an object after all.

If we add elements from other works, such as *Beyond the Pleasure Principle* (1920) and *The Ego and the Id* (1923), we may say that there is some Trieb* fusion between Eros* and death Trieb*, a certain degree of admixture that also involves some degree of defusion. However, although the presence of the object is in reality unnecessary, ego* identification* with the object enables the superego to take advantage of this situation to punish the ego. Sometimes, the ego defends itself (obsessional neurosis) whereas at other times it surrenders meekly, as in melancholia*, the narcissistic neurosis *par excellence.*

SELF-REPROACH

Ger.: Selbstvorwürfe. – Sp.: autoreproches. – Fr.: auto-reproches. – It.: autorimproveri. – Port.: autoacusações.

This reproach is addressed to the ego* by the superego*, especially in the case of obsessional neurosis or in the neuroses* in general, for not being like the ego ideal* as demanded by the superego. In obsessional neurosis, self-reproach is particularly sadistic since libido has returned (cf. regression*) to the phase of anal-sadistic autoerotism* and has taken the ego and superego back as well. The ego's attitude is submission to the superego, albeit under protest (ambivalence), always awaiting a distraction of the superego to rebel. The result is the complaint (the ego's complaint addressed to its oppressive superego), a typical element in the discourse of the obsessional character*.

In melancholia*, self-reproach is almost pathognomonic. Its presence enables us to differentiate melancholia from mourning*. It corresponds to withdrawal of libido from the object, an aggressive libidinal break from it, the decathectization* of its unconscious (Inc) presentation* and the ego's identification with the object as in the phase of the pleasure ego*. The previous tie of hate with the object now becomes the same tie with the ego, now identified with this object; for this reason it is reproached by the superego. In this picture, the ego does not rebel against the punitory superego, which may lead the patient to suicide since it imaginarily corresponds to murder of the object, now identified with the ego.

SENSE OF INFERIORITY

Ger.: Minderwertigkeitsgefühl. – Sp.: sentimiento de inferioridad. – Fr.: sentiment d'infériorité. – It.: senso d'inferiorità. – Port.: sentimento de inferioridade.

An implicit decrease in self-esteem* is often suffered by patients with transference neurosis*, generated by the difference between their ego ideal* and ego*, a gap that provokes a sense of guilt*.

It also results from the lack of love* of the individual's objects*.

The latter is usually produced by the patient's inability to love, a product of repressions* with their libidinal introversion, and of taking refuge in the world of phantasy* (which increase the sense of guilt because they are usually beautified disguises of incestuous or parricidal scenes).

These causes intertwine with each other, since growing distance from object wishes* in reality and their transfer to phantasies leads to more distance from demands of the ego ideal in relation to specific actions* the ego needs to exert according to the ideal.

We may go back to earlier periods of life. For example, to an unresolved castration* complex, a typically feminine situation (in both men and women) which leads to phallic fixations* in the period of the first levels of recognition of sexual difference, which is phallic–castrated. The sense of inferiority is produced by the feeling of being castrated, of being deprived of the organ of love. Then, the facts and their metapsychological explanation become more complicated, since narcissistic libidinal withdrawal* may ensue, cathecting the ego. If libidinal withdrawal is successful, defensive ego traits against the sense of inferiority appear instead, such as arrogance or even delusions* of grandeur in psychotic clinical pictures.

Melancholia* is a narcissistic clinical picture presenting features of the sense of inferiority: regressive hate* towards the object* is aimed by identification* at the ego, and the superego* consequently gluts its cruelty on the ego.

In these cases, the sense of guilt* predominates, acquiring delusional characteristics. The feeling of inferiority has a more aggressive nuance, is more heavily charged with hate: hate for the ego (in which the object is camouflaged), related to the degree of regression* and therefore, to defusion of death Trieb*.

> The sense of inferiority has strong erotic roots. A child feels inferior if he notices that he is not loved, and so does an adult. The only bodily organ which is really regarded as inferior is the atrophied penis, a girl's clitoris. But the major part of the sense of inferiority derives from the ego's relation to its superego; like the sense of guilt it is an expression of the tension between them. Altogether, it is hard to separate the sense of inferiority and the sense of guilt. It would perhaps be right to regard the former as the erotic complement to the moral sense of inferiority.
>
> (*New Introductory Lectures on Psycho-Analysis*, 1933, pp. 65–6)

SEPARATE PSYCHICAL GROUP

Ger.: separaten psychischen Gruppe. – Sp.: grupo psíquico separado. – Fr.: groupe psychique séparé. – It.: gruppo psichico separato. – Port.: grupo psíquico separado.

This is one of Freud's first approximations to the concept of repressed unconscious* or repressed presentation. This approximation stems in part from concepts presented by Pierre Janet, a disciple of Charcot, regarding the splitting of consciousness in hysteria*. Freud considered that hysteria is not caused by a problem of degeneration preventing the ego* from performing its synthetic function, but rather a psychical problem: since certain wish* presentations* are irreconcilable with the patient's conscious ego, it defends itself against them by separating them from associative commerce or thought* activity. It removes libidinal cathexis* from the words necessary for access to consciousness, and consequently unacceptable impulses cannot be put into action.

If the original cathexis of the psychical group cathects a muscular or sensory innervation, a conversion hysteria* is configured.

If the separate psychical group remains in the preconscious*; that is to say, possesses cathected word-presentations* (so long as they are isolated affectively or by associative bindings from the remaining preconscious presentations, unable to participate in associative commerce), obsessions, obsessional ideas and other symptoms of obsessional neurosis* are produced; the subject thinks them involuntarily and neither understands nor accepts them as belonging to the subject's own ego, despite the anxiety they cause.

SEXUALITY

Ger.: Sexualität. – Sp.: sexualidad. – Fr.: sexualité. – It.: sessualità. – Port.: sexualidade.

Freud's conception of sexuality, developed throughout his works, is one of his greatest contributions to our knowledge of human beings and their psyche.

The sexuality presented in Freudian thought is an expanded sexuality compared to what is commonly understood by it. In this sense and by virtue of its constant transformations, it extends to almost all phenomena of psychical life, although it simultaneously maintains its specificity.

This conception emerges from clinical experience with neurotic patients, the origin of whose symptoms* always includes unconscious sexual phantasies* which, when made conscious, drive back these symptoms.

However, they also exist in the origin of psychical structures such as the ego* and its character* and the superego*, which is in charge of the subject's behaviour in adult life. We try to produce changes in these structures through psychoanalysis; especially by making constructions* of the period in which they formed, which is the period of infantile sexuality* remaining in the adult's unconscious*.

Sexuality also participates in the origin of culture*. The latter is ultimately a vicissitude of human sexuality and the avatars of its history.

In the life of human beings, sexuality goes through diverse "libidinal phases". In each of these stages, certain sensations and a type of link with objects* corresponding to certain erotogenic zones* predominate. All this makes them appear to be different phenomena.

This also occurs in animal sexuality, but the difference in human beings is its development in two surges, separated by a latency* period when sexual development is "frozen" in favour of cultural progress. Acceptance of this conception involves the existence of infantile sexuality which does not include procreation but does include pleasure*.

Pleasure seeking is essential to all the phases of sexuality and is ultimately the thread that brings it together; it is therefore one of the principles governing the functioning of the entire psychical apparatus. We have mentioned several elements: the existence of sexuality that arises at the very first and develops until it reaches the possibility of procreation; this development takes place in several stages, but has basically two "high tides" which culminate in adolescence when it unfolds with all its capacity for action and therefore for pleasure seeking, which becomes essential for human sexuality.

Sexuality has different vicissitudes. It may be transformed into neurotic symptoms and creative activities, beginning with language*, by virtue of a psychical alchemy referred to by Freud as sublimation*.

The concept of Trieb* is associated with the concept of sexuality; it is the turning point at which human sexuality moves from the biological into the psychical. Other themes surround it turbulently: libido*, wish*, Trieb*, object*, narcissism*, and so on.

Then, human sexuality accompanies the vicissitudes of sexual Trieb*; it arises from bodily needs, but when they are connected with presentations* of experiences with objects, they become wishes (if we emphasize the presentational) and into libido (if the emphasis is placed on the energetic aspect); the essence of Trieb is the impulse (*Drang*) towards action to take with an object, the latter becoming the aim* of Trieb which discharges its source.

After 1920, in the "second Trieb theory", sexuality becomes life Trieb* *par excellence.* The tendency to repeat previous pleasurable experiences tames death Trieb* which tends to return to the inorganic.

The result is the essence of the phenomena of life: the longest delay possible on the path leading to death. This path must include the pleasure principle* and another element which perfects it: the reality principle*.

Now we have come to an apparent paradox: satisfaction of infantile and even adult sexual Trieb, although (as life Trieb) it supports cultural phenomena, is in itself anticultural. For this reason, infantile sexuality is mostly repressed and then constitutes the repressed unconscious. Its aim is partly inhibited, creating cultural ties such as tenderness, friendship, and others. It is also partly sublimated (cultural ties are also sublimations), becoming human creations to transform "the face of the earth".

The adult sexual couple is antisocial, since they do not want to share their partner (in non-perverse sexual acts, of course), but wish to master this partner. They do not want to share each other, at least during the period of previous courtship and after the moment of the pleasurable sexual link (*Group Psychology and the Analysis of the Ego*, 1921).

Culture establishes a representative in the psychical apparatus to ensure obedience to this cultural mandate and to defend itself from sexual Triebe (especially in children). This guard is a part of the ego called the superego, in charge of regulating, by watching the ego, different forms of satisfaction of sexual Trieb and wishes.

This superego may even, paradoxically, call upon death Triebe for help in order to keep sexuality in line.

Infantile sexuality is at first autoerotic. However, this autoerotism* (which is never absolute, except in the first levels of the ego when the object of pleasure is considered ego since the psyche functions only with the category of *being** and not with that of *having**) is inaugurated by the maternal object during caregiving of the infant. This generates the wish to repeat sensations perceived in these experiences, which may be satisfied immediately on account of autoerotism.

The advent of language enables a nearly limitless complexity of perception by consciousness of the different types of relations between presentations, since word-presentations* allow the ego's consciousness to perceive its own thought* chains.

Autoerotism also becomes wish-fulfilling phantasies* of wishes for different types of links with objects (sexual or desexualized) in thoughts that prepare the subject for action and the possibility of transforming these wishes into facts (by inhibition* of the hallucination* created by the incipient ego).

It becomes possible to think of this body called ego* as a unit. This is the seat of thought, which attains unimagined heights by virtue of language. This achievement is joined by the submission of the different bodily erotogenic zones to phallic supremacy*, which ultimately forms a unit with this body and its manner of feeling pleasure. From this a new psychical space is generated called ego (a definitive reality ego). Autoerotism thereby becomes narcissism (*On Narcissism: An Introduction*, 1914).

This narcissism is a different means of satisfaction of sexual Trieb, partly opposed to object Trieb, which comes to a new crossroads when the first level of recognition of sexual difference is reached (*From the History of an Infantile Neurosis*, 1918).

The phallic* period, in which the wish for recognition of sexual difference by object libido clashes with horror of it, since it is considered a danger by narcissism essentially based on the phallic, a dead-end that concludes with establishment of the superego and dissolution* and repression* of the Oedipus complex*, the zenith of the development and fall of the empire of infantile sexuality.

The latency* period ensues, an apparent suspension of sexual development until puberty, when it resurges with all its strength and conflictive problems, now with a body that has developed and is able to put it into action.

In the course of this process, neurosis*, sexual perversions*, psychosis*, or character* disorders may be formed, or a more normal ego may be created leading wishes through many positions encountered within and outside the psychical apparatus whose structuring improves depending on their synthesis.

This explanation of the development of sexuality, so complex and described so succinctly in this text, contains Freud's very original proposal regarding this subject; in it, he is able to intimately interrelate the bodily biological and the social, also explaining the way in which these two levels function together to structure everything psychical, human behaviour in general, and its pathology in particular.

SEXUAL PERVERSION

Ger.: sexuelle Perversion. – Sp. perversión sexual. – Fr.: perversion sexuelle. – It.: perversione sexuale. – Port.: perversão sexual.

This form of satisfaction of sexual Trieb* differs from those of neurosis*, psychosis*, and normality.

The term "perversion" antedates Freud, and has a denigrating connotation attributed to it by a moral evaluation of sexuality* which indicates that sexual perversions have been and for the most part continue to be condemned by society.

Freud utilizes a photographic metaphor to describe them as the "negative" of the neuroses. Unconscious phantasies* generate symptoms* in neurotics; however, they become real facts in perverse individuals. They are forms of infantile sexual satisfaction*, both pre-oedipal and oedipal. They originate in traumatic or hereditary fixation points which in neuroses are repressed and produce anxiety*, whereas in perversions they are a source of pleasure*.

In *Three Essays on Sexual Theory* (1905), Freud classifies them phenomenologically:

Deviations concerning the sexual object. This is the case in homosexuality, of which there are three types: absolute, bisexual, or occasional;

Deviations concerning the sexual aim. Anatomical violations, fetishism, sadism-masochism, voyeurism-exhibitionism, for example, are considered perversions;

All these cases are considered perversions when they become necessary conditions for sexual excitation and orgasm and are preferred over "genital" or "normal" sexuality. In normal adult sexuality they may be part of fore-pleasure* leading to the genital aim.

Human sexual development involves so many vicissitudes that the idea that fixation points generating perverse or neurotic tendencies might not be generated in its course responds to an ideal rather than to reality.

Freud outlines different metapsychological explanations (which may be articulated) of the phenomenon of homosexuality and perversion in general. In this direction, in *Leonardo da Vinci and a Memory of His Childhood* (1910), he explains:

> In all our male homosexual cases the subjects had had a very intense erotic attachment to a female person, as a rule their mother, during the first period of childhood, which is afterwards forgotten; this attachment was evoked or encouraged by too much tenderness on the part of the mother herself, and further reinforced by the small part played by the father during their childhood. Sadger emphasizes the fact that the

mothers of his homosexual patients were frequently masculine women, women with energetic traits of character, who were able to push the father out of his proper place. I have occasionally seen the same thing, but I was more strongly impressed by cases in which the father was absent from the beginning or left the scene at an early date, so that the boy found himself left entirely under feminine influence. Indeed it almost seems as though the presence of a strong father would ensure that the son made the correct decision in his choice of object, namely someone of the opposite sex.

After this preliminary stage a transformation sets in whose mechanism is known to us but whose motive forces we do not yet understand. The child's love for his mother cannot continue to develop consciously any further; it succumbs to repression. The boy represses his love for his mother: he puts himself in her place, identifies himself with her, and takes his own person as a model in whose likeness he chooses the new object of his love. In this way he has become a homosexual. What he has in fact done is to slip back to autoerotism: for the boys whom he now loves as he grows up are after all only substitutive figures and revivals of himself in childhood – boys whom he loves in the way in which his mother loved him when he was a child.

(pp. 99–100)

In *A Child Is Being Beaten* (1919) he adds:

The most obvious result of such a discussion is its application to the origin of the perversions. The view which brought into the foreground in this connection the constitutional reinforcement or premature growth of a single sexual component is not shaken, indeed; but it is seen not to comprise the whole truth. The perversion is no longer an isolated fact in the child's sexual life, but falls into its place among the typical, not to say normal, processes of development which are familiar to us. It is brought into relation with the child's incestuous love-object, with its Oedipus complex. It first comes into prominence in the sphere of this complex, and after the complex has broken down it remains over, often quite by itself, the inheritor of the charge of libido from that complex and weighed down by the sense of guilt that was attached to it.

(pp. 191–2)

In this last passage, he shows us the participation of the superego* in perverse masochistic pleasure, to which repression* of the genital is added, as well as regression to the stage of predominant anal-sadistic* erotism and the transformation of sadism* into masochism*, which also involves the sense of guilt*. We could say that the central problem of perversions centres upon sexual difference; that is to say, its non-recognition by perverse individuals. "Object libido" strictly speaking is what is satisfied with a sexual object different from the subject, possessing a different sex. Any relationship with objects of the same sex or who are not recognized as belonging to a different sex is formed with "homosexual libido". Infantile sexuality is provided basically with homosexual libido since it does not recognize sexual differences, which emerge only with the appearance of phallic problems in the Oedipus complex (phallic–castrated), culminating in adolescence (masculine–feminine).

Homosexual libido is an intermediate step between object and narcissistic libido; intermediate not in the developmental sense but rather considering its location in relation to the ego* and the object*. It is object libido since it recognizes the object as a source of pleasure, but is also narcissistic since sexual difference is not recognized; some object choices* are based on the subject's own attributes, whether actual or from childhood. Sexual differences are disavowed as a means of defence* against castration anxiety* felt in the period of the Oedipus complex. However, since disavowal* was unsuccessful, it generated splitting in the ego* by which castration anxiety was able to enter and, with it, implicit recognition of this difference.

In perversions the unconscious object presentation*. is cathected* and the preconscious word-presentation as well. The object is narcissistic, either representing the ego or alternatively, presentations of the ego are mixed in specific aspects with those of the object. Whether the object is mixed or identified with the ego or not, there is object desire; this object is recognized as such in every way except in connection with the object's sex; narcissism* would face terrible danger if it were otherwise.

These characteristics of object choice place perversions within narcissistic pathology. They are non-psychotic narcissistic affections.

SEXUAL TRIEB

Ger.: Sexualtrieb. – Sp.: pulsión sexual. – Fr.: pulsion sexuelle. – It.: istinto o pulsione sessuale. – Port.: pulsão sexual.

This is life Trieb* *par excellence* whose ultimate aim is preservation of the species, especially from the biological viewpoint. In this sense it also creates progressively larger units, constantly making the inorganic and life itself more complex. Thus, it is also opposed to death Triebe* which tend to disaggregation, to separation of these complexities created by life, in order to return to the inorganic.

It is guided by the pleasure principle*, the search for perceptual identity* with pleasurable experiences in the object* link through the erotogenic zones*, especially in the period of infantile defencelessness, most of which are repressed in the unconscious*.

Sexual Triebe develop in a complex manner until the possibility of procreation is reached; at that moment they coincide with the maximum capacity for pleasure: genital pleasure*, which is added to the previous pleasures corresponding to each erotogenic zone or developmental phase in which each of these zones predominates and later subordinated to this greater pleasure.

These erotogenic zones are awakened from the outset in the object link through caregiving showered by the object on the defenceless human infant; in this way, attraction to the object is born, with wishes* for it and sexual Triebe aimed towards pleasure already obtained and potentially obtained with it. Their anaclisis is self-preservative Triebe* with the pleasurable sensations awakened by caregiving of the erotogenic zones, a plus of pleasure following satisfaction which slowly becomes independent of it.

These Triebe are less willing to recognize reality than self-preservative Triebe, since the object of pleasure is variable from the outset, even autoerotic, and for this reason recognition of reality becomes less indispensable for satisfaction of this Trieb or some part of it.

However, the part of sexual Trieb first attracted by the object, together with self-preservative Trieb, soon need the reality principle*, and must aim towards its recognition (initial reality ego*).

Sexual Trieb is the best type of taming of death Trieb, with which it is always fused to diverse degrees. The higher sexual evolution is, the greater degree of fusion there will be. For this reason, in diverse libidinal regressions* which may appear in pathology, Trieb defusions may be produced which liberate death Trieb.

Although the development of libido* has individual aspects, it also follows a path left by the species on its road towards culture*.

In the oral* phase, the aim is to incorporate the object (model of identification*), and its pleasure is derived from sucking on the mother's breast, which may be extended to any zones of the baby's own body which stimulate labial mucous membranes in a rhythmic manner (autoerotism*).

Afterwards, when the anal* zone predominates, the muscular apparatus is dominated and sadism* and Trieb for mastery* may be discharged more effectively. The active pleasure of this phase resides in discharge of the muscular apparatus; its passive pleasure resides in the pleasure of anal mucous membranes by means of retention of faeces. In this phase, the object is starting to be recognized as the source of pleasure (forced by reality), and with it the first level of anxiety signal* arises; fear of object loss*.

With mastery of the muscles, the first playing is possible, which enables a symbolic level of mastery of the object, thereby partly attenuating fear of object loss.

However, the main event is the beginning of language* acquisition, which forms the basis for many other consequences and for culture in general, the erect position also cooperating, as well as mastery of sphincters and muscles (weapons for action), control of urination to extinguish fire, and especially, the central cause generating culture: the prohibition of incest and parricide. The formation of a speaking, thinking ego* arises with language, with word-presentations that may be utilized to symbolize or think about the object (infantile sexual theories*), and also to reach it, but especially to be able to think about it and even to think about the child's own self, to think about the ego.

The subject brings all this baggage to the phallic phase (former levels included the pleasures of seeing and being seen, touching and being touched, sadism and masochism*, for example), a phase that inaugurates the first level of recognition of sexual difference (although certain differences were already recognized), and roads are opened which distinguish girls from boys in human culture. This first level of recognition of sexual difference coincides with the second level of object choice* and the second level of infantile masturbation* (presentational and incestuous).

In boys with a predominantly positive Oedipus complex*, the object, predestined due to its anaclisis* in self-preservative Trieb, becomes incestuous. The father with whom he seeks to identify because he loves him acquires the characteristics of a rival, and this identification takes on a hostile tone.

Henceforward the greatest trauma* of infantile sexuality* develops, leading to definitive passage into culture by establishment in the psychical apparatus of a structure, a product of secondary identifications*, a specialized part of the ego: the superego*.

This superego is from that time forward dedicated to watching over the ego from within the subject's psychical apparatus to ensure that it complies with the basic requisites of human culture: the prohibition of incest and parricide.

Following establishment of the superego – a commemorative monument to the Oedipus complex in the psychical apparatus – sexuality* enters a period of latency*, specific to the human species, in which sexuality is as if suspended in time, expressed by sublimations, their derivatives, or inhibitions of its sexual aim (tenderness, friendship, social sentiments).

Sublimation* and suppression* of Trieb in this period are exerted in exchange for maternal and paternal affection, which calms the oedipal storm.

Therefore, human sexuality develops in two separate periods. It reappears with all its force and drama in puberty and adolescence, transformed into exogamic* sexuality.

Thus, the history of infantile sexuality left in the unconscious continues, revealing its effectiveness in repetition compulsions* of situations in the vicissitudes of subsequent histories with objects.

The case is different when sexuality in object links was not essentially satisfactory or was traumatic early in life. This may have generated the circumstance that sexual Trieb continues to be satisfied autoerotically and narcissistically, that object choices are predominantly narcissistic, or that narcissistic wounds are not tolerated from that time forward. For example, if sexual difference cannot be accepted in the phallic phase (phallic–castrated), it must be disavowed. This may generate splitting in the ego*, one of the characteristics of sexual perversions* such as fetishism* and homosexuality* in which the Oedipus complex acquires a predominantly negative characteristic (homosexual, narcissistic).

Here, sexual Trieb adopts perverse characteristics and falls within narcissistic pathology; that is to say, ego defences against sexual Trieb acquire this characteristic.

In girls the road of Trieb is complex. The girl establishes a more prolonged pre-oedipal link with her mother in the oral, anal, and phallic phases; in the third, substantial differences from boys appear.

In all the phases, forms of satisfaction are both active and passive in relation to the aim. Sexual Trieb is essentially active, since it is "tendency".

The part of phallic activity corresponds to clitoral masturbation associated with more or less conscious, more or less disguised phantasies* of making the mother have a child. These phantasies may sometimes be partly corroborated or also reinforced by the birth of a sibling. Another form of expression may be playing with dolls.

The passive form tends to be expressed by phantasies of maternal seduction*, supported by historical truth* of the mother's caregiving and washing of her infant daughter, which awaken pleasurable sensations in the erotogenic zones.

This maternal link is later observed as the negative Oedipus rather than pre-oedipal, phallic castration now evident although it had been perceived before by observation of a brother or felt in the ambivalence* of her mother's link with her in comparison to her brother (existing or wished for).

The girl therefore confronts the castration complex* which produces deep feelings of being handicapped, hatred towards her mother who is considered guilty of this fact, and envy of boys for the penis they possess (cf. penis envy), for example.

This complexity of deeply painful feelings may leave traces, in some cases indelible, in her character*, including defence* against them. By virtue of the hate-filled break from her mother, she changes object and then expects to get a child (by the symbolic equation: penis=child) from her father, then enters the positive Oedipus which continues until puberty, when she also changes her predominant erotogenic zone, passing to the vagina and displacing paternal object choice onto an exogamic object choice. The latency period in girls is less manifest, repression* is more moderate, and establishment of the superego takes longer than in boys.

We could advance the idea that in the structure of the female psychical apparatus the ego's masochism predominates over the superego's sadism. The opposite would be true for the male psychical apparatus in which the superego's sadism predominates over the ego's masochism. This could be attributed to the way the superego is structured in males which gives it sadistic characteristics, not usually observed in women; despite the existence in men of feminine masochism. We could also consider a predominance of sadism in the female ego ideal* in cases where it is structured (phallic fixations) as masculine. We propose all these ideas in general terms and as lines for investigation.

Sexual Trieb's aim is discharge, accomplished through an object, towards which it is impelled by its somatic source (cf. Trieb*). Its purpose is to reach the Trieb aim* and carry out specific action* although it may have variations since the object is variable (fixations* deprive it of variability). Its aim is sometimes active and sometimes passive; this aspect also possesses some variability, at least developmental.

Sexual Trieb may also be successfully repressed and remain dissolved (cf. dissolution*) in the unconscious (boys' incestuous desire for their mother, for example), or may return from it and generate neurosis* (when repression fails). It may be sublimated, a product of culture, and may also generate culture. In this case, taming* of death Trieb is not as successful, since it inhibits the sexual aim, leaving Trieb desexualized, and consequently, a larger proportion of death Trieb is left free.

The conscious ego may also tame sexual Trieb, knowing its thing-presentation* by virtue of the word that represents it. Then it binds it with other presentations, giving it 'associative commerce' and thereby use of thought* activity, or even a possibility to apply judgement of condemnation*.

SHAME

Ger.: Scham / Ischande. – Sp.: vergüenza. – Fr.: honte. – It.: vergogna. – Port.: vergonha.

One of the dams of infantile sexuality*, it is formed as an anticathexis* of the Trieb* pleasure of looking and the reversal into the opposite*, the pleasure of being looked at (exhibitionism).

Both types of satisfaction of this Trieb undergo a first level of repression*, "primal repression"*, which changes the affect* into possible Trieb satisfaction by transforming it from pleasurable into anxiety-producing. Shame is one form of this anxiety*. It is usually felt in response to the sight of the object's* nudity or to exposure of the subject's own nudity. These scenes may acquire more or less symbolic characteristics (for example, shame for "dirty words" or dirty jokes: a symbolic form of exhibitionism, being undressed or undressing).

Shame is an important, even indispensable requisite for access to culture*.

It acts in a psychoanalysis at first as an obstacle to free association*; since shame is a conscious affect that may sometimes be consciously suppressed, the analyst suggests that patients leave it aside and give free rein to whatever comes to mind. It is easier for patients to do so when they are in sublimated positive transference*, when shame originates mainly in conscious or preconscious causes, than when they proceed from unconscious primal repressions which lie beyond conscious will*.

A child's scopophilia is closely related with its infantile sexual curiosity, which is related with the Trieb for knowledge*. These Triebe are associated with inherited primal phantasies* such as the primal scene*. All this stimulation leads to infantile eagerness for knowledge which inevitably leads towards the Oedipus complex* and all its dramatic problems. The latter include recognition of sexual difference followed by the definitive establishment of primal repression and the superego*.

From that point on, shame acquires an oedipal tinge related with meanings of this type or referring to this theme. In the absence of excessive traumatic situations*, shame is useful as an adaptive cultural manner to approach the object. Otherwise, depending on the type of fixation* produced, it may be too intense and too difficult to overcome.

Neuroses may then be originated with heavy degrees of repression and libidinal introversion; or the opposite: shame may be too weak or also be anticathected or suppressed, thereby indirectly contributing an important element ("brazenness" on account of its lack) to narcissistic disorders and perversions*, psychopathic disorders, and even psychosis*.

SOCIAL FEELINGS

Ger.: Sozialgefühle. – Sp.: sentimientos sociales. – Fr.: sentiments sociaux. – It.: sentimenti sociali. – Port.: sentimentos sociais.

These feelings may be attributed to attraction exerted by the object*, removed from a sexual or erotic aim: friendship, tenderness, solidarity, altruism, family ties, and so on. Concern for the object predominates, and they constitute social links, buttressing culture*.

They proceed from sublimation transformations of sexual libido* on which they are based, their aim inhibited. The same type of libido links the group*, the origin of paternal-filial ties following the dissolution of the Oedipus complex* and establishment of the superego* in the psychical apparatus.

They are therefore homosexual, and since sexual difference is unrelated to them, recognition of sexual difference is unnecessary for their existence.

> After the stage of heterosexual object choice has been reached, the homosexual tendencies are not, as might be supposed, done away with or brought to a stop; they are merely deflected from their sexual aim and applied to fresh uses. They now combine with portions of the ego-instincts and, as "attached" components, help to constitute the social instincts, thus contributing an erotic factor to friendship and comradeship, to *esprit de corps* and to the love of mankind in general. How large a contribution is in fact derived from erotic sources (with the sexual aim inhibited) could scarcely be guessed from the normal social relations of mankind. But it is not irrelevant to note that it is precisely manifest homosexuals, and among them again precisely those that set themselves against an indulgence in sensual acts, who are

distinguished by taking a particularly active share in the general interests of humanity.

(*Psycho-Analytic Notes on an Autobiographical Account of a Case of Paranoia (Dementia Paranoides)*, 1911, p. 61)

Even today the social feelings arise in the individual as a superstructure built upon impulses of jealous rivalry against his brothers and sisters. Since the hostility cannot be satisfied, identification with the former rival develops. The study of mild cases of homosexuality confirms the suspicion that in this instance, too, the identification is a substitute for an affectionate object choice which has taken the place of the aggressive, hostile attitude.

(*The Ego and the Id*, 1923, p. 37)

Especially by virtue of these sentiments, lasting love links are established, since their form of discharge is attenuated and never total as in sexuality* not inhibited in its aim. When these links are lost on account of frustrations* in social relations, for example, Trieb* loses opportunities for sublimation, which may give rise to pathological formations through libidinal introversion which sometimes extends to narcissistic* withdrawal.

In contrast, belonging to a certain type of institution or artificial group* (religious institutions are a good example) helps some kinds of symptoms to disappear, mainly those of transference neuroses.

"Thus the fact which is characteristic of the neurosis is the preponderance of the sexual over the social instinctual elements" (*Totem and Taboo*, 1913, p. 73).

SOMATIC COMPLIANCE

Ger.: somatisches Entgegenkommen. – Sp.: solicitación somática. – Fr.: complaisance somatique. – It.: complacenza somatica. – Port.: solicitação somática.

The concept of *somatic compliance* arises in Freud when he asks "whether the symptoms of hysteria are of psychical or of somatic origin, or whether, if the former is granted, they are necessarily all of them psychically determined" (*Fragment of an Analysis of a Case of Hysteria*, 1905, p. 40). Freud answers himself: "every hysterical symptom involves the participation of both sides. It cannot occur without the presence of a certain degree of somatic compliance offered by some normal or pathological process in or connected with one of the bodily organs" (Ibid.). He even states that, if this compliance does not exist, the symptom is different from a hysterical symptom; perhaps it would be a phobia or an obsessional idea; that is to say, an entirely psychical symptom.

Somatic compliance therefore resides in the facility of the subject's body to be utilized to express the meaning of a psychical symptom. All the same, the source of this facility is unclear: whether it resides in some previous or simultaneous bodily affection, a mimicking propensity in the subject or some part of the body, organic background, the excitability and concomitant defence of the erotogenic zones, or something else. What is quite clear is that Freud considers the hysterical possible not only because of the nature or presentational content of the repressed phantasy but also because the subject's somatic compliance enables it.

SOUL

Ger.: Seele. – Sp.: alma. – Fr.: âme. – It.: anima. – Port.: alma.

Freud never wrote about the soul as a subject in particular, although he referred to it repeatedly. The theme of the soul is traditionally subject-matter for religion or philosophy. Freud did not consider himself a philosopher and at a certain point even rejected any type of philosophical speculation of his own, instead following Charcot's motto: *Observe until the phenomena speak*. He always considered that his field of thinking was science. This does not mean, of course, that beyond his conscious intentions, but consistent with the very nucleus of his thought, he may not somehow have practised philosophy. He also admitted his affinity for philosophy, an attraction from which he said he defended himself in order to dedicate himself entirely to science. In his time (dominated by positivism, which is in reality a philosophical position) and in the scientific circle in which he was trained, philosophical speculation, especially metaphysics, were considered unclear and lacking in positive results. Science was obliged to be the child of empirical observation, although of course, Freudian empirical observation, following Kant, includes speculation; further, in some cases, he himself mentioned that he departs from the observational in order to resort to the terrain of speculation; one example is his explanation of the origin of what he called death Trieb*. Although Freudian metapsychology is part of observation, it sometimes reaches such a high level of abstraction that it becomes difficult to relate it to its subject, even though this relation exists and is quite intimate.

Freud used the word "soul" in an Aristotelian sense, as a synonym of the psyche or the psychical apparatus in general. Therefore, a Freud scholar could presumably tell us something about his conception of the soul because his scientific activity addressed the psyche. This was his subject. Perhaps we could say something about the subject of the soul in relation to the nucleus of Freudian thought, which is more akin to scientific description but not closely related to any philosophical description, even though this posture itself involves a philosophical position. Of course, what we describe here is in no way influenced by or connected with any kind of religious belief.

What, then, does Freud consider the psyche to be? If we were forced to decide in favour of a central concept for it, we would choose the presentation* together with energy (as a quantity of excitation which cathects and is cathected by presentations, through which it circulates on its path towards action). It goes without saying that Freud's concept of the presentation is not the same as the concepts of other thinkers, Schopenhauer's for example. Freud considers the presentation a memory or trace of perception*. In the famous Chapter 7 of *The Interpretation of Dreams* (1900) he calls it a "mnemic trace"*. This does not mean that the presentation is a simple register of reality; it is a processing of reality, but we could say that its place of origin is perception. Therefore it is the processing of what was a perception. What does this processing comprise? First, perception as he described it is selective; this selection is related with both what is wished for and also what is feared. This relation is dynamic: what was satisfactory is wished for and what was painful or traumatic is feared; that is to say, the same wish that was once a perception is now a presentation that seeks identical repetition: it seeks identity. Memory is also selective; it recalls what is satisfactory and forgets what is painful or traumatic; repression is its offspring. Presentational processing therefore starts with reality but departs from it, although it must still guide the search for action in order to reach a certain identity through action. This process becomes increasingly complex.

Human beings form two types of presentations: those that recall things, objects, and each individual's concepts regarding them, and also everything perceived and felt in relation to a certain perception which went through the entire sensory apparatus with them; the others are those that recall words that speak about these things, symbolizing them, language* no less; at a certain point, this language becomes so important in the human psyche that it is nearly synonymous with the psyche and therefore also of the soul. Both the problem and the virtue of words is that, as words in themselves, they may be presentations of something not experienced by the subject, but may provide something which enables the subject to speak (or think). This is possible because the subject may accumulate experiences of others through words which influence and become part of the soul. However, it is obviously not the same to speak about Spain as it is described in books as to know about it by going there. What is experienced, the mark left in the soul by experience* is referred to by Freud as the thing-presentation*. The language that speaks of it (making it even more complex, words also have their history in each individual's life; they are experiences in themselves, something different) is the word-presentation. Further, there are pleasant and unpleasant experiences; the soul seeks to repeat the pleasant ones by virtue of the pleasure principle* and the unpleasant ones by means of the Nirvana principle. Trieb seeks to repeat whereas thought* strives to find similarities in the differences between what is sought and what is repeated. In the process of this task, it creates.

However this may be, once words are attained, they are used for thinking, although thought in words always refers to thing-presentations, previous to and simultaneous with words, and to the idea the individual has acquired about them. Thought* with words may in turn establish logical connections between presentations of things that exceed those of analogy*, contiguity* and the search for perceptual identity*, going on to others that are more complex and in some way include them in this search for perceptual identity*. However, the soul is also identification*, an original Freudian concept, which although it could be described as an extension of the concept of presentation, is also new and expands the capacity of the psyche in general and the way to understand it in particular. The same may be said of psychical structuring which Freud refers to as the psychical apparatus; it includes repression* with its effects of presentational forgetting and the consequent stiffening and "shrinking" of the soul familiar to the subject; superego guilt, aspiration to ideals and so on: the rest of Freud's works. All this is the legacy of both parents, of experiences with them, experience in which the subject was not of course simply passive; that is to say, the ordering of the psyche based on presentations and identifications which model the possibility of action carried out at first by the body*. Somatic memory circulates throughout these presentations; depending on its relation with them, it acquires the name of libido*, Trieb* or wish*.

Summarizing, we have a body with memories of things that happen to it; these are presentations in general, cathected by quantity of energy, and which in turn also cathect (cf. cathexis*). The action of this body springs from this process, either directed by thought* produced by language* and consciousness*, or directly, by thing-presentations relegated to the unconscious* at the moment of structuring of the psychical apparatus. Another ingredient, also presentational, in this complex network with its psychical structures is the inherited presentations or primal phantasies which were also perceptions of experiences, foundational but pertaining not to the subject but rather to the human species. These phylogenetic phantasies act as categories that need to be filled with individual experience, which is summed up in Goethe's dictum from *Faust*, quoted by Freud: "What thou hast inherited from thy fathers, acquire it to make it thine" (*An Outline of Psycho-Analysis*, 1940, p. 207, *n.* 1).

The soul completes its circle when the body's life ends. The quota of immortality that the soul may access lies in its attributes which may be perpetuated through identifications of offspring, even in contents of some presentations of their psyche, whether pleasant or unpleasant; also in works accomplished by each subject in a lifetime, and in the memory of those still alive, all elements contributing to this measure of possible immortality. With the passing of generations and with repression, mortal histories* may sometimes be transmitted through words, thereby attaining the category of myths* or history*. In other cases they may be transmitted through unconscious mechanisms such as identification* and then simply be repeated.

SPECIFIC ACTION

Ger.: Spezifische Aktion. – Sp.: acción específica (o acorde a un fin). – Fr.: action spécifique. – It.: azione specifica. – Port.: ação específica.

This action adequate to an aim is performed by the subject in the external world; the subject changes the latter in some way, by virtue of which a lasting discharge is produced in the source of Trieb*. It is the opposite (in its relation to reality*) of internal change* (expression of emotions) and hallucinatory satisfaction of wishes*, neither of which produces discharge in the Trieb source.

Freud mentioned this concept in his *Project for a Scientific Psychology* (1950*a*) and *The*

Interpretation of Dreams (1900*a*), but it is also implicit in many other works, from the paper on anxiety neurosis (1895), through *Repression* (1915*d*), and finally in *Civilization and its Discontents* (1930*a*).

For example, in *Instincts and Their Vicissitudes* (1915*c*) he states that physiology

> has given us the concept of a "stimulus" and the pattern of the reflex, according to which a stimulus applied to living tissue (nervous substance) from the outside is discharged by action to the outside. This action is expedient in so far as it withdraws the stimulated substance from the influence of the stimulus, removes it out of its range of operation.

A few lines below, he notes that an instinct is a stimulus for the psyche:

> an instinctual stimulus does not arise from the external world but from within the organism itself ... An instinct ... never operates as a force giving a momentary impact but always as a constant one ... A better term for an instinctual stimulus is a "need". What does away with a need is "satisfaction". This can be attained only by an appropriate ("adequate") alteration of the internal source of stimulation.
>
> (pp. 118–19)

Therefore, the specific action should be the end of the energetic path that begins at the perceptual end* when the stimulus (internal or external to the body) enters the psychical apparatus and is perceived as an unpleasurable sensation now called affect* (internal change, expression of emotions, screaming, vascular innervation) that passes through this apparatus, binding as it goes through with presentations that lead it to the motor end where it completes the specific action inscribed in these presentations*. The action to which it thus arrives lowers the feeling of tension produced when the stimulus entered the psychical apparatus.

The concept of specific action refers originally to self-preservative Trieb* (giving rise to the idea of "specific" as if it were "one" action in particular), but becomes far more complex when referring to sexual Trieb*, since conflict in its vicissitudes generates splitting, repressions, and confrontations between different psychic places. It becomes even more complex when we add the factor of death Trieb* and its deflection toward the subject's exterior by virtue of the muscular system (destructive Trieb*); further complexity may be added by re-introducing destructive Trieb turned against the ego* by the superego, or Trieb that remains "floating" in the psychical apparatus from the outset in the form of primary or erotogenic masochism*.

In all these cases, the action with which Trieb pressure (*Drang*) must conclude loses its specificity or becomes more relative. For example, may we consider sublimation* or perversion* a specific action? Trieb seeks discharge. In its confrontation with culture* (partly outside the psychical apparatus and partly inside, by virtue of action of the superego), it may "succumb", its presentation decathected (successful dissolution* or repression*), or may be satisfied by substitution as in sublimation (partial satisfaction but satisfaction after all, which includes narcissistic satisfaction that increases self-esteem*). Trieb may also take a path by which to achieve some discharge (in the manner of a valve) by virtue of internal change or as the expression of its affects, for example anxiety*. Other paths of discharge may be some neurotic symptoms such as hysterical symptoms. Trieb may obviously be discharged by sexual perversions. It may also do so in a "normal" way as in sexual actions permitted by culture in general and by each individual superego in particular. In sum: we consider that sublimation possesses the characteristics necessary to be considered a specific action; we could say that it adds complexity to the concept but is not different, at least in regard to the narcissistic satisfaction it produces and its effect on the subject's self-esteem*. We cannot say the same for neurotic symptoms which are a hurdle for sublimation or even for the perverse if it is not simply one of the steps on the path leading to sexuality*.

In general, the problem discussed up to now in regard to sexual Trieb centres upon object libido* and its conflicts. As for narcissistic libido, it also acquires its own set of problems when it is unable to become object libido. In the case of perversions, an intermediate space of libidinal satisfaction is achieved between narcissistic* and object* satisfaction ("object" because it is satisfied by an object and "narcissistic" because the object represents the ego*). If eroticized narcissistic Trieb is thereby satisfied, conflicts arise with human culture* or in social links, since the aim of homosexual Trieb is not inhibited (social Trieb). Some conflicts with the superego may in turn generate neurotic aspects (sense of guilt*) in a perversion.

Narcissistic libido is satisfied principally (in the adult) by pleasing the ego ideal* that demands sublimation. Therefore, action the ego will take must aim in this direction. Narcissistic libido is also satisfied by love from the object*.

In the psychoses*, libido is (generally) purely narcissistic and action is autoplastic*. In these clinical pictures, the aim is not to modify the real external world, and there is regression to autoerotism*. Given that action is pure or nearly pure repetition compulsion, it loses its characteristic of being "adequate to an aim".

As for our main possibilities of specific action: we have already mentioned sexual acts acceptable for human culture and the superego; also, essentially, ties with inhibited aims such as tenderness, friendship, group and social activities, and sublimational activities in general (homosexual libido). Since the aim is inhibited, a need is generated to vary the type of act, given the partial quality of its satisfaction which in turn enables and even imposes the creative and changing activity characteristic of culture but not of Trieb. Creation is thus an effect of culture on Trieb repetition compulsion.

In sum: specific or expedient action is action that produces partial or complete discharge of the source (depending on the degree to which Trieb is desexualized*) carried out by the ego in an adequate manner (in reality). This expediency is reached mainly when discharge action is accepted by the superego (representative of culture* and of narcissism*) and by culture (if not, its lack of cultural adequacy produces social anxiety).

These different and changing forms of Trieb discharge, though seriously limited by all these processes, produce well-being. They involve action in the external world (whose most important aspect is the object*) that "changes the face of the Earth", adequacy to the reality principle*, full functioning of secondary process* including a certain dose of aggression* (hate* carried into action pertaining to self-preservative Trieb*, sexual Trieb, and destructive Trieb); such extreme complexity is not always achieved in the subject's lifetime in view of the many and constantly opposing ego dependencies.

In any case, it is a constant aspiration and should be included in the concept of health.

SPLITTING OF THE EGO

Ger.: Ichspaltung. – Sp.: escisión del yo. – Fr.: clivage du moi. – It.: scissione dell'io. – Port.: clivagem do ego.

In this process produced in the preconscious ego* or more precisely, in its thought* activity (in secondary process*), contradictions are accepted in the ego when its synthetic function fails. Consequently, its thinking functions in relation to what is split off as if in primary process*.

This situation is rooted in a confrontation, during the period of the Oedipus complex, between sexual Triebe* of the id* seeking satisfaction and the superego seeking to block their satisfaction. The superego, posted in reality*, proves the existence of castration by the evidence of the female genital, a reality it utilizes as a threat when onanistic pleasure is satisfied.

The ego splits. On the one hand, it disavows* the existence of castration, the latter loses its dangerous quality, and therefore masturbation* may be resumed satisfactorily. On the other hand, it recognizes castration, inferred from anxiety* that appears in response to anything that might refer to it.

If disavowal leads to hallucination* the process is a psychosis*. If it is limited to displacement* of the value of the female penis to an item of underwear, a zone of the body, or others (which represent the female penis or a moment previous to discovery of castration), a more typical event of ego splitting, the vicissitudes of fetishism* ensue. This splitting is intra-ego. In the preconscious, some synthetic capability is lost; it could be said that each contradiction accepted by the ego produces splitting in it.

The ego's function is to obtain a synthesis between all the opposing forces of the psychical apparatus. When the ego splits, a large part of this capacity is lost, and the ego is also impoverished. Intra-ego splitting differs from intersystemic splitting (unconscious-preconscious) produced by repression* or defence mechanisms* in response to castration anxiety cultivated as a signal by the ego, by virtue of which the ego does not accept Trieb impulses presented by the id as its own.

Intra-ego splitting produces a fissure in the ego and its recognition of reality; in time, this crack may grow larger with each new splitting, allowing increasingly severe affections and their expanding rejection of reality.

STEP ASIDE

Ger.: Ausweichen. – Sp.: hacerse a un lado. – Fr.: se mettre de coté. – It.: farsi ad un lato. – Port.: arredar-se.

This unconscious ego mechanism, occasionally or partially described by Freud, consists basically in avoiding competition by leaving the "war booty" to the rival. It is a secondary or contributing cause of homosexuality*; for example, in women, to avoid rivalry with the mother or sister for the father's love* or that of men in general.

The same may occur in men with respect to their brothers or father in relation to the mother's or other women's preference; instead of fighting for it, they yield by "stepping aside".

This mechanism is common in twins. The ego* of each needs very much to differentiate itself. Often, if one twin develops a certain character trait*, the other takes the opposite, for example, if one is a womanizer, the other may be homosexual or shy with women).

In the case of brothers who are not twins, if one is a professional or a musician, the other may not want to compete and step aside, choosing a different type of road in life, mostly caused by this difficulty in competing, which may be preconscious* or unconscious*.

In deeper respects, we may observe the same mechanism in relation to ego characteristics or ways of being, for example: homosexuality. What is perceived in this mechanism is avoidance of competition and of expressions of aggression* in the struggle for ego affirmation. This may be related to death Trieb* not deflected into destructive Trieb*: so-called primary or erotogenic masochism* which Freud mentions as "mysterious masochistic tendencies of the ego" as a substrate of the future homosexual subject's difficulty to enter the positive Oedipus complex*, which involves acceptance of sexual difference, castration anxiety*, and development of rivalry with the father. All this may be avoided by stepping aside, identifying* with the mother (in the case of boys), disavowing* castration, and splitting of the ego*.

However, stepping aside is not in the category of an unconscious ego defence mechanism*. It is simply a clinically observable fact, the result of use of other defence mechanisms or their collaborator. It is not specific of homosexuality; at most, it is part of a certain passive characteristic of the personality. It is even unclear whether it is unconscious, and if so, to what degree it is. Probably, the more unconscious it is, the more neurotic it is, or alternatively, it may be a character pathology. However, when it is more conscious, it may be part of perversions* or narcissistic neuroses. In *The Psychogenesis of Homosexuality in a Woman* (1920) and in *Some Neurotic Mechanisms in Jealousy, Paranoia and Homosexuality* (1922), Freud considers it typical of homosexuality but not limited to it.

SUBLIMATION

Ger.: Sublimierung. – Sp.: sublimación. – Fr.: sublimation. – It.: sublimazione. – Port.: sublimação.

This is one of the vicissitudes of Trieb*. It consists principally in the desexualization* of its aim*, which is thereby accepted by culture* and its representative in the psychical apparatus, the superego*; this manoeuvre is also practised by the ego*, since it constitutes quite an effective way to discharge Trieb proceeding from the id*, though in a more attenuated form than the original one.

Therefore, it is a type of specific action* that "changes the face of the earth", generating culture and cultural ties.

Sublimation of sexual Trieb yields results, since it is not suppressed (cf. suppression*) but is instead aimed in directions different from the original one, and is included in a manner we could consider symbolic, which gives it new complexity and creates new levels of satisfaction, acquiring cultural characteristics.

All phenomena constituting products of culture are therefore sublimations, including the types of link with objects they involve (social ties such as friendship, tenderness, libidinal group* ties, and other phenomena). When these homosexual ties (homosexual in the sense that they ignore sexual difference) sublimated by libidinal withdrawal* are decathected, regression to narcissism* ensues and the ego is libidinally hyper-cathected, as for example in paranoia* and its delusion* of grandeur.

Satisfaction provided by sublimation is also narcissistic in character, even though it is a vicissitude of object libido, since the ego ideal* (which demands sublimation) is satisfied by it, and the recompense is its love* (observed clinically as self-esteem*). However, when it is impossible to sublimate and thereby meet the superego's* demands, a sense of guilt* is perceived. Therefore, sublimation is also a demand of the superego ("You ought to be like this (like your father) ... You may not be like this (like your father)") (*The Ego and the Id*, 1923, p. 34), but it cannot be attributed solely to this imperative. In reality, its existence depends more on the ego; the superego may demand it but cannot enforce it.

This level of superego exigency is similar to, mixes with, or is mistaken for a type of Trieb suppression similar to repression* in the manner of anticathexis* (for example, an individual may utilize work to reinforce repression of Triebe, but the arrival of the weekend is enough for the conflicts they generate to reappear).

However, the objective of repression, unless it fails as when the repressed returns* in the neuroses, is to block access of Trieb to the conscious level, in order to prevent it from reaching action.

Sublimation, however, is not a product of anticathexes. It is more like what Freud describes as collateral cathexes in the *Project for a Scientific Psychology*, 1895–1950) (although these not only explain sublimation but also the taming of Trieb in general, an ego function), or the mechanism of ego inhibition* of Trieb and its guidance into action in reality*.

Although a certain degree of ignorance of Trieb is implicit, especially in some types of sublimation, and in this aspect it is similar to repression, it is also true that only by virtue of the work of thought* activity is it possible to know Trieb, since thought itself is ultimately a product of language* and of the ego. All three are different levels of sublimation of Trieb.

We emphasize: thought, language, and even the ego are sublimations of Trieb or derivatives of them; sublimations of Trieb create the ego (by virtue of identification* and de-sexualization*) and are created by the ego (which defends itself in this way from demands of Trieb in response to the threat of punishment by the superego and anxiety produced by social factors: the need to be loved by one's fellow human beings).

These are sublimations achieved by humanity throughout the course of its history and by each subject during his or her individual life.

It is also the opposite of repression, since repressed Triebe, unable to access the ego, cannot be sublimated. Just the opposite: they remain eroticized or sexualized, although they are in the repressed unconscious and cannot be utilized by the ego. Since they are sexualized or their aim is uninhibited, the ego keeps them in the unconscious; when they return from the repressed they are sexualized, and therefore become neurotic symptoms* or some other production of the unconscious, since the ego is unable to include them in itself, in its desexualized libido.

Most sublimations may be attributed to the mechanism of identification; therefore, Trieb is desexualized and object libido* becomes narcissistic libido* (that is to say, what was an object cathexis becomes a characteristic of the ego):

> Indeed, the question arises, and deserves careful consideration, whether this is not the universal road to sublimation, whether all sublimation does not take place through the mediation of the ego, which begins by changing sexual object libido into narcissistic libido and then, perhaps, goes on to give it another aim.
>
> (*The Ego and the Id*, 1923, p. 30)

There is something more, in regard to death Trieb*: it is deflected and becomes aggression*, Trieb for mastery*, sadism*, fusing with sexual Trieb. This destructive Trieb, a product of this fusion, must be tamed in order to make it acceptable to culture; then, sublimation's participation is also essential, inhibiting the aim (always erotic) through cultural creations such as work, sports, and so on.

By virtue of different degrees of fusion, sexual Trieb is able to bind part of the tendency to return to the inorganic inherent to death Trieb.

However, when sublimation desexualizes it by inhibiting its aim, it produces the liberation of some death Trieb, generating the paradoxical effect that, besides originating increasingly complex life phenomena, it also includes free quantities of death Trieb.

As the levels of sublimation become more complex, the forms of destructivity are concomitantly more sophisticated. At times, through this Trieb defusion, the cultural process seems to be not only the creator of new levels of complexity of life, but also the destructive agent of death. This is the paradox.

SUBSTITUTE FORMATION

Ger.: Ersatzbildung. – Sp.: formación sustitutiva. – Fr.: formation substitutive. – It.: formazione sostitutiva. – Port.: formação substitutiva.

As a consequence of secondary repression, this preconscious word-presentation* replaces the original repressed presentation* or its derivative (when this presentation was repressed, it was left without its basic signifier; the thing-presentation* was still cathected but had no bridges to connect it with the word-presentation representing it to consciousness*.

A substitute formation involves return of the repressed*: the failure of repression* and symptom formation*, for example in hysteria*, whose conversion symptoms are substitute formations of repressed presentations. It also coincides with the anticathexis* of reaction formation* as in the anal character, although in this latter case it is not homologous with symptoms but with characteristics of the ego*. In a second step, in obsessional neuroses*; that is to say, with the failure of repression and return of the repressed through obsessions, these obsessions are again formed by substitute formation, growingly connected with the repressed of original presentations rather than with the repressor.

The mechanism of substitution of the presentation in substitute formations utilizes the laws of association* (contiguity* or simultaneity, analogy*, and opposition*) which go unnoticed by consciousness and logical thought* existing in the ego's preconscious.

Substitute formation is a compromise struck between the ego and Trieb*, not always becoming a neurotic symptom.

SUBSTITUTIVE SATISFACTIONS

Ger.: Erzatsbefriedigungen Leisten. – Sp.: satisfacciones sustitutivas. – It.: sodisfazioni sostitutivi. – Port.: satisfações sustitutivas.

These satisfactions may be provided by symptoms*, degraded forms of sexual satisfaction, or in Freud's terms, pleasures that cannot be felt as such. In the last case, repressed Trieb is partly satisfied (the symptom* is a product of return of the repressed*) and is partly a punishment for it.

However, the symptom is not the only form of substitutive satisfaction; repetitions which may even be produced at the outset of an analysis, a dangerous moment when libido is displaced from its symptoms (manifesting a false sensation of cure produced in positive transference) and may be put into action, for example, when the repressed has not been sufficiently worked through (cf. working through*) libido not sufficiently bound (cf. binding*), and for example hasty object* choices made which are destined to pay for repressed guilt associated with the wish for this choice. Freud adds that bitter marriages tend to be built upon acted out neuroses. This is the basis of one of his pieces of advice to the analyst: that when patients accept the analytic contract, they should also accept not to marry or make any other important decision during the treatment without having first analysed it thoroughly in this treatment.

SUPEREGO

Ger.: Über-Ich. – Sp.: superego. – Fr.: surmoi (o sur-moi). – It.: super-io. – Port.: superego.

This structure arises in the psychical apparatus in a deferred* manner following the period of the Oedipus complex* as a consequence of secondary identifications* (not directly following definitive recognition of objects* as the main source of pleasure and as a rival) with parental figures and especially the father, which enables the definitive entry of culture* into the individual's psychical apparatus and of the individual into culture.

Three aspects converge in it: phylogenetic inheritance, infantile narcissism, and the "commemorative monument" to the Oedipus complex.

Phylogenetic inheritance. Freud describes the origin of the superego as events reconstructed largely from his hypotheses in relation to the origin of the evolutionary process of hominization as he presented them in his work, *Totem and Taboo* (1912). In this text, Darwin's writings on the formation of groups of hominids, originarily in the form of primitive hordes* under the orders of a leader who possessed all the privileges including castration, murder, or exile of his sons from the horde. According to Freud, those who managed to survive succeeded at some point in establishing homosexual bonds in exile and, inventing a new weapon, rebelled against the father, killed him, and devoured him.

The fraternal alliance* or band of brothers* was thereby formed. Totemism* followed, in which the brothers' fear of their dead father was displaced onto an animal considered a forebear, which was then worshipped and felt to be sacred, this worship including offerings and the totem meal*, repeated as a periodic ritual.

The Freudian hypothesis is that after the parricide committed by the united brothers, and therefore during totemism, identification* with the paternal figure is produced, becoming a very important part of the ego* and the origin of the superego. The external father, with all his power, lost his strength (the consequences of the murder of the father were decisive, not this event itself), and this strength was passed on to the superego, an internal psychical structure of beings who began to be called humans. Later, this superego was established as the instrument of projection* onto the external world in the period when the animistic conception of the world predominated.

This new structure was dedicated to the enforcement of requisites that would inaugurate culture: repression of incest and parricide.

With the advent of the superego, what had been done only for the benefit of the father or the leader of the horde now sprang from within each man's psychical apparatus as his own internal impossibility.

We dedicate a paragraph to the *feminine superego*. It is formed partly by cross inheritance with the male, with phallic predominance; and also by inheritance from the matriarchy* predominant in the period between the primal horde and the fraternal alliance, as well as the maternal attitude of defending the smallest of her inoffensive young from the primal father in view of his need for power, which ultimately ensured, by virtue of her courage and protection of her narcissism*, the survival of the species.

Following this line, the feminine superego is doubtless much less demanding of sublimation*: narcissism is satisfied by bringing up her young; we could think that her "categorical imperative" is lower, which does not mean that she has none; it proceeds in part from phallic cross inheritance, from the period of matriarchy when she had to occupy the father's place as well as her maternal narcissistic links with her young.

Leaving aside phylogeny, we take up *ontogenetic narcissism* in which the ego ideal* is constituted: a substructure or function of the superego which demands sublimation but is incapable of forcing it. The ego, which must attain it, does not always succeed. When it is unable to reach it, a sense of guilt* ensues.

The feminine castration complex* is a typical example of the reduction of self-esteem* when the ego ideal is phallic and a fixation* is produced in this erotogenic zone*. As a result, many forms of defence against it may originate. If preconscious wishes connected with these erotogenic zones are repressed but succeed in returning from the repressed*, they generate neurosis. If what is repressed* (decathected*) are unconscious wishes, this repression may produce tendencies to depression* or narcissistic disorders ranging from sexual perversions* to psychoses*, in which lowered self-esteem tends to present as the opposite, as the defence against it, varying from haughtiness to delusions of grandeur.

The ego ideal demands perfection. This aspiration originates in the hedonistic conception of the ideal ego* or the pure pleasure ego* of infantile narcissism which considered everything pleasurable to be ego and was indifferent or hated the rest, considering it not-ego. Ultimately, the ego ideal wishes to refind what it once was, that delusion of grandeur it once had.

"To be their own ideal once more, in regard to sexual no less than other trends, as they were in childhood – this is what people strive to attain as their happiness" (*On Narcissism: An Introduction*, 1914, p. 100).

At the time that the individual enters the period when the phallic erotogenic zone predominates, the formation of the ego and narcissism is concluded; in this period it is essentially phallic, and therefore the predominant anxiety* in boys is castration* anxiety. In girls, it is anxiety for loss of the object's love*, which may restore what they feel is a narcissistic wound: castration. The notion of sexual difference on these levels is phallic–castrated.

The period between the discovery of sexual difference and adolescence is utilized by girls to work through and learn about their sex. If all goes well, they arrive at this phase with a superego structured similarly to a boy's, perhaps differing with respect to some values; perhaps also less rigid, without the urgency forced by castration anxiety. Girls must work through their mother complex* linked to castration, separate from their mother and pass to their father, and from him to another man, thereby gradually valuing their sex for itself rather than as a lack of the masculine.

However, a bedrock* remains in the ego*, and on its account sexual difference produces anxiety* and originates defence mechanisms* of the unconscious ego against this anxiety, which may lead to different types of alterations.

With the culmination of the Oedipus complex, the object is finally defined as the most important source of pleasure of sexual Trieb*, libido* therefore becomes essentially object libido, and wishes* are for objects with which actions related with the erotogenic zone predominating at the moment are desired; this zone unifies all the previous zones and gives them the dimension of an ego in the body (cf. body*).

By anaclisis* on self-preservative Triebe*, the object chosen is the mother, by both girls and boys. For this reason, boys generally begin with the positive Oedipus, which is later dissolved and reappears only through unconscious derivatives of some elements of it, never or very rarely linked to its original presentation* (incestuous after entering the Oedipus complex).

For girls, the mother (as an object) was at first pre-oedipal* but now becomes negative oedipal, the link with her tinged with hostility configuring the maternal complex. This dead-end street must lead to a passageway to the father, and from him to boys (in adolescence); however, this passageway on such a difficult road is either totally or partially blocked.

In boys, the road is apparently less tortuous, but they must go through castration anxiety originating in the phallic phase when reality* imposes sexual difference on the ego, and this is also difficult.

If previous vicissitudes of Trieb* have included passages from activity to passivity, the bases are laid for the establishment of a negative Oedipus, and homosexuality is sought in the father-complex*, producing disavowal* of sexual difference and return to the cloacal theory* with the masochistic* phantasy* of giving the father a child; this may proceed from a masochistic ego, along with a sadistic superego. In any case, the ego is split* since it partly accepts sexual difference and feels castration anxiety.

The ego in turn may defend itself from this level of Trieb working through (for example, by repressing it like the "Wolf Man" or by projecting it like "Schreber"), or may accept it with pleasure, as in the case of sexual perversions*, or even with some complaisance as in some neurotic symptoms of the "Wolf Man".

In the boy's positive Oedipus, the crossroads is that the object desired up to that time has now acquired incestuous characteristics from the viewpoint of what the ego wishes to do with it. The true meaning of the father's presence as the mother's sexual partner is also discovered; the boy understands, in a deferred* manner, the primal scene*, sexual difference, and the real impossibility of competing with his father in spite of an intense desire to do so at that time.

This catastrophe leads to the vicissitude of dissolution* in the unconscious. Primal repression* (the force of dislodgement) of infantile sexuality* culminates and is completely forgotten, the superego remaining as a commemorative tribute, a reaction formation* created by identification with the major characters in this drama, mainly the hated and loved rival, the father.

This superego is from this time forward in charge of controlling the ego, giving orders regarding what it "must be" and what it "must not be", in such a manner that it splits off from it, confronting and persecuting the ego. Its model of what it "must be" is the ego ideal originating in the ideal ego of infantile narcissism and, as a model of what it "must not be", in the conscience*.

To enforce these orders, it forces the ego to utilize unconscious defence mechanisms (secondary repression or "pressures to hunt") in response to Trieb, generating anxiety in the ego if it does not respond.

Part of the roots of the superego are in the id*; it is also the heir of phylogenetic experience and a reaction formation against it; therefore, although it is a force against Trieb, it is heavily cathected by it.

When the ego is unable to suppress* sexual Triebe, it calls upon death Triebe* bound by the superego.

Therefore, the superego may bind part of the death Triebe which were freed in the psychical apparatus when they were not deflected, and also acquire part of these destructive Triebe, now turned against the ego, and now punishing it in the best of cases.

The superego may also sometimes take charge of quantity of death Trieb liberated by each sublimation when a portion of Trieb fusion is left over.

All this involves discontent, generated by this structure and imposed on the psychical apparatus by culture (as its priest), but is also a product of its history. Therefore, not only is Trieb dissatisfaction produced, but it is "stricter than the strictest", the search for Trieb pleasure gradually becoming a need for punishment* and a conscious or even unconscious sense of guilt. The latter is quite probably one of the most resistant defenders of illness.

Therefore, the strength of the categorical imperative of this structure proceeds from its connections with Trieb, especially with quantum of aggression* liberated by Trieb defusion associated with sublimation, in turn demanded of the ego by the ego ideal.

The superego therefore has a conscious, a preconscious, and an unconscious part (*New Introductory Lectures on Psycho-Analysis*, 1932); the unconscious is the theory's most controversial part. It is probably here that punishment dreams*, unconscious sense of guilt*, its participation in masochism*, and the irrational aspects of this structure are produced: the expression of an external power within the apparatus.

This is not what is most desirable; it should be the guardian of reason.

SUPPRESSION

Ger.: Unterdrückung. – Sp.: sofocación. – Fr.: répression. – It.: repressione. – Port.: sufocação (da pulsão).

This action and effect results from the struggle between one part of the psychical apparatus and Trieb*, either in relation to the presentation* or to the *quantum* of affect*; through this mechanism, the aim proposed by Trieb to the knowledge and action of the ego* is thwarted. Trieb may be suppressed (one or both of its aspects) in diverse ways, some of which are unconscious and others conscious. Unconscious suppression originates in ego defence mechanisms* or repression* in the broad sense. These act directly on the presentation and indirectly on the *quantum* of affect. We identify three phases. Fixation* or primal repression* is the first dam established by anticathexes* which remove the initial freedom of sexual Trieb* in the form of satisfaction of the erotogenic zone*. It also generates the mode of choice of the object* of pleasure*.

The second is "repression proper", which adds fresh anticathexes to the previous anticathexis, especially those located in the perceptual apparatus where they function as resistance*. In transference neuroses*, it also removes cathexes from preconscious word-presentations* when they are attracted by the primarily repressed in the unconscious.

These three aspects of repression proper are different in each of the ego defence mechanisms corresponding to the different types of neurosis.

The third phase consists in failure of repression and return of the repressed* from the unconscious fixation by virtue of a substitute formation* of the original presentation which takes the form of a symptom*.

We have discussed suppression suffered by the Trieb* presentation due to repression in the broad sense and unconsciously, although conscious mechanisms also exist. One of these is negation* by which Trieb is not yet considered part of the ego, although its preconscious presentation would enable this recognition.

Another conscious mechanism is judgement of condemnation* or rejection, by which the ego is more accepting of Trieb as its own, without however allowing it to reach action, but condemning or rejecting it as being unadvisable, divorced from reality, or ethics, or otherwise unsuitable.

The affect* corresponding to Trieb, to longing* for the presence of the object of Trieb, or anxiety in response to danger of its loss, or of its punishment, may also be suppressed. This is also produced by conscious or unconscious mechanisms. The former consist strictly in suppression of the affect, as when laughter or sadness is inhibited at a certain moment. The others derive partly and indirectly from repressive mechanisms, and sometimes, as in dreams*, are the product of affective ambivalence* in which a pleasurable affect counteracts an unpleasurable affect in connection with this dream or a certain event.

SYMPTOM

Ger.: Symptom. – Sp.: síntoma. – Fr.: symptôme. – It.: sintoma. – Port.: sintoma.

All symptoms indicate a pathological process. Its phenomenology expresses an unaccustomed variation of a function, or the introduction of a new operation of it, apart from the compulsive characteristics inherent to all Trieb processes, not manageable by the ego's* conscious will.

They are an expression of return of the repressed* in transference neuroses*, failures of secondary repression. The repressed returns from fixation* points generated by primal repression*, with distortions produced by compromises with the ego from which substitute formations* arise, resulting in symptoms or arising from them.

Therefore, symptoms are degraded manifestations of sexuality, "pleasure that cannot be felt as such" (*Beyond the Pleasure Principle*, 1920, p. 11).

In paranoia* and paranoid schizophrenia*, they are the noisy part of the illness, although they result from attempts to cure itself, to reconstruct the object world. After decathexis* of the thing-presentation*, which by virtue of the word-presentations* utilized with the laws of primary process* produce delusions* that may be considered symptoms from our viewpoint, even though the paranoiac patient's ego would quite probably disagree with our opinion.

In actual neuroses* the symptom is caused by a quantity of somatic excitation* not bound to presentations* which automatically became anxiety*, resulting in a crisis of anxiety or its equivalents.

In traumatic neuroses*, symptoms are originated by a first effect of the actual trauma*; the quantity of excitation (in this case proceeding from outside the subject's body, from reality*) overwhelms the possibilities of the psychical apparatus* to bind* it with presentations and the amount of preparedness anxiety* corresponding to the protective shield against stimuli. For this reason, the psychical apparatus repeats the traumatic situation* in dreams* in order to redirect the facts to the reign of the principle of pleasure–unpleasure. The ego is thereby able to feel preparedness anxiety that could have created a means of defence against the dangers of reality and which, given the magnitude and the surprise, it could not feel at that moment.

Thus, it is able to bind some repressed and other preconscious thing-presentations. It is not always successful; it is sometimes defeated by the pure and simple tendency to repetition inherent to unconscious Triebe and especially to death Trieb.

Freud utilizes the term "symptom"* to refer to that of transference neuroses*. We discuss these in more detail. We said that they result from the return of the previously repressed* by primal repression*, proceeding from the fixation point it originated through a compromise between the ego and Trieb*. Thus, the latter is expressed as a substitute formation* and to a certain extent with some degree of action* (but not specific, only to the extent of an internal alteration* as described in the *Project for a Scientific Psychology*, 1895–1950), although the ego may overrule it. Then, the preconscious ego feels that it is extra-territorial, an "internal foreign land" (*New Introductory Lectures on Psycho-Analysis*, 1933).

Once Trieb*, proceeding from the id*is anticathected* by primal repression, it produces anxiety in the ego, which cultivates in it the memory of the traumatic* anxiety of birth and utilizes it as a danger signal (in its more elaborate forms, anxiety for object* loss, castration* and so on) against the possibility that it may be repeated in situations similar to others in the past that were traumatic, the main one being castration anxiety.

The unconscious part of the ego, governed by the pleasure principle*, and before feeling anxiety as a symptom, unconsciously creates defence mechanisms*. The different symptoms of the neuroses are produced in this way.

Symptoms are therefore a type of defence* against anxiety. In conversion hysteria*, the defence against anxiety for loss of the object's love predominates, in obsessional neurosis* the defence against anxiety before the superego* and in anxiety hysteria* the defence against castration anxiety (*Inhibitions, Symptoms and Anxiety*, 1925).

A symptom generally has several simultaneous meanings (especially in conversion hysteria), but they may also be successive (obsessional neurosis). When they become chronic, new facts, new experiences, new phantasies related with them are added, attracted by their existence, so long as they serve to express their new and former meanings.

In other cases, transformations are produced in the ego which originate character traits* (the classical example is reaction formation*), but these correspond to pathologies of the ego and not to neurotic symptoms.

At this point a complication arises. When symptoms become chronic, the ego sometimes attempts in the second place to include them as part of itself because of its tendency to synthesis (without understanding them and without accepting their Trieb origin, simply considering them as one more extravagance of the ego). In this way, symptoms come to be part of the ego's characteristics which are bothersome but are now accepted as its own.

In time, the presence of the symptom brings secondary gain* (protection and caregiving by the object, for example), besides being the best topical, dynamic, and economic solution the ego has found to rid itself of the conflict (primary gain from illness*). In both cases, ego resistance* presents obstacles that must be worked through if a cure is to be achieved.

The appearance of a symptom is an indicator of pathological decompensation. It may be neurotic (transference neurosis* or others) or psychotic (melancholia*, acute hallucinatory confusion*, hysterical psychosis*, schizophrenia* and its different clinical forms).

Psychoanalytic theory explains the mechanism of formation of all these clinical pictures, but refers especially to transference neuroses when it theorizes on symptoms in the broad sense. In this disorder, and also in others, symptoms have an unconscious meaning and in this sense, like dreams, they are another *via regia* to access the unconscious.

Analysis seeks the meaning or diverse meanings based on the patient's associations* and any mnemic symbols*, represented in this particular substitute formation*, of the "genuine" representation of the Trieb.

This unveiling of the meaning of symptoms is essential in Freudian theory from the outset; it lost some of its value with more knowledge of the psychical apparatus and of the ego when the aim to change the ego pushed the former aim into second place. It would perhaps be a good idea to revise this point. Knowledge of the meaning of a symptom and its consequent cure is not opposed to further deepening of knowledge of the ego but precisely the opposite: the ego, or an important part of it, is configured in the same way, and sometimes utilizes the same mechanisms as the symptoms.

Therefore, the revelation of the meaning of a symptom may bring to light aspects that would otherwise remain hidden from the ego, or may awaken others that had never been found. Therefore, given the interweaving of a person's representational fabric, it is advisable to go deeply in every possible direction. Symptoms are a preferential direction, since they are often what causes patients to suffer and brings them to analysis.

SYMPTOM FORMATION

Ger.: Symptombildung. – Sp.: formación de síntoma. – Fr.: formation de symptôme. – It.: formazione di sintomo. – Port.: formação de sintoma.

Symptoms* always result from return of the repressed* and therefore from failure of repression*. It manifests a Trieb* impulse that causes the ego* anxiety*; the ego defends itself from it, but not entirely efficiently, since this anxiety may be part of the symptom or continue to be expressed by it. It is also a hidden form of sexual satisfaction that the ego cannot feel unless it first degrades it to the category of symptom. Symptom formation expresses conflict among Triebe*, the superego*, and reality*.

The ego resorts to symptom formation when it cannot achieve an effective synthesis between all these opposing elements in order to think and attain (or not attain) action. We could also say that the synthesis thereby achieved by the ego is precisely the symptom, but this synthesis loses effectiveness because it hides its contents from consciousness*, thereby preventing thought and action that might result from it. However, it is also effective since it ignores and paralyzes Trieb.

Neurotic symptoms are always substitute formations* of repressed Trieb, although this Trieb is not always constituted as such. Symptom formation is aided by regression* and predispositional fixation*. Regression goes back to the fixation and emerges from that point, returning from the repressed.

In anxiety hysteria*, in particular in the second and third phases (formation of phobia* of the object onto which the anxiety was displaced*, or phobia generating object and its surroundings), symptom formation coincides with substitute formation and anticathexis*. The preconscious presentation* onto which castration anxiety* was displaced is a substitute formation of the original repressed presentation, a symptom (Little Hans's fear of being bitten by a horse) and is anticathexis, or alternatively, the ego places an anticathexis of attention* in the perceptual-consciousness system in response to possible perception* of the phobia producing substitute object.

Vigilance is extended to anything associated with the original repressed presentation to ensure that neither it nor any of its derivatives return from the repressed.

T

TABOO

Ger.: Tabu. – Sp.: tabú. – Fr.: tabou. – It.: tabù. – Port.: tabu.

This social formation produces a status in certain persons, words, events, texts, situations, and other phenomena by which they become sacred and impure, idealized and hated, sought out and avoided, familiar and uncanny, a mixture of something heavily charged with affective ambivalence*, highly desired and severely forbidden, in which the last factor predominates; therefore, disobedience of a taboo produces great anxiety.

This mechanism is typical of the thought* of primitive beings, and is part of the modes of thought of neurotics in the present day, as for example, obsessional neurotics* whose illness is usually called the "illness of taboos", even though it also exists in some phobias*, in conversion hysteria* and even as social customs.

Taboos have been described with respect to the deceased, the dead person's name, the taboo on this person's survivors, widowers, and widows. Taboos fall upon rulers, enemies, animals (the core of totemism*), adolescents before sexual initiation, menstruation, women in delivery, new-born babies, sick persons, anything contagious (for example, fatal illnesses such as cancer whose name is avoided, AIDS, mental illness and other types of socially unacceptable illnesses, generally associated with poverty), as well as houses, plants, places, and other things.

Wundt considers the taboo humanity's oldest, unwritten legal code. The taboo is estimated to be older than the gods, reaching back to epochs previous to any type of religion.

The person who breaks a taboo becomes taboo, since this individual becomes contagious and tempting (given the ambivalence at the root of the taboo), therefore dangerous, as if to incite others to break this kind of "natural law".

Obsessional neurosis and taboo are "equally lacking in motive and equally puzzling in their origin. Having made their appearance at some unspecified moment, they are forcibly maintained by an irresistible fear" (*Totem and Taboo*, 1912, p. 26).

The guiding prohibition in both cases is against touching, which in obsessional neurosis may reach the "*délire de toucher*". This illness is part of the essence of one of the defence mechanisms*: isolation*, which endeavours to interrupt contact between presentations* as well as with affects*.

Complicated evasive ceremonials* result from efforts to isolate for avoidance of contact; they sometimes extend to certain phobias of anxiety hysteria*.

Obsessional neurosis endeavours to isolate presentations; displacement onto the trivial among presentations also characterizes it; both mechanisms touch on the theme of contact and contagion typical of taboos, since: "Obsessional patients behave as though the 'impossible' persons and things were carriers of a dangerous infection liable to be spread by contact on to everything in their neighbourhood" (Ibid., p. 27).

In the taboo, repressed unconscious wishes* struggle against social prohibitions which try to foil free displacement* by means of association*; therefore, social customs reinforce their defences* against those wishes. These defences* against anything taboo constitute the foundation of a future conscience*.

> Taboo is a primaeval prohibition forcibly imposed (by some authority) from outside, and directed against the most powerful longings to which human beings are subject. The desire to violate it persists in their unconscious; those who obey the taboo have an ambivalent attitude to what the taboo prohibits. The magical power that is attributed to taboo is based on the capacity for arousing temptation; and it acts like a contagion because examples are contagious and because the prohibited desire in the unconscious shifts from one thing to another. The fact that the violation of a taboo can be atoned for by a renunciation shows that renunciation lies at the basis of obedience to taboo.
>
> (Ibid., pp. 34–5)

TAMING OF TRIEB

Ger.: Triebbändigung / Bändigung von Triebsansprüchen. – Sp.: domeñamiento pulsional. – Fr.: domination pulsionel. – It.: dominazione pulsionale. – Port.: sujeição da pulsão.

We say that Trieb* is tamed by the ego* when the latter is able to "drive with its own reins": it recognizes this Trieb as its own, accepts it as a wish*, now the ego's* own, which the ego would like to fulfil, but which it may renounce or postpone in pursuit of other variables that come into its consideration and are more or less important to it at the moment.

Taming involves a cathected word-presentation* representing the thing-presentation* (also cathected) to the ego's preconscious. Therefore, tamed Trieb or its aim is accepted as a wish, although action on it is inhibited (cf. inhibition*) momentarily pending a final decision to transform it into action or not. Perhaps the most important aspect of taming of Trieb is the possibility to choose that it gives this ego by virtue of relations between word-presentations of thought* activity belonging to the preconscious ego. The latter has come to know Trieb well, can speak to it, find a place for it in the logic of thought, and thereby moderate its passage into action. In other words, the thing-presentation belonging to the unconscious wish formerly in primary process* is able to enter secondary process*. Taming therefore begins with knowledge of Trieb, and from that point plans its guidance or not into specific action*. It is one of the essential objectives of the psychoanalytic cure.

It is quite different from what produces the process of repression*; this mechanism generates ignorance with respect to Trieb and its transformation into something else (symptoms*, parapraxes*, forgetting*) which is compulsive and unstoppable for the ego; thus, the ego apparently achieves the objective of blocking the passage of Trieb into specific action* but the cost is heavy: ignorance, consequent impoverishment, and loss of the ego's freedom. The ego is enriched by knowledge of Trieb and by taming it with thought activity and the desexualization* (leading to sublimation*) it involves, and is simultaneously relieved of the pressure of anticathexis demanded by repression.

As Freud explains it in *Analysis Terminable and Interminable* (1937):

> To avoid misunderstanding it is not unnecessary, perhaps, to explain more exactly what is meant by "permanently disposing of an instinctual demand". Certainly not "causing the demand to disappear so that nothing more is every heard from it again". This is in general impossible, nor is it at all to be desired. No, we mean something else, something which may be roughly described as a "taming" of the instinct. That is to say, the instinct is brought completely into the harmony of the ego, becomes accessible to all the influences of the other trends in the ego and no longer seeks to go its independent way to satisfaction.
>
> (S.E., pp. 224–5)

TERROR

Ger.: Terror / Schrecken. – Sp.: terror. – Fr.: terreur. – It.: terrore. – Port.: terror.

This unpleasurable affect is produced by a sudden invasion of large quantities of excitation from the exterior: external and current traumatic events overwhelm the protective shield* and the psychical apparatus does not have time to establish some type of defence* in the form of escape or even a defensive reflex, or at least a certain cathexis of attention* to enable preparedness anxiety* with all presentations* available for binding. The psychical apparatus thus taken unawares is invaded by quantity of excitation* which produces terror during the traumatic event. Afterwards, it will endeavour to forget this event during the day, but the memory of this traumatic event reappears in spite of the subject's preconscious ego in the dreams* of traumatic neurosis*.

This is generated in part by simple repetition compulsion* beyond the pleasure principle* and in part because the psychical apparatus wants to bring the presentation* of the memory* of the traumatic situation* into the pleasure principle through its mitigated repetition by which it becomes thinkable and may be related with others. This may provide an opportunity to feel preparedness anxiety instead of terror and to gradually succeed in binding to other presentations. In this way, the pleasure principle of at least one of the systems may be accessed, and traumatic dreams* may be transformed into anxiety dreams* or even punishment dreams*.

THING (OF THE WORLD)

Ger.: Ding. – Sp.: cosa (del mundo). – Fr.: chose (du monde). – It.: cosa (del mondo). – Port.: coisa (do mundo).

A thing of the world refers to the external world, to reality* outside the psychical apparatus, where the object*, the fellow human being, occupies a privileged place but which also includes nature and the biological body.

In his *Project for a Scientific Psychology* (1950), Freud describes the external world as composed of "masses in motion and nothing else" (p. 308). Our perceptual apparatus gives them quality* when it perceives them; it perceives a temporal characteristic of their motions (their period*) as this quality. A thing of the world is therefore an objective thing perceived by us in a subjective manner. Science endeavours to learn more and more about this objective thing, or perhaps it is satisfied with a coherent and rational way to subjectivize it.

The perceptual complexes we receive, among which the object is privileged since it is the most directly related to wish fulfilment*, are composed of a central part and attributes. The central part is repeated since it is intrinsic to the thing: we cannot understand* it. The attributes are the other part, the varying part. We may understand attributes. We are able to apprehend them and make them ours; they are the thing's attributes. We do this when we imitate movements (Freud considers attributes the thing's movement), upon which we understand them. We know what it means to move our hand when we do so. We understand the meaning of laughter when we laugh, of the scream or pain (this is so true that in order to feel sadistic pleasure, the subject must first go through the experience masochistically, know what is felt; the sadist enjoys the masochist's pleasure* by identification). We understand our fellow human being when we put that individual's attributes through our own body by means of the cathexis* of a certain body movement. Therefore, the parts we cannot process in this way – features, what is inherent to this individual but does not correspond to his or her way of moving – corresponds to a thing nucleus intrinsic to the person and incomprehensible to us.

These incomprehensible things of the world that we cannot process by a body cathexis therefore remain objective, a quantity of excitation* that cannot be bound by the psychical apparatus beyond it. This is what Kant would describe as the "thing in itself". Although Freud adds nothing theoretical to this Kantian concept, he borrows it in order to mark the limits of the field of his theory which end at this point. He does not propose to study the thing but only to mention it. We could also pinpoint this as the place that separates metapsychology from metaphysics. Further, he does so in part explicitly in *Beyond the Pleasure Principle* (1920) since the incomprehensible parts are the traumatic parts which remain, a quantity that cannot be bound to a presentation. This concept of trauma is related in this text to death Trieb* striving for repetition beyond the pleasure principle*.

The world within the psychical apparatus starts out with thing-presentations, not things in themselves but their subjective traces.

In essence, these presentations are traces of objects; we could also say that the history of the link with objects is in the thing-presentation. This link was formed by the perceptual apparatus (erotogenic zones) which subjectivized it at the very moment of perception*, and then much more in a deferred* manner. Experiences that could not be subjectivized and qualified remained "things of the world", "masses in motion", quantities of excitation – therefore traumatic – which may now push the psychical apparatus to repeat them in an attempt to understand them or may ally with death Trieb, in which case they remain mere repetition compulsion*.

THING-PRESENTATION

Ger.: Sachvorstellung (or Dingvorstellung). – Sp.: representación de cosa. – Fr.: représentation de chose. – It.: rappresentazione di cosa. – Port.: representação de coisa.

This results from the processing of traces left in the psychical apparatus by experiences in life which form, together with quantity of excitation* or *quantum* of affect* cathecting them (cf. cathexis*), libidinal Triebe*, wishes*, and libido* itself (the phenomenon constituted depends on the aspects of this union emphasized).

Since they are traces of experiences, they are therefore traces of the entire perceptual apparatus* and of all the erotogenic zones* (since experiences with the object take place through them). Sight is the principal sense, and therefore visual images are the characteristic component of thing-presentations.

How are they formed? The best model is found in Freud's description of the experience of satisfaction* (*Project for a Scientific Psychology*, 1895–1950; *The Interpretation of Dreams*, 1900). It refers to a hypothetical first experience, although it also applies to all subsequent experiences which are "filed" in order of quality*, importance, and other features. Some are heads of a series including many others, to which the latter subsequently refer.

In adults, the psychical apparatus is also split into id*, ego*, and superego*, and these in turn into unconscious, preconscious, and consciousness, which further complicates localization of the "placement" of registers of new experiences and to which of these previous experiences they are referring. The experience of satisfaction leaves the image of an object* registered in the apparatus, movements performed during this experience by object and subject (these movements configuring the attributes of the thing-presentation), together with the pleasurable sensation (the core of the thing in the thing-presentation: what is most deeply desired).

The thing-presentation is therefore of experiences with the object through the perceptual apparatus (erotogenic zones), which leave traces. These become presentations* which when recathected acquire characteristics of wishes, and therefore wishes for objects, since the subject has learned that the desired sensation may be obtained through the link with them.

These object wishes are impregnated with object libido developed from both the link with the object itself and also the mark it left in the psyche. Therefore, thing-presentations are essentially object presentations of what is experienced with objects.

With changes in the predominance of the different erotogenic zones, traces are left in the psyche of experiences with objects through these zones. Inevitable traumatic events generate fixations* when they require defensive anticathexes* which configure the first primal repressions*. These repressions are brought together when they go through the most important traumatic event in infantile sexuality*: the Oedipus complex* which leaves definitive primal repression* ("after-pressure"), the origin of infantile amnesia*, and the dissolution* of all infantile sexuality*, henceforth commemorated by a monument installed upon it, called the superego*.

Therefore, what is dissolved are essentially thing-presentations of this infantile sexuality, since they have become incestuous during the period of the Oedipus complex; incest and parricide make culture* impossible.

Thing-presentations of infantile sexuality are relegated to the unconscious or the id. Since they are not given words, they cannot access the preconscious of the ego, which would experience anxiety in their presence. However, they are nonetheless cathected in the unconscious, searching for chinks in the ego with this "after-pressure" (secondary repression), the state in which they are forced to remain. They sometimes succeed in accessing consciousness (through neurotic symptoms*, dreams*, parapraxes*, and other phenomena).

Although adult experiences therefore have their own characteristics in part, thing-presentations of unconscious wishes inevitably pressure for expression through them, sometimes producing a return of the repressed*, and even transference neuroses*. If they remain definitively repressed in the unconscious, the ego is somewhat impoverished, and its ability to experience and to complete specific actions* is diminished.

New experiences in life, resembling and thereby achieving some perceptual identity* with repressed thing-presentations, may produce anxiety* in the ego. In a dynamic process, the ego sometimes succeeds in differentiating what is desired and unconscious from what is perceived, but at other times its ability to distinguish them is lowered (in transference* itself, for example).

When thing-presentations are decathected* as a result of deep frustrations* with the first objects or other causes, these objects are no longer wished for, and ego presentations are cathected instead, configuring narcissism*. In this process, object libido is transformed into narcissistic libido, since the incentive to "refind the object" is quite poor and does not stimulate the psychical apparatus; however, an ego wounded by the object does need this narcissistic libido, especially when infantile frustration is revived by something actual. This is the situation of so-called "narcissistic pathologies".

THOSE WRECKED BY SUCCESS

Ger.: Die am erfolge scheiten. – Sp.: los que fracasan al triunfar. – Fr.: ceux qui échouent devant le succès. – It.: quelli che falliscono al trionfare. – Port.: os que fracassam ao triunfar.

This type of character* types is identified when "the illness followed close upon the fulfilment of a wish and put an end to all enjoyment of it" (1916, p. 317).

The precipitating factor of the disorder (neurosis*, organic illness, accidents, psychosis) is not frustration* but rather the opposite: satisfaction, fulfilment of a long-desired preconscious wish*. In a classical example, Schreber's *dementia paranoides* is produced shortly after his designation as President of the Dresden Supreme Court.

We find some points of similarity with the "negative therapeutic reaction", observed when progress in the analytic process (understanding of a symptom*, a dream*, the culmination of a construction*) produces a worsening of pathology and symptoms (if transitory, it could be normal, a "for the last time"). It is also similar to "superego resistance" to the cure*: punishment meted out by the superego to expiate the sense of guilt*, the debt the ego* must pay, and its need for punishment*. In this specific case, an unconscious need for punishment is manifested in behaviour and even in the ego's character, which the superego prevents from reaching success despite demands from the ideal to do so, probably because success implies parricide stemming from the Oedipus complex*.

In these conditions, the sense of guilt is unconscious*. It is inferred from the attainability of aims versus the suffering the subject must go through when they are satisfied. This terrain seems to belong to the unconscious superego.

We may also say that this type of character probably has important fixation* points produced by anticathexes* based on disavowal* of sexual difference, which were later repressed in the unconscious. Triumph is therefore unconsciously felt to be a triumph over the parent of the same sex (positive Oedipus), followed by regression to the negative Oedipus, which is satisfied by failure (masochistic-homosexual submission to the superego-father).

THOUGHT

Ger.: Gedanke / Denken. – Sp.: pensamiento. – Fr.: pensée. – It.: pensiero. – Port.: pensamento.
This type of relation between presentations* inherent to secondary process* and therefore a function of the preconscious ego* utilizes the reality principle* with desexualized cathexes* less intense than those needed for action but stronger than those utilized in phantasy (these precisely may be sexualized). These quantities of energy necessarily undergo severe processing for displacement* from one presentation to another. In other words, they require strong cathexis and weak displacement*.

Thought utilizes presentations to probe reality*. These presentations are constituted by processing traces left by experience. This probe is followed by continuing to specific action* which demands a much larger quantity of energy. It is mental planning aimed at reaching action.

The aim of thought is to achieve identity or some degree of it in order to comply in part with the pleasure principle* by inhibiting it to a reality principle. When the pleasure principle was invaded by the entry of stimulus into the psychical apparatus* (external or proceeding from Trieb), the apparatus then sought thought identity*: identity between what is wished for and what is perceived by utilizing thought to obtain it. Identity is not found, and only with shades of it will be found since thought activity is governed by a derivative of the pleasure principle which is the reality principle.

The seat of thought is the ego: both preconscious and conscious ego. Therefore, it utilizes word-presentations* although another type of thought in images with some level of binding exists previous to the appearance of words; Freud calls it reproductive thought. When we refer to thought, we "think" in word-presentations which, because they signify unconscious thing-presentations, involve the highest level of binding or taming of Trieb*, which may be processed in this way through its link with other word-presentations, gradually conforming the fabric of the ego which keeps it constant, tamed (principle of constancy*), and apt for use in specific action.

With respect to reality testing* accomplished by the ego utilizing thought, Freud's description of cognitive thought* is interesting. He defines three types of experiences in perception*, and for this purpose he subdivides the perceived into two parts: one that does not change since it is inherent to the object*, called the thing*, and the other that does change (the way it moves and what it does), which are attributes of the thing. The object's thing belongs to the object; we can neither have it nor be it; however, we may make the object's attributes go through our body: we may understand* it (we may for example move like it, the basis of identification*).

In the first of these three types of experiences, what is wished for and perceived are identical (some for example are autoerotic), and therefore have no need of thought to find identity since they already have it and are not enriching for the ego.

In the second type, the object may also be the same although it may also show us unknown attributes. These attributes demand thought through presentations until we discover the wished-for object with a new attribute. In order to understand it we needed to repeat it, imitate it, identify with it, and materialize it really or imaginarily. The third type of experience results from encountering something totally new: a different object and different attributes. In this case, by hyper-cathecting* the perception, we seek something similar to what was being sought and perhaps find attributes similar to what is wished for and through them, even similar aspects in the thing.

The aim of thought is always to search for identity between what is desired and what is perceived, and therefore its activity continues until it is found, at least different degrees of it imposed by recognition of the reality implicit in it (although there may be exceptions as occurs in ego splitting*); superego demands must also be met. In these difficulties and in the quantity of unrepressed and therefore desexualized preconscious word-presentations (representatives of unconscious thing-presentations) which may be interrelated resides their complexity.

In adults, the ability to think is restricted by repression* since it generates forgetting*: decathexis* of repressed preconscious presentations which the preconscious ego is therefore unable to utilize for thinking.

The ego ideal* demands new complexities (sublimations* which may or may not be reached by the ego) on the one hand, and on the other, predominantly demands repression, thereby decreasing thought activity.

Thought is governed by the laws of secondary process; for this reason, it is difficult for cathexis to pass from one presentation to another. In its search for identity, libido* must comply with certain conditions: the principle of non-contradiction, notions of time and space. These conditions emerge along with recognition of reality; contact with reality creates the ego which is what thinks, plans, and postpones action in order to execute it at the appropriate moment, and is also able to think about itself by virtue of the word-presentation by which it succeeds even in naming itself and becoming an object of Trieb (which is thereupon no longer autoerotic but becomes narcissistic).

All these conceptions add complexity to the concept of thought, although it is precisely this greater complexity that makes the cure possible. When repressions are lifted we bring word-presentations into the preconscious ego where they become part of its capital which the ego was unable to utilize when they were repressed. The ego may now include them in its "associative commerce" to think, compare, and evaluate them, then decide whether to put them into action. This ego is thereby enriched by experience and gradual binding of libidinal Triebe. It may even work through unconscious traumatic facts by detaching them from the present, and interrupt the repetition compulsion* or generate more complex levels of it (repetition compulsion, after all, is not always the same, in spite of its definition; what is repeated may vary and become more complex even though it is repetition).

Thought is an ego function which utilizes the reality principle and secondary process which binds word-presentations, representatives or signifiers of thing-presentations, in consciousness: unconscious residues of experiences with objects through the erotogenic zones*, the origin of unconscious wishes*. Thought utilizes desexualized libido which composes the preconscious and conscious ego. However, it sometimes occurs otherwise: thought is eroticized, typical in obsessional neurosis* which utilizes thinking not as preparation for action but instead to replace action, even the erotic charge corresponding to action.

Freud describes several types of thought in his *Project* ... (1895) such as reproductive, cognitive, critical*, practical* and others, differentiating between unintentional errors of thought and parapraxes; however, as he himself reformulates it, the unconscious* takes advantage of errors of thought in order to find expression.

Before accessing the preconscious, a repressed unconscious presentation tends to wait in the ante-chamber of the "no" of negation* where it already acquires word-presentation. Then it may be thought and thereby enter the preconscious ego and its collateral chains of thought, accessing a higher level of binding or Trieb taming where it chooses whether to execute, reject or postpone action.

THOUGHT IDENTITY

Ger.: Denkidentität. – Sp.: identidad de pensamiento. – Fr.: identité de pensée. – It.: identità di pensiero. – Port.: identidade de pensamento.

The psychical apparatus* seeks this objective when it already possesses secondary process* and a preconscious ego*, its headquarters. It then becomes an objective of the preconscious ego and its thought* activity. What is sought is identity with what is desired, however partial it may be. To attain it, the ego must ascertain this identity in the diverse attributes of the object* perceived by comparing them with properties of the desired object.

Therefore, it must test reality*, study what is perceived and the desired presentation*, and find similarities and differences.

In reality, the psychical apparatus is moved to think in order to find similarities or identities, and will endeavour to "refind such an object, to convince oneself that it is still there" (1925, pp. 237–8). However, in order to avoid frustration (as it has learned by utilizing experience with perceptual identity* in primary process*), it must accept reality* and evaluate the quantity of identity.

This activity is possible only through an ego* capable of inhibiting hallucination* by placing chains of thought between it and discharge. These chains of thought grow more and more complex, acquiring their definitive form with the advent of the word-presentation*. Then, the degree of binding* of quantity of excitation* reaches its highest level. We succeed in taming Trieb* when, having a thing-presentation* cathected with quantity of excitation (now libido* configuring an unconscious* wish*), this presentation accesses consciousness by virtue of closely interlinked word-presentations* utilized by the ego for its thought activity as preparations for action.

This action may be carried out when, once thought activity is completed, the ego concludes that the object perceived is the one desired or possesses attributes to make it similar enough or close to it. Sometimes action is postponed in search of the right moment. It may also not be carried out because of a judgement of condemnation* (not involving repression* but sometimes based on it).

The action to be performed is the "specific action"* which involves the existence of an ego with thought activity and which therefore seeks thought identity. Thought identity is based on the distinction between desire and perception*.

The ego must also distinguish identity from analogy*, contiguity*, and even opposition, and determine the associative path to which the perceived and its attributes belong. It might think, for example: this is similar but not the same, or it is next to it, which does not mean it is the same, or perhaps it sometimes does.

In sum, it must utilize the reality principle*.

TOTEMISM

Ger.: Totemismus. – Sp.: totemismo. – Fr.: totémisme. – It.: totemismo. – Port.: totemismo.

In this social system, described by the ethnologist, Robertson Smith, some primitive tribes attribute the ancestry of the clan to a certain animal which they worship and may not harm or eat, except at certain times when the totem meal* is celebrated with specific rituals. It is a phase in humanity's evolution towards culture.

In the Freudian hypothesis, totemism is instated subsequent to the primal horde* and concurrently with the establishment of the fraternal alliance or band of brothers* after the events in connection with parricide, a time when exogamy* is being practised.

The ambivalent emotional attitude of the sons to their father remained in force during the whole of later development. A particular animal was set up in the father's place as a totem. It was regarded as ancestor and protective spirit and might not be injured or killed. But once a year the whole male community came together to a ceremonial meal at which the totem animal (worshipped at all other times) was torn to pieces and devoured in common. No one might absent himself from this meal; it was the ceremonial repetition of the killing of the father, with which social order, moral laws and religion had taken their start (*Moses and Monotheism: Three Essays*, 1939, p. 131).

It therefore results from displacement* of the father-complex* and guilt* for parricide on to an animal which acquires characteristics of the father of the primal horde who is considered sacred, a protector, and its ancestor. However, his murder and ritual consumption are ceremonially and periodically repeated.

Totemism is not a religion in the evolution of human thought, but does contain its seeds.

A relic of this "stage" (not a chronological stage from one given year to another given year, but a logical stage which quite probably exists, even in the present, in some places on our planet) of humanity persists as a tendency in infantile sexuality* to be attracted by animals, even in infantile phobias which are nearly always zoophobias* whose forms are quite similar to those of the totemism of primitive peoples.

TOTEM MEAL

Ger.: Totemmahlzeit. – Sp.: banquete totémico. – Fr.: banquet totémique. – It.: convitto totémico. – Port.: banquete totêmico.

Freud adopted this concept, developed by William Robertson Smith, as part of his theoretical construction (which he himself referred to as a "scientific myth") regarding the origins of human culture* in general and of totemism* in particular.

Robertson Smith, quoted by Freud, formulated "the hypothesis that a peculiar ceremony known as the 'totem meal' had from the very first formed an integral part of the totemic system" (*Totem and Taboo*, 1912–13, p. 132). At this feast, held on certain dates, animals were sacrificed whose meat and blood were consumed by the god and his worshippers. This type of sacrifice was a public ceremony and a festivity for an entire clan.

"The ethical force of the public sacrificial meal rested upon very ancient ideas of the significance of eating and drinking together. Eating and drinking with a man was a symbol and a confirmation of fellowship and mutual social obligations" (Ibid., p. 134); "the sacrificial animal was treated as a member of the tribe; the sacrificing community, the god and the sacrificial animal were of the same blood and members of one clan" (Ibid., p. 136).

Robertson Smith provides abundant proof that the sacrificial animal is the equivalent of the ancient totemic animal. All sacrificial animals were originally sacred: only on festive occasions and with the participation of the entire clan was it permissible to eat its meat.

> The clan is celebrating the ceremonial occasion by the cruel slaughter of its totem animal and is devouring it raw – blood, flesh and bones. The clansmen are there, dressed in the likeness of the totem and imitating it in sound and movement, as though they are seeking to stress their identity with it ... When the deed is done, the slaughtered animal is lamented and bewailed. The mourning is obligatory, imposed by dread of a threatened retribution ... its chief purpose is to disclaim responsibility for the killing.

After this, the festival continues which is "a permitted, or rather an obligatory, excess, a solemn breach of a prohibition" (Ibid., p. 140).

For Freud, the totem meal, perhaps humanity's first festivity, is the repetition and commemorative celebration of the moment in which, in Darwin's primal horde*, all the exiled sons allied with each other and murdered the father, after which they ate him. This event generated and was generated by the band of brothers* that later produced social bonds. The prohibition of incest and parricide appeared from their midst as a product of longing* for the father and their guilt* for having killed him, thereby generating the superego in their psychical apparatuses.

This feast, now displaced on to the totem animal, repeats this memorable and criminal feat that set so much into motion: social organizations, ethical limitations, and religion.

TRANSFERENCE

Ger.: Übertragung. – Sp.: transferencia. – Fr.: transfert. – It.: traslazione o transfert. – Port.: transferência.

Transference, an observable phenomenon in psychoanalytic clinical work, has a phenomenological and a metapsychological explanation. The phenomenological explanation is that affect* corresponding to experiences of the past is brought into the present, in this case with the psychoanalyst. Therefore, scenes of the past or their corresponding affects are experienced in present-day scenes.

It also has a metapsychological explanation. We may begin by saying that the *quantum* of libidinal energy corresponding to a repressed unconscious object wish* presentation* is brought towards a preconscious word-presentation* with which it maintains an associative type of relation (by contiguity*, analogy*, or opposition) unknown to the preconscious ego. Consequently, the *quantum* of affect* corresponds to the repressed thing-presentation* pertaining to events of infantile sexuality* but is in preconscious object presentations in present-day life; they are consequently unusual and generally out of place. Although the preconscious ego does not know their cause, it is sometimes able to justify them in the manner of the secondary revision* of dreams*; that is to say, through rationalizations*.

In the phenomenon of transference, the infantile event and its affective intensity is brought into the present where the scene is re-experienced but not remembered by the activity of conscious memory. Trieb*, the repressed wish* and their histories of formation are not tamed, but rather simply displaced on to a present-day event which by some law of association* revives these Trieb or wish histories as if they were in the present.

In transference, repressed unconscious object wish presentations are cathected, a cathexis* which succeeds in returning from the repressed* by means of displacement* of libidinal energy on to a preconscious presentation which is thereby also cathected. We would say that it is hyper-cathected*, also bearing the characteristics of Trieb; that is to say, compulsive, peremptory, and repetitive.

Although there is unconscious and preconscious cathexis, the latter does not bind with the former since it does not in reality belong to it; it is simply a figurehead for a different presentation which remains unconscious and therefore unknown. Then, however, the opposite occurs: the preconscious presentation acquires the intensity and free displacement of the unconscious one.

Transference unfolds from neurotic links, of course, and participates in all links between human beings. It is governed partly by the pleasure principle* (included in the reality principle*), and partly by a tendency beyond it, ruled by the Nirvana principle*, which repeats the traumatic event of infantile sexuality.

Transference of affects corresponding to object* cathexes of repressed infantile sexuality on to the preconscious presentation of the psychoanalyst is a clinical observation in all psychoanalytic processes; since it was also discovered in them, its description derives from them.

Patients consult for their symptoms* because they perturb them, are perceived as being foreign to their preconscious ego, and unmanageable by it. The unconscious ego defends itself from the anxiety signal* caused by the infantile Trieb wish, displacing it onto the preconscious presentation of the analyst without the knowledge of the preconscious ego. Then, the neurosis experienced symptomatically is experienced during the treatment in the link with the analyst. It is now a transference neurosis*; in its course, the patients' symptoms usually improve, in contrast with the link with their psychoanalyst which deteriorates notably, and may therefore become a strong resistance* to the advance of the treatment.

In this case, the transference is analysed as resistance; in it, constructions* made previously are corroborated vividly and affectively, or new indicators may lead to new constructions, or new interpretations* with the very appreciable addition of vividness of the phenomenon which transforms it into a full truth.

Analysis of transference neurosis is possible if it is allowed to emerge but not to develop into another repetition; if it may be transformed into words that give the phenomenon binding and understanding*, not only will one of the most tenacious resistances have been overcome but the matter will also have been reversed, converting analysis of transference into a complete, enriching therapeutic weapon of the preconscious ego, its ability to think and to think about itself, to understand and understand itself, to feel and understand its sentiments, which adds meaning to all the previous process.

Before the negative transference neurosis there is positive sublimated transference which it is not necessary to analyse although it is not forbidden to do so. It enables the establishment of the link of the "therapeutic alliance" in which construction may continue, since the patient associates, brings in dreams, and other work. In it, the continuity of the patient's interest in investigating him- or herself is sustained and therefore also the continuity of the treatment; however, it is advisable to bear in mind the possibility that negative transference may reemerge.

Therefore, transference may acquire diverse aspects: sublimated positive transference is the base of the therapeutic alliance necessary for the patient to associate in the freest way possible and thereby enable the constructions of the deepest possible facts of infantile sexuality. When transference is eroticized, it becomes negative transference, the patient's associations are interrupted, and transference love* originates, an ego resistance that may also be difficult to overcome if it is not grasped in time and interpreted, inserting it into the understanding of repetition, which is accomplished through construction, the lifting of repression*, and the revelation of historical truth*, thereby filling in previous mnemic lacunae with the "worked through" construction of infantile sexuality.

Finally, transference may be directly hostile and lead to confrontations that repeat others experienced or wished for during infantile prehistory. Throughout all, the analyst preserves an investigative and understanding attitude in order to help the patient to understand him- or herself, to understand these compulsive attitudes in the present which proceed from repetitions of the history of the patient's links with the first object: history and prehistory forgotten up to this moment.

Analysis of transference thus becomes one of the distinctive characteristics of psychoanalytic treatment and a curative weapon *par excellence,* although it also has limitations. This process as described above is usually produced in the neuroses.

In character disorders, transference does not unfold with the magnitude of a neurosis (so long as the character* dominates the scene); we could say that it is nearly always kept attenuated and therefore interferes with free association. However, we would say that the link with the analyst repeats the history of the explanation of the character of the patient's ego, and therefore analysis of transference may also become essential in these cases.

In narcissistic disorders, the problem is different: in this type of patients, a more or less intense decathexis* of the unconscious object wish has taken place, and this libidinal cathexis has been sent to fill in the ego's gaping wounds by hyper-cathecting it. Therefore, when these forms of defence* are successful, the link with the object is fairly unimportant to the narcissistic subject.

It could be thought that these patients do not form transferences. We would say instead that their transferences are more difficult, more painful, burdened with fear of object loss* and even automatic anxiety* or the feeling of helplessness*. For this reason, Freud considered it difficult or even impossible to treat them.

In these cases, other resources are called for: hospitalization, psychiatric medication, daytime hospital treatment, therapeutic companions, and other resources, to help the patient's ego to bear these anxieties* originating in the object link and to construct their explanation, originating in the earliest links which are repeated in the same modality and require treatment.

When it is possible to break down the narcissistic barrier in this way, the links produced are of course transferences: repetitions of history and also prehistory, in which repetition compulsion* beyond the pleasure principle predominates.

In persecutory paranoia*, sublimations and social ties are eroticized (all with homosexual libido), and the unconscious wish is projected into the unconscious of the wished-for object and turned into its opposite; therefore, the transference link may quite easily become a persecutory delusion*, which makes this work very arduous and difficult. Perhaps what is important is to maintain the ideal distance to enable the therapeutic link while preserving it from becoming so eroticized that it has to be discontinued. If this ideal distance is maintained, it may be desexualized (the ego functions with desexualized libido), allowing the return of a certain capacity for sublimation with which social ties thereby improve.

TRANSFERENCE LOVE

Ger.: übertragungs Liebe. – Sp.: amor de transferencia. – Fr.: amour de transfert. – It.: amore di transfert. – Port.: amor de transferência.

This is a situation which some psychoanalytic treatments may go through. According to the Freudian example, it consists in a patient falling in what is basically sensual love with the therapist. In the case that it is the therapist that falls in love, it is a counter-transference* phenomenon. When patient and therapist are the same sex, the libido* involved is homosexual, an intermediate point between object libido and narcissistic libido, and the pathology of the phenomenon therefore exceeds the limits of typical neurosis and enters those of narcissism. Everything then becomes even more complex since the therapist may be representing, on different levels, the father or the mother.

The phenomenon described is of course considered an obstacle to analysis. It is part of negative transference* and as such an expression of resistance* of the patient's ego* with serious risks for the continuation of the treatment.

Although in the last analysis all love* is transference love, on these occasions what tends to be involved is more transference than love, apart from the fact that the objective of the treatment, the patient's cure, becomes relegated. Each case has its specificity and each therapist must call upon his or her creativity to save the situation, but basically the attitude should be the usual: the analytic attitude; that is to say, to analyse, neither rejecting the patient nor of course accepting his or her amorous proposals. These are simply taken as emergents of the unconscious* that is being repeated vividly in transference and is trying to force an action; therefore it is difficult to bind it with word-presentations that would enable it to be thought about, but it should be attempted. Correct analysis and construction* of the facts being repeated and their relation to the present and actual (thereby differentiating between the past that is making itself present and actual in order to return this fact to the past and to its original place in memory, now conscious, and in this way to succeed in stopping it from repeating in the present) enable the subject to advance further in knowledge of the ego. A certain degree of "falling in love" with the therapist is found in every analysis, and like any other love of this type, it involves the phenomenon of idealization* which gradually vanishes with the progress of the treatment; however, this "falling in love" is generally desexualized and therefore more manageable, thinkable, and less compulsive. There may even be moments or a certain degree of non desexualization with participation in positive transference for love of the therapist as the subject once did with the parents of infancy. In this case "improvements" will be for love of the therapist. If the unconscious meaning of this fact is not revealed during treatment, there will be no changes in the ego; this passing improvement will simply be a repetition of history and nothing more.

Psychoanalytic treatment seeks to learn historical truth* (the truth that in this case is repeated) of the ego* and of the history of the patient's Trieb; on this path psychoanalysts may encounter situations that put their own ego and affects* to the test. The need to institute training analysis in psychoanalytic institutions was born out of these and other types of situations.

TRANSFERENCE NEUROSIS

Ger.: Übertragungsneurose. – Sp.: neurosis de transferencia. – Fr.: névrose de transfert. – It.: nevrosi di transfert. – Port.: neurose de transferência.

Psychoanalysis has always worked especially on this group of neuroses, and has had its greatest success in treating them. They are obsessional neurosis*, conversion hysteria*, and anxiety hysteria* or phobia*. These neuroses are produced as an effect of defects of secondary repression exerted by the unconscious ego* against Triebe* of the id*. Since secondary repression is not totally effective, id Triebe (unconscious wishes formed by their presentational cathexis, which provokes their repression) sometimes manage to return from the repressed*; by means of a disguise (a substitute formation*) they originate symptoms, ("foreigners inside" the ego which it is unable to dominate and therefore appear compulsively.

Repression* withdraws cathexis* from the (preconscious) word-presentation*, but cathexis remains in the unconscious thing-presentation*, which therefore struggles constantly to access the preconscious. To block it by withdrawing cathexis from the word-presentation requires the help of an anticathexis* to impede its access to the preconscious.

This describes defence mechanisms*. One mechanism or another predominates depending on fixation* points of Trieb and the ego. Each fixation point may originate different transference neuroses: the major mechanisms are: conversion* (repression proper) in hysteria; displacement* in anxiety hysteria*; reaction formation* (the origin of anal character* more than of obsessional neurosis itself, although the latter is built upon it); undoing (what has been done)* and isolation* in obsessional neurosis.

The term "transference neurosis" is derived from clinical practice, since the repressed seeks to return by transferring itself on to available preconscious presentations*, and the presentation of the analyst is one of these. Therefore, during treatment an artificial "re-experiencing" of the phenomena which originated the neurosis is produced. They are repeated in the analytic link, sometimes as ego resistance* to continuation of the treatment, which Freud refers to as a repetition. The patient repeats in order not to remember.

However, this resistance becomes what is perhaps the major weapon in the cure and gives psychoanalytic treatment its identity: analysis of the transference neurosis of forgotten infantile sexuality*, now transferred on to the link with the analyst. In the experienced clarification of transference* and logical historical reconstruction of what is transferred on to actual links, mainly the link with the analyst, is one of the major possibilities of a cure, the lifting of repression, re-cathectization of preconscious presentations against which the ego has been defending itself but which it no longer fears. They now become thinkable, enriching the ego, and become part of its wealth. Since anticathexes are also needed less, the ego is freer to use its own energy.

The notion of transference involves repression and also, consequently, transference of cathexis from a repressed unconscious thing-presentation to a preconscious presentation which acts as a disguise of the former while preserving all the affective current.

In transference neuroses, object libido* is introverted (cf. libidinal introversion); cathexis passes from real objects* to those of phantasy*, a phantasy that may also then be repressed and, if it returns from the repressed, may generate symptoms or transferences.

Therefore, transference neuroses are unlike narcissistic neuroses in the sense that in the latter, object libido is withdrawn, not into phantasy but onto the ego. It thereby becomes narcissistic libido and may produce what are called narcissistic neuroses in which cathexis is withdrawn from the thing-presentation, the unconscious presentation of the object. In this way the unconscious object wish is lost. Unlike transference neuroses, in narcissistic neuroses we observe phenomena of restitution* but not transference.

TRAUMA

Ger.: Trauma. – Sp.: trauma. – Fr.: trauma. – It.: trauma. – Port.: trauma.

The trauma theory has had an intricate development in Freud's works. At one point, Freud recants it, but it re-emerges later, refreshed, with new and previous levels of complexity.

Our description is not a simple sequence of the turns Freud takes in his thinking about it, although this is partly inevitable, but we try to present a global conceptualization that contains, in a dynamic way, the direction we consider the most important one in Freudian thought on this subject.

Any stimulus surpassing the capacity of the psychical apparatus to bind it with presentations*, in the best of cases with word-presentations*, is traumatic; if not, at least with unconscious thing-presentations*, the latter a primary process type of "binding", not real binding*. However, since there is a presentation, the pleasure principle* is involved, and therefore it remains within its realm.

During the traumatic situation*, quantity of excitation* rules, entering the psychical apparatus and leaving it just as it entered, without leaving any presentational trace or only sketchy ones, perhaps the painful sensation corresponding to physical trauma. What remains of this painful sensation is, on the one hand, a facilitation* in the psychical apparatus which leads it to repeat it; on the other hand, defensive anticathexes* leading to the opposite, generating fixations* which thereafter tend to be repeated.

Since the trauma destroyed the presentations, no register of them remains or else they are not the important part of the trace left behind; what is more important is the painful passage of quantity of unbindable excitation, not bindable at least at that moment. This tends to be repeated and is located beyond the pleasure principle.

In any case, the psychical apparatus also seeks to re-establish its functions, trying first to reinstate the protective shield*. For this purpose, in traumatic dreams*, it feels the preparedness anxiety that the trauma left it no time to feel. Later, it simply repeats in part and tries to reconstruct the facts with thing-presentations in the unconscious through these traumatic dreams*, and therefore they are sometimes transformed into anxiety* dreams or punishment dreams which continue to be transformed and made more complex; now they are constituted as wishes* or punishment for them, and therefore function within the pleasure principle. From this point, binding may be sought with preconscious word-presentations. This is the objective of psychoanalysis, the highest level of binding.

What is the attitude of the preconscious ego* towards the trauma? On the one hand, it tries to maintain defensive anticathexes, especially if they had to be extreme, which it utilizes and sometimes succeeds in "forgetting"* the trauma, sending it into the state of repression*. On the other hand, it seeks the best binding possible with word-presentations of the preconscious ego by utilizing thought* activity to enable the best affective and Trieb binding and decrease the tendency to repetition.

Summarizing: we have three types of effects of trauma on the psychical apparatus. (The difference between a present-day traumatic situation and one corresponding to infantile sexuality* was described in Traumatic situation*.) One effect is repetition compulsion*. There is compulsion because there is facilitation produced by the sudden passage of quantity of excitation through the psychical apparatus when the latter is unable to obtain a predominant presentational register of it. What tends to be repeated is therefore the suffering itself (if there is any presentation, it only lends a scene to this suffering), automatic anxiety*. Traumas of infantile sexuality create difficulties for the ego to establish anxiety signals* or increase their magnitude, leading in the latter cases to defence mechanisms* befitting the magnitude of anxiety (the greater the anxiety, the more extreme the defence, unless it is automatic anxiety, against which there is no effective defence mechanism).

When trauma leaves a presentational level with at least unconscious thing-presentations, its levels of binding will be the type of defence mechanisms utilized in response to anxiety signals such as castration anxiety* or those which repeat phenomena instead of remembering them, as in transference*. These are products of Trieb fusions; they may partly be simple repetitions, but they do provide an opportunity to obtain word-presentations by means of psychoanalysis, and thereby to become a part of the preconscious ego and its thought activity; this enables them to stop being mere repetitions or to produce something new with what is now thinkable, tamed by the ego.

The latter is the objective to be attained: it is what we call the "working through of trauma". We endeavour to bring it into thought activity, in order to understand the reasons behind fixation points*, repetition compulsions, automatic anxieties, the structuring of the ego by now binding thing-presentations with word-presentations and thereby bringing them into secondary process*.

TRAUMATIC DREAMS

Ger.: traumatische Träume. – Sp.: sueños traumáticos. – Fr.: rêves traumatiques. – It.: sogni traumatici. – Port.: sonhos traumáticos.

These are recurrent dreams* following a traumatic situation* that is re-experienced in the dream's content. This generates even more anxiety* in the dreamer until they disappear, once the period of the traumatic neurosis* has concluded.

They are produced partly by repetition compulsion* beyond the pleasure principle*, which simply seeks to repeat the traumatic experience as a shortcut to return to the inorganic; but also because the psychical apparatus attempts to reinsert the experience of the traumatic situation into the pleasure principle. Then, reconstruction of the protective shield* is attempted to restore protection overwhelmed during the traumatic situation, which it must now repeat (by dreaming about it), basically until the ego is able to feel preparedness anxiety*, the last line of defence against stimuli whose magnitude, associated with the surprise of the traumatic situation, left no possibility to feel and then to find bindings with presentations* of the past.

If this binding is achieved, the dream is no longer traumatic and becomes an anxiety dream*; it is therefore ruled again by the pleasure–unpleasure principle.

It thus belongs once more to the theory of wish fulfilment*, having a "capitalist partner" to which it is bound (a cathected thing-presentation* of a repressed wish of infantile sexuality*; that is to say, an unconscious wish), whereas the formerly traumatic event (now a danger-situation*) becomes the "industrial partner".

If it is unable to achieve this binding, it remains beyond the pleasure principle as repetition compulsion.

Fixation* to the trauma*: trauma or quantity of excitation* without binding or with only one presentation (that of the traumatic scene), which therefore tends to be repeated (but may eventually not be limited to dreams, carrying over into events), facilitated by this traumatic quantity, so intense that it is consequently unable to achieve better representational quality*.

TRAUMATIC NEUROSIS

Ger.: Traumatische Neurose. – Sp.: neurosis traumática. – Fr.: névrose traumatique. – It.: nevrosi traumatica. – Port.: neurose traumática.

This type of psychical affection occurs following mechanical forces, shocks, and other accidents occurring in the subject's present life (not in infantile history as in historical neuroses) representing a risk of death. The clinical picture may be similar to that of hysteria

> in the wealth of its similar motor symptoms, but surpasses it as a rule in its strongly marked signs of subjective ailment (in which it resembles hypochondria or melancholia) as well as in the evidence it gives of a far more comprehensive general enfeeblement and disturbance of the mental capacities.
>
> (1920, p. 12).

In common traumatic neurosis, two features are prominent: the centre of gravity of the cause seems to be the factor of surprise or terror*. Also, in most cases, simultaneous physical damage or a wound offsets the production of neurosis. Also:

> dreams occurring in traumatic neuroses have the characteristic of repeatedly bringing the patient back into the situation of his accident, a situation from which he wakes up in another fright … the patient is, as one might say, fixated to his trauma.
>
> (Ibid., p. 13)

According to Freud's explanation, traumatic neuroses refer to external excitations whose force has been so great that it has breached the protective shield against stimuli*. They result from vast destruction of this barrier: anxious expectation* and its hyper-cathexis* of the perceptual apparatus "constitute the last line of defence of the shield against stimuli"

(Ibid., p. 31). The traumatic event in this case is quantity of external excitation* which, acting by surprise, produced terror in the absence of previous anxious expectation* in the ego* which could bind the quantity of excitation and transform it into quiescent or bound energy*. An enormous disturbance of psychical energetic economy* was produced in the organism: it was inundated by large volumes of stimulus. Originally, the pleasure principle* was abolished.

> But it is not in the service of that principle that the dreams of patients suffering from traumatic neuroses lead them back with such regularity to the situation in which the trauma occurred. We may assume, rather, that dreams are here helping to carry out another task, which must be accomplished before the dominance of the pleasure principle can even begin. These dreams are endeavouring to master the stimulus retrospectively, by developing the anxiety whose omission was the cause of the traumatic neurosis.
>
> (Ibid., p. 32)

Recovery of mastery is a function of the psychical apparatus which, though not contradicting the principle of pleasure, is independent of it. The dreams* of traumatic neurosis limit the theory that dreams are wish fulfilment*, since they obey repetition compulsion* which is more primitive.

TRAUMATIC SITUATION

Ger.: traumatische Zustand. – Sp.: situación traumática. – Fr.: situation traumatique. – It.: situazione traumatica. – Port.: situação traumática.

A situation is traumatic when it possesses a sufficiently high level of excitation and takes the psychical apparatus* by surprise (without preparedness anxiety*, for example), piercing the protective shield* against stimuli and thereby overwhelming the representational level that was functioning previously, ruled by the pleasure principle*. Since the traumatic situation cannot be bound to presentations* (unconscious thing-presentations* or, of course, preconscious word-presentations*), it is left out of this principle and lies beyond it.

Then the quantity of excitation* that entered the psychical apparatus is ruled by the Nirvana principle*, and therefore tends to traumatic repetition, essentially the painful part of the situation, not the presentation itself, although in this way it may come to achieve some level of representation. Other traumatic events – perhaps the most common – are able to leave a precarious representation, since what is essential is not the fact but rather the pain caused by the trauma*, which is what in reality is endeavoured to be repeated as a kind of shortcut to return to the inorganic.

Therefore, what defines the traumatic situation is the quantity of external excitation and the psychical apparatus' difficulty to handle it.

Some traumatic situations depend not only on external quantities but also on internal Trieb quantities. On account of sexual Triebe*, the ego* has a complex link with objects* of the external world. The effects on sexual Triebe travel through deferred* time, repetition compulsion*, inherent to all Triebe and especially to death Trieb*, joining them. The traumatic events of infantile sexuality* are a good example. During this period they could be simple stimulations of erotogenic zones*; at that time they were not traumatic; at most they may have produced some irritation in the erotogenic zone involved, but there were no presentations with which to bind them because of previous ignorance or even foreclosure* of them (as might occur with phallic stimulation of a baby in the midst of oral or anal development). They become traumatic in a deferred* manner in the period of predominance of the corresponding erotogenic zone. Then, the level of excitation is the same as in the (past) traumatic event, originating defence mechanisms as if the traumatic situations* were actual. These traumatic events belonging to moments of development of infantile sexuality are another cause of the formation of fixations* or primal repressions* whose only mechanism is untimely anticathexis* of Trieb inflow, anticathexis that must be maintained with constant expenditure of energy from that moment forward and which attracts unconscious derivatives to return, to make their position strong, then to attempt to return from the repressed* by diverting repression*.

With respect to sexual Trieb, the concept of traumatic situation is more complex, since it involves several factors: quantity of external excitation, the period of the subject's sexual development at the time of the trauma*; also, perhaps a distinctive and major fact, its movement through time, the participation in it of history; however, something else makes it even more complex: this history is forgotten and sent to the unconscious, although it is re-experienced in repetitions, for example, in transference*, as if they were actual events. In this phenomenon, life Triebe* are without a doubt fused with death Triebe, the latter even predominating. The birth trauma, prototype of all subsequent traumatic situations, consists of quantities of excitation that invade a psychical apparatus lacking any possibility to bind them to any presentation.

The danger-situation* consists in fear of the traumatic situation. Angel Garma developed Freud's line of thought and, taking it to its last consequences, introduced the theory that all dreams are ultimately an attempt to work through a traumatic situation.

TRIEB (PLURAL: TRIEBE)

(See: Strachey, J., 1962, Notes on some technical terms whose translation calls for comment, in *The Standard Edition of the Complete Psychological Works of Sigmund Freud*, Vol. 1, pp. xxiv–vi.)

Ger.: Trieb. – Sp.: pulsión. – Fr.: pulsion. – It.: istinto o pulsione. – Port.: pulsão.

This psychical stimulus proceeding from inside the subject's own body is produced by bodily needs produced constantly; but only periodically, after passing a certain threshold, it enters the psychical apparatus where, with the first levels of binding with presentations* (thing-presentations in the unconscious), it acquires the name of Trieb. At this point it is no longer simply a biological stimulus, having now acquired psychical characteristics from the presentation.

On this first level of binding between energy and presentations (primary process* free energy* able to condense and displace itself easily among presentations is guided by the laws of association* which it utilizes to search for perceptual identity*), we find a substantial difference compared to the concept of instinct* (*Instinkt*) in which presentations are inherited (for this reason Freud states that inherited protophantasies are what most resembles animal instinct in our psyche (*From the History of an Infantile Neurosis*, 1918), and it seems that from the outset they are fixed and immutable, produced by the experience of our species.

In this regard, Trieb is a more dynamic concept, a product of the individual's ontogenetic history, the subject's own experience, since presentations in the person's psychical apparatus are ultimately its traces.

However, since these concepts include each other, they are not easily distinguished. Inherited presentations act similarly to Kantian philosophical "categories", providing order for the way we understand (the *a priori* of) our perceptions*. However, we need the latter, which are the subject's own experiences. We must acquire for ourselves what we have inherited.

This "category" must take a different plotline for each individual, including the person's history, sealed within presentations of the psychical apparatus, in order to become Trieb.

Trieb, we understand, is at first nothing more than the psychical representative agency (*Repräsentanz*) of a source of intrasomatic stimuli in continuous flow; this is unlike the "stimulus" produced by singular excitations proceeding from the outside. Therefore, "Trieb" is one of the concepts that separate the psychical from the bodily. The simplest and most obvious hypothesis on the nature of Triebe is this: they have no quality in themselves whatsoever and must be considered as only a measure of demand of work for mental life. What distinguishes Triebe from each other and gives them specific properties is their relation with their somatic *sources* and their *aims*. The Trieb source is an excitatory process inside an organ, its immediate aim consisting in cancellation of this organ stimulus.

> There is a further provisional assumption that we cannot escape in the theory of the instincts. It is to the effect that excitations of two kinds arise from the somatic organs, based upon differences of a chemical nature. One of these kinds of excitation we describe as being specifically sexual, and we speak of the organ concerned as the "erotogenic zone" of the sexual component instinct arising from it.
>
> (*Three Essays on the Theory of Sexuality*, 1905, p. 168)

> [A]n "instinct" appears to us as a concept on the frontier between the mental and the somatic, as the psychical representative (*Repräsentanz*) of the stimuli originating from within the organism and reaching the mind, as a measure of the demand made upon the mind for work in consequence of its connection with the body.
>
> (*Instincts and Their Vicissitudes*, 1915, pp. 121–2)

The Trieb theory is part of the base of Freudian thought although it never achieved absolute conceptual clarity. Freud humorously referred to it as "our mythology" (*New Introductory Lectures on Psycho-Analysis*, 1933, p. 95). This theory gradually grew more complex in the course of his works and with the advance of his discoveries.

At first, he described the existence of two basic Triebe: self-preservative Triebe of the ego* whose model is hunger and sexual Triebe* which are not limited to the preservation of the species but instead search for pleasure*; their model is love* and their evolution is far more complex than the previous Triebe which form their anaclisis.

Progressively, based on the description of infantile sexuality* in *Three Essays on Sexual Theory* (1905) and by virtue of the participation of this infantile sexuality fixated* in adult sexual perversions* and in the neuroses*, and also because it constitutes the trunk of the repressed unconscious*, sexual Trieb becomes the main figure generating what is most complex in psychical problems: its presentations of object* wishes* and its conflicts which Freud at first considers principally related to self-preservative Triebe.

Following his description of narcissism*, the description of sexual problems becomes even more complex. At first, infantile sexuality is predominantly autoerotic (although this autoerotism* originates in the object link, since this object is associated with care given the baby, awakening erotogenic zones* (*Three Essays on Sexual Theory*, 1905), it is composed of part Triebe* which gradually constitute a unit. This unit's first level of culmination is the phallic phase in which the Oedipus complex* develops and the object is definitively considered the main source of pleasure. At the same time, all the isolated erotogenic zones come together under phallic* supremacy to form a new institution called the ego* which is thereby born from the body and from marks left in the subject by history (experienced with the object and autoerotically). Libido*, which now seeks satisfaction or pleasure in the object link, is called object libido, and what gives the ego pleasure is narcissistic libido (*On Narcissism: An Introduction*, 1914).

This organization becomes even more complex. The object* has a new part, intrinsically its own (the thing*), and attributes of this thing. These attributes may constitute what is mainly sought in the object and may also be similar to attributes of other objects in the subject's history or similar to the subject's own attributes.

Object choice* may take place by anaclisis* on attributes of objects of history or on the subject's own characteristics. In the latter case, a narcissistic object choice, it is an intermediate step between narcissism and object choice. This is homosexual object choice which disavows the existence of sexual difference sought by object libido but feared by narcissistic libido because of the resemblance, for a child between four and six years of age, between the female genital and a castrated male genital, the only genital considered to exist at that time.

Therefore, object libido comes into conflict with narcissistic libido, a conflict between two modes of sexual Trieb. If pleasurable experiences in the object link (including traumatic oedipal problems) predominate, the object's attraction overcomes narcissism and sexual Trieb is satisfied, especially in the object link; if not, the subject needs to devote him or herself to stanching wounded narcissism by overloading the ego with libido and taking refuge in it.

Trieb possesses pressure, aim, object, and source. Pressure (*Drang*) is "its motor factor, the amount of force or the measure of the demand for work which it represents (*Instincts and Their Vicissitudes*, 1915, p. 122): it is the essence of Trieb, its factor pressuring towards action.

The aim (*Ziel*) of Trieb consists in its satisfaction, reached when stimulus produced in the Trieb source is cancelled. Sexual Triebe are able to change their aims or to inhibit them partly; therefore, aim-inhibited Triebe are created such as those satisfied, for example, by tenderness and friendship.

The object (*Objekt*) is that by which Trieb reaches its aim. In sexual Trieb it is most variable, since it is not originally connected with it; it is instead a product of the subject's history with the object and with the subject's own body; presentations of wished-for objects and their attributes originate on the basis of these histories leading to the aim.

When traumatic situations* occur with objects as a product of history, their presentations are fixated by anticathexes*; through this mechanism they lose their variability.

The source (*Quelle*) of Trieb is the somatic process inside an organ or body part, an erotogenic zone, whose stimulus becomes Trieb when it is bound to a psychical presentation.

The schema presented above becomes more complex in 1920 with the addition of new elements to the Trieb theory which complicate it so greatly that it becomes a new Trieb theory.

In the first place, we have

> a universal attribute of instincts and perhaps of organic life in general which has not hitherto been clearly recognized or at least not explicitly stressed. *It seems, then, that an instinct is an urge inherent in organic life to restore an earlier state of things* which the living entity has been obliged to abandon under the pressure of external disturbing forces; that is, it is a kind of organic elasticity, or, to put it another way, the expression of the inertia inherent to organic life.
>
> (*Beyond the Pleasure Principle*, 1920, p. 36)

Therefore, Trieb is not only stimulus for the mind, obliging the psyche to work to find an outlet for it, but also repeats a previous state or diverse previous states.

Until 1920, early moments experienced long ago with the object, now endeavoured to be "refound" are experiences of satisfaction* or pleasure (both self-preservative and sexual Trieb seeking at first to avoid experiences of pain*). In this way, the reign of the pleasure principle* is constituted, although it needs the reality principle* to seek its aim in a real and substantial way.

This first type of repetition, whose most important clinical expressions constitute both great therapeutic difficulties and also major weapons (transference* and transference neurosis*), remains mainly within the pleasure principle. At least, events pleasurable for one of the systems are repeated although they may generate anxiety in another system.

However, Freud also observes repetitions of events that were never pleasurable for any system of the psychical apparatus (purely traumatic events). Therefore, they represent a more fundamental, more daemonic tendency to repetition which is not part of the pleasure principle but is beyond it.

In a daring proposal, Freud states (*Beyond the Pleasure Principle*, 1920) that there is a type of Trieb which seeks to repeat the state previous to the existence of life, to return to the inorganic: death Triebe*. In spite of being self-preservative Triebe *par excellence*, they are different from the others, now grouped under the term of life Triebe* because they aim to preserve something different. The former endeavour to preserve what is before life (death Triebe) and the latter to preserve past, pleasurable moments in life (life Triebe), thereby becoming opposites.

This type of opposition is extremely complex. We now have life Triebe which seek to repeat a previous pleasurable state experienced in the object link, which left presentations of this event in the psychical apparatus, and consequently acquired the characteristics of both Trieb and object wish, lending what was previously perceptual quality* to quantity of bodily excitation, now producing the memory of and desire for it: presentational quality.

For their part, death Triebe endeavour to regress to the inorganic, to pure quantity, and reject the world of quality.

These two types of Trieb intermix to different degrees. They are found in the diverse forms of life Triebe or Eros*, in erotogenic zones (and through them the history of the object link) evolutionally higher than sexual Trieb, with a larger degree of Trieb fusion and therefore better taming of death Triebe. The latter are deflected to the exterior by virtue of muscular action, becoming destructive Triebe*. They then join sexual Trieb in diverse proportions of fusion (sadism* and Trieb for mastery, for example). Death Trieb ultimately seeks to defuse binding between quantity of excitation and presentations (thing-presentations* and word-presentations*) achieved by life Triebe, in order to regress to pure quantity, the world of the inorganic.

The phenomenon generated by this mechanism is repetition compulsion* which seeks to repeat a basically quantitative traumatic event. A small proportion of death Trieb remains free in the psychical apparatus as primary erotogenic masochism* (*The Economic Problem of Masochism*, 1924). Another part is deflected to the exterior as aggression and, lastly, part of the latter returns to the psychical apparatus by means of the superego* which binds it and utilizes it to suppress* sexual and aggressive Triebe which have become antisocial in the adult, also producing phenomena such as moral masochism and need for punishment*.

TRIEB AIM

Ger.: Triebziel. – Sp.: meta pulsional. – Fr.: but pulsionnel. – It.: meta pulsionale. – Port.: meta pulsional.

This is the end point of the arc initiated (in sexual Trieb*) when quantity of excitation* proceeding from the body and its erotogenic zones* (the source of Trieb*) enters the psychical apparatus and binds initially with a thing-presentation*. It thereupon becomes libido* and configures an unconscious* object wish*. If this wish is to reach consciousness* and to be put into action, it must be bound to word-presentations* and be thought. When the specific action* is performed, Trieb satisfaction or pleasure* is reached as soon as the state of stimulation at the Trieb source is cancelled. Hence, the aim of Trieb is its satisfaction.

"[T]here may yet be different paths leading to the same ultimate aim; so that an instinct may be found to have various nearer or intermediate aims, which are combined or interchanged with one another" (*Instincts and their Vicissitudes*, p. 122).

Some sexual Triebe have an "inhibited aim" which implies partial but more lasting satisfaction. "Aim-inhibited" Trieb enables friendship, tenderness, and sublimation in general; however, this process is also a product since it generates culture*; when Freud includes death Trieb* in his theorization, he notes that it generates a certain defusion of Treibe*. This defusion is produced when higher levels of fusion are inhibited (more precisely: the genital* aim) with consequent liberation of extra death Trieb. The latter is strictly tamed when sexual Trieb is able to take this fusion to its original (genital) aim. This situation creates the paradox in which desexualized or aim-inhibited libido, one of the origins of cultural ties, must pay for it. This payment is made by freeing extra death Trieb (self-destruction) in some cases, or of destructive*, aggressive* or mastery* Trieb, all enemies of culture.

TRIEB FOR KNOWLEDGE

Ger.: Wissbegierde. – Sp.: pulsión de saber. – Fr.: pulsion de savoir. – It.: pulsione di sapere. – Port.: pulsão de saber.

This is a sublimated form of the Trieb for mastery* to which the part sexual Trieb* for seeing is added.

In this way, infantile curiosity is born, leading to the construction of infantile sexual theories* (the phallic mother* and the cloacal theory* for example), also to discovery and understanding of the primal scene* and the first conception of sexual difference involved (phallic–castrated).

This Trieb* fails at this first infantile level because the idea of castration* cannot be worked through by the child's psychical apparatus due to narcissism*; therefore, all presentations of infantile sexuality are repressed along with the Trieb for knowledge associated with them.

Sometimes this loss is nearly definitive and therefore the egos formed are poor in presentations and conceptions of reality*. In other cases, Trieb for knowledge is eroticized and replaces sexual excitation (the obsessional neurotic's erotization of thought); it may also produce sexual excitation (generating, on the one hand, diverse forms of perversion* or, on the other hand, neurotic learning impediments due to anxiety in relation to knowing); finally, it is sublimated as the thirst for knowledge of scientists, for example. In this case it is utilized by the ego* in its thought* activity to progressively learn about different levels of reality of the external world and of the subject's own reality. To carry out a psychoanalytic treatment, the analyst needs the patient's thirst for knowledge as an ally (as well as the patient's desire to be free of neurotic suffering), the patient's eagerness to investigate about him or herself, which lead to different levels of working through of historical truth*, with which the patient is able to clearly differentiate this type of truth from actual reality.

TRIEB FOR MASTERY

Ger.: Bemächtigungstrieb. – Sp.: pulsión de apoderamiento. – Fr.: pulsion d'emprise. – It.: istinto o pulsione d'impossessamento. – Port.: pulsão de apoderar.

This Trieb is a product of fusión of sexual Triebe* and death Triebe*. Its form of expression is through sexual Trieb as a need to possess the object*; this need may be physical or psychical, and may even involve destruction of the object (for example, the wish to devour the object). It appears in the oral* cannibalistic phase when the aim is incorporation of the object (which will serve as a model for identification*), although this aim involves its destruction.

It develops further in the anal* phase together with the first levels of recognition of the object as the main source of pleasure and the consequent appearance of fear of object loss from which mastery of the object protects the subject.

In the anal phase, the child's incipient ego* begins to dominate the muscular system and the child thereby learns to control its sphincters (one of the basic conditions for access to culture*), and also deflects death Trieb, transforming it into aggression*, sadism*, and Trieb for mastery*, which have similarities and differences. The subject's sadism takes pleasure in the object's suffering when mastering it and exerting power over it, and in having the object in the subject's possession. Although each aspect involves the other, in some cases, the difference is important. The masochist enjoys pain inflicted on him or her by the sadistic subject, but also exerts power over the latter. Normal jealousy* also involves a quota of Trieb for mastery in all love links.

With the phallic phase, struggle with the rival for possession of the object appears. In this sense, the need for mastery separates from love*, and is now expressed nearly purely in the fight with the rival, which is therefore a conflict for possession of the object.

Both phases involve ambivalence*, although it predominates in the anal, in the link with the chosen object.

This Trieb is not autonomous but rather an expression of Trieb fusion; death Trieb is part of aggression, and is even implicit in hate*; sexual Trieb in the fact that it may be part of love, of object wishes and also of narcissism* (love of the ego*), in the loving link itself and also in the struggle with the rival.

It is a part Trieb* which gradually falls (although never entirely) first to phallic supremacy and then to the genital, becoming part of sexual Trieb as a whole.

On its highest genital* level, the subject does not want to share the partner, but wants to possess him or her (as the subject's territory). In this sense sexual Trieb is antisocial.

Trieb for mastery participates in many other types of unions. Together with the Trieb for seeing, it forms Trieb for knowledge* or infantile sexual curiosity. It leads the subject to develop the first infantile sexual theories* and to grasp the primal scene* towards which the child is also impelled by phylogenetic primal phantasies*.

Its sublimation* in adults generates the need for knowledge common to all human beings, especially scientists.

It also participates in children's play as symbolic mastery of reality* with a certain level of action that differentiates it from mere phantasy. It is also involved in art* which originates from a wish to possess objects of reality, which is fulfilled symbolically by virtue of artistic creation.

All these latter examples involve sublimation* of sexual Trieb* and, in part, of Trieb for mastery.

TRIEB FUSION AND DEFUSION

Ger.: Triebmischung / Triebentmischung. – Sp. mezcla y desmezcla pulsional. – Fr.: union-désunion pulsionnel. – It.: fusione e defusione pulsionale. – Port.: fusão e defusão pulsional.

These terms are Freud's presentation of relations between life Triebe* and death Triebe* in his last Trieb theory.

Death Trieb is a tendency of all living matter to return to the inorganic state. Life Trieb* is the tendency to return to moments before life (experiences of satisfaction/pleasure).

Death itself has no unconscious thing-presentation*, does not belong to unconscious* presentations*, is not experienced and therefore is not wished for in the period of infantile sexuality*. Lacking any presentation, it cannot be repressed*.

Therefore, the presentation of one's own death is not part of the unconscious but is acquired later by the ego's* preconscious* through the incorporation of speech*, which adds an unsuspected dimension to thought* activity, enabling among other things a presentation of the subject's own death in words by understanding another's death, concomitantly with the culmination of structuring of the psychical apparatus into an id*, an ego, and a superego*.

What we are unable to acquire is any experiential presentation or sensation of it, which the thing-presentation requires. At most, a preconscious word-presentation of death may refer to similar unconscious infantile experiences (castration, fear of the superego, and behind it, of the father, felt in the form of punishment by destiny).

Therefore, death Trieb lacks a thing-presentation and is unable to configure an unconscious wish* for the subject's own death. For this reason we say that death Trieb is Trieb by virtue of its tendency, but that lacking unconscious presentation, it acts mutely, utilizing thing-presentations of life Trieb or Eros* to lead them towards its aim. For this reason, Freud introduced fusion. All Eros Trieb is mixed with a quantity of tendency to return to the inorganic. The more Trieb fusion and synthesis there is in object* relations through the erotogenic zones*, the more Trieb fusion and therefore more taming* there will be of the tendency to return to the inorganic. In contrast, when Trieb regresses* to previous stages of libidinal evolution, either more defusion or less fusion results.

At this point we devote a separate point to sublimation*, both the child and mother of culture*. When Trieb fusion decreases due to its essential desexualization*, it generates Trieb defusion and a consequent liberation of death Trieb.

Therefore, everything whose thing-presentation corresponds to Eros is part of the pleasure principle* although it more or less subtly includes a beyond the pleasure principle which may lead to situations increasingly similar to something akin to the inorganic.

In another vicissitude, cathexis* is withdrawn from the thing-presentation (as in the psychoses*, for example, schizophrenia*), and then death Trieb and its repetition compulsion* in search of an "eternal return" to the inorganic dominates the scene.

Previous degrees of defusion also exist. Sadism* results from a deflection of death Trieb onto the external world of objects which may produce erotic pleasure*. This erotic fusion with the tendency to destruction is also a defusion of erotism which liberates destructivity.

The opposite is feminine masochism*, secondary to erotogenic (primary) masochism. In this case, sexual pleasure is obtained through pain, suffering or humiliation (nearing presentations of death). In moral masochism, the aim is suffering itself even without erotic reward, and defusion is even greater.

In absolutely desexualized sadistic or destructive pleasure (the pleasure of killing), the fusion is with narcissistic sexual Trieb pleased by the ego's sensation of omnipotence (*Civilization and its Discontents,* 1930) when it is able to decide whether others will live or die.

Concerning suicide, Freud demonstrated in melancholia* (of which melancholic suicide is a prototype) a fantasy* of hate* or revenge against an object cathected with libido* (this hate is a regression of love*) and therefore as a liberation of death Trieb through a libidinal presentation: it is the superego's hate aimed at the ego or at the object of the ego's identification (cf. identification*).

Repetition compulsion corresponds to the preservative tendency of all Triebe; they differ in what they wish to repeat: Eros wants to repeat pleasurable situations which therefore include a larger proportion of libido in their fusion, whereas death Trieb wants to return to nothingness. The former seeks increasingly greater complexities and the latter, absolute rest (*Beyond the Pleasure Principle*, 1920). Repetition compulsion contains both, in different proportions, beyond or closer than the pleasure principle.

All pleasure-seeking repetition tending towards complexity falls mainly within this principle. When it seeks or finds unpleasure* and pain without achieving new syntheses, it has gone beyond.

In clinical work, dynamically interwoven quantities, fixation* points, and traumatic events defeat all simplification.

TRUTH, HISTORICAL

Ger.: historische Wahrheit. – Sp.: verdad histórica (verdad vivencial). – Fr.: vérité historique. – It.: verità storica. – Port.: verdade histórica.

Traditionally, the concept of truth is the opposite of falsehood and is homologous to reality*. Historical truth in both regards (as opposed to falsehood and homologous to reality; that is to say, psychical reality) and in reference to historical and prehistoric events of infantile sexuality*, is one of the aims we seek during psychoanalytic treatment.

The truth of unconscious thing-presentations*, hidden beneath a disguise of compromises, substitute formations*, or unconscious derivatives of repressed presentations* in the preconscious, recovers these repressed thing-presentations for the preconscious ego; this gives them the word that names them, thereby improving the ego's distinction between its own wish* and what belongs to external reality.

In this regard, historical truth is opposed to the falsehood in substitutive compromise formations; it therefore enables more adequate reality testing through better differentiation based on knowledge of the truth of the subject's own history, as well as connections with present-day reality by the examination of similarities and differences between the two.

If the repressed wish is more fully known, it is differentiated from reality and may be tamed (cf. taming); if not, the ego is dominated by it.

Repressed unconscious presentations originate in the perception* of experiences; although these experiences were grasped and interpreted by individual subjectivity, re-conceptualized and distorted in a deferred* manner, they contain remnants of these original experiences which differ from the way they are remembered: by conscious memory or by other types of remembering such as repetition compulsion*, symptoms* (mnemic symbols*), and other phenomena.

Analytic work seeks the truth concealed by all these processes the presentations have undergone, since they or their interrelations with other presentations contain meanings of symptoms*, fixation* points, ego character traits*, repetition compulsions* and other vicissitudes.

It is preferable to speak in terms of levels, since what is true on one level is not true on another. However, a more encompassing global truth in a person's life lends its own meaning to its small truths which are sometimes mutually opposite but not in relation to the global truth.

Historical truth sought by psychoanalysis is the truth of events of infantile sexuality, essentially of its traumatic situations*. The aim is to find the patiently assembled construction* of events in the subject's life, partly through memories*, now arranged in a new order with a different logic and new meanings, discovered and yet to be discovered; also by the decoding of dreams*, screen memories*, linguistic constructions, parapraxes*, and transference* repetitions.

Summarizing, historical truth is the truth of events exactly as they were experienced by the subject when they occurred. The main facts are traumas* of infantile sexuality which originated fixation points of the subject's sexuality*. Their interpretation involves subjectivity as does any perception, since the perceptual-conscious system contains branches of the unconscious that influence perception; that is to say, the mode of perception of the "moving masses" of the external world and their secondary revision* and also the way they are stored in memory.

The latter factor (memory and its relation with repression*) is perhaps the most specific mechanism capable of modification by psychoanalysis. Repression (broadly, all ego defence mechanisms responding to anxiety signals*) acts by preventing presentations of the traces of what the subject experienced and remembered from accessing the ego's preconscious by decathecting the corresponding word-presentations* that would enable it.

When repression* fails, the repressed returns*. This return is only possible through a compromise, a substitute formation* that disguises the memory that was already disguised at the moment of its perception when it was perceptual quality.

This failure of repression (the return of the repressed*) may be partly decoded through psychoanalysis; this decodification may be utilized to reconstruct the truth of the facts from a different, less obscurantist perspective than the patient's unconscious repression. Although material truth* is inaccessible, a truth nearing the facts as they occurred may be reconstructed; at least a truth involving the most logics possible, enough to access understanding of the meaning of a symptom, a character trait or a repetition compulsion.

Historical truth is at the root of neurotic symptoms, characteristics of the ego, and delusions*. In the last of these we may find their "seed" of truth, which sometimes enables us to propose an attempt to understand their meaning. This resource may be utilized during a treatment (recalling all the limitations of treatments of patients with narcissistic psychoses*; cf. psychoanalytic technique*) at certain moments when positive transference* is established with the patient's neurotic aspects; these truths help the subject to understand psychotic moments and dispense with delusions or hallucinations* for the reconstruction of the object world. This reconstruction re-converts unconscious thing-presentations. These patients are those most exposed to repetition of the traumatic event in their personal history, an event involving a huge quantity of automatic anxiety* when the ego was unable to generate more sophisticated anxiety signals.

Freud also applies the concept of historical-experiential truth, not to reveal it in a patient but for a historical-social reconstruction in *Moses and Monotheism: Three Essays* (1939). He was discussing the difference between religious illusion* and the existence of one god, based according to his hypothesis on the truth of the existence of the father of the primal horde*, considered omnipotent by its members; the one god referred to that father in humanity's prehistory.

TURNING ROUND UPON THE SUBJECT'S OWN SELF

Ger.: Wendung gegen die eigene Person. – Sp.: vuelta contra la persona propia. – Fr.: retournement sur la personne propre. – It.: riflessione sulla propria persona. – Port.: volta contra si mesmo.

This is one of the vicissitudes of sexual Trieb* previous to establishment of oedipal primal repression* or anticathexis*. The object of Trieb changes its path whereas the aim remains unchanged.

The object, by definition, returns to the subject without changing the characteristic of the Trieb aim*, which continues to be active.

It is intimately connected with "reversal into the opposite"*. It is even another way to explain or to focus on these Trieb vicissitudes from a different perspective.

First, Freud describes masochism* as sadism* turning round upon the subject's own self, one of its vicissitudes: "the masochist shares in the enjoyment of the assault upon himself, and … the exhibitionist shares in the enjoyment of [the sight of] his exposure" (*Instincts and Their Vicissitudes*, 1915, p. 127).

The same phenomenon as the one explaining the notion of reversal into the opposite is investigated from the perspective of opposition between ego and not-ego.

In reversal into the opposite, the perspective was placed on the notion of the Trieb aim which was active and became passive. Although the result is the same, they are two different perspectives of the metapsychological explanation which address different theoretical problems.

Turning round upon the subject's own self occurs with the murderous portion of the Oedipus complex* in the case of phobia*, for example Little Hans's, in which hostility was displaced from the father on to horses, after which hostility from horses was feared.

TYPICAL DREAMS

Ger.: typische Träume. – Sp.: sueños típicos. – Fr.: rêves typiques. – It.: sogni tipici. – Port.: sonhos típicos.

Freud gives this term to certain dreams* which almost all human beings have had in the same way, and which we tend to assume also have the same meaning. It may be thought, considering their universality, that they spring from the same sources in all individuals.

Freud conceptualized typical dreams before he described universal symbols* with which they are closely related, and which he added after *The Interpretation of Dreams* (1900) when he continued to discuss them in his *Introductory Lectures on Psycho-Analysis* (1916–17), and further explained his hypothesis on the origins of universal symbolism in *Moses and Monotheism: Three Essays* (1939).

> If we attempt to interpret a typical dream, the dreamer fails as a rule to produce the associations which would in other cases have led us to understand it, or else his associations become obscure and insufficient so that we cannot solve our problem with their help.
> (*The Interpretation of Dreams*, 1900, p. 241)

They are usually anxiety dreams* in which an ambivalent wish* is partly expressed, causing sensations found to be universal in human beings and symbolic in general (dreams of falling as falling into temptation, or of flying as a symbol of erection, and so on). The most typical are dreams of embarrassment at one's own nudity, the death of loved ones, flying, falling, vertigo, the examination dream, and others).

U

UNCANNY, THE

Ger.: Unheimlich. – Sp.: lo siniestro (ominoso). – Fr.: sinistre (inquiétant). – It.: sinistro (perturbante). – Port.: sinistro (ominoso).

Uncanny situations, personal or not, are sometimes produced in the subject. An uncanny feeling is a special type of anxious sensation whose qualitative characteristics are in the order of terror and horror; it is produced in some typical situations experienced either because of phantasies of them or deriving from them.

Psychoanalysis attributes the origin of this type of unpleasurable affect* to these particular representations, qualitatively different, whose specific characteristics transform them into a special aesthetic phenomenon in a manner opposite to that of humour* which utilizes pleasurable affects.

The uncanny is described in diverse ways: it is something familiar which becomes terrifying, something inanimate that becomes something animate; for example, an automaton or a doll that suddenly springs to life; it may be an unexpected encounter with a deceased person or someone identical to that person. Another situation that provokes the sensation of the uncanny is the presence of the "double",

> which appears in every shape and degree of development: figures considered identical because they look alike. This relation is accentuated when mental processes leap from one of these figures to another – by what we could call telepathy –, so that one possesses the same knowledge, feelings, and experience as the other. Or it is when the subject identifies himself with someone else, generating a doubt as to which self he or she is, or substitutes the extraneous self for his or her own. In other words, it involves a doubling, dividing, or exchanging of the self. And finally, it is a constant recurrence of the same thing – the repetition of the same features or character traits or vicissitudes, of the same crimes, or even the same names through several consecutive generations.
>
> (*The Uncanny*, 1919, p. 234)

It is also a special type of castration* anxiety (the representation of being deprived of one's eyes in the story by E. Hoffmann, *The Sand-Man*).

Other factors associated with the area of the uncanny are: animism*, magic* and enchantment, omnipotence of thought*, all of which give hyper-cathected psychical activity priority over the facts of reality*.

Therefore, we have a special unpleasurable affect whose quality is unpleasure* but with a specific quality (terror or horror); that is to say, the perceptual quality* of the unpleasurable affect has a meaning; other ingredients are the perceptual quality of whatever is being experienced and the representational quality of preconscious presentations* (representatives of unconscious thing-presentations*in consciousness) to which they refer, the greatest generators of this affect.

It is even produced sometimes almost solely by preconscious presentations in the order of mixed phantasies* or daydreams*, or by fancied interpretations of reality, or by inexplicable facts, or by all of these, intermingled in diverse ways.

The central affect is anxiety*, the specificity of this type of anxiety produced by the special type of relation between presentations resulting in this complexity and sophistication of anxiety and of its cause by which the feeling of the uncanny is generated.

Preconscious presentations represent unconscious id* thing-presentations* to consciousness; these thing-presentations include those of repressed infantile sexuality*. All the presentations from which the feeling of the uncanny originates refer to this sexuality.

The impression of the familiar that has become terrifying is the mark of infantile sexual trauma (the protagonists, both of the primal scene* and of seduction*, are the parents or their representatives). The traumatic event tends to be attributed to familiar persons. This appears so frequently in memories "forgotten" by his patients that Freud sometimes denies their existence.

The perception of the primal scene and all its accessory elements may be uncanny to the infantile mind. For example, in boys, the idealized father figure with whom he identified primarily was extremely familiar in the period when he even wanted to be like him. However, during the Oedipus complex* he is terrifying.

Identification* and the fact that the ego* is formed mainly through it lends much strength to the figure of the double, apart from the narcissism* involved, in the formation of situations felt to be uncanny. In the period of primary narcissism, during the "reign" of the pure pleasure ego*, the object *was* the ego and the ego *was* the object, to the extent that it produced pleasure. If this situation reappears in adult life and is utilized for return of the repressed*, it may acquire uncanny attributes.

The same may occur in relation to the mother or a sister (prototypes of familiar objects) for a boy who is beginning to discover sexual difference and encounters the female genital (a terrifying organ for him in the throes of the Oedipus complex), which he understands (cf. Understanding*) as a lack of the male organ.

Animism, magic, and omnipotence of thought* are typical of infantile thought, which includes the phantasy that an inanimate being may spring to life; this is similar to disavowal* of the death of a loved one in particular and as an abstraction in general.

The thought of one's own death is an idea that the preconscious works through gradually through language* acquisition and the ability to think about the ego in time and space, and therefore possessing finitude and fear of it, which in the unconscious is registered as castration* anxiety* or a sense of guilt* before the superego*.

The feeling of the uncanny arises from an imperfectly defined assemblage, mainly qualitative (its connection with castration* anxiety, anxiety signal*, and situation of danger* relates it more closely to the representational than to the quantitative aspect of any affect: with its mnemic symbol*), of all those situations of infantile sexuality. In the adult, the feeling of the uncanny arises from this complex assemblage of all these situations proceeding from the unconscious and their connection with facts of reality. This of course includes the repetition compulsion* characteristic of all Triebe*, but which practically defines death Trieb*, which is thereby able to fuse with Eros.

UNCONSCIOUS

Ger.: Das Unbewußte. – Sp.: inconciente. – Fr.: inconscient. – It.: inconscio. – Port.: inconsciente.

The unconscious is one of Freud's crucial discoveries, perhaps the most important. Although it is a concept mentioned in philosophy, it had never been conceptualized with Freud's scientific precision. We could say that it gave birth to metapsychology, a field of psychology that includes the unconscious within its conception of psychical phenomena, and a theoretical branch of psychoanalysis.

Unconscious has several meanings. As a noun, it is a place in the psychical apparatus described by Freud in his first topic, a place nearly limited at that theoretical moment to repressed wishes* and the hereditary, ruled by primary process* and the pleasure principle*. The second topic, rather than replacing the first, makes it more complex. In our view, it adds new levels to the former; the previous levels do not disappear; all to the contrary, they are enriched by the new ones, and phenomena not included in the first topic (such as concepts of the ego*, conscience*, superego*, and sense of guilt) become explainable.

With the complexities Freud added in the second topic, we may partly think of the unconscious as a simple attribute of the new psychical structures (and we do, partly), but we may also preserve its characteristic as a noun. Thus, it has its own mechanisms, forms of functioning, and its own laws (primary process ruled by the pleasure principle, mechanisms of condensation* and displacement* of libido* among thing-presentations* in order to reach perceptual identity* rapidly). In this line of thought, the second topic of the psychical apparatus adds to the concept of unconscious: Triebe* of the id* (all of the id), ego defence mechanisms* or the ego's unconscious part, and the unconscious part of the superego. Thus the theory progresses from an unconscious with not only Triebe and libidinal wishes (including fusions* and defusions* with death Trieb*, but also part of the structures defending against them.

Historically, Freud's first approximations to the concept of unconscious are the "separate psychical groups"* (separated from its relation to or from belonging to conscious thought*), the origin of neurotic symptoms*, which could be brought to consciousness* (or put into words) by hypnosis. Later, "irreconcilable presentations" are the second conceptual step towards what would eventually be the repressed unconscious. Conceptualization, therefore, developed gradually as a theoretical need to ground curative action on neurotic symptoms, and from there, psychoanalysis was born as a new science of the psyche, a "new psychology". As always in Freud, theory grew out of practice, the latter grounding the former, in some cases opening new roads.

The unconscious is populated by thing-presentations; when they reach a certain level of cathexis*, they become wishes. Thing-presentations are able, at the beginning of life, to access consciousness directly through reproductive thought which enables the ego to notice differences between wishes and perceptions* (secondary process), and also through hallucinatory wish* fulfilment (primary process). Reproductive thought thereby enables some recognition of the difference between a memory* now desired and a perception belonging to reality* (the baby distinguishes its mother from strangers), a level of ego functioning that inhibits hallucination, differentiated from another previous type and from which it defends itself in order to avoid frustration*; the latter (the first in logical time) consists of hallucinatory wish fulfilment, and gives credit to hallucinations* of wishes, thereby drawing away from reality testing* and from reality itself. Shortly afterwards, the language* of words is learned, with which a fundamental qualitative leap enables thinking not only in images but also, through words, to represent thing-presentations and relations among them before consciousness. This type of relation among presentations* is then called thought* in the strict sense. This is a preparation for the ego to enter into action, allows it to know reality and its attributes better, and even to think about itself. The ego may be an object of thought starting with the existence of language with words since the moment it can name itself and take it as an object (narcissism*).

Practically starting with language acquisition, thinking (a fact of the preconscious ego and consciousness) is done with words. In order to make a wish conscious, therefore, the wish needs a word-presentation* to represent it before consciousness.

However, there are no words in the unconscious (which does not mean that they do not exist), and thing-presentations belonging to the unconscious need to obtain them in order to reach consciousness. Secondary repression takes advantage of this state of things by decathecting (cf. Decathexis*) word-presentations representing thing-presentations to keep them from accessing consciousness.

We shall see exactly how this takes place.

Beginning with the establishment of primary repression* of infantile sexuality* and secondary repression of its derivatives, "prehistorical" thing-presentations are kept outside the limits of the ego. Hence, access of unconscious thing-presentations to the preconscious ego in their "crude" form is made more complex until it becomes more and more impossible.

Then the need of a representative to access the preconscious increases. It is the word-presentation, which inaugurates what has been called the "symbolic order".

After the Oedipus complex*, the cathexis of the word-presentation (of incest and parricide or rather its derivatives) is the main target of attacks by secondary repression, at least the repression by the unconscious ego by trying to withdraw from it its cathexis and thereby to impede access of Triebe of infantile sexuality to the preconscious ego, which are also mixed with destructive and antisocial Triebe.

The suppression* of Trieb achieved in this way enables the structuring of a psychical apparatus less harassed by Triebe, which it is thereby able to hold at bay almost without realizing it, although not without cost, and of course not without consequences, some of these more or less severe.

The unconscious is therefore a star figure in the psychical apparatus, although by definition it is not recognized by the subject as participating in the official cast.

The concept of unconscious seems to lose vigour with the new territorial division: id/ego/superego. Now it seems to be a quality, an adjective: unconscious ego, unconscious superego. This is partly true, but only if we consider the second Freudian topic a correction that invalidates the first topic rather than a further complexity that includes it. If we view it in the latter way, the concept of unconscious does not lose its substantiality. If we also consider it a structure, a complexity of them, their ranks grow, since other structures, substructures forming part of the central structure, the unconscious, enter the unconscious condition. In fact, as we said, the unconscious has grown.

If we write unconscious with its abbreviation Ucs., we do so with the intention of underscoring its structural characteristics, with its own laws such as that of atemporality, condensation* and displacement*, perceptual identity seeking, all belonging to the pleasure principle and ruled by primary process; which in this line of reasoning rule important parts of the ego and superego besides the id.

The presentations of things are traces left in the psychical apparatus by experiences with them, mainly with objects*. For this reason, they are generally object presentations or refer to experiences with objects, since what is important happened with them, which is what makes them important. Thing-presentations are also unconscious (not absolutely: the reproductive thought mentioned above under this term to a certain extent contradicts the following reasoning).

Consciousness is an apparatus perceptor of qualities; if memory traces* now become presentations are to be registered by consciousness, they must be perceived as such.

Words also came into being in this way, followed by language. Words, representing the presentations of things before consciousness, gave birth to a different and specifically human universe, when consciousness was able, through them, to perceive its wish-presentations cathected and related among themselves in order to carry them to a good end through action, following reality testing.

Therefore, we conclude that memory traces or presentations of objects are in themselves unconscious. In order to access consciousness in a psychical apparatus that never stops growing more complex, they need more and more words, as well as a different type of hypercathexis* such as that of attention*.

Consciousness perceives words and their interrelations, their attributes, through other words. These words are also perceptions and leave a trace, becoming word-presentations, memories of sounds with meaning and therefore signifiers. We refer to the word-presentations when we speak of conscious memory, since they are the ones that, in their most complex and elevated form – and at this moment of cultural evolution, nearly unique – may be best registered by consciousness.

We therefore have representations of things, of experiences with them and word-presentations; the latter represent or signify or symbolize the thing-presentations before consciousness. They also connect them and connect among themselves through complex combinations.

In evolution, the different periods have left traces in the psychical apparatus. These traces become identifications* (the origin of the ego) and presentations (of wishes of objects). Anticathexes* also form, generating fixations* (primary repressions) when stimuli become too intense (traumatic), really or relatively, given the immaturity of the psychical apparatus. This sometimes occurs during passages of predominance from one erotogenic zone* to another. For example, weaning may become traumatic (more so if a sibling has been born) and may create oral fixation points.

All this produces changes in Triebe and their vicissitudes. For example, concerning the way of satisfying themselves, they may go from active to passive aims. Or satisfaction may be thwarted. The main obstacle impeding satisfaction results from a change of affect generated by the anticathexis whose paradigm is reaction formation*, which turns what was pleasurable into something disgusting, shameful or immoral. Since the mastery of the muscular apparatus is also greater, it is utilized in order to dominate the former to avoid suffering fear of object loss which starts to become manifest. In the meantime, the first games begin, a magical and symbolic expression of control of the object; what is most important is the appearance of spoken language by virtue of word-presentations learned in the link with the mother.

Very soon afterwards, in the phallic phase, the Oedipus complex develops. In its course, the previous anticathexes are consolidated, acquiring a tone connected with oedipal problems. New fixations appear and the former ones are reinforced in the erotogenic zones and object presentations corresponding to their histories in the link with objects, experienced through them. Thus, primary repression is finally established and split off from the psychical apparatus into an unconscious and a preconscious-conscious that gradually separates increasingly (especially the unconscious from the preconscious).

Incestuous and parricidal presentations* of the Oedipus complex are "dissolved" in the unconscious, and they appear in the preconscious (at least cathected as wishes) through their derivatives, sometimes an origin of sublimations* and other times of return of the repressed*, a cause of neurotic symptoms, dreams*, parapraxes*, or jokes*.

Following the "dissolution" of the Oedipus complex, the psychical apparatus consolidates its constitution and therefore the repressed unconscious as well; from this moment on, later repressions are secondary, reinforcements of the basic primary repressions.

The major function of secondary repression is to impede access of object wish presentations of infantile sexuality (which are now incestuous) to consciousness, so that they may not in turn come to actions.

The cathexis is removed from the word-presentation, a cathexis displaced on to another word-presentation or to the presentation of a bodily innervation, or to some other, and new anticathexes are put into place to impede progress toward words. These anticathexes may be composed of the same words or innervation to which the cathexis was displaced (substitute formations*) or may establish themselves in perception (the hysteric does not see the sexual but "scotomizes" it). "Tertiary" defences* such as obsessional ceremonials* or phobic ramparts* are also formed.

This anticathexis of secondary repression is expressed clinically as ego resistance to the progress of the analysis, a constant and sometimes very sophisticated obstaculization.

Primary repression cooperates with secondary repression (with which it forms part of its mechanism) by attracting derivatives like a magnet from the unconscious. The unconscious archetypes do the same, which tend to be repeated and to become clinical resistances* to the cure, resistances therefore coming from the unconscious itself.

Products of secondary repression, presentations whose access to words was removed are added to the unconscious where they are part of the repressed unconscious. This is what is behind neurotic symptoms, dreams, parapraxes, and so on.

When Freud escribes his second topic or structural theory, with the id, the ego, and the superego, the unconscious remains in the id; we could say that its name changes, although the ego and the superego, also having unconscious parts, make everything more complex. The id, in turn, which in itself is unconscious, now contains the repressed unconscious but also the primal phantasies* originating in phylogeny, universal symbols*, also phylogenetic, and the thing-presentations of ontogeny, previous to words. We said that part of the superego-ego ideal is also unconscious, which comes from phylogeny, from infantile narcissism and from secondary identifications* with paternal images causing the unconscious sense of guilt* or need for punishment*.

The unconscious (composed of thing-presentations of the id, of ego defence mechanisms, and of the unconscious part of the superego, apart from the phylogenetic) possesses its own laws. The interrelations among thing-presentations are subject to primary process. Libidinal energy passes freely among them. Therefore the unconscious works with free energy* or at least with an extremely loose level of binding. Thing-presentations are not univocal but may be condensed, being identified by their attributes.

That is to say, we have a system that works with condensation and displacement that is also ruled by the pleasure principle, which therefore utilizes perceptual identity by virtue of which the discharge* is effected in response simply to reactivation of the level of stimulus in the nucleus coming from the Trieb source, with no regard for reality* and the consequent frustration*.

Frustration is clearer in relation to self-preservative Triebe*. However, the sexual Triebe* – some of which are supported by the former – are more independent of reality, since at least in principle they may be satisfied autoerotically and, in this sense, are less frustratable.

In this system, there is no "perhaps", there is no room for doubt in it; there is no notion of time, nor a before nor an after, everything is present. Neither is there negation*; there is no "no", and therefore there are no contradictions in it: one and its opposite are the same thing, and their identity is rapidly found. It would be interesting to find these laws and characteristics functioning in the ego and the superego. This is not so difficult to conceive of if we think of all the unconscious phenomena, some studied in depth and other studied by Freud after 1920, such as resistances to the cure, masochism*, the negative therapeutic reaction, the unconscious sense of guilt, the repetition compulsion*, punitory dreams and many others.

UNCONSCIOUS FEELINGS

Ger.: Unbewusste Affekte / Gefühle / Empfidungen. – Sp.: sentimientos inconscientes. – Fr.: sentiments inconscients. – It.: sentimenti inconsci. – Port.: sentimentos inconscientes.

By definition, feelings are "felt", perceived by the perceptual apparatus, which is consciousness or preconscious. They are conscious. Therefore, it is paradoxical and even contradictory to refer to unconscious feelings. However, the paradox is not an error: it indicates the limits of theoretical discourse, of conscious discourse.

Feelings, emotions, and affects* are usually considered synonyms. It is what the perceptual-conscious system perceives: perceptive qualities it receives regarding the inside of the body, apart from those corresponding to perceptions* of the world outside the body.

In Freudian metapsychology, these feelings have a basically economic explanation. They are a first level of discharge of quantity of excitation* that enters the psychical apparatus from the body, as we said.

They may also participate in the main level of discharge of excitation produced when specific action* is carried out. Then, they are pleasurable. In the former cases they function as a safety valve when there is an increase of excitation, and are therefore qualified by the preconscious as unpleasurable.

Some "feelings" (anxiety signals*) need no economic explanation because they are in reality danger signals, memories of traumatic events, re-created by the ego* in order to prevent them by automatically and unconsciously applying ego defence mechanisms.

A further complication is that anxiety* (perhaps the prototypical affect), for example, is considered by Freud to have a bodily component (tachycardia, excessive sweating, and other signs) and the perception of this type of discharge, in addition to the unpleasurable feeling of anxiety.

In his clinical description of anxiety neurosis*, he presents the differences between attacks of anxiety. He refers to one of these as "equivalents of anxiety"; in these episodes, only the bodily component of the clinical picture is manifested, without the typical feeling that characterizes anxiety as an affect and sometimes prevents the subject from becoming aware of this anxiety. In these cases, is the feeling conscious or unconscious? If it were unconscious, by what hypothetical mechanism does it originate? Or is it simply a bodily reaction?

Defence mechanisms*, or repression* in the broad sense, act on presentations*. The latter may generate feelings; the ego defends itself from them if they are unpleasurable, and therefore represses some presentations.

At the outset of some neuroses such as obsessional neurosis* and anxiety hysteria*, this objective is not reached, and other mechanisms are needed to achieve some kind of affective stability. Also, more or less traumatic events of "actual" life may cause affects, one of which is anxiety.

A specialization of this anxiety (preparedness anxiety*) is one of the levels of protection against stimulus, by which presentations more or less traumatizing in reality* may be bound and included in secondary process* and thought* activity, which enlarges the ego's experience. If it is overloaded or if the protective shield was absent at the moment of the experience, it becomes a traumatic situation*.

Perhaps the best known of these paradoxical unconscious feelings is guilt*: the analyst does not find it in the patients' discourse but infers it from their behaviour. If they live in a state of constant suffering generated by attitudes of obvious self-punishment* and do everything possible to avoid escaping it, in spite of doors that opening make it possible, it is because there is an internal "need for punishment" that is relieved by expiation of guilt. Since this guilt is unknown to consciousness and the preconscious ego, it is inferred to be unconscious.

All these facts add complexity to the concept of unconscious feeling, which refers to quantity of excitation cathecting presentations, which as thing-presentations* remain forever cathected in the unconscious* (except in narcissistic affections). When this cathexis* increases beyond a certain *quantum*, it is registered by the perceptual-conscious system as unpleasure*.

The cathected thing-presentation (the unconscious wish*) needs to find a word-presentation* in the ego's preconscious. For this purpose, it must overcome several barriers, one of them unconscious (ego defence mechanisms or repression in response to anxiety signals), the most unmanageable for the ego's preconscious.

If it obtains a word-presentation it may enter thought activity, be compared with reality*, and even judged. In the last case in which all the parts of the psychical apparatus agree (when there are contradiction in the ego it may undergo splitting), it may reach action, and discharge of the energy cathexis that was cathecting presentations may become a pleasurable feeling. This complex path includes detours, shortcuts and so on, even different kinds of obstacles. The feeling may be suppressed* in various ways. If it is suppressed consciously, the feeling is known – we could say even felt – in an attenuated way, as sometimes occurs in mourning* or at moments in mourning when thought activity is temporarily able to dominate affective expression.

If it is suppressed unconsciously, repression is indirect. The original presentation is suppressed. Any unconscious thing-presentation that remains cathected may potentially generate affect. These are the formations of affect* described by Freud in *The Unconscious* (1915).

However, the affect is still somewhat independent of the presentation, as soon as it is perceived as such by the perceptual-conscious system, when it acquires a certain magnitude and does not need, as thought* activity does, the preconscious presentation in order to reach it. In actual neuroses*, anxiety, especially the equivalents of anxiety, may also be a particular form of expression of affect or may establish mixed neuroses in which the above described mechanisms also intervene.

In narcissistic pathology, especially schizophrenia*, a dulling of affect is produced, probably by decathexis* of the unconscious thing-presentation where the object wish is born, and subsequent passage of libidinal cathexis to the ego in order to stanch narcissism. Therefore, little or no feeling appears because the deepest wish for the object (the unconscious wish) has been lost. Libido* is almost entirely occupied with providing for the narcissistic refuge by hyper-cathecting the wounded ego. The subject is seemingly indifferent, as if devoid of feelings. Then they cannot manage to form unconscious "formations of affect", since object wishes are simply not cathected (although they may also "resuscitate" when they are given blood to drink", like the ghosts in *The Odyssey*).

UNDERSTANDING

Ger.: Verständnis. – Sp.: comprensión. – Fr.: compréhension. – It.: comprenzione. – Port.: comprensão.

This human activity in relation to fellow human beings encompasses affects and thought: by virtue of understanding, a person understands what is occurring to another person by "putting him or herself in the other's place", feeling what the other feels or doing what the other does, by means of a body cathexis* of the subject's own (all this in a manner mitigated and controlled by the ego*).

It is part of the complex of the fellow human being* by which babies understand their mother by imitating her actions (the mother in turn understands* her baby's helplessness by virtue of the baby's screaming). If the mother moves her hand, the baby understands what this means by moving his or her own hand; if she weeps, the baby understands by weeping, and if she laughs, by laughing. From then on, it is one of the forms of human learning.

It therefore corresponds to secondary process*, to thought activity*, by which the other person's attributes become ego attributes. In this form of thought we observe "the imitation-value of a perception" (*Project for a Scientific Psychology*, 1895–1950, p. 333). Although it is an unconscious mechanism, it is intimately related to identification* (even to direct primary identification* since the baby repeats what the mother does without necessarily considering her an object* separate from the ego). Understanding involves not only the intellectual but also feelings (identification is also the first type of love) and curiosity inherent to infantile sexual Trieb*. It is precisely infantile sexual curiosity that allows the baby to discover sexual difference as he or she nears the phallic phase. Then, children understand primal scenes* between their parents and the trauma they suffered from them, and also other traumatic moments in relation to sex suffered both previously and afterwards. They understand them in a deferred manner since they are now able to feel them bodily.

When boys discover the female genital wished for by object libido*, they cannot easily understand it; they cannot put themselves in its place since this requires their narcissism to accept the possibility of loss of their penis: nothing less than the loss of the seat of all the pleasurable feelings that lent unity to their ego.

Infantile curiosity then succumbs to repression*. In this way the latency period is generated, remaining triumphant until puberty, when the "file" is re-opened. By virtue of the new burst of object libido, the boy is gradually able to be close to women and to understand them as beings with genitals different from his own: an active process carried out by the preconscious ego with thought activity and reality testing*. Boys must overcome infantile fears of castration, repressed and therefore able to return and again become effective.

Understanding is utilized by adults (we already mentioned the baby's mother) although in this case the requirement of action for understanding is mitigated. Adults call up memories* in images and connect their attributes by applying the symbolic universe of words or their presentations: in sum, they think. However, this thinking includes affect* (expression of emotions). Understanding is therefore not simply intellectual understanding. It means putting oneself in the other's place; it is not indifferent, but instead moving, and the subject's own body participates heavily (its actions and reactions) in it. In Freud's words, "seeks it with a psychical cathexis of one's own (an experience of one's own)" (Ibid., p. 332).

UNDOING (WHAT HAS BEEN DONE)

Ger.: Ungeschehenmachen. – Sp.: anulación de lo acontecido – Fr.: annulation rétroactive. – It.: rendere non accaduto o annullamento retroattivo. – Port.: anulação do acontecido.

In this defence mechanism* or form of secondary repression, magical thought* is utilized in order to make something that has happened "disappear", this usually being something the subject did or fancied having done.

Undoing what has been done is an unconscious* ego mechanism typical of obsessional neurosis*; it usually produces "symptoms in two acts" in which the second cancels the first with the odd idea that by doing so it will disappear and everything will then be as if nothing had happened. It also generates obsessional ceremonials*. Both acts are compulsive, even though the subject's ego* attempts to explain them with rationalizations.

The thing-presentation* of the id* Trieb* prohibited by the superego* receives preconscious* word cathexis* (not the original one but cathexis that was displaced from it and disguised) despite the fact that it was never accepted by the ego as its own.

Therefore we have a presentation of a preconscious wish*not accepted by the ego as its own but which imposes itself on it as a compulsive thought; this may even lead to compulsive action (cf. compulsion*). This is the compromise the ego strikes with Trieb* when it receives an anxiety signal* in response to the superego. In order to justify itself to the latter, it must carry out the second act which is the undoing; by utilizing magic*, the ego makes the action or the actionless fantasy "disappear" as if nothing had happened.

Undoing what has been done is the origin of many symptoms of obsessional neurosis: (a) two-step symptoms: dirtying and washing hands, opening and shutting the gas valve, the "Rat Man's" famous removing and replacing of the stone, and (b) one step symptoms in which one step involves action whereas the "first" remains in phantasy. This last case is the basis of many obsessional ceremonials.

The two-step symptom is an expression in turn of affective ambivalence*, the expression of love*-hate* at two different moments.

This technique also has a salient role in enchantment practices in the myths* of peoples and in religious ceremonies, since it springs from the primitive animistic attitude towards the surrounding world.

We can say that undoing has relatively little success in repressing Trieb which, especially in two-step symptoms, may be carried into action in a more or less symbolized form, even though it is later undone. It also tends to need to extend itself in the manner of the phobic rampart*.

During all this lapse of time, until undoing is successful, anxiety* is present.

UNIVERSAL SYMBOLS

Ger.: Universalsymbol. – Sp.: símbolos universales. – Fr.: symboles universels. – It.: simboli universali. – Port.: símbolos universais.

These forms inherited from the experience of our species gives us the possibility to substitute or replace one thing-presentation* for another after language* acquisition but separate from it (in humanity and in individual experience), belonging to the unconscious*.

Universal symbolism is a way to replace one thing with another (which symbolizes it) that is more primitive, more archaic than the symbolic created by the language of words. It is part of the id's* phylogenetic heritage. It is universal, not related to different languages but rather previous to them.

> It is a question of an original knowledge which adults afterwards forget … Moreover, symbolism disregards differences of language … Here, then, we seem to have an assured instance of an archaic heritage dating from the period at which language developed … It might be said that we are dealing with thought connections between ideas – connections which had been established during the historical development of speech and which have to be repeated now every time the development of speech has to be gone through in an individual. It would thus be a case of the inheritance of an intellectual disposition similar to the ordinary inheritance of an instinctual disposition.
>
> (*Moses and Monotheism: Three Essays*, 1939, pp. 98–9)

Universal symbolism was studied first by the philosopher K. Scherner, although incompletely, since he accounted only for symbols of the body. Freud took up what he had presented and extended it to other meanings which he observed, especially in his studies on dreams* and also in myths*, symptoms*, jokes*, and in everyday life.

They are formed as a result of a comparison centred on a relation of analogy*, mainly formal, between one visual image and another. This mechanism is unknown to secondary process* and its word-presentations*: the preconscious ego and therefore the ego* does not understand it. The mechanism of dreams takes advantage of this situation and sometimes utilizes it to represent images proceeding from a presentation* of fulfilment of unconscious wishes*. Universal symbols do not usually generate the dreamer's associations since they are not a part of the day's residues*; in this sense they are "mute", since they are more related to experiences of the species than to the individual's, although they may include them partly, since they extend and broaden along with changes in humanity, new symbols appearing, always governed by the same mechanisms. The individual may also have had individual experiences with things that unconsciously symbolize something universal and may then associate with these experiences. In any case, it subtracts nothing from the valuable concept Freud describes.

"A constant relation of this kind between a dream-element and its translation is described by us as a 'symbolic' one, and the dream-element itself as a 'symbol' of the unconscious dream-thought" (*Introductory Lectures on Psychoanalysis*, 1916, p. 150).

The variety of things figured symbolically in dreams is not large: the human body as a whole, the subject's parents or children, siblings, birth, nudity, female or male genitals, and so on.

The human body is represented by the house, especially the female body. The parents by the king, queen, or other important persons: the dreamer's children or siblings by small animals or vermin; birth by water, or getting into or out of it. Dying is symbolized by leaving or travelling; male genitals by an umbrella, knife, revolver, or anything predominantly convex in form. Female genitals, however, are represented by containing or concave objects, and also by those used for entering or leaving such as doors and windows, sometimes by a chapel. An airplane's take-off symbolizes an erection.

> The very great majority of symbols in dreams are sexual symbols … The topics I have mentioned are few, but the symbols for them are extremely numerous, so that each of these things can be expressed by numbers of almost equivalent symbols.
>
> (Ibid., p. 153)

> [W]e are faced by the fact that the dreamer has a symbolic mode of expression at his disposal which he does not know in waking life and does not recognize … We can only say that the knowledge of symbolism is unconscious to the dreamer, that it belongs to his unconscious mental life … Now, however, it is a question of more than this, of unconscious pieces of knowledge, of connections of thought, of comparisons between different objects which result in its being possible for one of them to be regularly put in place of the other. These comparisons are not freshly made on each occasion; they lie

ready to hand and are complete, once and for all. This is implied by the fact of their agreeing in the case of different individuals – possibly, indeed, agreeing in spite of differences of language.

(Ibid, p. 165)

We also find universal symbols in myths and traditional tales, popular sayings, and folk songs, also in current linguistic uses and poetic phantasy; in these cases it is mistaken for allusion, and therefore also for the figure of the metaphor whose meaning is usually known by the preconscious. They also intervene in the formation of paranoid delusions* as in the "Schreber" case.

Although this concept is interesting for theoretical conception and discussions it may generate in the development of linguistics as a science, its importance in psychoanalytic practice is relative; however, its study is important.

Symbols are utilized as a complement to dream analysis when the dreamer's associations are exhausted; their universal meaning is integrated with global interpretations of the dream centring mainly on associations, but only experimentally, and actually with less certainty, than the results of "associative interpretation" based on the patient's associations. In any case, it is sometimes useful, besides the interesting study of its origin, especially on account of its relation to language.

UNPLEASURE

Ger.: Unlust. – Sp.: displacer. – Fr.: déplaisir. – It.: dispiacere. – Port.: desprazer.

This disagreeable sensation is perceived in the perceptual-conscious system (Pcpt.-Cs) when quantity of excitation* increases. The time lapse in which this increase occurs is important: the shorter it is, the greater the unpleasure. Rhythm is also important. Of course, some increases of excitation are pleasurable, for example, of sexual excitation. This probably relates to small discharges being produced through each erotogenic zone* (fore-pleasure*) and to pursuit of the reward of final pleasure.

Unpleasure generates the tendency to escape from it. Unpleasure may be experienced in different ways. The most common way, on which all the others are hinged, is anxiety*. Anxiety is generated by an increase in quantity of excitation, except that which the ego* utilizes as the anxiety signal in order to marshal defence mechanisms* against Triebe* to avoid automatic anxiety*, a previous anxiety and unpleasure *par excellence* due to its increase of quantity of excitation.

Another unpleasurable sensation is physical pain, caused by an accumulation of excitation in the psychical apparatus due to an alteration in the protective shield*. In psychical pain or mourning, the cathexis of longing* is hypercathected in response to each evidence of object loss in reality*, giving rise to this painful sensation each time reality demonstrates that its satisfaction is impossible. What can we say about masochism? Apparently, especially in moral masochism and the negative therapeutic reaction that tends to accompany it, provoked by the sadism of the unconscious superego* and the ego's masochism, the psychical apparatus is seeking unpleasure: punishment to satisfy or expiate guilt* through suffering, especially the suffering produced by psychical illness, but also by psychosomatic affections and even by a certain propensity to accidents.

All these forms present the greatest and most complex resistances* to the cure.

In general, the rules of functioning of psychical apparatus obey the pleasure principle*; that is to say, pursuit of pleasure and escape from unpleasure; however, something beyond this attracts it towards the inorganic, thereby opposing the previous principle, and consequently generated by death Trieb*; as a result of this opposition produced in the form of Trieb fusion and defusion* the subject is led to seek unpleasure, repeating situations that guide the subject compulsively and even diabolically in that direction.

V

VERTIGO

Ger.: Schwindel. – Sp.: vértigo. – Fr.: vertige. – It.: vertigine. – Port.: vertigem.

This is a special type of anxiety* or phobia* of falling from heights or abnormal fear that this might happen to another person.

This symptom* results from a transformation of the affect* originated by anticathexes* repressing infantile pleasures produced by stimulation of the ear's vestibular apparatus, such as those caused by the parents' game of throwing the baby into the air, the pleasure of rocking or swinging, climbing trees, and other pleasures. It may be part of anxiety hysterias* and the origin of phobias or inhibitions* of the ego* which more or less restrict the subject's activity.

Vertigo may also indicate masochistic tendencies of feminine-type masochism* (in men and women) including unconscious suicidal tendencies that produce the ego's anxiety (castration anxiety*; the suicidal phantasy* may substitute homosexual wishes* involving castration anxiety); when the ego feels anxiety it creates the phobia to defend itself from it, predictably gaining the meagre success of all phobias but which is concealed by the ego's inhibition* to access heights, for example.

VIOLENCE

Ger.: Gewaltsamkeit. – Sp.: violencia. – Fr.: violence. – It.: violenza. – Port.: violência.

An attempt to define a concept such as violence metapsychologically may be quite difficult, although we all know what we mean when we mention it. We could mention that it is a characteristic of certain human relations, of people towards nature, or of persons towards themselves, all this being related in some way.

What is this characteristic? We could refer to aggression*, cruelty, mastery*, sadism*, masochism*, debasement of fellow human beings, destruction of their dignity, and perhaps many other forms. However, none of these concepts defines violence, although they may participate in it. Degrees of violence exist in nearly all aspects of behaviour. Even love may be violent. We could in any case state that any act may acquire violent characteristics when it surpasses certain limits of intensity. This does not exclude "soft" violence; this type occurs when it proceeds from a threat, in which case it is moved into the future, issued to the object of violence, a loved one, or some other complexity of it, or it may be metaphoric, although it always involves magnitude. Its definition is therefore close to the quantitative, which implies representational weakness and the Trieb's *Drang*: the "essence" of Trieb which, when not sufficiently joined with a presentation to bind it, becomes death Trieb*. In this sense, the violent approaches the concept of the traumatic without necessarily being the same. Violence is what traumatizes, whereas the traumatic is what this violence produces.

In *Beyond the Pleasure Principle* (1920), Freud formulates a hypothesis on the origin of life, stating that in some way all living beings, human beings included, contain violence (the tendency to return to the inanimate), and therefore must deflect their death Trieb, their principle of inertia, in order for their life to continue. In men, extra violence is determined by their Oedipus complex. The struggle between the father and his son determines the struggle between men which always involves a dominator and a dominated: this is violence. Sublimation* itself generates extra violence by inhibiting the Trieb aim, thereby liberating a remnant of death Trieb. This is expressed in some cultural products (for example, war power on which power relations between nations are established) and in culture itself. Domination of nature produces an increase in population, which increases the magnitudes in conflict; violence increases disequality among people and consequently injustice as well.

All this produces spiralling violence which could exterminate our species and even the existence of life on Earth. Although Freud did not live to see the atomic bomb, his reasoning, expressed in *Civilization and its Discontents* (1930), makes it foreseeable. Is there no remedy? In spite of everything, the creator of psychoanalysis considers that culture itself and the reason it contains has the remedy; however, this reason must know and bind its Trieb origin and the history of its Trieb, rather than simply repress and ignore it, thereby becoming a caricature of reason: rationalization*. Very little room is left for caricatures.

W

WILL

Ger.: Wille. – Sp.: voluntad. – Fr.: volonté. – It.: volontà. – Port.: vontade.

Since this function derives from Triebe* in the preconscious ego*, the latter is therefore familiar with it; the preconscious ego must decide whether to carry these Triebe into action or not, how, and when.

In the Freudian hypothesis of the origin of human groups, the leader of the primal horde* monopolized the decision regarding actions to be carried out by its members. The members of the group* had no will, or had only enough to obey the leader.

The will proceeds from unconscious Trieb, especially from its pressure (*Drang*). With the acquisition of language*, it receives an addition: words to represent it before consciousness and through which the preconscious ego is able to think about it and possibly reach action. Will is therefore a conscious psychical process which at first knows nothing about unconscious wishes; if they return from the repressed*, they impose themselves on it compulsively, beyond the ego's domains. Freud's discovery of the repressed unconscious* produced a narcissistic wound in the human ego which up to then had equated psyche to will; his discovery demonstrated that a large part of psyche escapes will, which may partly be reclaimed for the realm of the subject's preconscious ego by psychoanalytic treatment.

WISH

Ger.: Wunsch (Begierde o Lust). – Sp.: deseo. – Fr.: désir. – It.: desiderio. – Port.: desejo.

In Freudian theory, a wish is a psychical proposal seeking to be gratified. This is one way to introduce the subject. Actually, no definition of wish in the theory is what we could consider very rigorous or strict, even though the whole Freudian theory is in general. However, the concept is still fairly clear and concise. Freud utilizes it more at some moments of his theoretical development than at others, but he never discards it. He utilizes it to explain some phenomena, or some of their subtleties, more than others. But he never developed a specific theory of wishes as he did for closely associated concepts such as Trieb* and libido*.

In vague terms, we could say that the concept of the wish moves more comfortably within what is called the "first topic", because in it, Freud developed his presentational theory, and the wish is, as we shall see, intimately related to cathexis* of the presentation*. However, nobody could say that in the "structural theory" Freud dropped the theme of presentation. All to the contrary, it continues to be a theme as late as *Moses and Monotheism: Three Essays* (1936).

In this text he did develop something new which we could consider to derive from the theme of presentation: the theory of identification; however, this addition simply makes the theory more complex rather than replacing it.

Whenever Freud explains something new or a new level of a problem, the theorist has no need to repeat what he has already said. Also, how do we explain dreams* if not by presentational theory? It is clear that the structures of the second topic are presentational structures. The id*, the ego* and the superego* are psychical structures, and what makes a phenomenon psychical is precisely presentation. Therefore, explicitly or implicitly, wishes are always present in Freudian theory.

It is true that sometimes, when new concepts arise, different nuances or fresh angles may appear which generate new complexities, and on this road, confusions arise and interfere. For example, it is not always easy to differentiate between wish and libido in some aspects, and especially between wish and Trieb.

The wish is born in the formative moments of the psychical apparatus following the first experiences of satisfaction*. From then on, bodily necessity arises joined to presentations left in the psychical apparatus by these experiences. Necessity has therefore achieved psychical presentation. When this presentation, originating in the memory trace* left by experience, is recathected, it becomes a wish. It is the motion aimed toward this presentation, the link established between bodily necessity and presentation. The advent of the wish inaugurates the psyche and is the motor of the psychical apparatus.

The experience of satisfaction in reality leaves a presentational complex that includes three types of presentations: (1) the one activated first when the wish is revived: the cathected presentation of the satisfying object*; (2) presentation of movements made with this object and those the object made, and (3) presentations of the feeling of discharge in the nucleus of the ego (*Project for a Scientific Psychology*, 1950). The wish is therefore a wish for the object with which the ego seeks to act; the ego also endeavours to induce the object to effect other actions.

> A change can only come about if in some way or other (in the case of the baby, through outside help) an "experience of satisfaction" can be achieved which puts an end to the internal stimulus. An essential component of this experience of satisfaction is a particular perception (that of nourishment, in our example) the mnemic image of which remains associated thenceforward with the memory trace of the excitation produced by the necessity. As a result of the link that has thus been established, next time this necessity arises a psychical impulse will at once emerge which will seek to re-cathect the mnemic image of the perception and to re-evoke the perception itself, that is to say, to re-establish the situation of the original satisfaction. An impulse of this kind is what we call a wish; the reappearance of the perception is the fulfillment of the wish; and the shortest path to the fulfillment of the wish is a path leading direct from the excitation produced by the necessity to a complete cathexis of the perception.
>
> (*The Interpretation of Dreams*, 1900, pp. 565–6)

Therefore, the wish is a wish to repeat the experience of satisfaction felt in the link with whoever provided extraneous help* and has become the wished-for object. Each experience of satisfaction leaves new wishes; self-preservative Triebe* are more repetitive, the object is more fixed, and the object is not only wished for (it cannot be renounced without endangering continuity of the subject's own life, for example), but is also a necessity. Sexual Triebe*, however, generate different types of wishes depending on the predominant erotogenic zones*, at least until phallic supremacy organizes all of them under its direction and until object choice*, having become incestuous, is repressed (cf. repression*). The object of sexual Triebe is much more changeable, a characteristic that decreases with the production of fixations*. These Triebe may also gratify themselves by means of the subject's own body.

Choice of sexual object is anaclitic*, based on satisfactions partly of self-preservation and partly of the subject's own body, for whose feelings the object is still a determinant factor. For this reason, the object is chosen depending on fixations left in the body by its history with the object (the body's history and its presentations gradually become the ego).

In this pre-Oedipal* period the infant learns to talk by practicing language*. Unconscious wishes for objects may reach the preconscious, link to word-presentations*, and thereby generate preconscious wishes.

After going through the Oedipus complex* the psychical apparatus splits, and many wishes are repressed (the incestuous, the parricidal, and with them nearly all infantile wishes), become unconscious* and belong to the id*. They are no longer considered part of the ego, which denies them entry and removes its preconscious cathexis from them: the cathexis of their word-presentations.

These repressed wishes never give up their wish to return directly (cf. return of the repressed*) or by way of preconscious derivatives of the unconscious that represent them and evade censorship*. This return generates dreams*, parapraxes*, neurotic symptoms*, and so on.

Sometimes, unconscious wishes may also overcome censorship (by desexualization* for example) and become preconscious wishes which are therefore felt to belong to the ego and whose satisfaction is sought. What is important here, aside from real external factors, is their degree of proximity to prohibited incestuous and parricidal wishes (the closer they are, the smaller the possibility of satisfaction, at least in the terrain of "normality" and neurosis).

Preconscious ego wishes not repressed by it are those of its self-preservation in part (the wish to sleep, for example) whereas others configure aim-inhibited wishes such as tenderness and friendship or desexualized wishes. Another part consists of sexual wishes coming from the id and accepted by the ego, probably because they apparently do not create conflict or because they are able to dodge a clash with the superego and reality*. Then they may be fancied or acted upon (with the guidance of the reality principle*). They may also be condemned by judgement if they generate conscious conflict, whenever the ego considers it necessary. However, sometimes the ego may simultaneously adopt them and also hold them in the terrain of phantasy without acting upon them. When they end in action at the cost of a certain type of splitting in the ego*, we observe "eccentricities of normal persons". In any case, the wish is a preconscious wish, generally with more binding and passage to secondary process, although its deeper meaning always lies in the unconscious repressed wish.

Freud also mentions superego wishes when he attributes wishes of punishment* and self-punishment* dreams to this agency. They are explained as fulfilment of superego wishes (*New Introductory Lectures on Psycho-Analysis*, 1933). In some way, unconscious sense of guilt* or need for punishment*, in general terms and referring to wishes, are references to sexual desire (not to be confused with genital*), although the possession of presentations (thing and word) may give self-preservative Trieb a wishful characteristic. However, when we refer to unconscious wishes, they are sexual.

Does any pure wish correspond to death Trieb? Freud thinks that this is not possible since there is no thing-presentation of the individual's own death in the unconscious. It is contradictory to refer to any "experience of death" that leaves a trace in the psychical apparatus. However, there is a wish for others' death; when cathected, it is called destructive Trieb.

We could add sadism* or mastery*, as well as hate* and aggression*; all these possibilities are diverse degrees of fusion* with Eros and carry presentations corresponding to sexual fixations of each individual history. In this sense, they are sexual wishes. Even the pleasure of killing is narcissistic sexual pleasure, a phantasy of omnipotence that may even have an object. Although there may be an unconscious need for punishment that comes from the superego; although the latter cultivates it pure in its seedbed, it is no longer a wish or Trieb but has become anticathexis* and also psychical processing of an erotic link with the parents (in which hate and the struggle for Oedipal power, etc. predominate), consequently leading to identifications* with them and thing-presentations* of them.

Paradoxically, we know that "there is" a "mute" death Trieb. If it speaks, it is through presentations (thing and word) of sexual wishes with which it is fused. Therefore, we can say that we see it indirectly in the above-mentioned examples of aggression, hate, sadism, and mastery.

The concept of the wish is superimposed on the concepts of Trieb and even libido. They sometimes seem to be synonyms or different levels of the same phenomenon; at others, different things.

The concept of Trieb is a frontier concept between the somatic and the psychical. It is probably closer to the somatic and pressure (*Drang*) towards action, whereas the wish is closer to the presentational side. This is why Freud describes "hallucinatory wish fulfilment"* rather than "hallucinatory Trieb fulfilment", and speaks of wishes when he needs to explain dreams, fantasies, and even symptoms; that is to say, when the emphasis is on presentational content. However, when he needs to explain ego defence mechanisms* in response to anxiety signals* in the face of Trieb dangers, or when he explains the id, he speaks of exigencies of Trieb exerted on the ego, as well as in the search for Trieb satisfaction which is ultimately the same as that of wishes.

Now we shall examine the differences between wishes and libido. Somatic sexual energy is called libido when it is bound to a presentation; it is the energy that cathects it, whereas the wish resides more in presentation (cathected by libido); therefore, although they are different, these two phenomena are too close to each other for us to distinguish them entirely clearly.

In *The Interpretation of Dreams* (1900), Freud speaks of wishes; in *Three Essays on Sexual Theory* (1905) he mentions Trieb; in the metapsychological writings of 1915 the concept of Trieb predominates, although he also speaks of wishes, especially in relation to dreams; in *The Ego and the Id* (1923) he refers almost only to id Triebe, and again in *Inhibitions, Symptoms and Anxiety* (1925). The concept of libido is found throughout his works.

However, important features differentiate these concepts. For example, although wishes may be preconscious, Trieb is an unconscious concept.

Also, we identify object libido and narcissistic libido, but in relation to wishes, although we may speak of object wishes, it is more difficult to speak of narcissistic wishes, at least in any pure form; they may be an extension of the concept of homosexual wishes which therefore refer to an object.

For example, children are so dependent on the object's love* in the period of latency* that they may adopt the object's wishes as their own. Upbringing is based on these principles: children give up their Triebe in exchange for maternal love, sometimes in such a radical way that they become preconscious wishes through identifications in the ego and principally in the superego: in the latter, generally in opposition to unconscious wishes and therefore supporting unconscious repression that holds back emergence of repressed wishes. We could therefore think that need for the object's love is narcissistic, and it is to some extent, but not in the strictest sense of libido coming from the id to cathect the ego. Individuals cannot desire themselves because they have themselves. They may wish to be loved by the object or wish to reach the ideal, but this ideal consists of traces left by the object in the infantile past: the wish to return to lost infantile omnipotence. In this sense they are narcissistic wishes, but the object's trace is never missing in all these complex developments of desire that sometimes confuse our thought*. Ultimately, the definitive difference between these concepts is not totally clear but rather "*non liquet*", as Freud so often said.

May we speak of narcissistic Trieb? Yes, but only of sexual Trieb with autoerotic satisfaction. When we speak of narcissism in the strict sense, we speak of libido in the ego.

Finally, our grounding is Freud's explanation in Chapter 7 of *The Unconscious* (1915) in relation to cathexis of the presentation in order to justify a preconscious wish for the object. When both the unconscious thing-presentation and the preconscious word-presentation are cathected, the latter means or represents the former in consciousness. If preconscious cathexis is withdrawn, the wish enters a state of repression in the unconscious. In transference neuroses*, the unconscious thing-presentation is cathected and perhaps too highly, but it has no preconscious word-presentation in order to access consciousness. In other words, a wish for the object exists but is unknown to the subject; it may be discovered in dreams, symptoms, and so on. One of the objectives of psychoanalytical treatment is to recover libidinal energy needed to cathect the preconscious word-presentation. As long as the wish remains repressed, that energy belongs only to the unconscious thing-presentation.

In these neuroses, cathexis has been displaced or transferred (cf. transference*) onto other preconscious presentations; in anxiety hysteria* this has occurred to the point of constituting phobias*. In obsessional neurosis* its associative and affective connections with the rest of the preconscious presentations have been isolated*, or magical mechanisms have been called upon to avoid feeling that they belong to the ego; ultimately, anxiety develops in regard to these obsessions, never accepted as wishes of the preconscious ego* even though they are located in it topically. In conversion hysteria*, the wish has found expression by virtue of bodily cathexes chosen by association* with laws of contiguity*, analogy*, and others and has become, in the case of associations by analogy, a mnemic symbol* of thing-presentations now repressed and fighting to return from that state. In narcissistic disorders (especially psychoses such as schizophrenia*) the thing-presentation of the object is decathected, and this unconscious cathexis is diverted to the ego. This process is narcissism* *par excellence* since the unconscious wish for the object is decathected. We repeat: in simple schizophrenia there is no unconscious wish for the object. Cathexis is withdrawn from the unconscious thing-presentation (which configures the unconscious wish for the object which is the motor of the psychical apparatus). However, the remaining preconscious presentations no longer represent unconscious presentations but only occupy the empty place left by the latter when they were decathected. Therefore, these preconscious cathexes (word-presentations) are governed by the same laws as the others (primary process*). In this way, organ speech* and paranoid delusions* are configured: the latter could be described, perhaps by exaggerating a bit, as preconscious wishes for the object not supported by any unconscious wish. They are in reality attempts to reconstruct wishes for the object world, not from the depths of the psychical apparatus but only out of words. These words are no longer signifiers and only imitate the signified.

WORD-PRESENTATION

Ger.: Wortvorstellung. – Sp.: representación de palabra. – Fr.: représentation de mot. – It.: rappresentazione di parola. – Port.: representação de palavra.

Infants learn this special form of memory trace* in the link with their mother as a product of the transformation of the "internal alteration"* (expression of emotions, screaming, vascular innervation).

On account of the response of "extraneous help" (the mother figure), this simple form of affective discharge becomes an appeal, thereby acquiring meaning, and the infant may notice its own scream; the experience of pain* may also arise; the ground is thereby formed on which language* proper gradually originates.

It arises in the psychical apparatus at first to perfect and later to enable perception* of thing-presentations* by consciousness* by transforming them into a perception (auditory, signifier of a signified); thus, these sounds first reach perception and then become memory traces*. Once they have been processed into presentations*, they are utilized by the psychical apparatus to enable the conscious to access knowledge of its unconscious wishes*, not only presentations themselves but also their interrelations. Interrelations between presentations (logical relations, for example) can very slightly and only ambiguously be represented by visual images; they need words, some for greater precision and others simply in order to be represented. (In dreams*, logical relations are expressed only by contiguity in time and in space: *The Interpretation of Dreams*, 1900.)

In this way logical relations between presentations succeed in entering thought, which enables new reasoning, new levels of complexity, more Trieb binding, greater differentiation between wishes and reality*, and better examination of each of these; also, the ability to think about oneself, the ego, and other matters.

> We learn that what becomes conscious in [visual thinking] is as a rule only the concrete subject-matter of the thought, and that the relations between the various elements of this subject-matter, which is what specially characterizes thoughts, cannot be given visual expression. Thinking in pictures, is, therefore, only a very incomplete form of becoming conscious.
> (*The Ego and the Id*, 1923, p. 21)

This is the origin of all the possibilities opened to human beings by the creation of thought* activity, the fruit of the creation of language and of its corresponding word-presentations whose residence in the psychical apparatus is in the preconscious ego, and which may access consciousness when they overcome conscious censorship* through the addition of cathexis* of attention*.

"From the point of view of psychology the unit of the function of speech is the 'word', a complex presentation, which proves to be a combination put together from auditory, visual, and kinaesthetic elements" (*On Aphasia,* 1891, in Appendix C, *The Unconscious*, 1913, p. 210).

> [T]here corresponds to the word a complicated associative process into which the elements of visual, acoustic and kinaesthetic origin enumerated above enter together. A word, however, acquires its meaning by being linked to an "object presentation", at all events if we restrict ourselves to a consideration of substantives. The object presentation itself is once again a complex of associations made up of the greatest variety of visual, acoustic, tactile, kinaesthetic and other presentations.
> (Ibid., p. 213)

The word-presentation is the representative before consciousness of the thing-presentation when it is linked to it directly as its signifier. This signification is also worked through by the link with many other words or signifiers of other thing-presentations. In this fabric governed by the preconscious ego which has now developed, it is possible to tame Trieb*, and the ego is more capable of making decisions with respect to specific action*.

Repression* takes a different course. It tries to break the link between the word-presentation and the thing-presentation; in transference neuroses it withdraws cathexis from word-presentations (secondary repression) and displaces* it, cathecting a different word or a muscle innervation, etc., which then act as new anticathexes* whose unconscious meanings include Trieb satisfaction and even punishment for it.

In narcissistic psychoses*, cathexis is withdrawn from the thing-presentation, thereby removing the word's meaning. Now, it is no longer a signifier and becomes in practice the thing-presentation with the concrete meaning it had early in life when the child was learning language; therefore, it is treated with primary process* which generates delusions*, among other manifestations: these are autoplastic* endeavours towards restitution* with links with the world, now emptied of meaning and far removed from reality, since the thing-presentation is cathected neither definitively nor for the moment.

WORKING THROUGH

Ger.: Durcharbeitung. – Sp.: trabajo elaborativo o elaboración. – Fr.: perlaboration. – It.: elaborazione. – Port.: perlaboração.

This part of the process of taming Trieb* takes place during analytic work; through it, the patient recognizes repressed unconscious presentations of the id* and ego* resistance* anticathexes*, consequently placed into "associative commerce" and the activity of judging, and therefore, into thought* and therefore secondary process*.

However, in this working through, knowledge of cathexes* of id presentations becomes particularly important. These presentations resist relinquishing the presentations to which they are fixated, a phenomenon related to psychical inertia* (*The Ego and the Id*, 1923), compulsion repetition* inherent to Triebe* in general, and death Triebe* in particular (although death Triebe, instead of forcing the fixation*, act by separating the cathexis from the presentation, thereby removing its psychical quality*, and consequently, presentational libido becomes mere quantity: pure and nearly biological repetition).

What is worked through is therefore the memory* itself (memorized or acted on through repetition [*Remembering, Repeating and Working-Through*, 1914]), whatever is opposed to it, and Trieb's intrinsic tendency to repeat (*Inhibition, Symptoms and Anxiety*, 1925).

Therefore, working through is a means to open new roads for the ego, new possibilities and facilitations by virtue of new facts guided by it and the feeling of new experiences by which it may also be attracted.

Therefore, we seek more plasticity, to overcome archaic fixations through knowledge of the ego; an ego which, by acquiring greater plasticity in its knowledge, is able to tame them and to choose better the timing and manner of putting them into action in order to convert them into facts.

Presentations accessing the ego's consciousness* through this process are word-presentations belonging to the ego's preconscious.

Through them, the ego is enriched, accessing the possibility of the highest level of Trieb binding in the psychical apparatus, provided by thought activity ruled by the reality principle*, by which the ego is progressively differentiated from the object*, and what is real – even when unpleasurable – from what is desired. If the latter cannot become reality*, it leads directly to frustration*, although intermediate satisfactions also exist. The ego's definitive characteristics now become part of what is real, and may consequently be managed better by the preconscious ego since it knows them, as well as the id impulses from which the ego defends itself in an unconscious manner, but no longer needs as much.

The process of working through takes place gradually and slowly, as does the activity of secondary process in general, transforming compulsive id cathexes into quiescent cathexes, possessing a wide preconscious* network of signification, and therefore easily accessible to the ego's consciousness.

WORK OF MOURNING

Ger.: Trauerarbeit. – Sp.: trabajo de duelo. – Fr.: travail du deuil. – It.: lavoro di lutto. – Port.: trabalho de luto.

Mourning the loss of something previously possessed or even desired, especially the death of a loved one, demands arduous work of the ego, at times absorbing all its energy and capacity. This work in part produces narcissistic withdrawal during the process of the work of mourning. Its labour during mourning must aim to recognize this loss; that is to say, recognize that wishes once satisfied in the link with the lost object will no longer be satisfied; now, however, psychical pain appears whenever a perception refers to it. The work of mourning must remove libidinal cathexis from the presentation of this newly lost object in the psychical apparatus, a situation that reappears in each detail of the subject's life that refers to the object, provoking the pain of recognition of its definitive absence. At first, this work is intense. Gradually, when the presentation of the object is no longer hyper-cathected as it was, it becomes a less painful, tolerable memory. The energy of libidinal cathexis is then directed towards a new object in search of a fresh possibility of satisfaction. The ego has then concluded its work of mourning.

Since this process is so psychically painful, the subject's ego may sometimes utilize defence mechanisms against this pain, which may in turn produce an inadequate conclusion to this work, establishing what may become pathological mourning. In this case, mourning causes neurotic symptoms in an over-determined* manner; it must be made conscious along with all the determining elements of the symptom. Freud explains:

Reality testing has shown that the loved object no longer exists, and it proceeds to demand that all libido shall be withdrawn from its attachments to that object. This demand arouses understandable opposition – it is a matter of general observation that people never willingly abandon a libidinal position, not even, indeed, when a substitute is already beckoning to them … Normally, respect for reality gains the day. Nevertheless its orders cannot be obeyed at once. They are carried out bit by bit, at great expense of time and cathectic energy, and in the meantime the existence of the lost object is psychically prolonged. Each single one of the memories and expectations in which the libido is bound to the object is brought up and hyper-cathected, and detachment of the libido is accomplished in respect of it. Why this compromise by which the command of reality is carried out piecemeal should be so extraordinarily painful is not at all easy to explain in terms of economics. It is remarkable that this painful unpleasure is taken as a matter of course by us. The fact is, however, that when the work of mourning is completed the ego becomes free and uninhibited again.

(*Mourning and Melancholia*, 1917, pp. 244–5)

Z

ZOOPHOBIA

Ger.: Tierphobien. – Sp.: zoofobia. – Fr.: zoophobie. – It.: zoofobia. – Port.: zoofobia.

This phobia* is typically infantile, manifesting during the period of the Oedipus complex*, which results from displacement* of the father figure on to a certain animal which is feared, thereby successfully avoiding conflict with the father.

It is a relic of the totemism* of primitive peoples which emerged following the murder of the father by the sons of the primal horde*, a father they then feared and worshipped, in spite of his periodical ritual sacrifice. In these cases, the animal is considered a tribal ancestor, just as the father was in reality.

The repressed Oedipus complex in these phobias may be positive or negative. In both cases, castration by the father is feared, phylogenetic residues participating in this fear.

Another type of zoophobia exists in adults (usually feminine phobias): nearly universal fear of or aversion for snakes, rats, cats, and other animals on account of their phallic symbolism and the sexual temptation produced by the phallus, generating anxiety for the ego*. They are sometimes part of sensations and situations related with the uncanny* and they have the peculiar feature of being isolated, presenting in patients with certain hysterical characteristics (not of anxiety hysteria*) for whom it is not as indispensable to generate the rampart characteristic of phobia.

Reference

Reik, T. (1953) *The Haunting Melody: Psychoanalytic Experiences in Life and Music*. New York: Farrar, Straus & Young.

INDEX